ESSENTIAL HYPERTENSION AND ITS CAUSES

ESSENTIAL HYPERTENSION AND ITS CAUSES

Neural and Non-Neural Mechanisms

Paul Korner

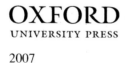
UNIVERSITY PRESS

2007

OXFORD
UNIVERSITY PRESS

Oxford University Press, Inc., publishes works that further
Oxford University's objective of excellence
in research, scholarship, and education.

Oxford   New York
Auckland   Cape Town   Dar es Salaam   Hong Kong   Karachi
Kuala Lumpur   Madrid   Melbourne   Mexico City   Nairobi
New Delhi   Shanghai   Taipei   Toronto

With offices in
Argentina   Austria   Brazil   Chile   Czech Republic   France   Greece
Guatemala   Hungary   Italy   Japan   Poland   Portugal   Singapore
South Korea   Switzerland   Thailand   Turkey   Ukraine   Vietnam

Library of Congress Cataloging-in-Publication Data
Korner, Paul I.
Essential hypertension and its causes : neural and
non-neural mechanisms / Paul Korner.
    p. ; cm.
Includes bibliographical references and index.
ISBN 978-0-19-509483-1
1. Essential hypertension. I. Title.
[DNLM: 1. Hypertension—etiology. WG 340 K843e 2006]
RC685.H8K672 2006
616.1'32—dc22   2006023747

9 8 7 6 5 4 3 2 1

Printed in the United States of America
on acid-free paper

This book is dedicated to
Björn Folkow
a dear friend and stimulating colleague

Our many intense debates and arguments about
integrative biology and medicine
helped shape the approach used in this book
and probably doubled the time for its completion.

Preface

Essential hypertension (EH) is the commonest type of high blood pressure and is responsible for many deaths and much serious illness, which has been the reason for the huge research effort to determine its causes. However, countless scientific articles still keep proclaiming that "the causes of essential hypertension remain unknown." In view of the number of publications that descend on the hypertension specialist like a waterfall, such proclamations seem to overlook the considerable amount of knowledge that we already have about the etiology of EH. The problem may be a lack of synthesis rather than a lack of information.

This book brings together some of this knowledge into a coherent and clinically relevant account of the pathogenesis of EH. At present, the great advances of molecular biology are not being utilized to the best advantage in hypertension research. It is like navigating across the tricky waters of the circulatory control system with the aid of a high-resolution microscope, without having first examined the physiological properties of the system at relatively low-power resolution. For example, the remarkable dearth of progress in identifying the "blood pressure genes" that give rise to EH has been the lack of focus on the central nervous system (CNS), which is the initial source of the elevation of blood pressure (BP). Accordingly, the aim of the book has been to define the main initiating causes of EH, the early mechanisms by which BP is raised, and the additional factors that contribute to the progressive elevation of BP over a period of several years.

Richard Bright discovered renal hypertension in the middle of the 19th century, and for many years afterward few doubted that all hypertension was of renal origin. However, by the start of the 20th century, a number of physicians had become convinced that many types of high BP had nonrenal causes. Today the research court remains evenly divided between those who still believe that renal dysfunction is the source of EH and those who emphasize a number of nonrenal causes.

Clinicians may ask whether we need to know the causes of EH. After all, currently available antihypertensive drugs diminish the risk of its serious complications. However, rational measures for its prevention are dependent on understanding the causes of this disorder and the physiological basis of its complications. This requires analysis of how the control system works in those that develop EH and in persons with normal BP. This has meant looking afresh at many areas of circulatory control.

Chapter 1 gives a brief account of the history and clinical features of EH and of various experimental approaches that have improved our understanding of hypertension. The nature of the circulatory control system itself is examined in chapter 2, beginning with a brief account of the generic features of control systems. Linear control systems have fixed regulatory parameters and set points, while "adaptive" nonlinear systems have parameters that alter automatically when the operating conditions exceed certain limits. The linear model has been favored by most cardiovascular physiologists, whereas those in fields such as somatic motor control have opted for the more realistic adaptive systems. Current evidence suggests that adaptive systems provide more appropriate models for mammalian circulatory control. Changes in parameters that cause an increase in resting BP under the environmental circumstances that give rise to EH are part of the adaptive system's normal operation. Once the adaptive nature of the control system has been recognized, many otherwise puzzling circulatory responses can be related to long-term alterations in system properties. Chapter 2 also discusses the general approach employed for defining the inputs and outputs that give rise to EH, with the latter providing clues about more proximal regulatory processes.

Guyton's theory of hypertension, first proposed some 40 years ago, is briefly considered. The theory makes a case for the renal origin of all hypertension. Guyton thought that this was due to salt overload when renal dysfunction limited salt excretion. There are many discrepancies between the theory's predictions and critical experimental findings in various types of hypertension. This is partly due to Guyton's use of a linear model of circulatory control and partly due to inadequacies of the biological analysis, particularly in the area of neural regulation. Guyton was correct in his emphasis that there is renal impairment in most types of chronic hypertension. However, in EH the kidney is the long-term victim of nonrenal influences and is not the initial source of hypertension.

As with so many disorders, genetic and environmental factors are both important in the development of EH. Biometrical geneticists have shown that inheritance is polygenic and that environmental factors also make a large contribution to the rise in BP (chapter 3). An animal model with genetic properties resembling those of persons with EH is the so-called borderline hypertensive rat (BHR), which is a hybrid of normotensive rats and rats with spontaneously developing genetic hypertension. In a neutral environment BHR have normal BPs, but when exposed to chronic stress or a high-salt diet, they develop sustained hypertension. Advances in the area of molecular BP genetics have been mainly technological and as yet none of the genes important in EH have been definitively identified. What has redeemed the field have been the spectacular successes in several rare monogenic types of hypertension in which single gene abnormalities have been identified, with their effects on function explaining the largely renal pathophysiological mechanisms that cause the elevation of BP. It has been argued that EH must also be due to the same mutant genes, but this is simply wishful thinking.

Chapter 4 considers the contribution of four conditions to the rise in BP in EH: psychosocial and mental stress, high dietary salt intake, obesity, and obstructive sleep apnea. These are the main environmental causes of EH. All of them also increase BP in normotensive subjects, but persons with EH are more susceptible to some of the stimuli. The long-term effects of regular exercise training are antihypertensive and may also reduce stress.

Analysis of the hemodynamic and autonomic output patterns in EH indicates that there is an early tonic increase in sympathetic neural activity (SNA) and a phasic rise in adrenaline secretion (chapter 5). The autonomic pattern resembles the hypothalamic defense response, normally evoked by stress. Gradually, nonneural factors including the characteristic structural and functional changes of the peripheral vasculature come into play, contributing increasingly to the rise in BP.

The tone of the vascular smooth muscle (VSM) of the small arteries and arterioles depends on the net effect of local metabolic activity, changes in blood flow and BP, and neurohumoral constrictor influences (chapter 6). When structural changes develop in the resistance vessels, the altered vessel geometry confers a mechanical advantage on the force developed during contraction, which amplifies the elevation of BP. In turn, this is also the cause of deterioration of organ function.

In hypertension, the heart has to work harder against the high BP (chapter 7). This is achieved through several mechanisms, including elevation of cardiac SNA and development of concentric left ventricular hypertrophy (LVH). However, structural changes in the coronary vasculature and the extent of myocyte enlargement eventually set the limit to the heart's pumping capacity. Once this has been exceeded, focal myocardial damage develops, sometimes giving rise to cardiac failure.

Chapters 8 to 14 consider the mechanisms by which BP is raised by the individual environmental and lifestyle causes of EH. By way of introduction, chapter 8 considers the major neural pathways contributing to cardiovascular regulation by the CNS and the role of neurons that release generically different transmitters at their endings. The major autonomic effector responses are mediated through fast transmitter neurons, so called because the transmitter (e.g., glutamate) exerts its full effect in 1–2 ms. In contrast, the changes evoked by slow transmitter neurons are of slow onset and longer duration (100 ms). The slow transmitter neurons are interneurons that carry information from one neuron population to another. They release various monoamines or peptides from their endings, through which they modulate the responsiveness of fast transmitter neurons. For example, information about stress from the prefrontal cortex is transmitted to the hypothalamic defense area through dopaminergic (DA) neurons. An increase in DA neuron activity evokes the defense response. Moreover, destruction of DA neurons in young spontaneously hypertensive rats (SHR) attenuates this neural type of hypertension, which resembles EH. It is envisaged that in EH the DA neurons are important in increasing the defense pathway's responsiveness to stress. This is called sensitization and ensures that repeated stimulation of the pathway makes it respond to ever milder stresses, so that hypertension eventually becomes permanent. The molecular mechanisms were discovered by Eric Kandel, who first studied this type of strengthening of synaptic transmission during aversive conditioning in the sea snail *Aplysia* (Kandel, 2001). It is assumed that marked strengthening of synaptic transmission of the defense pathway occurs only in persons genetically susceptible to EH, so that the high BP is maintained by ever smaller levels of stress.

Chapter 9 discusses the properties of whole-organism baroreflexes, which perform moment-to-moment adjustments to minimize the acute effects on BP of various circulatory perturbations. The "whole organism" designation indicates that in the intact organism these reflexes arise through the combined profile of inputs due to changes in arterial, cardiac, and pulmonary baroreceptor activity, rather than through three or more independent baroreceptor sources. Disturbances tend to alter arterial, cardiac, and pulmonary pressures in different proportions and sometimes in different direction, which affects the efficiency with which baroreflexes maintain BP. The neurons associated with baroreflex pathways have connections to virtually all cardiovascular neuron populations in the CNS. Hence, when the state of the adaptive circulatory control system changes, so often do the baroreflex parameters. For example, the BP sensitivity of sympathetic constrictor baroreflexes is greater in persons with EH than in normotensives, reflecting their greater hypothalamic responsiveness. However, the cardiac vagal baroreflex is depressed due to the raised cardiopulmonary load in EH. The change in properties of each baroreflex is mediated through distinctive slow transmitter neurons.

During exercise, there is a work-related substantial rise in BP, and the autonomic changes are a variant pattern of the defense response (chapter 10). The sources of regulatory drive come from the cortex, afferent nerves from the active skeletal muscles, and from baroreflexes. The cerebellum coordinates the autonomic changes closely with active skeletal muscle contraction. It relates actual motor performance to that desired by central command, making appropriate adjustments to both motor and autonomic activity.

Regularly repeated submaximal exercise has the opposite long-term effects on BP and the autonomic pattern. BP falls between bouts and remains low for days to weeks. This is partly due to expansion of the vascular bed of the previously active muscle, and partly to tonic depression of sympathetic baroreflexes, which reduces cardiac SNA and R_1 vessel constrictor tone.

Chapter 11 considers how stress is perceived by the brain. This is a highly individual matter, with strong subjective elements. Stress may be felt in response to a number of mental and occupational challenges, adversarial confrontation, socioeconomic hardship, and many others, and the resulting responses have autonomic, emotional, and often somatic motor components. In turn the responses are not just dependent on events of the moment but depend on memory of previous analogous events. Persons with EH often feel more anxious and depressed than normal individuals, so the intensity of stress may appear greater than in normal subjects. In both humans and animals there are excellent case control studies conducted over long periods, showing that stress gives rise to chronic elevation of BP. When stress is substantial, the BP rises in everyone. The high BP normally subsides rapidly once the source of the stress has disappeared. However, in persons genetically susceptible to EH, exposure to chronic stress sensitizes the defense pathway, which is ultimately responsible for BP remaining high at minimal levels of environmental stimulation. In humans, the elevation of BP through sensitization is gradual because a powerful forebrain inhibitory system limits hypothalamic hyperresponsiveness.

High dietary salt is another factor that contributes to the elevation of BP (chapter 12). Normally, body salt composition is safeguarded by at least five major homeostatic systems. Such tight regulation of sodium chloride makes it difficult to evaluate how salt affects BP in the intact organism. In healthy normotensive animals, BP is very insensitive to elevation of salt intake, but salt sensitivity develops when renovascular hypertension is induced in the same species. The Dahl-S rat is an extreme genetic variant of high BP sensitivity to salt, where an increase in salt intake markedly raises BP. In contrast, in the Dahl-R rat, the same change in salt intake has no effect on BP. The difference in responses is due to the high sodium permeability of the blood-brain barrier, so that elevation of brain sodium raises BP through stimulation of brain ouabain neurons and the defense area. In human populations, there is also a range of BP sensitivities to salt, with salt sensitivity greater in those genetically susceptible to EH. In salt-sensitive individuals, an increase in salt intake raises SNA, which is probably mediated through ouabain neurons.

The prevalence of obesity has been increasing in many countries (chapter 13). In some obese individuals, excessive food consumption appears to be an attempt to alleviate stress, with eating providing relief from stress-related anxiety. Unfortunately, the resulting obesity is injurious to health, largely due to the development of non-insulin-dependent diabetes mellitus (NIDDM). However, the rise in BP due to chronic obesity is only small, remaining within the normal range of BP in about 50% of obese persons. This is because the neural pressor effect of the adiposity hormone leptin is largely offset by the peripheral vasodilator effect of hyperinsulinemia. The remainder of obese individuals have hypertensive obesity due to the superposition of the autonomic defense pattern on normotensive obesity.

Obstructive sleep apnea (OSA) is a secondary hypertension in which nocturnal nasopharyngeal obstruction of the upper airway evokes an oxygen-conserving variant of the defense response (chapter 14). About 70% of sufferers from OSA are obese, which accentuates their respiratory problems. The phasic airway obstruction triggers the cardiovascular changes, which are the result of apnea plus increased arterial chemoreceptor activity, followed by hyperventilation. A proportion of OSA sufferers also develop rises in daytime BP. This is related to the repeated nocturnal arousals after each apneic episode. Both nocturnal and diurnal rises in BP are prevented by applying continuous positive airway pressure through a face mask during sleep.

Chapter 15 addresses three questions about the role of the kidney in hypertension: (1) the significance of the results of experimental renal transplantation; (2) why nephron numbers are low in chronic EH; and (3) differences in the role of the kidney in renal hypertension and EH.

Transplantation of the kidney from a Dahl-S rat or SHR into a normotensive recipient raises the latter's BP, while a graft from a normotensive donor into a hypertensive recipient lowers BP. This has been regarded as proof that hypertension is due to genetically determined renal tubular dysfunction, probably related to sodium transport. However, the evidence about tubular dysfunction may not be as strong as was once thought: The rise in BP is at least partly due to presence in the graft of structurally remodeled resistance vessels, which raise vascular resistance. Another factor is new evidence demonstrating a definite extrarenal source of BP rise.

One hypothesis about the low nephron numbers in chronic EH is that this is a long-term legacy of the effect of fetal stress on renal development. There is some support for this, but it probably accounts for only a small proportion of persons with EH. Most individuals have normal nephron numbers at the start of EH, which decrease as a consequence of chronic vasoconstriction.

In renal hypertension, the kidney is the source of the high BP, which only rises when substantial renal vascular changes and ischemia occur. The changes include redistribution of renal blood flow due to the actions of both renin-angiotensin and autonomic nervous systems. These are illustrated in an analysis of the mechanisms in renal artery stenosis, renal cellophane wrap hypertension, and low-renal-mass hypertension. In all of them, nephropathy occurs much earlier than in EH, where the brain is the source of the initial renal changes. In mild and moderate EH the nephropathy is small; it increases considerably as EH becomes severe, when it resembles the changes in renovascular hypertension. In all types of hypertension including EH, sufficient loss of renal parenchyma results in either malignant hypertension or renal failure.

Chapter 16 discusses the pathogenesis of SHR hypertension, in which the defense pathway is sensitized in neonatal life as a result of increased DA neuron activity and remains permanently hyperresponsive to stress. Another factor contributing to the hypertension is the early BP-independent structural narrowing of the immature resistance vessels in response to elevation of circulating catecholamines. This ensures a very rapid rise in BP as soon as most of the VSM cells have become contractile by 4–5 weeks of age. SHR hypertension is completely prevented by neonatal sympathoadrenalectomy. Early inactivation of the renin-angiotensin system also attenuates SHR hypertension, largely through peripheral vascular remodeling, with widening of R_1 vessels.

The last chapter summarizes the two major syndromes of EH: (1) stress-and-salt-related EH (SSR-EH) in lean or only slightly overweight persons; and (2) hypertensive obesity, that is, SSR-EH plus obesity. In both syndromes, sensitization of the defense pathway is the key initiator of elevation of BP. This affects DA neuron synapses linking cortex to hypothalamus. Sensitizable synapses are an attribute of thalamocortical and memory neurons and are not normally found in the autonomic nervous system. The synaptic sensitization is responsible for hypothalamic hyperresponsiveness to environmental stimuli. In mild EH, it accounts for the elevation of SNA and associated rise in BP. As BP rises further, the SNA-mediated constrictor effects on TPR are gradually reinforced by the vascular amplifier and changes in NO and other peripheral regulatory molecules. These not only raise BP further but bring about deterioration of vital organs and the other complications of EH.

The last part of the chapter discusses the potential of various nonpharmacological measures in programs designed to reduce the prevalence of EH. Some of the forms of treatment are relatively specific antagonists to the early changes that occur in EH. Their use in established EH in conjunction with antihypertensive drugs is also considered briefly. The drugs mainly produce relatively nonspecific reduction in BP, which has been highly beneficial. The nonpharmacological interventions will ameliorate some of the early changes in EH that initiate the elevation of hypertension, while some of the drugs could be highly effective in reversing some of the secondary changes that keep BP high.

Acknowledgments

The present synthesis is based on the work of many authors from all over the world. They have made a substantial contribution to the book, which has been gratefully acknowledged throughout the text. In addition, each figure and table based on previously published work gives the relevant reference and, where appropriate, acknowledges the publisher's kind permission to use the material.

I owe a great deal to the stimulus provided by my students and collaborators over a period of nearly 40 years when I worked at the University of New South Wales, the University of Sydney, and the Baker Medical Research Institute in Melbourne.

It is a pleasure to acknowledge the support I received from John Chalmers, John Uther, Saxon White, Malcolm West, John Shaw, Peter Fletcher, Peter Blombery, and Gordon Stokes during the earlier period. Subsequently in Melbourne, I received tremendous support from Garry Jennings, Murray Esler, James Angus, Warwick Anderson, Alex Bobik, Julie Campbell, John Ludbrook, the late Patricia Dorward, Sandra Burke, Geoff Head, Emilio Badoer, Duncan Blake, Ian Meredith, Arch Broughton, Joe Smolich, Gillian Deakin, Robyn Woods, Kate Denton, Christopher Reid, Krishna Sudhir, Barbara Evans, Rod Dilley, Judy Oliver, and Judy Segal.

Our international visitors increased the research skills of our group and brought in many new ideas. I want to express my grateful thanks to Masami Iriki, Michael de Burgh Daly, Peter Friberg, Michael Adams, Michael Andresen, Walter Riedel, Jean-Luc Elghozi, Jennifer Angell-James, Carol-Ann Courneya, Peter Weissberg and Martha Weinstock, John Manning, and Martin Evans.

I am grateful to Professor Yukio Yamori, who introduced me to the world of the Japanese spontaneously hypertensive rat, which has turned out to be a most valuable model of genetic hypertension of neural origin. Professor Barry Thornton helped me to understand the properties of adaptive control systems and their significance in biology.

The final version of the manuscript was read in its entirety by my son, Dr. Anthony Korner, and I am most grateful to him for all his work. He made many invaluable suggestions about behavioral mechanisms and learning. His comments helped to lighten the style of some of the chapters and to explain the clinical relevance of some of the physiology. Professors John Chalmers, James Angus, Robert Graham, Eugenie Lumbers, Roger Dampney, Margaret Morris, Barrie Thornton, and Brian Andersons read some of the chapters and made valuable comments.

I want to express my deep appreciation to Marcus Cremonese, who produced all the illustrations for the book. I greatly admire his professional skills and his unflappable good humor that have made him such an agreeable collaborator. I hope the figures will make the text more digestible. Rosemary Coucouvinis performed the secretarial work much of the time, transcribing the innumerable corrections in fairly illegible handwriting to produce the final version of the manuscript.

I cannot speak highly enough about the great help that I received from Oxford University Press through my first editor, Jeffrey House, whose patience and constructive suggestions were of the utmost value and have, I hope, made the book more readable. In the final editing, the constructive comments of Regan Hofmann and Carrie Pedersen, and William Lamsback have been much appreciated. Last, the excellent work of the copy-editor, Karen Fisher, and the production team led by Keith Faivre and Sheryl Rowe greatly contributed to the accuracy and clarity of the text.

The start of this project was facilitated by grants from the Clive and Vera Ramaciotti Foundation, the High Blod Pressure Council of Australia Foundation, and Merck, Sharp and Dohme (Australia).

Last, I want to acknowledge the great support I have had from all my family and friends. I am particularly grateful to my dear wife, Jennifer, for her help and encouragement for more than 50 years, which made it all possible.

Contents

VIII   Synthesis

Abbreviations

ACE, angiotensin-converting enzyme
ACh, acetylcholine
ACTH, adrenocorticotrophic hormone
ADP, adenosine diphosphate
AgRP, agouti-related peptide
AHI, apnea-hypopnea index
AMP, adenosine monophosphate
Ang I, angiotensin I
Ang II, angiotensin II
ANP, atrial natriuretic peptide
ANS, autonomic nervous system
AR, adrenoceptor
ATP, adenosine triphosphate
A-V, atrioventricular
AVP, arginine vasopressin
BF, blood flow
BHR, borderline hypertensive rat
BMI, body mass index
BMR, basal metabolic rate
BNP, brain natriuretic peptide
BP, blood pressure
BRS, baroreflex sensitivity
BW/BWt, body weight
CA, catecholamine

cGMP, cyclic guanylyl monophosphate
CI, cardiac index
CNS, central nervous system
CO, cardiac output
CRH, corticotropin-releasing hormone
CSF, cerebrospinal fluid
DA, dopamine
DASH (diet), Dietary Approaches to Stop Hypertension
DBP, diastolic blood pressure
DGD, degree of genetic determination
DMHN, dorsomedial hypothalamic nucleus
DOC, deoxycorticosterone
ECG, electrocardiogram
EDHF, endothelium-derived hyperpolarizing factor
EDRF, endothelium-dependent relaxing factor
EEG, electroencephalogram
EF, ejection fraction
EGF, epidermal growth factor
EH, essential hypertension
EJP, excitatory junction potential
eNOS, endothelial NOS
EO, endogenous ouabain
EPSP, excitatory postsynaptic potential
ET, endothelin
FF, filtration fraction
FFA, free fatty acid
FGF, fibroblast growth factor
G_{av}, average gain
GABA, gamma-aminobutyric acid
GDNF, glial cell line–derived neurotrophic factor
GFR, glomerular filtration rate
GRA, glucocorticoid-remediable aldosteronism
HB-EGF, heparin binding EGF
HP, heart period
HP-axis, hypothalamopituitary axis
HPR, heart period range
HQ, hindquarter
HR, heart rate
HRR, heart rate range
HT, see 5-HT
HW/BW, heart weight:body weight ratio
i.c.v., intracerebroventricular
IGF, insulinlike growth factor
IPSP, inhibiting postsynaptic potential
IV, intravenous
JGA, juxtaglomerular apparatus

LAP, left atrial pressure
LC, locus ceruleus
LHA, lateral hypothalamic area
LOD, logarithm of the odds
LTD, long-term depression
LTP, long-term potentiation
LV, left ventricle
LV/BW, left ventricle:body weight
LVH, left ventricular hypertrophy
LVMI, left ventricular mass index
LVP, left ventricular pressure
MAP, mean arterial pressure
MBG, marinobufagenin
MD, methyldopa
MLC, myosin light chain
MSH, melanocyte-stimulating hormone
MSNA, muscle sympathetic nerve activity
NA, noradrenaline
nCPAP, nasal continuous positive airway pressure
NEAT, nonexercise activity thermogenesis
NGF, nerve growth factor
NHB, neurohumoral blockade
NIDDM, non-insulin-dependent diabetes mellitus
NMDA, N-methyl-D-aspartate (glutamate receptor)
NMRI, nuclear magnetic resonance imaging
NO, nitric oxide
NOS, nitric oxide synthase
NPY, neuropeptide Y
NREM, non-rapid eye movement
NTS, nucleus tractus solitarii
OSA, obstructive sleep apnea
PAG, periaqueductal gray
PDGF, platelet-derived growth factor
PGI_2, prostacyclin
POMC, proopiomelanocortin
PRA, plasma renin activity
PRC, plasma renin concentration
PVN, paraventricular nucleus
Q, blood flow
QTL, quantitative trait locus
r_i, internal radius
RA, right atrium
RAA, renin-angiotensin-aldosterone system
RAP, right atrial pressure
R-AS, renin-angiotensin system
RBF, renal blood flow

REM, rapid eye movement (sleep)
RenVH, renovascular hypertension
RFLP, restriction fragment length polymorphism
RQ, respiratory quotient
RSNA, renal sympathetic nerve activity
RV, right ventricle
RVH, right ventricular hypertrophy
RVLM, rostral ventrolateral medulla
S, slope
S-A, sinoatrial
SAD, sinoaortic denervation
SBP, systolic blood pressure
SHR, spontaneously hypertensive rat
SHR.SP, stroke-prone SHR
SNA, sympathetic nerve activity
SR, sarcoplasmic reticulum
SSR-EH, stress-and-salt-related EH
TAB, total autonomic blockade
TEF, thermogenesis expended on food
TGF, transforming growth factor
TPC, total peripheral conductance
TPR, total peripheral resistance
TPRI, total peripheral resistance index
Vas R, vascular resistance
VEGF, vascular endothelial growth factor
VO_2, oxygen consumption
VO_2 max, maximum oxygen consumption
VSM, vascular smooth muscle
w/r_i, wall thickness to internal radius ratio
WKY, Wistar Kyoto rat
Wmax, maximum work capacity
1K-1C, one-kidney, one-clip
2K-1C, two-kidney, one-clip
5-HT, 5-hydroxytryptamine (serotonin)
5,6-DHT, 5,6-dihydroxytryptamine
6-OHDA, 6-hydroxydopamine

PART I

INTRODUCTION

1

A Short History and Some Clinical Aspects

Essential hypertension (EH) was recognized as a specific disorder a little more than 100 years ago, not long after accurate methods for measuring blood pressure (BP) were first developed. Tests for distinguishing EH from the various types of secondary hypertension are even more recent. The clinical definition of *hypertension* as distinct from *normotension* is arbitrary and is based on epidemiological analysis of cardiovascular risk. Effective antihypertensive drug treatment reduces this risk.

A Short History

Traditionally the discovery of hypertension is attributed to Richard Bright (1836), who found an association between renal disease and left ventricular hypertrophy (LVH). His speculation that LVH was a consequence of high BP turned out to be correct. However, verification had to wait until methods for the clinical measurement of BP became available, as described by Janeway (1904).

In fact, at the time of Bright's publication, BP could not be easily measured in either the clinic or the laboratory. Laboratory studies began from about the middle of the 19th century, following the invention of the mercury manometer by J.-M. Poiseuille, which permitted measurement of mean arterial pressure (MAP). Later instruments developed by Marey in France and Mahomed in England provided some information about the shape of the arterial pulse wave (O'Rourke, 1982a), but high-fidelity optical manometers and electrical strain gauges were not developed until the first half of the 20th century. It was only with these techniques that it became possible to characterize the arterial pressure pulse in health and various pathological conditions such as hypertension (Milnor, 1982; O'Rourke, 1982a).

The water-filled sphygmomanometer was the first practical clinical instrument for measuring blood pressure. It was developed in Germany in the 1880s by von Basch and von Recklinghausen, who defined the circumstances under which cuff pressure equalled that in the underlying artery (Janeway, 1904). A few years later Riva-Rocci (1896) developed an air-filled sphygmomanometer, similar to the modern instrument, which consisted of a pneumatic cuff around the arm, connected to a mercury manometer and to a hand pump and valve that permitted inflation and deflation. The cuff was first inflated to occlude the brachial artery, as indicated by the disappearance of the radial pulse. It was then slowly deflated until the pulse reappeared, which corresponded to the systolic BP. Some 10 years later, the Russian military physician Korotkoff (1905) worked out the significance of the auscultatory arterial sounds, which allowed estimation of both diastolic and systolic BP (Segall, 1985).

For nearly 50 years after Bright, all hypertension was thought to be caused by renal disease, but doubts gradually emerged as to whether this really was the case. By the latter part of the 19th century, physicians in Germany (von Basch), France (Huchard), and Britain (Allbutt) made a compelling case that some types of hypertension were of nonrenal origin (Janeway, 1904; Pickering, 1968).

Allbutt (1915) described many of the clinical features of EH, but his term for the disorder, hyperpiesis, was never popular. It was replaced by Eberhard Frank's term Essentielle Hypertonie, which became essential hypertension in the English translation (Frank, 1911). According to the *Oxford English Dictionary, essential* in a medical context means idiopathic, that is, of unknown cause, rather than something indispensable. A more recent synonym is *primary hypertension*, which has been used to distinguish EH from secondary hypertension in humans. In this book I use the term *essential hypertension*.

In EH, the BP level is a good predictor of future death or serious illness from stroke, myocardial infarction and failure, arrhythmias, renal impairment, and so on. This was first recognized through the work of two outstanding demographers, L. I. Dublin and A. J. Lotka, who worked for the life insurance industry in the United States. The prognostic implications were spelled out in their report to the Metropolitan Life offices in 1926 (Dublin et al., 1949). At that time, no effective drug treatment of hypertension was available and there were quite a few physicians who went into a state of denial about the implications of the report. However, later studies (e.g., at Framingham) showed that EH has the same adverse prognosis in the general population and not just in those able to afford life insurance (Kannel, 1990).

Volhard and Fahr (1914) used clinical and pathological criteria to differentiate EH from hypertension due to nephritis and other renal disorders. Volhard also described malignant hypertension—a rapidly progressing lethal type of high BP, which can occur as a complication in all forms of hypertension (Luft and Dietz, 1993).

Since then, many types of secondary hypertension have been described, apart from those related to renal disease (see below). From the early 1930s on it became possible to induce hypertension experimentally in animals, which opened up the era of pathophysiological analysis of the causes of the various types of hypertension.

Experimental Hypertension

Historically, the experimental induction of renovascular hypertension and genetic hypertension in inbred rats were landmark events in hypertension research.

Renovascular Hypertension

The first to develop a reliable method for experimentally inducing high BP was Goldblatt, who induced severe renal artery stenosis in dogs in which one kidney had been removed earlier (Goldblatt et al., 1934). The stenosis increases renin release from the kidney, which raises systemic BP by increasing the plasma concentration of the pressor hormone angiotensin II (Ang II;[1] Braun-Menendez et al., 1939; Page and Helmer, 1939; Page and McCubbin, 1968; Ferrario and McCubbin, 1973; Page, 1987). For many years this was regarded as the major cause of renal hypertension, until it gradually became clear that this did not adequately explain this condition (chapter 15).

Other types of experimental renal hypertension were soon developed, including renal artery stenosis with the other kidney left intact and chronic hypertension produced by wrapping the kidney in cellophane. These studies revived the original idea of a primary renal origin of EH. A major theory favoring this viewpoint was formulated by Arthur Guyton and is still popular today despite its numerous shortcomings (chapter 2).

Genetic Rat Hypertension

By the 1950s and 1960s, a role for genetic mechanisms in the pathogenesis of EH had been firmly established (Pickering, 1961, 1968). This provided the stimulus for the breeding of rat strains in which hypertension developed spontaneously without apparent cause, as in EH. The first strain to be produced was the New Zealand Genetic Hypertensive Rat (GH; Smirk and Hall, 1958), which was followed by the Japanese Spontaneously Hypertensive Rat (SHR; Okamoto and Aoki, 1963; Yamori, 1983). In addition, the Dahl-S (salt-sensitive) and Dahl-R (salt-resistant) rats were bred to simulate the variation in BP responsiveness to a high salt intake in human populations (Dahl, 1961; Rapp, 1994).

These and other strains were produced by classic animal husbandry techniques. However, to date only a few genes linked to hypertension in rats have been identified, and their physiological modus operandi is largely unknown. Indeed, our understanding of the pathophysiology of hypertension in each of the rat strains is just as unsatisfactory as that of EH. A huge amount of pathophysiological data has accumulated and awaits integration. A hypothesis about the operation of the circulatory control system in SHR is presented in chapter 16.

Clinical Hypertension

The diagnosis of EH depends on (1) determining whether and by how much the BP is permanently raised, and (2) excluding secondary causes of hypertension.

Essential Hypertension

EH accounts for about 90% of all hypertension in industrialized societies. These estimates have altered little over the years, despite improvements in the diagnosis of the various types of secondary hypertension (Lever and Swales, 1994; Kaplan, 2002).

EH is rare before 20–25 years of age, but its prevalence increases with age (Pickering, 1961). The present consensus is that the role of both genes and environmental factors is significant in the elevation of BP. In most patients with EH, hypertension is said to be benign, which means that serious organ damage develops gradually over a period of 10–20 years. This contrasts with the rapidly progressing malignant hypertension, where the progression of benign hypertension suddenly accelerates. Its signs include severe retinopathy, renal impairment, and widespread damage to other organs, which may develop over weeks or months.

Treatment of Hypertension

Until the 1950s, there was no effective antihypertensive treatment. Before then, heroic and mostly unsuccessful therapeutic measures were tried, such as the Smithwick sympathectomy (Smithwick, 1940; White, 1947) and the Kempner low-salt rice diet. These halted the progression of severe hypertension in some individuals, but mostly had little effect. The prognosis for severe hypertension was bad and its progression to the malignant phase was common.

Against this dismal background came the first effective treatment of high BP by administering ganglion-blocking drugs, such as hexamethonium or pentolinium (Paton and Zaimis, 1952). The clinical application was pioneered by Horace Smirk, assisted by Austin Doyle, in one of the world's first hypertension clinics in Dunedin, New Zealand. Smirk treated the patients with a strategy similar to that used by insulin-dependent diabetics and trained them to give themselves subcutaneous injections several times each day. His clinic served as a model for other centers throughout the world. Because of the unpleasant side effects of these drugs, only the most severely hypertensive patients were treated. The reduction in BP was often followed by dramatic clinical improvement and prolongation of life (Smirk, 1957; Kincaid-Smith et al., 1958).

Other drugs with more tolerable side effects soon followed, permitting treatment of patients with less severe hypertension. The drugs included the thiazide diuretics, rauwolfia, guanethidine, α-methyldopa, and clonidine. By the mid-1960s, the β-blockers and α-methyldopa (± diuretics) had become the drugs of choice. Today's therapeutic armamentarium is much larger and includes calcium antagonists, angiotensin-converting enzyme (ACE) inhibitors, angiotensin receptor antagonists, and many others. More is also known about nonpharmacological treatment of hypertension, including the antihypertensive effect of regular exercise.

The development of effective antihypertensive drugs was one of the truly dramatic therapeutic events in the 20th century, given the poor outlook before 1950. However, there is considerable evidence that even in well-controlled EH, the long-term prognosis is less favorable than in matched normotensive subjects (Bulpitt et al., 1986, 1988). There is therefore little cause for clinical complacency about the idea that we do not need to understand the causes of EH.

Secondary Hypertension

Together the various secondary types of hypertension account for about 10% of human high BP. They include hypertension due to different types of renal disease, aortic coarctation, excess production of aldosterone, excess secretion of cortisol, pheochromocytoma, several rare types of hypertension due to abnormalities of a single gene, and several other conditions (Swales, 1994a, c).

In these disorders, the pathology or physiological abnormality indicates the source of each type of hypertension. In a proportion of individuals a cure may be effected by surgical removal of the pathology or, in some of the disorders, by specific pharmacological treatment. However, BP recovery may only be partial or may be transient or absent.

Differentiating patients with EH from those with secondary hypertension involves special laboratory screening procedures. Some are simple and usually provide a clear answer, but occasionally more elaborate procedures are necessary to establish the diagnosis (Kaplan, 2002).

Severity of Hypertension and Future Risk

Routine clinical measurement of BP by physicians is the key to the detection of hypertension. International guidelines for grading hypertension are now widely used and there is considerable information on the relationship between the elevation of BP and future risk of cardiovascular disease.

BP Measurement

Many of the recommendations that were made some 100 years ago for the sphygmomanometric measurement of BP still apply today (table 1.1) (Janeway, 1904; O'Brien, 1994). Usually Korotkoff's phase 3 (muffling of sound) correlates best with simultaneous measurement of intraarterial diastolic BP (DBP), but in some individuals intraarterially measured DBP is more closely related to phase 5 (disappearance of sound).

Table 1.1. Technical Points to be Considered when Performing Clinical Sphygmomanometry

- Arm should be at heart level and relaxed
- Cuff deflation 1–2 mmHg/sec
- Armlet width 12 cm (wider with big arms)
- Sources of observer error: e.g., digit preference, prejudice, choice of Korotkoff phase for diastolic BP
- Standardized procedures and repeated measurements to reduce variability
- Calibrate research sphygmomanometers
- Home BP measurements by subject
- Ambulatory BP investigations

One of the big changes in medical practice over the last 50 years is the routine measurement of BP at the first examination of every patient. This is the key to detecting hypertension in the community. For many years, until the first large therapeutic drug trials were completed, doctors wondered whether patients who were often symptomless should be subjected to the worry of a lifetime of drug treatment. Today it is widely recognized that the latter is by far the lesser evil (figure 1.1).

In general, measurements should be performed under standardized conditions. In those with some elevation of BP, measurements should be repeated over a period of several weeks to help decide whether the elevation is sustained. BP levels are usually higher in the BP clinic or the physician's office than when measured at home or with ambulatory recording apparatus under less stressful conditions (Ayman and Goldshine, 1940; Hinman et al., 1962; Sokolow et al., 1966; Pickering et al., 1988; O'Brien, 1994; Pickering, 1995).

When first introduced, ambulatory BP was measured for 24 hours with a fine catheter inserted into the brachial artery, while the subject went about normal activities (Bevan et al., 1969). Over the last few years, instruments have become available for reliable noninvasive BP measurements (O'Brien, 1994, 2003). In a large study in treated hypertensives, the average ambulatory BP measured over 24 hours was found to be an independent risk predictor of future cardiovascular events, even after allowing for many other factors including clinic BP (Clement et al., 2003). Ambulatory BP

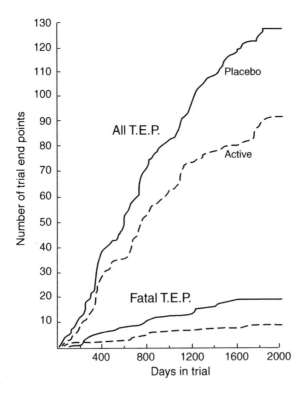

Figure 1.1. Results from Australian National Blood Pressure Study from subjects with mild to moderate hypertension, which show cumulative total trial endpoints (All T.E.P.) and fatal trial end points (Fatal T.E.P.); including 1721 subjects who received active antihypertensive treatment, while 1706 received a placebo. From Reader (1980), with permission of *The Lancet* and Elsevier.

measurements are more reproducible than those obtained intermittently in a clinic or laboratory setting, and ambulatory BP devices are finding increasing use in epidemiological, physiological, and clinical settings. They provide the most integrative measurement of the effect of daily life on a patient's BP.

Arterial Pressure Pulses

Clinical sphygmomanometry measures brachial artery systolic blood pressure (SBP) and diastolic blood pressure (DBP), from which MAP is calculated. MAP and DBP are closely similar in all conduit arteries, while SBP differs in the various conduit arteries because of differences in the pulse waveforms (figure 1.2; McDonald, 1960). The arterial pulse wave in any conduit artery is a compound pressure wave, which is the sum of the pressure waves leaving the heart and those reflected from the peripheral arterioles. Normally this summation is greatest in peripheral conduit arteries, which are closer to the reflecting site in the lower part of the body (McDonald and Taylor, 1959; O'Rourke, 1982b, 1995).

When the arteries have become stiffer, as in long-standing hypertension, the velocity of each wave is greater and the reflected wave is attenuated less on its voyage toward the central aorta. The central aortic pulse amplitude depends on the wave leaving the heart and on the reflected waves from the arterioles in the upper and lower parts of the body. In a stiffer arterial system, the wave leaving the heart and the reflected waves summate earlier, which accounts for the greater pulse amplitude of the central aorta,

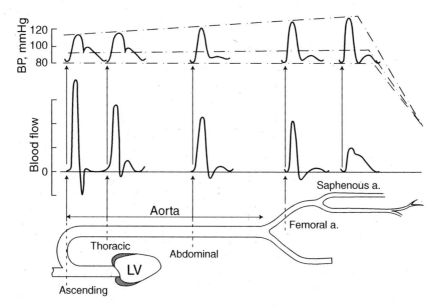

Figure 1.2. Arterial pressure and flow pulses in various conduit arteries from ascending aorta to saphenous artery. Note enhanced magnitude of pulse pressure in the peripheral vessels where sum of pulse wave emanating from heart and wave reflected from resistance vasculature is greatest. After McDonald (1960), with permission of Edward Arnold Publishers and Hodder Education.

which is almost as large as in the abdominal aorta. Hence, the greater increase in SBP compared to DBP is a sign of a stiffer arterial tree (chapter 6; O'Rourke, 2002).

Definitions of Hypertension and Future Risk

Table 1.2 gives the average BPs and ranges of various grades of hypertension based on the guidelines of the World Health Organization and the International Society of Hypertension (Chalmers, 1999). Sometimes the categories of borderline and grade 1 hypertension have been used interchangeably, since the risk of cardiovascular complications is rather similar (Julius, Jamerson et al., 1990) and this practice has been followed in this book. Mild hypertension usually represents an earlier stage in the natural history and it progresses to more severe grades of hypertension over a period of years. Isolated systolic hypertension sometimes occurs in older persons without preceding hypertension.

Guidelines of the International Society of Hypertension have been reviewed and updated every few years since the 1960s. The arbitrary dividing line between hypertension and normotension has been gradually lowered, which automatically increases the known prevalence of hypertension. The objective of this, of course, is to diminish future cardiovascular risk in the population. The rationale stems from the near-linear association between the level of BP and risk of complications of hypertension (figure 1.3; MacMahon, 1994; Collins et al., 1990). Reducing average resting BP by subjecting more people to antihypertensive treatment reduces the risk of stroke and other complications, such as cardiac failure, ischemic heart disease, and renal impairment. Even in mild hypertension, treatment confers a rapid benefit (figure 1.1; Reader et al., 1980). The risk associated with more severe hypertension is increased further by evidence of preexisting organ damage or other cardiovascular disorders at the time hypertension is diagnosed (table 1.3).

Table 1.2. Values of Systolic and Diastolic BPs (SBP, DBP, mmHg) and Mean Arterial Pressure (MAP, mmHg) in the Normal BP Range and in the Different Grades of Hypertension

Grade	MAP, mmHg (median)	SBP, mmHg	DBP, mmHg
Optimum	88	<120	<80
Average normal	96	<130	<85
High normal	103	130–139	85–89
Mild (grade 1)	112	140–159	90–99
Moderate (grade 2)	127	160–179	100–109
Severe (grade 3)	~150	≥180	≥110
Isolated systolic hypertension	~112	≥150	<90

Source: Chalmers, J., for the World Health Organization-International Society of Hypertension 1999 Guidelines for the Management of Hypertension, with permission of *Journal of Hypertension* and Lippincott, Williams and Wilkins.

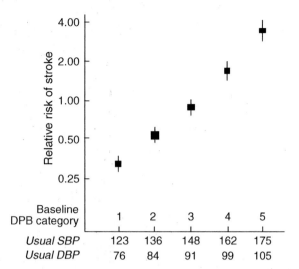

Figure 1.3. Relationship between systolic and diastolic BPs as measured in the clinic and the relative risk of stroke. From MacMahon (1994), with permission of Blackwell, Oxford.

Baseline DPB category	1	2	3	4	5
Usual SBP	123	136	148	162	175
Usual DBP	76	84	91	99	105

Over the last 30–40 years, information about epidemiology and management of hypertension has been rapidly disseminated to physicians by the international and national hypertension organizations. This has contributed to the large reduction in cardiovascular mortality and morbidity. Whether the lower risk is due solely to reduction of BP or whether additional factors play a role is still unresolved (ALLHAT Collaborative Research Group, 2002; Wing et al., 2003). One problem in the design of an increasing number of clinical trials is that the study populations selected are getting older and older: This results in a greater number of trial end points, yet the studies are getting more remote from the factors that initiate EH.

Table 1.3. Relationship between Grade of Hypertension and Future Cardiovascular Risk (Prognosis), and the Influence of Other Risk Factors

	SBP and DBP, mmHg		
Other Risk Factors	Grade 1 SBP 140–159, or DBP 90–99	Grade 2 SBP 160–179, or DBP, 100–109	Grade 3 SBP ≥ 180, or DBP ≥ 110
None	Low risk	Medium risk	High risk
1–2 factors	Medium risk	High risk	Very high risk
3 or more, or TOD and diabetes	High risk	High risk	Very high risk
Associated clinical conditions	Very high risk	Very high risk	Very high risk

Notes: Risk factors other than BP: smoking, total cholesterol, diabetes, family history of premature cardiovascular disease. Other factors adversely affecting prognosis: LDL, HDL, glucose tolerance, obesity, sedentary life style, socioeconomic, etc. TOD (target organ damage): LVH, proteinuria, ↑ plasma creatinine, retinopathy, etc. Associated clinical conditions: stroke, myocardial infarction, congestive heart failure, coronary revascularization, vascular disease.

Source: Chalmers, J., for the World Health Organization-International Society of Hypertension 1999 Guidelines for the Management of Hypertension, with permission of *Journal of Hypertension* and Lippincott, Williams and Wilkins.

The good news is that the number of those actually receiving therapy has more than doubled over the last two decades. The bad news is that about 50–60% of hypertensives who should have been treated receive either inadequate therapy or no treatment (Chalmers, 1999).

Concluding Remarks

All hypertension was originally regarded as of primary renal origin, but by the start of the 20th century it was widely recognized that this did not apply to EH, by far the most common type of hypertension. Epidemiological studies have indicated a strong correlation between the elevation of BP and future cardiovascular morbidity and mortality. The risk of the latter is greatly reduced by effective BP lowering with antihypertensive drugs.

If EH is to be prevented, it becomes important to know what causes EH and the physiological mechanisms through which BP is raised. Both genetic and environmental factors are involved in the development of EH. The environmental factors include psychosocial and other types of mental stress, high dietary salt intake, obstructive sleep apnea, and lack of exercise, all of which affect BP through their actions on the central nervous system (CNS). They affect both hypertensive and normotensive subjects, but the former become more susceptible to some of these stimuli. The next chapter considers the nature of the control system and how to study the mechanisms that raise BP.

PART II

BIOLOGICAL CONTROL

2

The Nature of the Cardiovascular Control System

M any ideas about biological control came from the field of industrial engineering. Accordingly, the first part of the chapter considers the generic features of man-made linear and nonlinear "adaptive" control systems. Circulatory physiologists still tend to use linear control systems, but there is little doubt that the system subserving circulatory regulation resembles a man-made adaptive control system rather than a linear system. In an adaptive system, the set point for resting BP alters under certain circumstances as part of its normal behavior, while under linear control theory the system would be regarded as dysfunctional. The approach used to provide a working model of how the circulatory control system works in EH is considered next. The last section considers briefly the "unifying" theories of hypertension, which tried to explain all hypertension by a single mechanism. For example, Page considered all hypertension as due to disordered tissue perfusion. Later, Guyton formulated a theory in which hypertension was considered to be a compensatory response to the limited capacity of the kidney to excrete salt.

Man-Made Control Systems

The science of control engineering is generally regarded as beginning in the 1780s with James Watt's invention of the fly ball governor for regulating the speed of steam engines. Many advances followed during the 19th and 20th centuries, mostly in response to the practical demands of industry in the fields of precision manufacturing, and more recently in electronics and computer and information technology (Wiener, 1961; Milsum, 1966; Thornton, 1971; Anderson, 1992). These were all linear feedback systems and the advances in control theory led to the development of a large range of linear devices, which improved responses to transient and steady-state perturbations.

The development of adaptive control systems began in the 1950s as a natural extension of linear feedback control (Aström, 1995). Theoretical analysis of these systems intensified between 1960 and 1980 and was helped by the advances in microprocessors and computers. The first commercial systems for process control appeared in the early 1980s, and initially adjusted the parameters of simple controllers automatically. Later they were used in flight control systems, automatic pilots, biomedical systems, robots, and artificial intelligence.

Linear Control Systems

A system is any collection of communicating materials and processes that together perform some function (Milsum, 1966). Figure 2.1 illustrates three types of control (from above): (1) open-loop control without feedback, where an increase in the input X (due to some outside factor) brings about a change in output Y, which has no effect on X; (2) negative feedback, when a change in X causes a change in Y, which then reduces the initial change in X; and (3) positive feedback, where X causes an increase in Y, which then causes X to increase, so that Y keeps getting larger and larger.

The basic components of a linear negative feedback control system include a controller and plant, which is the process being controlled (figure 2.2). The plant's output variable is measured by a feedback transducer, which conveys this information back to the controller. The output is compared to the reference signal, also known as the set point or desired output.

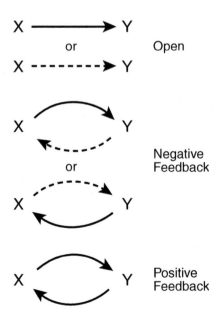

Figure 2.1. Symbol and arrow diagrams indicating relationships between variables X and Y; a solid line and arrow denotes an increase in variable, while a dashed line and arrow denotes a decrease. Top panel, in an open-loop system a change in X causes a change in Y, but the latter has no effect on X. Middle panel, negative feedback system, where X causes an increase (or a decrease) in Y, and the latter minimizes the original change in X. Lower panel, positive feedback, where an increase in X causes an increase in Y, which causes X to increase further. Based on Riggs (1963), with permission of Lippincott, Williams and Wilkins.

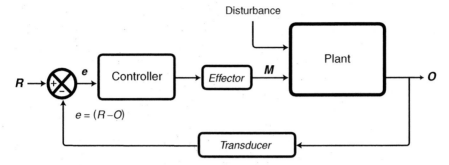

Figure 2.2. Negative feedback system, in which a disturbance acts on the plant and affects its output variable O; R is the reference input to the system's controller, e is the error signal, which is $(R - O)$; M is the magnitude of the effector response from the controller to the plant. Based on Milsum (1966), with permission of McGraw-Hill Book Company.

When a disturbance alters the plant's output, the error signal e is the difference between output and reference levels. If the controller is a regulator, the system minimizes disturbance-induced changes in plant output (figure 2.3, top). But when it is a servocontroller, the output follows the changes in input and the reference signal changes correspondingly (figure 2.3, bottom). An example is the power steering machinery of a ship's rudder, which follows the steering wheel when the navigator changes course.

An engineer generally applies different types of inputs (e.g., impulse functions, step or ramp functions, or oscillatory input) to study the dynamic (time-dependent) responses of the system. Simple linear first-order systems are classified according to the relationship between the controller's effector response (M) and the error signal (e). These are set out in table 2.1 and include (1) proportional control systems, (2) proportional plus time-derivative control systems, and (3) proportional plus integral control systems. The size of the error term is related to the performance of each system, and this type of control is often termed *feedback through error correction*.

When the feedback loop is opened (i.e., interrupted), the system responds without feedback. The ratio of the open- and closed-loop responses is a measure of how effectively the feedback has minimized the changes in plant output (Milhorn, 1966; Riggs, 1963). Clynes (1960) performed an ingenious study of the pupillary light reflex, which illustrates the distinction between the two types of control. Exposing the pupil to a wide beam of light elicits reflex pupillary constriction, which restores retinal illumination toward normal. The system becomes open-loop if the beam is made so narrow that it cannot be obstructed by maximum pupillary constriction.

A cardiovascular example of a physiological response that is adequately modeled by a linear control system is BP regulation through the arterial baroreflex during small respiratory perturbations. However, nonlinearities may develop when there are interactions between inputs, for example, between arterial and nonarterial baroreceptors.

Feed-Forward Systems

Feed-forward systems were developed to overcome problems of sluggish feedback control. They produce anticipatory responses ahead of an expected stimulus, but for

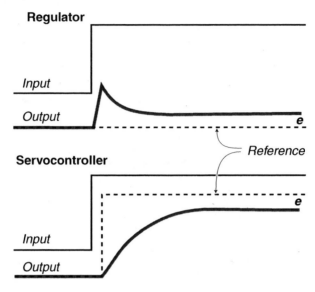

Figure 2.3. Top, in a regulator, a step change in input causes an initial transient increase, which is restored close to the reference level (i.e., the set point) due to negative feedback. Bottom, when the system operates as a servocontroller, the output follows the input with a time course that depends on the gain of the controller and other system properties; *e* is the error signal. Based on Korner (1971a), with permission of *Physiological Reviews* and the American Physiological Society.

them to work requires a good understanding of the normal relationship between input and output. After a disturbance is applied to the input, it normally takes time before the controller corrects a change in plant output through normal feedback. In a feed-forward system, a special controller detects the start of the disturbance and initiates the correction to almost coincide with the start of the change in the output. How well this works depends on how well the algorithm used in the feed-forward controller describes the system's normal performance. Feed-forward systems have fixed parameters, like normal linear feedback systems.

At first sight, some biological responses resemble those of feed-forward systems, such as the early heart rate rise at the start of exercise. But this no longer applies in successive sessions of exercise training, when the response is modeled more appropriately through nonlinear systems.

Table 2.1. Some Properties of Different Types of Linear Control Systems

Type of Control	Function	Effect
Proportional	$M = k_1 \times e$	
Proportional + derivative	$M = k_1 \times e + k_2 \times \partial e/\partial t$	Reduces hunting
Proportional + integral	$M = k_1 \times e + k_2 \int e \partial t$	No S–S error

Note: M = effector response of controller; *e* = error signal; S–S, steady state.

Nonlinear Adaptive Control Systems

Nonlinear adaptive control systems are multivariate systems, known as *adaptive* or *cybernetic* control systems (Wiener, 1954, 1961; Milsum, 1966; Thornton, 1971; Anderson, 1992; Arbib, 1995; Bar-Yam, 1997). This type of system has a particular set of *state variables*, where for each set of inputs there is a set of preferred outputs (Rosen, 1967). When the environment changes in a particular way, the controller's parameters are actively altered to provide the output desired by the engineer, which is called *feedback through parameters*.

An adaptive control system has a conventional feedback loop as in figure 2.2, and an outer adaptive loop (figure 2.4). The conventional loop has a controller, plant, and feedback sensor. The adaptive loop has sensors that continuously examine plant performance, which is called system identification and provides information about the state of the system. For optimum stability, several test stimuli are used for system identification, which reduces errors in estimating the state of the system and improves subsequent performance (Anderson, 1985, 1992). The controller's parameters are continuously recalculated and the parameters are changed when desired in relation to the function of the particular system, for example, in relation to weather conditions in an automatic pilot, which permits maintenance of desired performance. Under these conditions, the steady-state output value often alters from its previous level.

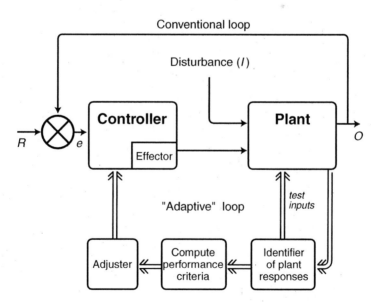

Figure 2.4. An adaptive control system has (1) a conventional negative feedback loop, with input *I*, output *O*, and error *e*; and (2) an adaptive loop, with a mechanism for testing the plant (system identification), a computer for calculating required changes in parameters to maintain output, and an adjuster that alters the controller's parameter. The diagram has only a single input and output, but adaptive control systems are usually multivariate with several inputs and outputs. Modified from Milsum (1966), with permission of McGraw-Hill Book Company.

The adaptive loop provides the system with a hierarchical configuration. The non-linearity arises from the adjustments made in the parameters.[1] Adaptive control systems have memory and logic circuits, which permit comparisons of present and earlier performance. Between parameter adjustments, moment-to-moment feedback is provided to the output through the conventional loop, as in a linear system.

System identification and parameter adjustment have an obvious resemblance to operations in the CNS. The CNS identifies complex inputs, some of which affect BP. Changes in the parameters of baroreflexes often serve as markers for alterations in the state of the control system.

The Mammalian Circulatory Control System

A historical introduction is followed by a short discussion of the cardiovascular control system during fetal development and some of the evidence that the adult cardiovascular control system behaves like an adaptive control system.

Early Ideas on Biological Control

Initially, ideas of biological control were rather independent of what was happening in industry. Claude Bernard (1878) was the first to point out that constancy and stability of the composition of the cells and body fluids was crucial for the proper functioning of higher organisms. These ideas were extended by Walter Cannon, who recognized that active regulation, often through the autonomic nervous system (ANS), was required to maintain the stability of variables such as BP and blood sugar. He termed the overall process *homeostasis*, derived from *homeo*, which means like or similar but admitting of some variation, while *stasis* was derived from statics, a branch of mechanics (Cannon, 1929a; Yates, 1982). In his 1929 article Cannon wrote, "the factors which operate in the body to maintain uniformity are often so peculiarly physiological that any hint of immediate explanation in terms of relatively simple mechanics is misleading" (p. 401).

Ever since, many have wondered what he meant by "so peculiarly physiological" (Yates, 1982; Benison et al., 1987). Cannon probably regarded the regulatory mechanisms underlying homeostasis as more complex than those of industrial control systems, which at that time were all linear with fixed set points. As a supporter of Darwin, he saw higher organisms not as a machine in the manner of the physicalists (Mayr, 1997),[2] but as the product of evolutionary experimentation over millions of years, as a result of which their regulatory attributes had gradually improved. He would probably have seen similarities to adaptive control systems which had not then been invented.

Eberhard Koch (1931) was one of the first cardiovascular physiologists to make use of concepts of control engineering. He proposed that regulation of arterial BP through the arterial baroreceptor reflex resembled that of a man-made linear regulator. Since then, others have extended the use of linear control theory in exploring performance of baroreflexes (Sagawa, 1965, 1972; Allison et al., 1969; Scher et al., 1991), regulation of cardiac output (CO; Guyton, 1955; Noordergraaf, 1963; Grodins and

Buoncristiani, 1967; Sagawa, 1967), some of the effects of exercise (Topham and Warner, 1967; Rowell, 1983), and so on. The feeling that these linear models were adequate was probably reinforced by their use in Guyton's theory on hypertension (Guyton and Coleman, 1967; Chau et al., 1979).

The shunning of adaptive control systems by cardiovascular physiologists and neuroscientists has not been mirrored in other areas of biology. Many other neuroscientists have readily embraced adaptive control systems, for example, in the fields of somatic motor control and learning (Ghez, 1991; Elbert et al., 1994; Arbib, 1995). Some nonlinear neural properties have also been described in the cardiovascular field (Korner, 1979a; Korner, Shaw et al., 1973; Dorward et al., 1985; Persson et al., 1993; Wagner et al., 1996). They have sometimes been treated as though the system were linear except for its set point, which was "reset" (Korner, 1970; Hollenberg, 1980; Persson et al., 1993). This disregards the main message, that linear models are inappropriate and that a more suitable regulatory model should be sought.

Embryo and Fetus

In the embryo and fetus, the major task is the rapid development of the cardiovascular system. The heart is the first organ to function in the organism, and its development and that of the primitive vasculature is one of the organism's highest priorities. Control is largely open, as in figure 2.1, and the developmental processes occur in response to the prerecorded instructions of specific genes (de Pomerai, 1986; Griffiths et al., 1993). Major mutations in these genes are usually lethal (Campbell, 1968; Rossant, 1996). However, some mutations may result in variation in organ size (e.g., of the kidney) which may have implications for BP in later life (chapter 15).

In the second half of fetal life, placental and fetal hormones and later the ANS take over some of the functions of the genes in relation to cellular differentiation and growth, but cardiovascular regulation is on a modest scale compared to what happens in adults (Thorburn and Harding, 1994; Thornburg and Morton, 1994). Epidemiological evidence suggests that adverse maternal influences reprogram the developing neuroendocrine systems, which affect the prevalence of cardiovascular disease in later life (Barker et al., 1990; Gluckman and Hanson, 2005). Indeed, some genetically hypertensive rat strains are specially susceptible to increases in maternal intake of salt (Zicha and Kuneš, 1999). These actions on the fetus could contribute to adult hypertension, but current epidemiological evidence suggests their effect on adult BP is small (chapter 4). Hence, EH is best regarded as a disorder of adults.

Regulatory Mechanisms in Adults

Adult regulatory mechanisms include the brain and its vagal and sympathoadrenal effectors and the local control mechanisms in the peripheral vasculature.

The CNS Controller

The CNS controller in figure 2.5 has attributes similar to the controller of man-made adaptive systems (figure 2.4). System identification by the brain takes place through

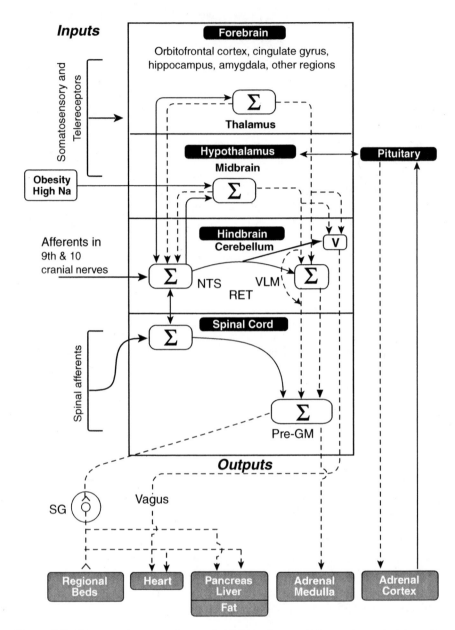

Figure 2.5. Diagram of main cardiovascular CNS pathways. Afferents from arterial, cardiac, and pulmonary baroreceptors reach nucleus of tractus solitarius (NTS) via the 9th and 10th cranial nerves. Somatosensory receptors and telereceptors signal environmental and dietary changes. Afferents from viscera, skin, and muscle enter spinal cord segmentally. Inputs are processed in spinal cord, NTS, and reticular formation (RET) where monoaminergic and serotonergic neuron groups are located. Obesity-related signals and Na$^+$ signals affect hypothalamic neurons. Note hypothalamopituitary connections. Autonomic outputs: vagus (V), preganglionic sympathetic motoneurons (pre-GM), sympathetic ganglia (SG), and postganglionic fibers. Integration (Σ) occurs at all levels of neuraxis, including spinal cord, ventrolateral medulla (VLM), cerebellum, hypothalamus, thalamus, and forebrain.

an elaborate sensory apparatus, which provides information about events in the outside world and within the body. This is further modulated by the circadian rest-activity cycle, itself an indicator of the complex nature of the control system (Yates, 1982, 1983). Factors such as stress, which evoke specific cardiovascular and emotional responses, are initially detected through visual, auditory, olfactory, and general somatosensory receptors. After processing by thalamus and cortex and after reference to past experience from neural memory circuits, the autonomic patterns are generated by neuron groups in the hypothalamus. Information about changes within the body comes from the arterial, cardiac, and pulmonary baroreceptors, arterial chemoreceptors, and various respiratory, visceral and somatosensory receptors, such as muscle chemoreceptors.

The controller consists of integrative centers in different parts of the neuraxis from cortex to spinal cord. Imaging techniques have shown that, in response to a complex afferent input profile, many areas of the brain alter their activity simultaneously. Performance of the task thus depends on networks of neuron populations.

The brain's parameter adjusters are groups of interneurons, some of which are located in the reticular formation of the brainstem. They convey information from neuron groups associated with the various afferent inputs to the target neurons that determine output patterns, which often have autonomic, behavioral, and somatomotor components. Their synaptic actions on various target neurons are through release of dopamine (DA), noradrenaline (NA), serotonin (5-HT), and various peptides. These interneurons release what have been called slow transmitters, because their action takes much longer than that of fast transmitters like glutamate. Slow transmitters act through second-messenger molecules, which alter target neuron responsiveness (chapter 8).

Most of the cardiovascular integrative centers affect the properties of baroreflexes. Hence, changes in baroreflex parameters often serve as markers of changes in the system's state. For example, in severe arterial hypoxia the gain of the renal sympathetic baroreflex is increased, while that of the cardiac sympathetic baroreflex is depressed (Iriki et al., 1977a).

CNS-Mediated Circulatory Control Is Adaptive

Two examples illustrate substantial parameter changes in which there are changes in resting BP and baroreflex properties. The first relates to the transition from the non-hypotensive to the hypotensive phase of hemorrhage, while the second is due to the long-term effects of exercise training. Both are discussed further in chapters 9 and 10. They suggest that the neural circulatory control system behaves like an adaptive system. Other examples will be encountered throughout the book.

Nonhypotensive and Hypotensive Phases of Hemorrhage

In hemorrhage, virtually all the afferent drive is due to simultaneous unloading of arterial, cardiac, and pulmonary baroreceptors (Korner et al., 1989; Oliver et al., 1990; Courneya et al., 1991). When blood is withdrawn at a constant rate in rabbits, BP alters very little from the previous resting value until 25–30% of the blood volume has been removed. The excellent BP maintenance is due to increased constrictor sympathetic neural activity (SNA), which compensates almost completely for the peripheral vasodilator effects of hemorrhage. Once the amount of blood removed has exceeded the above critical value, the BP drops suddenly by 40–50 mmHg, which is the start of the hypotensive phase of hemorrhage. The fall in BP and total peripheral resistance (TPR) is due to active reflex inhibition of SNA, in response to signals from specific LV receptors indicating that cardiac filling has become inadequate. The signals activate interneurons that release an opiatelike transmitter which affects target neurons in the hindbrain, causing inhibition of SNA (Thorén et al., 1976; Schadt and Ludbrook, 1991).[3] The transition from the nonhypotensive to the hypotensive phase of hemorrhage is associated with a major change in regulatory state: Before the switch, circulatory regulation is mainly through the ANS, while after the transition it is mainly through local peripheral regulators that cause vasodilation, thereby improving cardiac filling (chapter 9).

Exercise and Long-Term Effects of Training

Submaximal aerobic bicycle exercise performed for 30–40 minutes is a form of moderate stress, and the circulatory and autonomic responses are variants of the hypothalamic defense response. The pattern consists of rises in BP and CO, with marked vasodilation in the active muscles and vasoconstriction in renal, gastrointestinal, and nonactive muscle beds (chapter 10). BP is raised and the gain of sympathetic constrictor baroreflexes is increased and serves as a marker of the altered state of the system.

When the same level of exercise is repeated three times per week, the regimen causes long-term reduction in the resting BP between bouts. Generally this is associated with agreeable emotions, which is why regular recreational exercise is so addictive. The fall in BP is due to widening of the resting cross-sectional area of the active muscle bed, which in turn is due to training-induced hypertrophy of the skeletal muscle fibers. In addition, sympathetic constrictor baroreflexes are depressed between bouts, which limits their capacity to correct for the tendency for BP to fall (chapter 10).

Hemorrhage and exercise are examples of somewhat different types of adaptive control. The parameter changes related to hemorrhage occur automatically, like any reflex response. However, the performance of exercise is a voluntary activity, as is the decision to perform exercise regularly, while the parameter changes during and between bouts of exercise are automatic reflex events. These examples suggest that the CNS regulator is an adaptive nonlinear control system.

Peripheral Vasculature and Heart

The peripheral vasculature consists of numerous specialized peripheral beds arranged in parallel. Each bed has a branching network of large and small resistance vessels, followed by capillaries, venules, and veins (figure 2.6). The precapillary resistance vessels are important peripheral integrators of neurohumoral and local signals, which determine the changes in vascular smooth muscle (VSM) tone during a disturbance. The largest precapillary resistance vessels (R_1) make the greatest contribution to vascular resistance (Vas R), while the smaller precapillary vessels (R_2) are more susceptible to

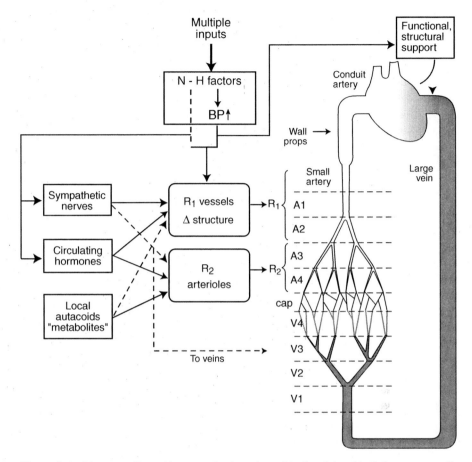

Figure 2.6. Diagram of branching organization of a regional peripheral bed. Larger precapillary resistance vessels (R_1) include small arteries and large arterioles; during stimulation by constrictor agonists, they contribute most to rise in Vas R, while the smaller R_2 arterioles are more susceptible to myogenic and metabolic stimuli. Structural changes in hypertension occur in R_1 but not R_2 vessels in response to hemodynamic and neurohumoral stimuli. In the conduit arteries, the wall becomes thicker and stiffer than normal. To maintain high BP requires the cardiac performance to match the high peripherally induced afterload.

local myogenic and metabolic stimuli (chapter 6). Other local determinants of VSM tone are local tissue metabolites and molecules with vasoactive properties produced by endothelium and other wall constituents. In the peripheral vasculature, parameter changes include alterations in nitric oxide (NO) and chronic structural changes.

Finding One's Way Around the Circulatory Control System in EH

The main environmental factors that give rise to EH include psychosocial and other types of mental stress, lack of exercise, high salt intake, obesity, and possibly obstructive sleep apnea (OSA; chapter 4). Genetic factors are a prerequisite for developing persistent elevation of BP, by increasing susceptibility to one or more of the above inputs.

Figure 2.7 is a schema of the system, with the CNS at the peak of the hierarchy. It is linked to subsystems regulating behavior, rest and activity, metabolism, and electrolyte and water balance, which in turn are linked to the circulation through the ANS, hormonal effectors, and local vascular regulators.

The results of case control and intervention studies suggest that the BP of persons with EH and normotensives usually responds to these stimuli. With stress, the BP responses are usually greater in persons with EH, while the changes in body weight

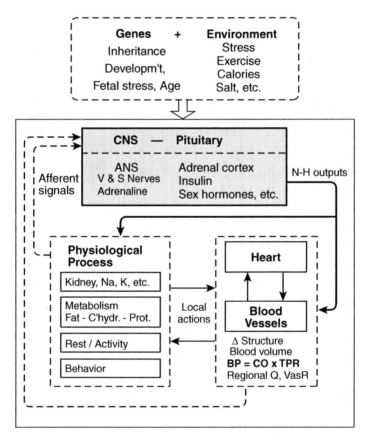

Figure 2.7. Schema of circulatory control system, emphasizing some main determinants of EH, including genetic and environmental factors, psychosocial stress, high dietary salt, obesity, and low physical activity. The CNS is at peak of the regulatory hierarchy with outputs through the autonomic nervous system (ANS) and hormones linked to the pituitary. The subsystems include renal function, metabolism, rest-activity functions, and behavior. All affect cardiovascular function. In chronic EH, structural cardiovascular changes develop and blood volume is generally low. N-H, neurohumoral; V, vagus; S, sympathetic; C'hydr, carbohydrate; Q, blood flow; Vas R, vascular resistance.

have similar effects on BP in both groups (chapter 13). The effects of salt on BP are more variable, but generally persons with EH are more responsive. This helps sort out which of the environmental inputs raise BP. However, the BP responses give few clues about the nature of the underlying mechanisms, because BP is affected by virtually all that goes on in the circulation.

To determine some of these mechanisms, it has been useful to examine the control system in the open form in figure 2.8 and compare the resting output patterns in the two groups, using variables that provide more specific information. Under steady-state conditions, each group's output is in equilibrium with its own inputs, which are usually not very different in the two groups. Hence, differences in output patterns point to differences in information processing by the control system. The procedure is the reverse of input-output analysis and is sometimes used by systems engineers when faced with a system of uncertain properties.

It soon became apparent that there were marked differences in the resting hemo-dynamic patterns between obese and nonobese individuals, both normotensives and hypertensives. This was largely due to the hyperinsulinemia associated with obesity, which causes peripheral vasodilation and increases renal reabsorption of sodium and water. The vasodilation lowers TPR in both obese groups, while the renal action

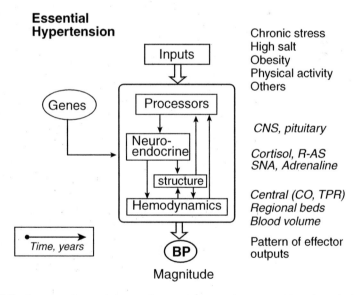

Figure 2.8. An open form of the cardiovascular control system. Alterations in input (top right) produce long-term BP changes in normotensives and persons with EH. To determine underlying mechanisms requires variables related to more specific functions than BP, which are shown on lower right of diagram. In lean persons with EH, the regional hemodynamic and neurohumoral patterns suggest activation of the hypothalamic defense response. It suggests that it may be important to focus on CNS mechanisms associated with perception and responses to stress, and to enquire why response threshold is reduced in EH.

Table 2.2. Vascular Resistance Patterns in Normotensive Controls and in Subjects with Mild and Moderate to Severe Essential Hypertension (EH)

Vas R	TPR	Renal	GI	Muscle	Other Beds
Normotensive	18.18	90.9	142.9	133.3	33.9
100 mmHg	(100%)	(100%)	(100%)	(100%)	(100%)
Mild EH	18.18	129.8	169.5	96.1	32.3
115 mmHg	(100%)	(143%)	(119%)	(72%)	(95%)
Moderate/Severe	24.5	217	220.3	152.9	39.9
EH 130 mmHg	(135%)	(238%)	(154%)	(114%)	(117%)

Note: Mean arterial pressure, mmHg; Vas R, vascular resistance; TPR, total peripheral resistance; GI, gastrointestinal bed. Percentage values under each resistance are percentages of normotensive controls.

increases their blood volume. It suggests that it is best to consider the differences between normotensives and hypertensives separately in lean and obese persons.

In lean individuals with moderate EH, the resting hemodynamic pattern resembles the defense response, with vasoconstriction in renal and gastrointestinal beds and vasodilation in the skeletal muscle bed (table 2.2). Resting SNA is raised in the various sympathetic outflows, while plasma adrenaline increases phasically during slight accentuation of stress, which causes vasodilation in skeletal muscle. The gain of the sympathetic constrictor baroreflex to skeletal muscle is raised, pointing to a chronic change in the system's state (chapters 5, 11).

What is striking is that in mild and moderate EH, the output pattern is similar to the autonomic response to stress. Moreover, its presence under resting conditions

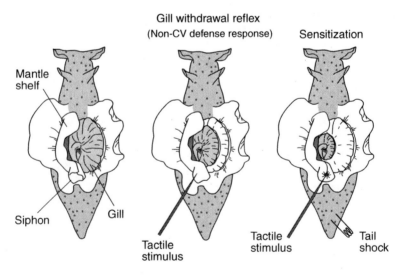

Figure 2.9. Left, dorsal view of the sea snail *Aplysia*. Middle, when skin of siphon is touched, gill and siphon are withdrawn reflexively into mantle cavity. Right, applying repeated electric shocks to the tail sensitizes the circuit activated in the reflex response, resulting in a lower threshold and a long-lasting response; see figure 2.10. From Kandel (2001), with permission of American Association for the Advancement of Science.

indicates that the stress intensity is too low to evoke the same response in normotensive subjects. Thus, the stress threshold in EH is reduced considerably.

A similar reduction in threshold has been found in borderline hypertensive rats (BHR) after prolonged exposure to stressful stimuli.[4] These rats have about half the SHR's number of high-BP genes, and only develop hypertension in an adverse environment (chapter 3). This is what generally happens in humans who are genetically predisposed to EH.

The reduction in threshold after frequently repeated exposure to stress has features in common with the learning process. The Canadian psychologist Donald Hebb (1949) was the first to suggest that learning involves strengthening of synaptic transmission. This is called synaptic sensitization. Kandel and colleagues were the first to identify the cellular mechanisms in the sea snail *Aplysia*, in which the neural processes are easier to analyze than in mammals, because of the simpler construction of its nervous system. Later the basic conclusions were also found to apply to the mammalian CNS (chapter 8; Kandel, 2001).

When the snail's skin is touched gently, it withdraws its siphon and gill reflexly into the mantle cavity for greater protection (figure 2.9). Sensitization develops after repeated application of painful electric shocks to the tail, which cause large increases in magnitude and duration of the reflex response (figure 2.10). The tail shocks raise the activity of a 5-HT interneuron, which increases the release of glutamate from sensory neurons that normally excite the motoneurons involved in the reflex. In addition, if the stimulus trains of electric shock are repeated regularly for several days they stimulate growth of synaptic varicosities, literally strengthening synaptic transmission.

The reduction in threshold raises *Aplysia's* readiness to respond to an aversive stimulus. The basic mechanism resembles the changes in humans susceptible to EH, in whom slow-transmitter dopaminergic neurons increase the responsiveness of the defense pathway.

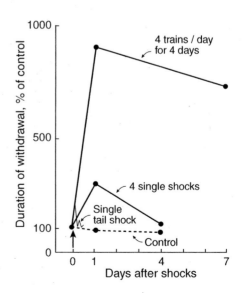

Figure 2.10. Effect of electric shocks on gill withdrawal reflex in *Aplysia*. After a single shock, the response to touch is prolonged for 1–2 hours; after four single shocks and four stimulus trains per day, there are further increases in amplitude and duration of withdrawal response. From Kandel (2001), with permission of American Association for the Advancement of Science.

Relating the output analysis to the various inputs suggests that stress is the main environmental factor that initiates the development of EH. High dietary salt intake potentiates the effects of stress, while hypertension in obese persons with EH appears to be due to the additive actions of obesity alone plus stress-related hypertension (see chapter 13).

Peripheral Parameter Changes in EH

The properties of the peripheral vasculature are altered from an early stage of EH. This is partly due to a rise in cortisol secretion, which inhibits endothelial nitric oxide synthase (NOS) and reduces local availability of NO in the vasculature, raising resting vascular tone.

Later on, the structural changes develop in the R_1 vessels due to growth of VSM cells, which narrows their lumen and raises the ratio of wall thickness to internal radius (w/r_i; figure 2.11; Folkow et al., 1958). This enhances the increase in Vas R produced by constrictor stimuli, thus enhancing the elevation of BP and TPR. As EH progresses, all the above factors contribute increasingly to the rise in BP. They also contribute to deterioration of organ function (chapter 6).

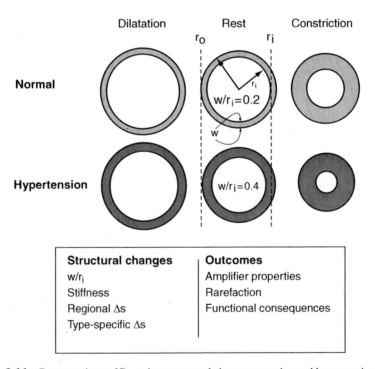

Structural changes	Outcomes
w/r_i	Amplifier properties
Stiffness	Rarefaction
Regional Δs	Functional consequences
Type-specific Δs	

Figure 2.11. Cross-sections of R_1 resistance vessels in normotensive and hypertensive circulation. In hypertension, internal radius (r_i) is narrower and ratio of wall thickness to r_i (w/r_i) is raised. Vascular narrowing in hypertensive circulation is present even when bed is fully dilated. Constrictor responses are enhanced in hypertension, hence the term Vas R amplifier.

Structural changes develop in the conduit arteries, which reduces their distensibility. The result is disproportionate elevation of SBP, particularly in older persons.

The left ventricle hypertrophies in EH, which is one mechanism by which the heart matches its performance to the continuously increasing peripheral afterload. What ultimately limits its performance, in the absence of atherosclerosis, is the hypertension-related changes in the coronary vasculature.

Page's Mosaic Theory and Guyton's Theory of Long-Term Blood Pressure Control

Both Page and Guyton tried to explain all hypertension through a common underlying mechanism. Hence their theories of hypertension are sometimes referred to as unifying theories.

Page's Mosaic Theory

Page regarded hypertension as a disorder of tissue perfusion (Page, 1949, 1987). The mosaic theory was modeled on renovascular hypertension, in which systemic high BP partially corrects the early low renal perfusion (Goldblatt et al., 1934; Page and Helmer, 1939, 1940). The early version of the mosaic theory lists the CNS, heart and vasculature, and renin-angiotensin system as playing a role in the elevation of BP (figure 2.12, top; Page, 1949, 1960, 1987; Page and McCubbin, 1965; Dustan, 1990). A decade later, these and some additional factors were presented in the famous octagon, with the mosaic arising from the interconnections of all its components (figure 2.12, bottom).

The mosaic theory makes the point that many factors are involved in hypertension (Page and McCubbin, 1965). However, there is no evidence about a defect in early tissue nutrition or perfusion, except in OSA. Nevertheless, the mosaic has become a hypertension icon.

Guyton's Theory of Long-Term Control of Arterial Pressure

Guyton's theory was developed nearly 40 years ago and tries to explain both normal and abnormal BP control (Hall, 2003a; Vatner, 2003). It still exerts considerable influence, and the frequency of its citation probably owes something to the popularity of his textbook of physiology (Guyton and Coleman, 1967; Guyton, Coleman, Cowley et al., 1972; Guyton, Coleman, and Granger, 1972; Guyton et al., 1974; Guyton, 1980, 1990; Cowley, 1992).

He selected a linear control model with fixed parameters and a fixed set point for arterial BP. The model has 15 major subsystems and includes some 400 functional relationships between variables, which were incorporated into a computer program.

The theory states that all hypertension is caused by a chronic salt load in excess of the kidney's excretory capacity. It derives from Lewis Dahl's concept about the role of salt in hypertension, which assumes a renal fault in salt handling (Dahl, 1961; Dahl et al., 1962). The Guyton system's main input is salt and water, while the arterial

Page Mosaic Theory

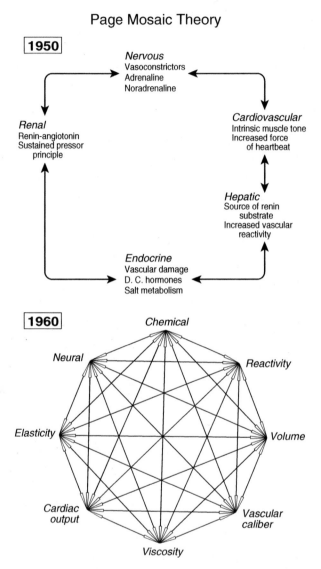

Figure 2.12. Two versions of Page's mosaic theory, published about 10 years apart (Page, 1949, 1960). The system's output is BP and interconnections and components are emphasized, rather than flow of information. From Dustan (1990), with permission of the *Journal of Hypertension*, and Lippincott, Williams and Wilkins.

BP level is determined by the kidney. Figure 2.13 is the critical feedback circuit, through the relationship between arterial BP and urinary output of salt and water. Guyton thought that the ANS played no role in long-term control of BP. His main reason for rejecting a role for the ANS was that arterial baroreceptors adapt rapidly

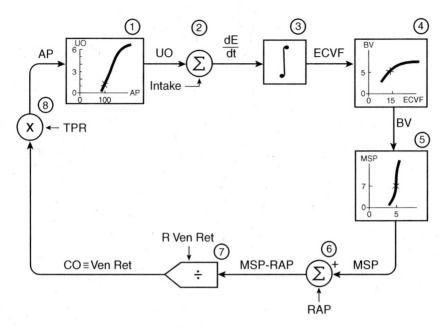

Figure 2.13. Critical feedback circuit in Guyton's theory: (1) relationship of arterial BP (AP) to urinary output of salt and water (UO); (2) summation point, where UO is subtracted from salt and water intake; (3) instantaneous accumulation of extracellular fluid volume (ECFV)(dE/dt); (4) relationship between ECFV and blood volume (BV); (5) relationship between BV and mean systemic pressure (MSP, mmHg); (6) summation point, where MSP is subtracted from right atrial pressure (RAP, mmHg), which equals gradient for venous return (Ven Ret); and (7) division of gradient for venous return by resistance to venous return (R Ven Ret), which equals Ven Ret (= CO, L/min); and (8) multiplier of CO × TPR equals AP. After Guyton and Coleman (1967), with permission of W. B. Saunders (Elsevier).

(Guyton and Coleman, 1967; Guyton, 1980). This is, as we shall see in later chapters, a very limited view of circulatory control involving the ANS.

In Guyton's opinion, the kidney is the main long-term controller of BP, through the BP-diuresis and BP-natriuresis relationships. He suggested that these disturbances of fluid and sodium balance are corrected within hours or days in normal individuals. However, when renal function is abnormal, restoration of the balance requires the development of hypertension.

An Early Discrepancy between Model and Experiment

To verify his hypothesis, Guyton initially used dogs in which renal mass had been reduced surgically to about 25–30% of normal (Guyton and Coleman, 1967). Remarkably, this did not affect BP until salt intake was raised two- to threefold, when severe hypertension developed (figure 2.14). Initially the BP rose due to elevation in CO, which was related to the rise in blood volume. Later TPR increased gradually

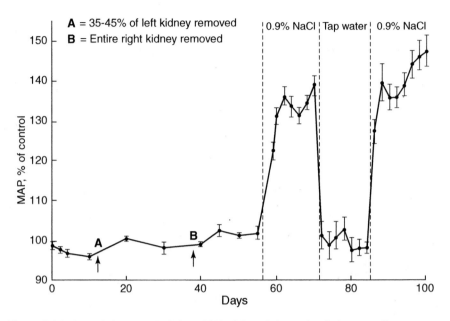

Figure 2.14. From left, removal of about 70% of the renal mass has little or no effect on mean arterial pressure (MAP, mmHg) until sodium intake is increased two- to threefold; note restoration to normal of MAP when tap water is substituted for high sodium. From Langston et al. (1963), with permission of *Circulation Research*, American Heart Association, and Lippincott, Williams and Wilkins.

and accounted for most of the rise in BP by the end of the second week of salt loading (figure 2.15; Guyton and Coleman, 1967; Coleman and Guyton, 1967; Guyton, 1980).

The basic feedback circuit in figure 2.13 predicts that CO and blood volume remain high without a change in TPR, instead of the elevation that actually occurs (figure 2.15). Having dismissed a long-term role for the ANS, Guyton's way of explaining the discrepancy between prediction and experiment was to invent a new mechanism, "long-term autoregulation," which was added to the model.

He and his colleagues have regarded long-term autoregulation as similar to normal autoregulation, where vascular tone is rapidly adjusted within seconds or minutes through myogenic and metabolic mechanisms. However, in his model long-term autoregulation only comes into play after a long latency, with the time course selected to accord with the experimental observations. A different time course suggests a different mechanism than normal autoregulation (Korner, 1980b, 1982). There has been endless discussion as to the role of long-term autoregulation in the elevation of TPR, or indeed whether it exists at all.[5]

One explanation not considered by Guyton or his critics is that the system is an adaptive control system rather than a linear system, and that the observed rise in TPR is due to a parameter change. The regulatory adjustments to a large salt and water load in the presence of a severely dysfunctional kidney take weeks to reach equilibrium.

Hence, Guyton's linear model may have correctly predicted the changes through the conventional loop shown in figure 2.4, during the early days of salt loading.

Sustained elevation of CO has been observed in the course of redevelopment of primary aldosteronism (Schalekamp et al., 1985) and in patients with severe renal impairment, in whom dietary sodium was raised while on fixed hemodialysis (McGrath et al., 1977; see chapter 15). However, in a group of anephric patients, the hemodynamic pattern was as in figure 2.15 (Coleman et al., 1970).

We now know that substantial ischemia develops in low-renal-mass hypertension, as the few remaining nephrons try to cope with high salt loads (Hostetter et al., 1981). The ischemia increases the activity of the renal chemoreceptors, which increases SNA after activating the hypothalamus (Campese and Kogosov, 1995).

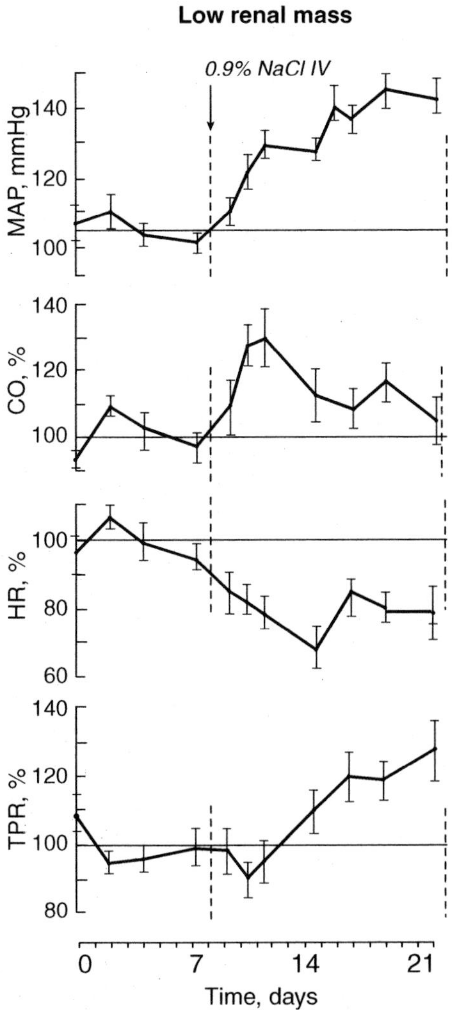

Low renal mass

Figure 2.15. Average changes in 6 dogs with low renal mass, when 0.9% NaCl IV was infused at arrow. Variables (% of baseline): mean arterial pressure (MAP), cardiac output (CO), heart rate (HR), and total peripheral resistance (TPR). Initial rise in MAP due to elevation in CO; later the rise in TPR accounts increasingly for rise in MAP. After Coleman and Guyton (1969), with permission of *Circulation Research*, American Heart Association, and Lippincott, Williams and Wilkins.

Thus, the irony after Guyton's dismissive view on neural autonomic control is that a neural mechanism arising from the kidney is responsible for the elevation in TPR in this type of hypertension, rather than long-term autoregulation (see chapter 15).

The idea of neural involvement is in accord with a study on the effects of salt loading on the regional blood flow and Vas R patterns, performed several years after the initial publication of Guyton's theory (Liard, 1981). On the first day after the start, Vas R had increased mainly in the renal and splanchnic and fallen in skeletal muscle, resembling the defense pattern, while after 5–7 days vasoconstriction was more general. The results suggest neurally induced changes rather than autoregulation, as had also been observed by Stekiel et al. (1981).

The Early High CO and Late High TPR Pattern

Guyton assumed that the early CO–late TPR pattern occurred in every type of hypertension. The high CO was thought to raise tissue perfusion above its metabolic requirements, triggering an autoregulatory rise in TPR, which restored CO and regional blood flows as tissue nutrition improved (Borst and Borst-de Geus, 1963; Ledingham and Cohen, 1964; Ledingham, 1989). However, the postulated sequence of hemodynamic changes is often absent, as indicated in the clinical studies of McGrath et al. (1977) and Schalekamp et al. (1985), and in many types of experimental hypertension (see chapter 15; Page and McCubbin, 1965; Conway, 1968; Ferrario et al., 1970; Freeman et al., 1977; Korner, Anderson et al., 1978).

Indeed, mild EH is the only type of high BP in which the rise in CO is regularly associated with the initiation of high BP. Several years later, as EH becomes more severe, the hypertension is due to elevation in TPR, with the latency excluding autoregulation. As discussed in chapter 5, the rise in CO and the elevation of TPR are both due to autonomic factors, while R_1 vessel structural changes contribute to the latter. Central blood volume is raised, while total blood volume falls with increasing severity of hypertension. Even Guyton had difficulty fitting EH into his schema of circulatory control, stating that "it is not possible to discuss the mechanisms of essential hypertension (EH) with a high degree of certainty. . . . In EH . . . blood volume or plasma volume are, if anything, slightly below normal" (Guyton, 1980, p. 457).

Thus, the idea that increased sympathetic activity plays no part in long-term regulation of BP is factually incorrect for EH, in which it is a major source of constrictor drive for several years.

Guyton's Theory in Retrospect

Guyton was a pioneer in cardiovascular systems analysis and his model is still admired for its mathematical form and the use of computers (Luft, 2004). He believed that long-term and short-term control of BP were mediated through different regulatory mechanisms. This is highly questionable, as are some of his ideas about the integral nature of long-term volume regulation by the kidney.

His group invented long-term autoregulation to explain the rise in TPR and spent much effort in demonstrating that an increase in blood volume could elicit normal autoregulatory responses (Granger and Guyton, 1969; Guyton, 1980; Cowley, 1992).

But they never explored whether this caused the rise in TPR in low-renal-mass hypertension, or whether there were alternative mechanisms. Another error is the assumption that all hypertension must be caused by excess salt intake and volume overload. This is not the case in early EH or even in renal artery stenosis hypertension.

His theory has received extensive criticism relating to all the above matters (e.g., Sapirstein, 1969; Sagawa, 1975; Fletcher et al., 1976; Freeman et al., 1977; Stephens et al., 1979; Korner, 1980, 1982), but this never made him reexamine the assumptions of his model or consider a better alternative model.

Undoubtedly the simpler mathematics was a major factor in Guyton and Coleman's decision to opt for a linear model. In man-made systems, mathematical modeling stands a better chance of being right, because the designer understands the system's purpose and the role of its components. However, when dealing with a complex system such as that regulating the circulation, the major challenge is to get the information flow right. If that is incorrect, a mathematical approach has little merit.

What Matters in Cardiovascular Systems Analysis?

It is a truism to affirm that biological systems analysis is about analysis of real systems rather than testing a priori hypotheses. Each type of hypertension has special features, as illustrated in later chapters. Hence, each type of hypertension merits detailed analysis of its underlying mechanisms.

The neural cardiovascular control system is a nonlinear adaptive system. Sometimes the neural parameter changes come automatically into play as a result of interactions between afferent signals, as in hemorrhage. However, because of the subject's voluntary efforts, regulation in exercise training or in EH is less deterministic. In both exercise training and EH, long-term parameter changes contribute to the maintenance of BP at a new level.

Disturbances of either short or long duration often elicit similar changes in neurohumoral and peripheral regulators and often similar changes in system parameters. It therefore seems unlikely that there are fundamental differences between long-term and short-term regulation, although the relative prominence of some of the effector mechanisms may differ.

Biological systems analysis, like integrative physiology, attempts to fit the function of components into the framework of the system's overall operation. In relation to EH, this involves studies in humans and experiments in animals, in vitro preparations and cellular systems. Fortunately, new methods for studying human neurohumoral function have greatly helped in understanding the macro aspects of cardiovascular regulation.

Sometimes it may be difficult to fit information about system components into the operation of the entire system, the properties of which often depend on the way the system is organized. For example, isolated vessels provide invaluable information about VSM contractile properties, but it is the organization of all the vascular branches and their innervation which determine whether autonomic, hormonal, and local factors are predominant. Similarly, in the intact organism neural cardiovascular control is about responses to interacting inputs, while isolated preparations are required to determine responses to individual stimuli. Yet both types of information are needed to understand how the intact system works.

The regulatory problems in EH relate to activities of everyday life, that is, stress, dietary factors, and the level of physical activity. All of them have long-term effects on BP in normotensives and hypertensives. In EH, the responses to the various environmental perturbations are qualitatively similar to those of normal persons, but a major quantitative variant is the lower threshold to stress. The parameter change results from biochemically and structurally induced strengthening of synaptic transmission, as illustrated in *Aplysia*. Analogous peripheral parameter changes are the structural changes in R_1 vessels. These changes add a dimension of permanence to the particular way the system works in hypertension, making the condition harder to reverse.

One consequence of the choice of linear models in circulatory control has been the intrusiveness at an early stage of the investigation of questions such as what variable is being controlled and what is the purpose of the regulation. This makes it difficult to perform the analysis without bias. It gives rise to a teleological pseudologic that A has to happen because of a change in B, which led both Page and Guyton to incorrectly conclude that hypertension was a compensatory response to dysfunctional components of the system.

Teleology plays a lesser role in the analysis of multivariate systems, partly because the analyst is usually not clever enough to work out all the interacting purposes and therefore performs the analysis without that knowledge. It is best to leave teleological speculations to the end of the analysis.

The hardest thing about biological systems analysis is to reinterpret data in the light of new evidence, which usually means abandoning preconceptions. I have always admired John Eccles for doing just that, when he abandoned his ideas on electrical transmission at synapses in favor of chemical transmission. This was in the best tradition of what should happen when a scientic hypothesis has been refuted (Popper, 1959, 1963). However, as Kuhn (1963) has pointed out, this is the exception rather than the rule. Adhering to unsustainable positions comes at a price. The long survival of the Guytonian dogmas has had an adverse effect on ideas on cardiovascular control and hypertension. However, it has had some benefit: Physiologists and physicians now think more deeply about control systems than they did in earlier times.

3

Blood Pressure Genetics

M uch of our understanding about inheritance of high BP and the role of the environment is based on biometrical partitioning of the BP variance into its component factors. However, to date the advances in the molecular genetics of hypertension have largely consisted of the development of new technologies. For example, we can dissect the genome and vary the extent to which particular genes are expressed, while the quest to identify the genes that cause EH or genetic rat hypertension has been largely unsuccessful. Only in several rare monogenic types of human hypertension have the mutant genes that cause the elevation of BP been identified, together with the mechanism of their action.

Background

A short account of the development of ideas on inheritance is followed by discussion of what determines the phenotype and polygenic inheritance. The section ends with a brief account of biometrical techniques for assessing heritability in humans and rats.

Ideas on Continuous and Particulate Inheritance

Two seminal papers on the nature of inheritance were published in the same year, 1865, by Francis Galton and Gregor Mendel, neither of whom was aware of the work of the other. Galton had concluded that talent was inherited from an evaluation of the biographies of outstanding men. He and his student Karl Pearson then went on to study traits such as height that varied continuously in the population, using the strength of the correlation between family members as a measure of hereditary transmission. Because the trait varied continuously, it was assumed that hereditary transmission was also continuous (Mather and Jinks, 1982).

Mendel's approach in his work on plants was completely different. He had shunned continuously varying traits and had concentrated on "true breeding" plants, with clearly recognizable characteristics that did not vary from generation to generation. After crossing different strains, he noted that the hybrids in succeeding generations segregate in what are now known as classic mendelian ratios. He therefore proposed that hereditary transmission was particulate and discontinuous.

This work had been reported to the Moravian Academy of Science in Brno (now in the Czech Republic) but went largely unnoticed for some 35 years. There it remained until 1900, when Correns, Tschermak, and de Vries independently rediscovered what Mendel had achieved (see Vogel and Motulsky, 1997). In the meantime, during the latter part of the 19th century, evidence had accumulated about the nature of cell division and what happened to chromosomes during mitosis and meiosis. In 1902, Walter Sutton in the United States and Theodor Boveri in Germany recognized independently that the behavior of chromosomes during meiosis paralleled the behavior of Mendel's particles. Hence their proposal that the chromosomes carried the genes, which became the term for Mendel's particles (Griffiths et al., 1993).

The same year saw the first application of Mendel's ideas to medicine. In a paper on the rare disorder alcaptonuria, Archibald Garrod (1902) noted that relatives of the patient either had the disorder or appeared to be normal. He was the first physician to explain hereditary transmission along mendelian lines and suggested a recessive mode of inheritance for this condition. Later he recognized a similar mode of inheritance in other disorders such as albinism and cystinuria. He termed the various genetic disorders "inborn errors of metabolism" (Garrod, 1923). He speculated that genetic factors probably also played a role in many other common diseases by increasing the body's susceptibility to these conditions.

At the time of Garrod's paper, the gulf between the Galtonians and Mendelians was still substantial. According to Mather and Jinks (1982), neither group appreciated the complexity of the relationship between genes and environment, that is, the phenotype. Such understanding was helped by two landmark discoveries. First, Johannsen (1909) showed in experiments in plants that any trait in an organism is never due to genes or environmental factors alone, but depends on interactions between genes and environment. Second, the studies of Nilsson-Ehle (1909) and later of East (1915) led them to propose the multiple-factor theory of genetic transmission, which became known as polygenic inheritance. This provides the genetic basis for continuous variation.

Over the next 30–40 years, R. A. Fisher and his collaborators greatly extended the statistical methodology used by Galton and Pearson in a manner that accorded with mendelian concepts (Fisher, 1918, 1930; Mather and Jinks, 1982; Cruz-Coke, 1983; Vogel and Motulsky, 1997). These were applied throughout the 20th century to determine heritability in EH and in various genetically hypertensive rat strains.

Relation between Phenotype and Genotype: The Norm of Reaction

The phenotype is the interaction between genes and environment, while the norm of reaction is the function that relates the environment to the genotype (Griffiths et al., 1993). To determine the norm of reaction experimentally requires organisms of uniform genotype, such as the fruit fly *Drosophila melanogaster*. One can then determine the effects of a large range of environmental factors on the phenotype, as indicated below.

Wild-type flies when bred in a cool environment have large eyes with some 1000 facets (figure 3.1), but at warmer temperatures the number of eye facets that they develop is smaller (Griffiths et al., 1993). In the cool environment, two *Drosophila* mutants, *Ultrabar* and *Infrabar*, have smaller eyes with fewer facets than the wild-type. However, at warmer breeding temperatures the number of facets is reduced in *Ultrabar* but increased in *Infrabar*.

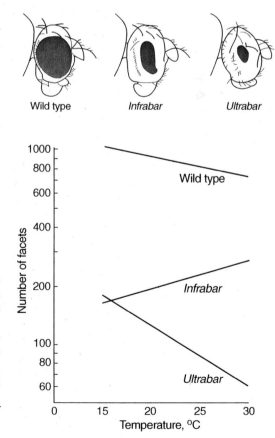

Figure 3.1. Top, eye size is a function of facet number in wild-type *Drosophila* and in the mutants *Infrabar* and *Ultrabar*. Bottom, relationship in the three sets of flies between eye facet number and environmental temperature (°C) for breeding and maintenance. From Griffiths et al. (1993), with permission of W. H. Freeman, New York.

From this one can conclude that *Infrabar* and *Ultrabar* have different norms of reaction, which sometimes reveal distinctive genotypes (figure 3.2). At cool breeding temperatures the two mutants have rather similar eye phenotypes, which makes it impossible to conjecture about differences in genotypes without genotyping their DNA. In contrast, the two phenotypes are distinctive at warm temperatures, which suggests an underlying difference in genotypes. Thus, a single genotype can produce different phenotypes, depending on the environment in which the organism develops. Furthermore, in some environments the same phenotype may result from different genotypes.

This type of analysis in insects can now also be performed in mammals, thanks to the development of recombinant inbred rat strains (see below). In relation to a human population, which consists of a mixture of genotypes, the norm of reaction can only be used notionally. However, in inbred rat populations and their F_1 hybrid, it helps to define the general nature of the genotype in which hypertension may develop during an exposure to an appropriate environment, as discussed later in the chapter.

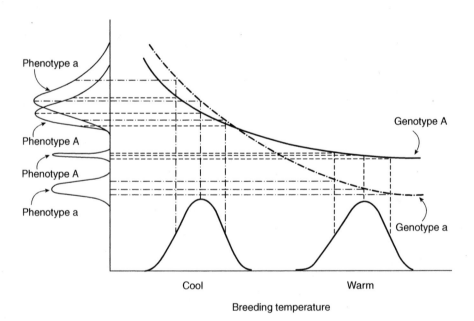

Figure 3.2. In a population consisting of two genotypes, the distribution of phenotypes depends on the environmental conditions. In one set of environments (*x* axis, right), phenotypes "A" and "a" are distinct (*y* axis, lower distributions), which suggests different genotypes. In the other environment (*x* axis, left) the two phenotypes overlap (*y* axis, upper distributions), and DNA genotyping is required. From Griffiths et al. (1993), with permission of W. H. Freeman, New York.

Polygenic Inheritance

The idea is that small actions on a trait such as BP by each of a large number of genes are responsible for its continuous variation in the population. In a given environment, the BP phenotype is the algebraic sum of the effects of all the genes.

In diploid organisms, each genetic locus has two alleles (genes): It is homozygous when the alleles are the same and heterozygous when they are different. Figure 3.3 shows the effects of genes at two loci on the BP phenotype (Rapp, 1983a). At locus A, the alleles are A_1 and A_2, while at locus B they are B_1 and B_2. A_1 and B_1 cause reduction in BP and are called minus alleles; A_2 and B_2 increase BP and are plus alleles. The progeny of the F_2 generation is produced by intercrossing animals from the F_1 generation, which are heterozygous at both loci ($A_1A_2B_1B_2 \times A_1A_2B_1B_2$). The 16 genotypes give rise to the five subclasses of phenotypes, due to differences in plus and minus alleles, suggesting that each is acting independently and additively.

In general, the frequency distribution has ($2k + 1$) classes, where k is the number of loci affecting BP. Each gene is inherited as a discontinuous mendelian trait. With two

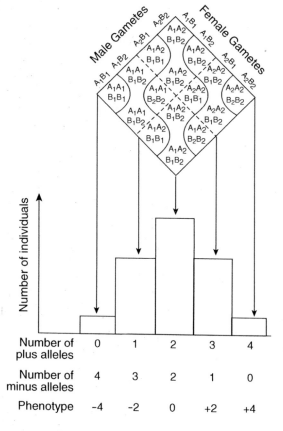

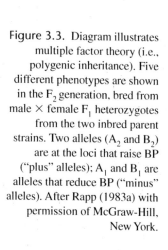

Figure 3.3. Diagram illustrates multiple factor theory (i.e., polygenic inheritance). Five different phenotypes are shown in the F_2 generation, bred from male × female F_1 heterozygotes from the two inbred parent strains. Two alleles (A_2 and B_2) are at the loci that raise BP ("plus" alleles); A_1 and B_1 are alleles that reduce BP ("minus" alleles). After Rapp (1983a) with permission of McGraw-Hill, New York.

Number of plus alleles	0	1	2	3	4
Number of minus alleles	4	3	2	1	0
Phenotype	-4	-2	0	+2	+4

genetic loci, the distribution is a symmetrical frequency histogram, but as the number of loci increases it approximates to a smooth curve. Nonheritable environmental factors sometimes mimic the effects attributed to polygenes (Mather and Jinks, 1982).

The idea of many small effects by a large number of genes works well for variables such as height or BP, which are determined by a large number of physiological factors. It is less obvious that this also applies to properties of individual components of the circulatory control system, for example, the activity of the defense pathway or the development of the resistance vasculature. These properties may be genetically determined, but probably by only a small number of genes.

Assessment of BP Heritability

Assessing heritability involves partitioning the BP variance in the population in a way that permits separating genetic and environmental components. This is well illustrated in hybrid populations derived from inbred hypertensive and normotensive rat strains.[1] In the parent population, the BP of such a strain becomes stable by about the twentieth generation of inbreeding when all the genes of the population, whether or not they affect BP, have become fixed, meaning that at least 99% of the alleles are homozygous.

One measure of heritability is the degree of genetic determination (DGD), also termed *broad heritability*. It is the genetic fraction of the total BP variance. Crossing an inbred hypertensive parent strain with an inbred normotensive strain gives rise to the F_1 hybrid population, the animals of which are intercrossed to produce an F_2 population (Rapp, 1983b; Kurtz et al., 1990). The average BP of F_1 animals is about halfway between those of the two parent strains (figure 3.4). Each parent strain is genetically uniform, so that its BP variance is due to environmental factors, which also applies to the variance of the uniformly heterozygous F_1 hybrid population. The breeding protocol for producing hybrids from two inbred rat strains, to determine the various components of BP variance in assessing heritability, is as follows. P_N and P_H are the inbred normotensive and hypertensive parent strains, while F_1 and F_2 are hybrid populations:

$$P_N \times P_H$$
$$\downarrow$$
$$F_1 \times F_1$$
$$\downarrow$$
$$F_2$$

In the F_2 population, 50% of genes come from each parent and the BP alleles segregate at random, as noted in figure 3.3. The total BP variance (V_T) is larger than in the parent and F_1 populations and is the sum of the environmental plus the genetic variance (V_E, V_G). Another way of producing segregated populations is by backcrossing F_1 animals with animals from one of the parent strains. This produces a population in which 25% of the genes come from one parent and 75% from the other.

Table 3.1 gives the formulas for partitioning the BP variance into genetic and environmental components and for calculating DGD and other indices of heritability

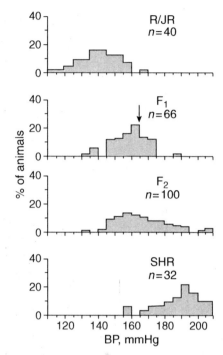

Figure 3.4. Frequency distribution of blood pressure for inbred R/JR and SHR parent populations, and for the F_1 and F_2 hybrids derived from them. The arrow over the F_1 distribution is the midparental value. The variance is largest in the F_2 population and is the sum of environmental and genetic variances. From Rapp (1983a), with permission of McGraw-Hill, New York.

(Griffiths et al., 1993; Vogel and Motulsky, 1997). In hypertensive rat strains, DGD ranges from 40% to 80%, indicating that a large part of the variation in BP is due to genetic factors, which therefore account for much of the average ΔBP between the parent strains (Kurtz et al., 1990).

Additive and Dominance Effects

In the F_1 population, the average BP is not exactly halfway between the parental BP values, which would be expected on the basis of independent action of each strain's

Table 3.1. Formulas for Partitioning of Total (i.e., Phenotypic) Variance and Genetic Variance of a Quantitative Trait and Related Genetic Parameters in the F_2 Generation Produced by Crossing an Inbred Hypertensive and Normotensive Strain

Variance Component/Parameter	Equation
Total (phenotypic)	$V_T = V_E + V_G$
Degree of genetic determination (broad heritability)	$DGD = V_G/(V_E + V_G)$
Additive and dominance components	$V_G = V_A + V_D$
h^2 (narrow heritability)	$h^2 = V_A/(V_A + V_D + V_E)$
Number of genetic loci	$n = R^2/8V_A$

Note: V_T, V_E, V_G, total, environmental, genetic variance; DGD, degree of genetic determination; V_A, V_D, additive and dominance components of variance; h^2, narrow heritability; n, number of genetic loci segregating independently; R, difference between mean BPs of parent strains.

BP genes. The discrepancy implies a role for other factors (Mather and Jinks, 1982; Rapp, 1983a; Griffiths et al., 1993).

An individual with alleles A and a at a particular genetic locus can belong to classes AA, Aa, or aa (figure 3.5). The phenotypes are specified by parameters d and h, where d is the deviation from the midpoint of phenotypes AA and aa, while h is the deviation of the heterozygote Aa from the midpoint.

The genetic variance V_G can now be partitioned into the additive variance (V_A) and the dominance variance (V_D; table 3.1). This leads to the definition of narrow heritability h^2:

$$h^2 = V_A/V_T = V_A/(V_A + V_D + V_E).$$

The greater h^2, the more characteristics of the parents are preserved in their offspring. Knowing h^2 gives an approximate estimate of the minimum number of genetic loci responsible for ΔBP between normotensive and hypertensive parents (table 3.1, equation 5; Falconer, 1960). The estimates in the various rat strains range from 2 to 6 loci, but this is probably an underestimate (Vogel and Motulsky, 1997). It suggests that the number of BP genes in these rats is smaller than is commonly associated with polygenic inheritance. However, the estimate is in accord with the idea that a relatively small number of genes may regulate a few critical components of the control system that affect BP. The properties of each component may be altered greatly by a mutation in a single or a small number of genes.

A third component of the genetic variance, called the *epistatic* component, arises from the interactions between aa and AA and genes from other loci. For example, the relationship between aa and AA may depend on whether the alleles at a second locus are BB, bb, or Bb. Such effects may contribute to nonlinearities in multivariate systems.

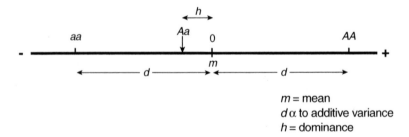

m = mean
$d\,\alpha$ to additive variance
h = dominance

Figure 3.5. An individual with alleles A and a at a particular locus can belong to classes AA, Aa, or aa. The parameter d is proportional to the difference between the two homozygotes and is the additive component of the variance; h measures departure of the heterozygote Aa from the mean value ($m = 0$) between homozygotes. From Mather and Jinks (1982), with permission of Chapman & Hall and Springer-Verlag.

Effect of Genes and Environment on Human Blood Pressure

In the 1940s, a number of investigators thought that the BP frequency distribution of the population was bimodal and suggested that EH was inherited as a single mendelian dominant gene (Platt, 1947; Sobye, 1948). EH was regarded as a condition qualitatively distinct from normotension. Subsequent work has not confirmed the bimodal nature of the distribution (Pickering, 1968; Ward, 1995). The latter is now regarded as a chance occurrence due to inadequate size of the population sample (Murphy, 1964). Furthermore, categorizing the population into only two groups leads to unrealistically large estimates of the strength of the genetic component of the BP variance within families.

All this was changed by the groundbreaking studies of G. W. Pickering and colleagues at St. Mary's Hospital in London, who were the first to show that there was no hard and fast dividing line between hypertension and normotension (chapter 4). They used larger and more representative population samples than in previous studies and were the first to consider the familial association of BP in solely quantitative terms (Hamilton et al., 1954a, 1954b; Pickering, 1961).

The BP distribution of the relatives of normotensives was found to be similar to that of the original subjects, while the relatives of hypertensives had significantly higher BPs (figure 3.6). The systolic and diastolic BPs of individual subjects were linearly related to the BPs of relatives except when the deviations from the mean were large (figure 3.7). They concluded that what is inherited is not hypertension, but the level of BP as such, be it high or low. A similar conclusion was reached in a number of subsequent North American and European studies (see review by Ward, 1995). Presumably the absence of correlation at the higher BPs of the subjects in figure 3.7 was due to random nonfamilial factors that raised the subjects' BP.

A history of hypertension in parents increases the chances that their children will be hypertensive (Shear et al., 1986; Hunt et al., 1991; Rebbeck et al., 1993). Some have found that the probability is greater when hypertension occurs in the father rather than the mother (Burke, Gracey et al., 1998).

In a population survey in Bergen, Norway, parental BP was measured in 1963–64 then followed some 30 years later by observations in their offspring (Mo et al., 1995). BP was highest in children of two hypertensive parents and lowest in children of two normotensive parents (table 3.2). Similar conclusions were reached in the British MRC trial for mild hypertension (Watt et al., 1991).

Multivariate Biometrical Estimates

Hamilton et al. (1954a) assessed the combined effects of genetic and shared environmental factors within families. More elaborate approaches have since been developed for assessing separately the magnitude of genetic, shared, and nonfamilial environmental factors (Rao et al., 1976; Annest et al., 1979b; Sing et al., 1986).

One model is based on the "family set" approach of Schull et al. (1970). This contrasts the resemblance of an individual to (1) a sibling and two biological relatives

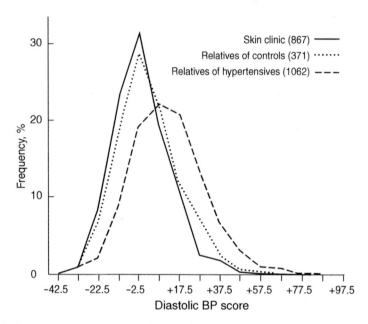

Figure 3.6. Frequency distribution curves of diastolic BP scores after adjustment for age and sex. Curves are from relatives of hypertensive propositi (dashed line), normotensive propositi (dotted line), and original St. Mary's Hospital population (solid line). BPs in relatives of hypertensive propositi were significantly higher. From Hamilton et al. (1954b), with permission of *Clinical Science,* the Biochemical Society, and the Medical Research Society.

(brother, cousin), and (2) two unrelated individuals (spouse and random control). Determining the relationships within and between households allows estimates of the role of the immediate family environment, the outside environment, and genetic factors.

Another approach has been path analysis, which assumes that the expected value of every observed correlation that influences family resemblance of BP can be defined in terms of underlying genetic, shared (sociocultural), and nonfamilial environmental factors. Interestingly, these estimates by different methods have all been close to Pickering's original estimates (Ward, 1995).

Adoption Studies

Adoption studies emphasize environmental factors that are independent of genetic factors. In the Montreal adoption study, all subjects came from French Canadian families to avoid confounding by ethnic heterogeneity (Biron et al., 1976; Annest et al., 1979a, 1979b). Three types of families were studied: those with only adopted children, those with both adopted and natural children, and those with only natural children. The BP variance within families was interpreted as dependent on the interaction between genetic factors and shared household environment, since family size and the mixture of adopted and natural children were without effect.

For systolic and diastolic BPs, the slopes (regression coefficients) of the relationship between parents and their natural children were about twice as great as those

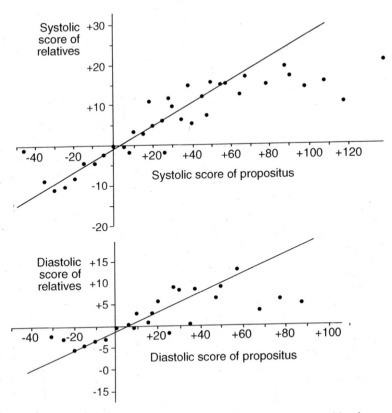

Figure 3.7. Age- and sex-adjusted systolic and diastolic BP scores of propositi and correspond-ing BP scores of relatives, with propositi coming from a mixed general population of hyper-tensives and normotensives. From Pickering (1968), with permission of Churchill-Elsevier.

Table 3.2. Blood Pressure and Heart Rate (Means ± SD) for Children of Two Normotensive Parents (−/−), One Hypertensive Parent (−/+), and Two Hypertensive Parents (+/+), Measured about 30 Years after the Initial Parental Screening Bergen Blood Pressure Study

Variable	Parent BP−/−	Parent BP−/+	Parent BP+/+
n	221	163	106
Age	34 ± 6	38 ± 7*	43 ± 6*.**
BP, mmHg			
SBP	121 ± 12	125 ± 12*	135 ± 15*.**
DBP	72 ± 10	76 ± 9*	85 ± 11*.**
Heart rate, bpm	71 ± 13	73 ± 11	77 ± 13*.**

Notes: n, number; SBP, DBP, systolic and diastolic BPs of offspring (bpm, beats/min); *p < .01 (−/− vs. +/+ or −/+); **p < .01 (−/+ vs. +/+). BP data not adjusted for age and sex.

Source: Mo et al. (1995), with permission of *Journal of Hypertension* and Lippincott, Williams and Wilkins.

Table 3.3. Components of BP Variance in the Population
Based on the Family Set Approach of Biometrical Analysis

Component	%
Genetic factors	30
Shared environment	15
Nonfamilial environment	55

between parents and their adopted children. Similarly, the coefficients between natural children were double those between adopted children. Lastly, the coefficients between children within the household (natural or adopted) were about twice the magnitude of the relationship between parents and children. It suggests that the shared household environment within a family has a significant effect on the children's BP.

Twins

Theoretically, monozygotic twins share 100% of their genes, while only 50% of genes are shared by dizygotic twins. It is usually assumed that environmental factors have similar effects on both types of twins. However, this has been questioned on the grounds that: (1) pairs of monozygotic twins and dizygotic twins usually come from different households, and (2) the family environment is more uniform for monozygotic than for dizygotic twins (Ward, 1995). The relationship between BPs of monozygotic twins has steeper slopes than that between dizygotic twins (e.g., 0.55 vs. 0.25), suggesting that twin studies overestimate the genetic effect on the BP variance (Ward, 1995). However, twin studies provide strong qualitative evidence that genetic factors play a role in the inheritance of some traits affecting BP, such as plasma catecholamine levels, aldosterone concentration, renin levels, and obesity (Grim, Miller et al., 1979; Hopkins et al., 1996; Luft, 2001).

Conclusion

The partititoning of BP variance into genetic and nongenetic components has been refined progressively since the method was first introduced by Fisher (1918; see Vogel and Motulsky, 1997). Table 3.3 gives the average estimates from several studies. Both genetic and environmental factors make highly significant contributions. The effect due to environmental factors is greater than that due to genes.

Genetic Basis for Trait Differences Between Hypertensives and Normotensives

We noted in chapter 2 that trait differences in output patterns between persons with EH and normotensives help define key differences in the control system's operation between the two groups. The question of whether genetic factors contribute to some of these trait differences that affect BP can be determined in rats with genetic hypertension by cosegregation analysis in F_2 or backcross populations. An analogous assessment in humans is based on classifying the groups according to the subjects' parental family history of hypertension.

Genetic Hypertension in Rats

For many years, much research on inbred rat strains documented trait differences between the hypertensive and normotensive strains ($\Delta trait_{h-n}$). Many of these were promoted as possible genetic causes of hypertension, even when there was only a tenuous connection with the cardiovascular system. These hypotheses ignored the phenomenon of genetic drift, which occurs due to random fixation of genes during inbreeding, including genes with no effect on the cardiovascular system.

This trait-collecting period came to an abrupt end with the publication of a paper by Rapp (1983b), which provided a logical basis for determining whether a given $\Delta trait_{h-n}$ was linked to BP. The Rapp paradigm on testing whether a between-strain trait difference is genetically determined is as follows:

1. There must be a difference in a physiological or biochemical trait between the hypertensive and normotensive strains.
2. The trait must follow Mendelian inheritance in an F_2 or backcross population derived from the parental strains.
3. The genes identified in criterion 2 must cosegregate with a significant increment in BP.
4. There must be a logical physiological or biochemical link between the trait and BP.

Given a significant difference in the trait between parent strains, its cosegregation with BP in F_2 or backcross populations strengthens the case that genetic factors play a role. This becomes incontrovertible if evidence of mendelian segregation can be demonstrated. The last point in the list above emphasizes the need to understand the trait's function in order to relate it to the genotype.

The Rapp paradigm was a major advance in genetic analysis of genetic rat hypertension. However, one should also bear in mind that genetically determined single trait differences are not likely likely to be of equal importance in the operation of the control system.

Some examples of trait differences between the Dahl-S and Dahl-R strains and between SHR and WKY strains follow and their significance is considered further in Chapters 12 and 16.

Steroid Profile in Dahl Rats

The differences in steroid patterns between salt-sensitive and salt-resistant Dahl rats (S, salt sensitive; R, salt resistant) show mendelian inheritance (Rapp and Dahl, 1971, 1972a, 1972b, 1976). In S rats, 18-hydroxylation of deoxycorticosterone (DOC) occurs at a greater rate than in R rats and accounts for the higher production of 18-hydroxydeoxycorticosterone (18-OH-DOC). This is offset by reduction in the 11β-hydroxylation of DOC to corticosterone (compound B), so that the sum of (18-OH-DOC + B) remains the same in both strains. The ratio 18-OH-DOC/(18-OH-DOC + B) provides the best discrimination between strains (figure 3.8). The magnitude

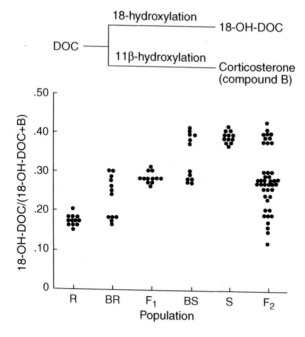

Figure 3.8. Scatter diagram of steroid ratio 18-OH-DOC/(18-OH-DOC + compound B) in different populations, obtained during in vitro incubation of rat adrenals in the presence of DOC precursor. R, Dahl salt-resistant rat; S, Dahl salt-sensitive rat; F_1, hybrid S × R; BR, backcross F_1 × R; BS, backcross F_1 × S; F_2, F_1 × F_1 cross. From Rapp (1995), based on Rapp and Dahl (1971, 1972a), with permission of Raven Press and Lippincott, Williams and Wilkins.

of the ratio between strains is unrelated to sodium intake with production of 18-OH-DOC not suppressed on high salt, while that of aldosterone is markedly suppressed.

In an F_2 population, the steroid ratios segregate close to the expected mendelian ratios of 1:2:1. The genotype was inferred from the phenotype on a high-salt diet and accounts for a ΔBP of ~16 mmHg between the putative SS and RR homozygotes. This is only a fraction of ΔBP between S and R rats on high salt (chapter 12), leaving the rest to be accounted for by other factors.

A similar analysis was repeated many years later, using the methods of molecular biology (Cicila et al., 1993). Both the 18- and 11β-hydroxylation of DOC is catalyzed by the enzyme 11β-hydroxylase, which is regulated by a single gene on chromosome 7. Restriction fragment length polymorphisms (RFLPs) for the 11β-hydroxylase gene have been found to cosegregate with the steroid ratio in F_2 rats and have helped identify the mutations that give rise to the abnormal steroid profiles.[2] The work has thus extended the initial conclusions.

Traits Contributing to SHR Hypertension

Resting renal SNA is higher in SHR than in normotensive WKY (chapter 16). In one of the first cosegregation studies, Judy et al. (1979) demonstrated a strong relationship between resting SNA and BP in a segregating backcross population (F_1 × SHR; figure 3.9), the progeny of which had on average 75% of genes from parent SHR.

After mating SHR × WKY, the F_1 hybrid has a BP at or slightly above that of WKY, which is why it is called the borderline hypertensive rat (BHR). In a backcross

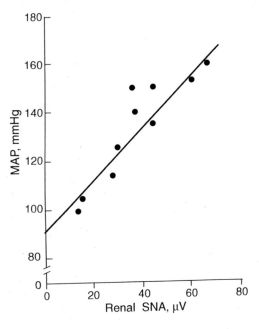

Figure 3.9. Relationship in 16-week-old rats between mean arterial pressure (MAP, mmHg) and resting renal sympathetic nerve activity (SNA, μV). The animals were from a backcross population originating from SHR and Wistar/Lewis rats. From Judy et al. (1979), with permission of *Hypertension*, American Heart Association, and Lippincott, Williams and Wilkins.

population (BHR × WKY) in which only 25% of genes came from the parent SHR, the renal SNA in response to air jet stress correlated closely with resting MAP (figure 3.10, top; Di Bona, 1991; Di Bona et al., 1996). In another study, intracerebroventricular (i.c.v.) guanabenz[3] lowered renal SNA, with the magnitude of the fall in SNA highly correlated to BP in the segregating population (figure 3.10, bottom). Thus, BP genes may determine renal SNA responsiveness and resting SNA in SHR.

Trait differences relating to the peripheral vasculature have also been studied by cosegregation. In F_2 rats derived from SHR and WKY, the diameter of the renal afferent arteriole at 7 weeks of age was closely related to BP at 23 weeks of age (figure 3.11; Norrelund et al., 1994). By 7 weeks, the VSM cell phenotype in SHR has only just become contractile, and the narrowing of the lumen is largely due to the CA-induced growth of the immature VSM cells during the neonatal period (chapter 16).

In contrast, the structural changes (medial thickness [m]/internal radius [r_i] ratio) in mesenteric R_1 vessels were not significantly related to BP in 14–16-week-old F_2 rats (Mulvany and Korsgaard, 1983; Mulvany, 1988). The reason for the different findings in the two beds is not clear. It may be due to developmental differences between beds; alternatively, the age at which the test was performed may be important, or the arteriolar narrowing may be a better index of genetic influences on structural changes than the m/r_i ratio. Genetic influences may be most obvious in young animals, while later superposition of nongenetically determined growth of the vessel wall may mask the earlier genetic changes. However, irrespective of a role of genetic factors, R_1 vessel structural changes are hemodynamically important as Vas R amplifiers of constrictor stimuli in all vascular beds (chapter 6).

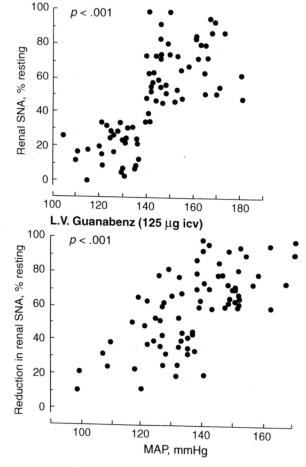

Figure 3.10. Backcross rat population (BHR × WKY), showing relationship of resting MAP (mmHg) to (top) air jet stress-induced increase in renal sympathetic nerve activity (SNA, % of resting) and (bottom) reduction in renal SNA after 125 μg i.c.v. guanabenz. From DiBona et al. (1996), with permission of *Hypertension*, American Heart Association, and Lippincott, Williams and Wilkins.

Unexpected Heterogeneity and Strange Attitudes

In an important paper, Kurtz and Morris (1987) described differences in resting BP and other traits in rats from nominally the same WKY strain bred by different commercial suppliers in the United States. The WKY turned out to be genetically heterogenous, as were SHR but to a lesser degree (Kurtz et al., 1989; Lindpaintner et al., 1992; St. Lezin et al., 1992). The nominally identical strains were in fact different substrains, raising doubts about the reproducibility of data from different laboratories.

The only surprising thing is that this result had not been anticipated. It was the inescapable legacy of the haste with which SHR and WKY had been introduced into the United States during the 1960s and 1970s (Nabika et al., 1991; Yamori, 1994; Yamori and Swales, 1994). The inbreeding of WKY had barely begun before they were shipped from Japan; the SHR breeding program, though incomplete, was more advanced. These problems were compounded by the premature release of stock to commercial suppliers by the U.S. National Institutes of Health.

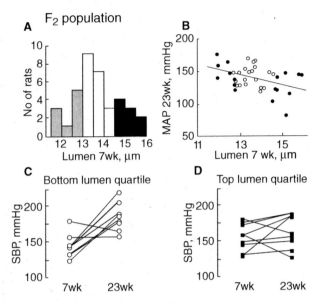

Figure 3.11. Relationship between renal afferent arteriolar lumen diameter (μm) at 7 weeks of age and mean arterial BP (MAP, mmHg) in same rats at 23 weeks of age, obtained from F$_2$ population derived from SHR and WKY. A, distribution of lumen diameters at 7 weeks; smallest quartile in gray; largest quartile in black. B, inverse relationship between lumen at 7 weeks and MAP at 23 weeks. Black circles are results from extreme quartiles; open circles data from remainder. Panels C and D show relationship of lumen diameter at 7 weeks to subsequent BP Adapted from Norrelund et al. (1994), with permission of *Hypertension*, American Heart Association, and Lippincott, Williams and Wilkins.

The question of reproducibility was a good reason for consternation. Nevertheless, the premature release of these rats was a once-off administrative bungle, which has not recurred since. If anything, it should have reinforced the need for high-quality experimental designs with adequate controls, to make the experiments of a given research group as self-sufficient as possible.

Instead, what was truly extraordinary was the raising of the question of whether trait comparisons between hypertensive and normotensive animals had any scientific value. Such a position not only weakens pathophysiological studies in rat hypertension but undermines a basic tenet of all clinical experimentation.

Raising the above question and downgrading the value of between-strain comparisons was encouraged by the geneticists on the grounds that not all $\Delta trait_{h-n}$ were due to genes (Kurtz and Morris, 1987; Rapp, 1987; Lindpaintner et al., 1992; Jacob, 1999). The following statement is typical:

Investigators have traditionally tried to exploit these etiological differences [between hypertensive and normotensive strains] to find the underlying causes of hypertension. Unfortunately, [many] of the . . . [experimental] designs used "control" strains such as the Wistar-Kyoto (WKY) rat, assuming that they differed from the spontaneously hypertensive rat (SHR) only at the "hypertension" genes. This has been shown not to be true because the strains used as "controls," even though they are normotensive, also exhibit many other phenotypic differences besides BP that were fixed during the process of inbreeding. Consequently investigators have made little headway in defining the causes of hypertension. (Jacob, 1999, p. 530)

This type of remark is characteristic of a grab for power by practitioners of an aspirant discipline, who feel undervalued because of their confidence that they have all the answers (Mayr, 1997). I do not know how many physiologists believed that every $\Delta \text{trait}_{h\text{-}n}$ was genetically determined. However, even if this belief was widespread, it is overly simplistic to suggest that not knowing about genetic drift was responsible for the lack of progress. Not that the physiologists have much to be proud of in collecting a huge data base of $\Delta \text{traits}_{h\text{-}n}$ as an end in itself, instead of spending time selecting the Δtraits that might help in determining the difference in operation of the control system, as has been done in chapter 16.

Nabika et al. (1991) noted that the DNA fingerprint patterns between the Japanese Izumo SHR and WKY strains are less diverse than in the U.S. strains. Similarly, the inbred Dahl S and R strains show greater genetic similarity than many other strains (Rapp, 1991, 1994, 2000). Given the concordance in DNA fingerprint patterns of the Japanese Izumo SHR and WKY strains and between inbred Dahl salt-sensitive and salt-resistant strains (S/JR, R/JR), there may be an advantage in using normotensive strains with a genetic background broadly similar to the hypertensive strain. As Rapp (1994) has stated, "genetic similarity is desirable for comparisons at the biochemical-physiological level, but each similarity makes it difficult to find genetic markers at the DNA level" (pp. 190–191).

Adequate controls are always necessary in experimental designs, as pointed out many years ago by R. A. Fisher (1947). They allow assessment of: (1) time-related cardiovascular and neuroendocrine changes, (2) between-strain differences in responsiveness to stimuli, and (3) the specificity of particular interventions.

Traits Contributing to EH

Mental Stress Test

Acute mental stress elicits greater rises in renal Vas R and plasma renin activity (PRA) in persons with mild EH than in normotensives with negative family hypertension, while the responses of normotensives with at least one hypertensive parent are of intermediate magnitude (figure 3.12; Hollenberg et al., 1981). This suggests that genetic factors enhance the renal vascular response to stress.

Modulator and Nonmodulator Responses

The test subdivides the population into "modulators" and "nonmodulators" on the basis of their aldosterone and renal Vas R responses to standard infusions of Ang II at two levels of salt intake (Hollenberg and Williams, 1995).

In modulators on low salt, Ang II enhances aldosterone production and blunts the rise in renal Vas R compared to the changes while on normal salt. On a high salt intake, Ang II blunts the aldosterone response, while the rise in renal Vas R is enhanced. In nonmodulators, the responses to Ang II are independent of salt intake, and both

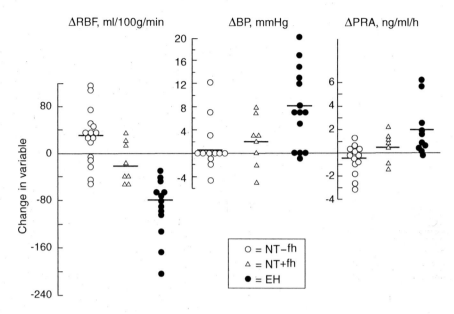

Figure 3.12. Changes evoked by mental stress test in renal blood flow (ΔRBF), mean arterial blood pressure (ΔMAP), and plasma renin activity (ΔPRA), in subjects with EH (black circles) and normotensives without a family history of hypertension (open circles) and with positive history (open triangles). From Hollenberg et al. (1981), with permission of *Hypertension*, American Heart Association, and Lippincott, Williams and Wilkins.

aldosterone production and the rise in renal Vas R are blunted. Modulators are more common in those with normal BP, but nonmodulators are more common in EH.

In nonmodulators, BP is more sensitive to alterations in salt intake. The test has been said to provide insights into the mechanisms of salt sensitivity. On a high-salt diet, the Ang II-induced rise in renal Vas R is reduced in nonmodulators who are homozygous to the T235 variant of the angiotensinogen gene (Hopkins et al., 1996). The test is difficult to relate to physiological perturbations; hence it is difficult to interpret.

Sodium-Lithium Countertransport

Cellular Na^+–Li^+ countertransport activity relates to cellular membrane functions. In EH, the maximum rate of countertransport in erythrocytes is almost double that in normotensives and appears to be specific for EH (Canessa et al., 1980; Sing et al., 1986; Rebbeck et al., 1993). The Na^+–Li^+ countertransporter resembles the Na^+–H^+ exchanger, which affects numerous cellular processes in brain, kidney, and VSM cells (Bobik et al., 1994).

There is undoubtedly a genetically determined difference in these transport systems between those with EH and matched normotensives. What is not known is whether this alone contributes to the BP rise in EH, or whether the effects only become manifest in the presence of the renal vascular changes, which appears to be what happens in Dahl-S rats (chapter 12).

BHR as a Model for the EH Phenotype

In a normal laboratory environment, the resting BP of BHR is the same or only slightly greater than in WKY. However, after a change to a high-salt diet or an increase in the level of stress, there are rises in resting BP and renal SNA (figure 3.13; Lawler et al., 1981; DiBona, 1991; Sanders and Lawler, 1992; DiBona et al., 1996). In WKY, stress and salt have minimal effects.

The likely norms of reaction in SHR, WKY, and BHR are indicated in figure 3.14. In SHR, the animals remain hypertensive in both healthy and adverse environments, while WKY remain normotensive. However, BHR are normotensive in a healthy environment but become hypertensive when this becomes adverse, when their BP reaches levels similar to those of SHR. BHR have fewer high BP genes than SHR, so that the implication is that the genetic determinants of sensitization of their defense pathway require reinforcement by the environmental inputs.

This is similar to the positions of humans who are genetically susceptible to EH, and in whom environmental reinforcement is needed to raise BP. It suggests a genotype

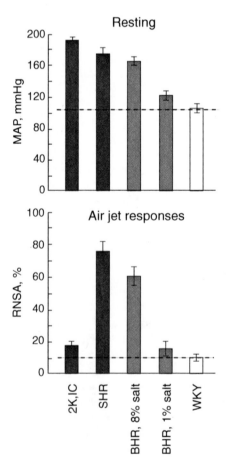

Figure 3.13. Resting MAP (mmHg) (top) and maximum RSNA response to acute air jet stress (% of resting) (bottom) in 16-week-old SHR, WKY, and BHR and in 10-week-old Sprague Dawley with 4 weeks' 2K-1C hypertension; BHR-8% salt, extra salt (wt/vol) in tap water; other rats received 1% NaCl in rat chow and tap water ad libitum. Adapted from DiBona et al. (1996), with permission of *Hypertension*, American Heart Association, and Lippincott, Williams and Wilkins.

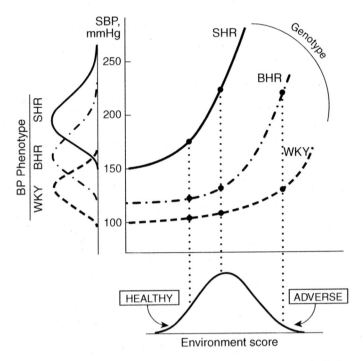

Figure 3.14. BP phenotype in SHR, WKY, and BHR, arising from hypothetical genotype × environment interactions. In these plots, the genotypic differences in susceptibility to environmental factors are determined by their slopes and intercepts.

similar to BHR, with a relatively low number of high-BP genes. In contrast, in those not susceptible to EH the genotype is resistant to salt and stress, as in WKY.

In EH, the low number of high-BP genes probably contributes to the late onset of hypertension in early adult life, contrasting with the childhood onset in SHR. This is suggested from the results in an F_2 population derived from SHR and WKY (figure 3.15; Harrap et al., 1986, 1988). In the parents, a significant ΔBP_{h-n} is apparent by 4–6 weeks of age. The F_2 population was classified into high- and low-BP rats at 16 weeks of age by selecting rats from the highest and lowest BP quartiles at that age. Their resting BPs had only begun to diverge when they were 12 weeks old (figure 3.15). This suggests that in high-BP rats there were fewer high-BP genes than the parent SHR, while low-BP rats had a greater number of high-BP genes than WKY. In a constant environment, there thus appears to be an inverse relationship between the number of high-BP genes and the time of onset of hypertension.

Molecular Genetics: Current Approaches to High-BP Genes

The discovery of the structure of DNA by Watson and Crick in 1953 marked the start of a revolution in biology and genetics. Like all revolutions, it has been exciting but

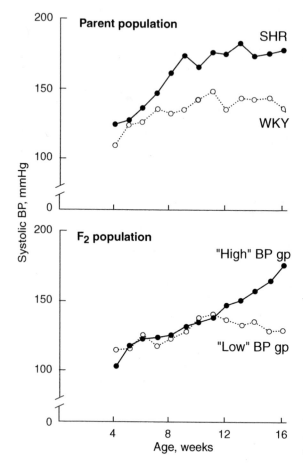

Figure 3.15. Age-systolic BP relationship in (top) parent SHR and WKY population, and (bottom) in F_2 rats categorized at 16 weeks of age into upper and lower BP quartiles. Data from Harrap (1986, 1988), with permission of *Clinical and Experimental Pharmacology and Physiology* and Blackwell.

not always comfortable. A huge number of new insights have been obtained into the way genes regulate cell functions (Alberts et al., 1989; Darnell et al., 1990; Cooper, 1997). In the hypertension field, there has been progress in the methodology of how to dissect the genome in animal models. However, to date the genes through which hypertension is inherited in EH or in hypertensive rats have for the most part not been definitively identified. In contrast, the role of the genetic mutation causing high BP has been fully elucidated in several rare types of human monogenic hypertension.

Quantitative Trait Loci Affecting BP

The various chromosomes have been systematically explored for quantitative trait loci (QTL), that is, segments of DNA that affect BP (Vogel and Motulsky, 1997; Rapp, 2000). When the gene location is already known, there are tests for determining the extent to which the observed mutation accounts for ΔBP.

Sometimes "candidate" genes are selected on the basis of their known role in cardiovascular regulation. If the gene's position on a genetic map is known, RFLPs are sought in the genomic DNA that distinguish between hypertensive and normotensive strains. If these are found, the relationship of the alleles to BP is determined in F_2 or backcross populations. Last, the mutant gene's protein product is determined, which permits study of its effects on the control system.

In the 22 chromosomes of the rat genome (2 sex chromosomes, 20 autosomes), all but 3 chromosomes have BP-QTLs (Rapp, 2000). Placing the BP-QTLs on linkage maps of particular chromosomes is usually accomplished with appropriate markers.[4] Marker alleles M_1 and M_2 are selected on the basis of linkage to BP alleles A_1 and A_2 in inbred parental strains P_1 and P_2. A_1 is a minus allelele ($\downarrow$BP) and A_2 a plus allelele ($\uparrow$BP). In the inbred strains, each marker and gene locus is homozygous for its respective alleles. The markers segregate in mendelian ratios in the F_2 population. The F_2 rats are phenotyped for BP and genotyped at the marker locus.

If locus M is close to A, the marker alleles M_1M_1, M_1M_2, and M_2M_2 rats will correspond to genotypes A_1A_1, A_1A_2, and A_2A_2 and ΔBP between classes reflects the genotype of A. But if the distance along the chromosomes between M and A is large, the recombination rate during meiosis often degrades the relationship between M, A, and BP.

With additional markers, a number of loci affecting BP can be studied along a chromosome, as illustrated in figure 3.16 for rat chromosome 9 (Rapp et al., 1998). At each locus, ΔBP is tested by one-way ANOVA over the three genotypic classes. The BP effect is greatest at locus Ae3 (anion exchange locus) and falls off on either side. A better test is to apply the method of maximum likelihood and calculate a statistic called the LOD (logarithm of the odds) score, that is, the ratio of the likelihood that there is a BP-QTL at the particular locus versus the likelihood that there is no QTL (Lander and Botstein, 1989; Liu, 1998). LOD scores ≥ 3.0 are generally regarded as statistically significant (Vogel and Motulsky, 1997).

When first identified, QTLs extend over rather long sections of DNA, each of which often includes a number of genes affecting BP. To dissect this into smaller segments requires additional markers used in conjunction with congenic strains and substrains.

Congenic and Recombinant Inbred Strains

Congenic strains and substrains help define whether a given QTL or a particular candidate gene influences the BP in the manner suspected. Congenic strains are genetically identical except for the segment of a particular chromosome (Kurtz et al., 1994; Rapp, 2000). Strains in which a whole chromosome has been substituted are known as consomic strains.

The latter have been used to investigate sexual BP dimorphism in SHR, in which BP is greater in males than in females, which occurs in many species, including humans. The dimorphism is dependent on the influence of both the Y chromosome and an autosome, as discussed for SHR and WKY in chapter 16.

The development of congenic strains involves moving a polymorphic marker gene from a donor to a recipient strain. After crossing the parent strains, the F_1 heterozygotes are backcrossed to the recipient strain for at least eight cycles. Then two offspring are bred which are homozygous for the original marker, in order to fix the latter on the genetic background of the recipient. If the QTL is closely linked to the marker,

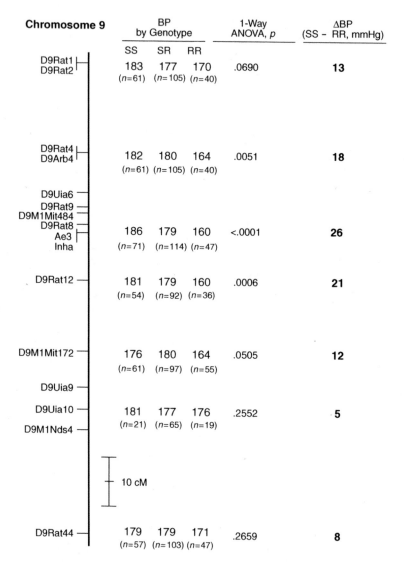

Figure 3.16. Linkage analysis of genetic markers to BP in chromosome 9 in F_2 rats, derived from Dahl S and R rats. Genetic linkage map is at left. Rats have been classified by marker genotype at each marker. S, allele from Dahl S rats; R, allele from Dahl R rats; n, number of rats; cM, centiMorgan. BP by the three genotypic classes has been compared by one-way ANOVA, with average ΔBP and p for significance between homozygotes in the two columns on right. From Rapp (2000), with permission of *Physiological Reviews* and American Physiological Society.

it becomes part of the congenic strain. Congenic substrains are constructed to include smaller and smaller sections of the original QTL.

Another novel preparation is the recombinant inbred (RI) strain. Each is generated from F_2 animals derived by crossing two inbred parent strains (Pravenec et al., 1989;

Kurtz et al., 1994). The F_2 animals are paired off at random and the progeny of each is inbred for 20 generations, creating a new inbred strain. The process allows alleles from different loci to recombine, forming new combinations in the line derived from each F_2 pair. Typically a panel of 10–40 RI strains is derived from the original parental cross, thereby simulating continuous variation over the BP range defined by the original parent strains. Each RI strain has a constant genotype and can be used to study the effect on the phenotype of a large number of perturbations, including environmental factors, aging, and drugs.

Transgenic Rats and Mice

New genetic material is introduced artificially into the genome through methods other than breeding, for example, by microinjecting an altered DNA construct into the pronucleus of a fertilized oocyte, or by infecting embryonic cells with material attached to a retroviral vector (Paul et al., 1994). After incorporation of the genetic material into the germ cells, the founder animals of the new line pass the transgene to their offspring.

This technology has produced novel types of hypertension. In the first transgenic rat preparation, the incorporation of the mouse renin-2 gene into the rat genome resulted in fulminant hypertension of 300 mmHg in 10-week-old rats (Mullins et al., 1990; Ganten et al., 1991; Paul et al., 1994). The mouse renin-2 gene is a foreign gene in rats, but plasma and tissue renins appeared to be under the control of rat renin. The mouse renin-2 gene is overexpressed in the inner layers of the adrenal cortex where it alters the profile of adrenal steroid production. This is responsible for the transgenic rat's pronounced sexual dimorphism, with BP much higher in males than in females.

Transgenic preparations often illuminate circumscribed functional mechanisms, such as signaling in cardiovascular hypertrophy (chapter 6). Sometimes genetic manipulation is restricted to a single tissue, for example, knocking out the insulin receptor on adipocytes (chapter 13).

Common gene manipulations include adding more copies or causing disruption of a gene, which often contribute to an understanding of its physiological role (Smithies and Kim, 1994; Smithies, 1997). Changes in either gain or loss of function induced by genetic manipulation are much more specific than the classic stimulation and ablation methods. Positive findings indicate a potential effect, but effects may be masked through compensatory changes in alternative pathways.

One example of the value of these preparations is the in vivo demonstration of a local role of the renin-angiotensin system in vascular hypertrophy. In some species, Ang II is produced not only through ACE but through the enzyme chymase, which plays the major role in the human heart (Dell'Italia and Husain, 2000). Recently a rat VSM chymase gene was introduced into the mouse genome in a manner by which its expression could be controlled (Ju et al., 2001). In the transgenic animal, the vascular walls of resistance and conduction arteries became thicker and their wall thickness/internal radius ratio increased. It suggests that the BP rise in these animals of 25 mmHg was due to increased chymase expression.

Positional Cloning

Prior to the above method, the objective was to detect biochemical differences between normal and mutant phenotypes and to relate them to differences in their protein products (Vogel and Motulsky, 1997). In positional cloning, the approach is reversed. A gene with an unknown mode of action is identified from studies of QTLs, and its DNA sequence is established. Its presence is inferred by finding open reading frames, which are long sequences that begin with a start codon and are not interrupted by a stop codon except at the termini. The sequences are compared with appropriate databases, permitting inferences about the gene's structure and its mRNA and protein product. This helps determine how a change in DNA sequence gives rise to a particular hereditary disease. One of the best-known medical applications has been in the identification of the mutation which gives rise to cystic fibrosis (Quinton, 1999; Reddy et al., 1999). This gene encodes a chloride channel, which is called the cystic fibrosis transmembrane regulator and plays a critical role for Cl⁻ and water secretion from various epithelia (e.g., in the lungs).

Human Monogenic Types of Hypertension

High BP caused by a mutation of a single gene includes glucocorticoid-remediable aldosteronism (GRA, familial hyperaldosteronism type I), apparent mineralocorticoid excess, and Liddle's syndrome. Other monogenic types of hypertension include autosomal dominant hypertension with brachydactyly (Schuster et al., 1996), autosomal dominant polycystic disease (Wang and Strandgaard, 1997), and Gordon's syndrome (familial hyperaldosteronism, type II; Jeunemaitre, Soubrier et al., 1992; Gordon et al., 1994; Stowasser and Gordon, 2000). Some features of the first three are briefly summarized below.

Glucocorticoid Remediable Aldosteronism

In this autosomal dominant hypertension, plasma aldosterone is raised, urinary outputs of 18-oxycortisol and 18-hydroxycortisol are increased, PRA is low, plasma volume is raised, and there may be metabolic alkalosis and hypokalemia (Lifton et al., 1992a, 1992b; Lifton, 1996; Luft, 1998; Stowasser and Gordon, 2000). Administration of glucocorticoids restores aldosterone production to normal. Aldosterone is normally regulated by the renin-angiotensin system, through the action of Ang II on cells in the adrenal zona glomerulosa, which express the gene for aldosterone synthase. In GRA, aldosterone is under the control of adrenocorticotrophic hormone (ACTH), which causes rises in the oxy- and hydroxycortisol derivatives that are normally produced in zona fasciculata cells.

It was the demonstration of these steroids in urine which provided the clue that aldosterone production in GRA took place at an ectopic site. The final steps in glucocorticoid and mineralocorticoid biosynthesis involves two enzymes, 11β-hydroxylase and aldosterone synthase, which are regulated by the genes CYP11B1 and CYP11B2. A linkage study in a large pedigree showed that the abnormal gene in GRA was on chromosome 8 (Lifton et al., 1992b). The abnormal gene lies between the two normal genes on the same chromosome. It is a chimeric gene that has the promoter region of the CYP11B1 (11β-hydroxylase gene) and the coding section of the CYP11B2 (aldosterone synthase gene; figure 3.17). The chimeric gene appears to be the result of unequal crossover during meoisis. The first section of the gene accounts for its increased expression in the ectopic site regulated by ACTH, while the coding section is responsible for the high aldosterone. It explains why glucocorticoid-induced suppression of ACTH normalizes aldosterone production through this gene.

Syndrome of Apparent Mineralocorticoid Excess

Apparent mineralocorticoid excess is an autosomal recessive type of hypertension, which is sensitive to the patient's salt intake. Plasma aldosterone and PRA are low, but plasma volume is raised. The condition is simulated by excessive intake of liquorice or its active principle, glycyrrhenitic acid. This inhibits 11β-hydroxysteroid dehydrogenase (11-β OHSD), which normally converts cortisol to inactive cortisone (Funder, 1994). Circulating cortisol has a high affinity for the mineralocorticoid receptor, which is normally "protected" by the enzyme (Funder et al., 1988; Funder, 1994). The hypertension is due to a mutation in the renal isoenzyme that reduces the activity of 11-β OHSD (Mune et al., 1995). Cortisol then stimulates mineralocorticoid receptors, causing hypertension through salt and water retention.

Liddle's Syndrome

Liddle's syndrome is an autosomal dominant hypertension. Plasma aldosterone and PRA are low and plasma volume is raised (Gordon et al., 1994; Luft, 1998). BP responds to thiazide diuretics and triamterene, but not to spironolactone. Liddle

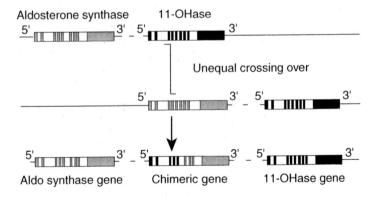

Figure 3.17. Diagram suggesting that chimeric gene duplication causing glucocorticoid-remediable aldosteronism (GRA) arises from unequal crossover between genes that encode aldosterone synthase and steroid 11-βhydroxylase, which are both on chromosome 8. The exons of the aldosterone synthase and steroid 11-βhydroxylase genes are shown, respectively, in gray and black. After Lifton et al. (1992a), with permission of *Nature* and Macmillan Publishers, Ltd.

thought that the patients had distal renal tubular defects that increased reabsorption of sodium and water. Indeed, in one patient the disease was cured by a renal transplant.

Linkage studies have localized the genetic mutations to a small section of chromosome 16, which affects the genes that encode the β and γ subunits of the amiloride-sensitive sodium channel (Hansson et al., 1995; Shimkets et al., 1995). For normal operation, the α subunit must also be functional; its gene is located on chromosome 12 (Lifton, 1996). Reabsorption of sodium through the channel is usually regulated by aldosterone. Mutations in the β or γ subunits cause it to remain on the apical surface instead of becoming internalized. The molecular change is due to an increase in proline in the COOH terminus. When the mutant channel is expressed in oocytes of *Xenopus*, whole-cell sodium current increases (Schild et al., 1995).

Essential Hypertension

According to Luft (1998):

> It is hard to pick up an issue of any hypertension-related journal without encountering reports on polymorphism and the confirmation or refutation of association studies. Nevertheless the results of this heady area of research are a little more sobering. Exactly how many genes have been found that are important in primary hypertension? . . . Sooner or later we shall be called to account for where all the money went. Perhaps we should start thinking of the answers (p. 1871).

Other geneticists have expressed similar sentiments, though perhaps not quite as directly. All have emphasized the difficulties of the task (Lifton and Jeunemaitre, 1993; Kurtz, 1995; Hamet et al., 1998; Corvol et al., 1999). In the three types of monogenic hypertension considered above, the mutants directly affect renal function. To believers in the renal origins of all hypertension, it has confirmed that the cause of EH must be renal. But this is simply wishful thinking.

Candidate genes that have been considered include genes regulating the renin-angiotensin system (e.g., angiotensinogen, ACE, aldosterone synthase); genes subserving renal tubular function (e.g., subunits of the epithelial sodium channel, α-adducin); the NOS gene; and several others (Luft, 1998; Corvol et al., 1999; Kato et al., 1999; Soubrier, 1999; Staessen et al., 2001). Many of them are involved in functions that are disturbed in EH. However, polymorphism in the above genes in EH has not been uniform, which makes their roles in EH uncertain.

Many geneticists think that the main limitation in EH is its multifactorial nature and the ambiguity of the BP phenotype (Lifton and Jeunemaitre, 1993; Corvol et al., 1999). From the viewpoint of defining underlying mechanisms, BP is not so much ambiguous as multifactorial, as discussed in chapter 2. For this purpose, output variables other than BP need to be employed so that the operation of the control system can be defined more specifically. In addition, current genetic studies do not differentiate between the genes likely to play a role in the initiation of EH which may be expressed in the CNS, and the genes regulating formation of structural vascular changes, which determine the long-term rise in BP and the degree of organ damage.

Markers and Candidate Genes

One of Pickering's legacies has been the idea that the number of genes contributing to EH is large (Lifton and Jeunemaitre, 1993; Harrap, 1994; Kurtz, 1995; Lifton, 1996; Hamet et al., 1998; Luft, 1998; Dominiczak et al., 2000). The unquestioning acceptance of this could be misplaced, at least with respect to the genes involved in the initiation of EH and SHR hypertension. In any event, the question is unanswerable in the absence of a hypothesis about the pathogenesis of EH.

Genetics and Systems Analysis

The importance of genetic inheritance in the pathogenesis of EH is now firmly established. The insights gained by family studies have been strengthened by the more direct assessment of heritability in hypertensive rat strains. In SHR, resting SNA and the response to stress are genetically determined and the enhanced SNA accounts for the elevation of BP, resembling what happens in EH.

The BHR has turned out to have a genotype resembling that of EH, where the rise in BP depends on both genetic and environmental factors. This contrasts with SHR, in which genetic factors sensitize the defense pathway sufficiently so that hypertension develops in virtually every environment. In contrast, in BHR extra environmental stimulation of the defense pathway becomes necessary to produce sensitization. Similarly, in the high-BP F_2 rats, the smaller number of mutant genes delays the onset of hypertension by 1–2 months compared to that in parent SHR in the same environment. In SHR, the early initiation of hypertension is not solely due to sensitization of the defense pathway, but is also due to the development of BP-independent changes in the larger resistance vessels (chapter 16). It raises the question whether the reduced number of regulatory genes that accounts for the delayed onset of hypertension affects one, the other, or both of the above functions.

In EH, the enhanced renal vascular response to stress is also genetically determined, probably mainly through greater CNS-mediated sympathetic responsiveness. Genetic factors also play a role in various cellular transport functions, of which the Na^+–Li^+ countertransport system is a marker. But what is not clear is how important this and related mechanisms are in the elevation of BP. It points to the need for genetic analysis to relate more directly to the cardiovascular control system.

Molecular BP genetics today is still at a stage where technology takes precedence over biological concepts. In EH or rat hypertension, the focus seems to be more on the genome than on the pathophysiological problems. Looking for BP-QTLs appears to be relatively random, resembling the collection of $\Delta traits_{h-n}$ in the pre-Rapp era.

The geneticists are correct in their assertion that BP differences provide no clue about underlying pathophysiology. Nor does BP provide a guide as to whether a lot of genes or only a few determine the inheritance of EH.

Looking for intermediate phenotypes that are regulated by single genes (Dominiczak et al., 1999) is not the same as looking for the $\Delta traits_{h-n}$ that distinguish between the way the control system operates in hypertensives and normotensives. From a physiologist's perspective, it seems highly likely that different genes are likely to regulate processes involved in the initiation of EH compared to those that determine its progression. All of this points to the need for more meaningful collaboration between physiologists and geneticists.

PART III

INPUT-OUTPUT ANALYSIS: POINTERS TO NEURAL INVOLVEMENT

4

Human Arterial Pressure

The BP is a highly multifactorial variable, meaning that it is influenced by virtually all that goes on in the circulation. This makes it of the utmost value as an indicator of future cardiovascular risk, assuming that it is measured by adequate methodology. Comparing the age-BP relationship between populations tells us that there are marked differences in prevalence of EH. Moreover, the prevalence of EH increases with age in populations in which EH is common. Specific intervention studies have helped to sort out the relative importance of mental stress, high dietary salt, obesity, and other factors as causes of EH. However, in all the above conditions additional analysis is required to indicate the physiological meaning of a given change in BP, as has been done in later chapters.

Blood Pressure Epidemiology

A famous controversy between Platt and Pickering in the 1940s and 1950s threw light on the nature of the BP frequency distribution in the population and on the nature of the inheritance of EH, as discussed briefly in chapter 3. Platt (1947, 1959) had suggested that the frequency distribution was bimodal and that EH was inherited as a mendelian dominant. On the other hand, Pickering (1961, 1968) showed convincingly that it was not bimodal and that there was no obvious demarcation between hypertension and normotension at any age (Hamilton et al., 1954a, 1954b, 1954c; Pickering et al., 1954; Oldham et al., 1960; Pickering, 1961, 1968). Hence, the famous aphorism "Hypertension is a quantity, not a disease."

71

Pickering (1961) went on to elaborate:

The old idea concerning the nature of essential hypertension is that the disease represents a qualitative deviation from the norm. Somewhere, if we could only find it, there is, according to this idea, a unique and specific fault which distinguishes those with the disease from those without it. This unique fault has a unique and specific cause. The new idea is that essential hypertension represents a quantitative deviation from the norm. The disease represents high arterial pressure without specific cause, and the harmful effects of this raised pressure. The difference between those with the disease and those without it is one of degree and not of kind. The differences are quantitative, not qualitative (p. 1).

Pickering sensed that hypertension called for a novel way of looking at some chronic diseases. However, I am not sure that he appreciated that it was the use of BP that was responsible for the quantitative nature of the difference between those with EH and those with normal BP. Certainly the environmental causes that raise BP also alter autonomic and hormonal effector activity and give rise to structural and functional vascular changes. These are absent in normotensives and can be regarded as qualitatively distinct. Nevertheless, the use of BP is indispensable in the medical management of EH and secondary types of hypertension. It is also an important first step in the physiological analysis of the underlying mechanisms.

The Age-BP Relationship

Pickering made extensive use of the age-BP relationship and found that the frequency distribution curve was unimodal at every age (figure 4.1); it was skewed toward high BP, with the tail becoming more prominent with age (Hamilton et al., 1954a). This has been confirmed in many subsequent studies (Miall and Oldham, 1958; Kannel, 1990; Staessen et al., 1990; Ward, 1995). Both systolic and diastolic pressures (SBP, DBP) increase with age. If the dividing line between hypertension and normotension for DBP is taken at ≥ 95 mmHg, the prevalence of EH at ages 25, 35, and 50 years is 3%, 10%, and 25% respectively; if the line is ≥ 90 mmHg, the prevalence is 5%, 13%, and 35%. The lower the dividing line, the lower the threshold for instituting antihypertensive treatment, which, if implemented, reduces future cardiovascular complications such as stroke (figure 1.3).

In figure 4.2, which is typical of industrialized Western communities, DBP reaches a plateau at about 60 years of age (Hamilton et al., 1954a; Staessen et al, 1990; Levy, 1999). In contrast, SBP rises throughout life, with the rate often increasing after 60–70 years of age. The different relationships suggest that the two BPs are influenced by different mechanisms (Oldham, 1968; Miall and Lovell, 1967; Miall and Brennan, 1981; Miall, 1982). Up to 60 years of age, SBP and DBP increase in parallel with the rises in SNA and TPR (chapter 5). However, in older people the continuing rise in SBP is due to a structurally induced decrease in distensibility of the large conduit arteries, which affects the shape of the arterial pulse.

In any conduit artery the pulse wave is a compound wave, which is the sum of the pressure wave leaving the heart and of waves reflected from the peripheral arterioles. Normally this summation is greatest in peripheral conduit arteries, which are closer to the reflecting site in the lower part of the body (figure 1.2). In hypertension, as the arteries become stiffer, the velocity of each wave is greater and there is less attenuation

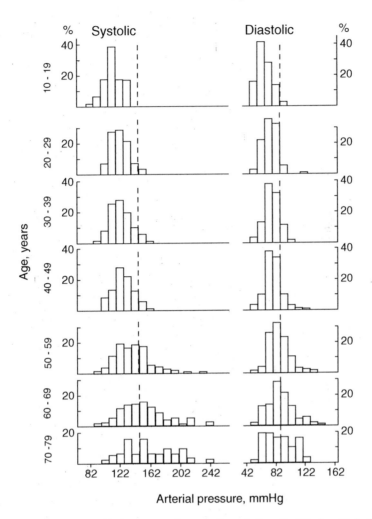

Figure 4.1. Frequency distribution curves for systolic and diastolic BPs (mmHg) of males in different age groups. Note increase in variance and greater skewing to right in older age groups. From Hamilton et al. (1954a), with permission of *Clinical Science*, the Biochemical Society, and the Medical Research Society.

of the reflected wave on its voyage toward the central aorta. O'Rourke found that the central aortic pulse amplitude depends on the summation of the wave leaving the heart and the reflected waves from arterioles in both upper and lower parts of the body (figure 4.3). With stiffer arteries, the wave leaving the heart and the two reflected waves summate earlier, which increases the pulse amplitude of the central aorta, so that it is almost as large as in more proximal conduit arteries (Taylor, 1965, 1966; O'Rourke and Taylor, 1966; O'Rourke, 1982b, 1995, 2002; Kelly and O'Rourke, 1995; Nichols and O'Rourke, 1997). The different factors responsible for the rises in SBP and DBP explain why each BP is an independent predictor of future risk (Kannel et al., 1981; Rutan et al., 1988; Levy, 1999).

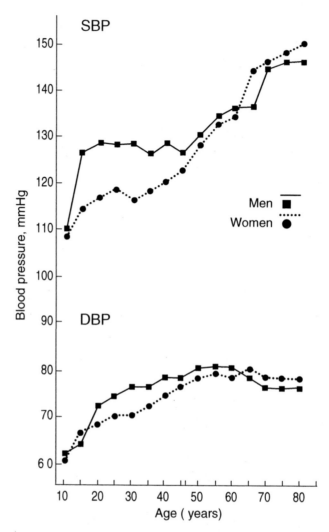

Figure 4.2. Relationship between age and systolic and diastolic BPs (SBP, DBP, mmHg) from Belgian males (*n* = 2044) and females (*n* = 2158) in 5-year age groupings. From Staessen et al. (1990), with permission of the *Journal of Hypertension* and Lippincott, Williams and Wilkins.

In older subjects, isolated systolic hypertension sometimes develops without preceding neural changes. This has been regarded as an exaggerated form of normal aging (Lakatta, 1987; Folkow and Svanborg, 1993). However, the risk of developing stroke or LV failure is similar to that in other types of EH.

Geographic, Ethnic, and Socioeconomic Differences

Epstein and Eckoff (1967) were the first to use the slope of the age-BP relationship as an indicator of the prevalence of EH in a population, and this is now used routinely in epidemiological investigations (Scotch, 1963; Epstein and Eckoff, 1967; Akinkugbe, 1985;

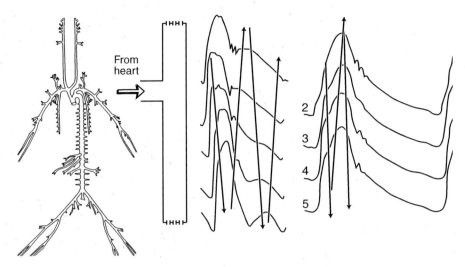

Figure 4.3. Left, O'Rourke's cathedral model of arterial system, which receives blood from heart one third along its length; an incompletely closed tube at head and tail ends are the two lumped sites of wave reflection. Middle, arterial pressure pulse tracings next to the tube were obtained from sites from aortic arch (top) to iliac artery (bottom). The line with downward arrow indicates compound pulse wave returning from upper reflecting site; line with upward arrow is pulse wave from lower reflecting site. Right, tracings from patient with stiff arteries. The greater pulse pressure in central aorta is due to more rapid wave travel. After O'Rourke (1982a, 1982b).

Poulter and Sever, 1994; Whelton et al., 1994; Henry, 1997a).[1] The steep slope in figure 4.2 is typical of populations from urban competitive societies, in which social tensions are rife and EH is common. On the other hand, BP does not alter with age at all in several rural societies, indicating a very low prevalence of EH (Cruz-Coke et al., 1964; Sinnett and Whyte, 1973; Poulter and Sever, 1994; James and Baker, 1995). The social organization, culture, and well-ordered lifestyle of these societies tends to reduce social tensions.

Scotch (1963) noted that the age-related rise in BP in Zulus who had moved to an urbanized community was greater than that encountered in their traditional habitat, and thought that this was due to greater psychosocial stress (figure 4.4). Similar BP differences have been observed in Pacific Island communities, in whom the slopes of the age-BP relationship differ markedly despite their similar ethnic background. For example, in Pukapuka, the lifestyle is traditional and BP changes little with age. In contrast, in Rarotonga, the administrative center of the islands, life is less cohesive socially and BP increases with age (Beaglehole, 1957; Prior et al., 1968). Similar changes have been observed when Easter Islanders have moved to mainland Chile (Cruz-Coke et al., 1964), in Tokelau Islanders who migrated to New Zealand (Beaglehole et al., 1977), and in rural families in Kenya who settled in nearby cities (Sever et al., 1980). All have migrated from traditional rural societies to more stressful urban communities, but greater consumption of salt, alcohol, and other dietary factors have probably also contributed to the BP rise.

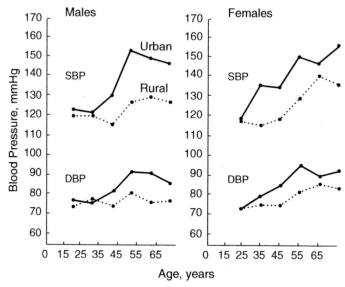

Figure 4.4. Relationships between age and systolic and diastolic BPs (SBP, DBP, mmHg) in urban and rural Zulu males and females. After Scotch (1963).

Henry analyzed age-BP relationships from 59 different ethnic and social groups. His six criteria for distinguishing between social cohesion and disharmony are summarized in table 4.1 (Henry et al., 1967; Henry, 1997a). From these a social tension score was derived for each group, which was related to the slopes of their age-SBP regression lines (figure 4.5).

Blood Pressure in African Americans

Hypertension is much more prevalent in adult African Americans than in whites (figure 4.6; Stamler et al., 1976; Akinkugbe, 1985; Prineas and Gillum, 1985; Whelton et al., 1994). The disparity starts at 20–25 years of age, with little difference before then (Prineas and Gillum, 1985; Prineas and Sinaiko, 1994).

The slave trade in the 18th and 19th centuries was one of the greatest involuntary population shifts in history. The effect on BP is still manifest in the descendants of this westward movement from Africa, in whom the resting BP rises progressively from Africa through the Carribean to the United States (Cooper and Rotimi, 1994; Cooper et al., 1999). One theory to explain the rise in BP is that it is a legacy of many years of racial, physical, and psychological abuse (Cooper and Rotimi, 1994). It is possible that this favored survival of persons with the EH genotype, who have a lower threshold for eliciting the defense response. Another theory is that the survivors of the slave ships had genes that gave them a survival advantage in conserving salt and water (Grim et al., 1995). In any event, African Americans still suffer relatively greater social disadvantage and stress compared to whites, which contributes to the greater prevalence of EH among them.

Table 4.1. Six Antithetical Attributes for Scoring Social Tension and Stress in Communities

Eunomy
  Agreed cultural standards, social harmony
	Anomy
	  Lack of standards, lawlessness

Social and cultural solidarity	Commercial and competitive culture

Extended family
  Several generations of relatives living in
  the same group of buildings
	Broken home
	  Broken family, separation, and divorce

Ancient homelands
  Land and buildings in a particular
  geographic region have belonged
  to the community
	Tenant expatriates
	  Without privileges that they took for granted until
	  recent translocation

Traditional culture
  Traditional coconut and taro cultivation;
  fishing; small-scale farming (e.g., Pacific
  islands, Chinese, Indian villages)
	Alien culture—New technology
	  U.S., European, Japanese, Australian agricultural,
	  fishing, industrial innovations; electronic age
	  for elderly

Domestic tranquility	Social violence Local violence (family, community), riots, war

Note: The total score for each community is related to slope of age-BP relationship. Each attribute has four scores: 0, +, ++, +++; 0 is harmonious. +++ the most stressful.

Source: Henry (1997a).

Fetal Determinants of Adult BP

Maternal (and infant) mortality correlates with cardiovascular mortality in later life, but the significance of this relationship is unclear. Barker and colleagues were the first to suggest that fetal development is retarded as a result of maternal ill health, as judged by low birth weight and thin habitus of the infants (Barker et al., 1990, 1992; Law and

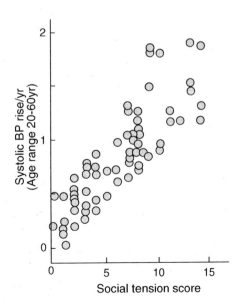

Figure 4.5. Relationship between slope of age-BP relationships and social tension scores in 65 populations and social groups. From Henry (1997a), with permission of LIT Verlag, Münster.

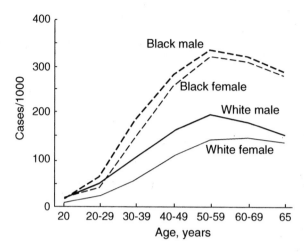

Figure 4.6. Prevalence of hypertension (defined as diastolic BP ≥ 95 mmHg) in black and white Americans. From Stamler et al. (1976), with permission of the *Journal of the American Medical Association.*

Barker, 1994; Barker, 1998). Low birth weight and other indices of growth retardation in infants correlate with greater adult mortality from stroke, coronary disease, and diabetes. Fetal stress may produce neuroendocrine reprogramming, affecting metabolism and increasing the chances of developing hypertension in later life. Here too there may be survival advantages to having a particular genotype (Gluckman and Hanson, 2005).

In the earlier studies, the BP of the low and high birth weight groups differed by 5–10 mmHg by the time they were 30–50 years old (Law et al., 1993; Nilsson et al., 1997; Moore et al., 1999). However, in larger subsequent series the magnitude of the change has diminished. The same has happened when BP has been measured at intervals between birth and adulthood (Falkner et al., 1998). One of the largest studies has been performed on 150,000 Swedish army recruits aged 18 years, in whom the BP difference between lowest and highest birth weight groups, although statistically significant, amounted to only 1.5 mmHg (Nilsson et al., 1997). Thus, fetal ill health probably has a definite effect on BP, but raises BP in only a small proportion of young adults with EH.

In animal experiments, inducing severe fetal stress or impairing placental blood flow resulted in rises in BP by 6–8 mmHg soon after birth, compared to controls (Robinson et al., 1995). Similarly, simulation of the prenatal steroid surge by injecting cortisol in fetal sheep raised BP by ∼10 mmHg after birth (Dodic et al., 1998). Higher BPs have also been observed in female offspring of rabbits with renovascular hypertension (Denton et al., 2003). However, it remains uncertain whether these substantial interventions simulate in vivo events in humans quantitatively.

Tracking of Blood Pressure

The extent to which a person maintains BP rank in the cohort as he or she becomes older is called tracking. Miall and Chinn (1973) studied this phenomenon in over 2000 subjects in two Welsh communities, measuring each subject's BP every 4 years for 16 years. In about two thirds, BP increased with age, while in the remainder

BP barely altered. The *tracking coefficient* is the same as a correlation coefficient of a subject's BP between two time points (Rosner et al., 1977; Clarke et al., 1978; Prineas and Sinaiko, 1994; Levy, 1999). After the age of 20, the coefficient is relatively large (0.5–0.6), indicating that many of those in a particular percentile of the frequency distribution maintain their rank. In children and adolescents, the tracking coefficient is low (0.1–0.2), suggesting that BP rank is not well maintained between childhood and adult life (Clarke et al., 1978; Hanis et al., 1983).

These results of BP tracking in adults may simply reflect that by then people have become more set in their ways. However, their resting BP is readily affected by stress, dietary changes, or exercise, as discusssed later in this chapter.

Diurnal Variation in Blood Pressure

BP has a regular circadian rhythm on which are superimposed fluctuations associated with various daytime activities.

Circadian and Activity-Related Changes

The circadian rhythm for BP is geared to the sleep/waking cycle and is regulated through a genetically controlled biological clock located bilaterally in the hypothalamus (Moore-Ede, 1986). The cycle begins with a decline in BP soon after falling asleep, and reaches a nadir about 2–3 hours later. On waking, the BP rises steeply and reaches a plateau after 1–2 hours on which fluctuations of varying magnitude and duration are superimposed (Mancia, 1990).

Ambulatory 24-hour BP measurements are used to relate the diurnal changes to the subject's activity (Baba et al., 1990; Harshfield et al., 1990; Pickering, 1995). This is illustrated in figure 4.7 in normal subjects and in those with mild and moderate EH, showing the average values at work, in the BP clinic, during home activities, and during sleep. The highest BPs were in the clinic and at work, while the minimum value occurred during sleep. $\Delta SBP_{(max-sleep)}$ and $\Delta DBP_{(max-sleep)}$ were 2–3 times as great in persons with moderate EH compared to normotensives, while the differences in mild EH were of intermediate magnitude. It indicates that work- and anxiety-induced stresses have greater effects on BP in persons with EH.

There has been controversy as to whether BP has a circadian rhythm or whether the changes are all due to the additional activity or stress during the day (Imai et al., 1990; Pickering, 1995). That there is a circadian component is suggested by: (1) changes in the timing of the rhythm in shift workers, (2) a latency between waking and falling asleep and the BP maxima and minima, and (3) alteration of rhythm by plasma glucocorticoids (Imai et al., 1990). Nevertheless, exercise and stress are superimposed on the circadian rhythm as unavoidable facts of life.

The nocturnal fall in BP is not present in all normal subjects or in all those with EH (Imai et al., 1990; Verdecchia et al., 1990; Minamisawa et al., 1994; O'Brien, 1994). It obviously is not present in those with nocturnal hypertension due to obstructive sleep apnea (OSA; chapter 14). The nocturnal fall tends to diminish in EH when cardiopulmonary load is high.

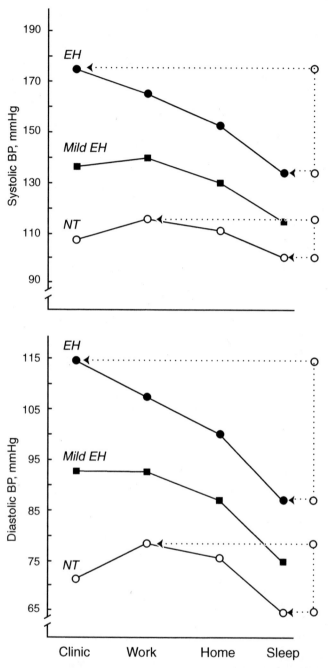

Figure 4.7. Mean systolic and diastolic BPs (mmHg) from ambulatory BP recordings in subjects with moderate EH (closed circles), mild EH (closed squares), and in normotensives (NT, open circles). Data for each subject are average BPs in BP clinic, at work, at home (normal activity), and during sleep. After Pickering (1995), with permission of Raven Press and Lippincott, Williams and Wilkins.

White-Coat Hypertension

So-called white-coat hypertension is one of the oldest stress tests in medical practice and develops almost always during a medical examination, when a physician measures a patient's BP for the first time and BP typically rises by 10–30 mmHg (Hinman et al., 1962; Pickering et al., 1988; Mancia, 1990; Pickering, 1995). The rise in BP is due to the patient's anxiety when confronting the physician, and it is usually absent when a nurse or technician make the measurements, but most subjects get accustomed to the procedure over a period of weeks, after which the BP reflects the true resting value.

Posture

On assuming the upright posture, MAP at heart level changes little and remains at ~100 mmHg. However, in the lower limbs it rises by ~60 mmHg due to the greater hydrostatic pressure, while cerebral MAP falls by ~20 mmHg (Rowell, 1986). Central arterial BP and CO remain close to the corresponding supine values because of a reflex increase in SNA and the massaging effect of the skeletal muscle pump on venous return.

The importance of reflex compensation through the ANS is evident from the responses of patients with severe autonomic neuropathy, in whom there is profound postural hypotension on assuming the upright posture (Bannister et al., 1977; Jennings et al., 1979; Esler, Jackman, Kelleher et al., 1980; Hilsted et al., 1981).[2] This also occurs in normal persons during pharmacological autonomic blockade (Korner, Shaw, West et al., 1973).

Some Factors Causing Long-Term Blood Pressure Changes

Factors causing long-term BP changes include psychosocial stress, exercise, dietary salt intake, OSA, and obesity. OSA is a complex type of stress and is considered in chapter 14.

Psychosocial (Mental) Stress

Both long-term and shorter studies in different social groups have been used to assess the magnitude and duration of BP responses to stress.

Age-BP Relationship in Distinctive Social Groups

These were studied in nuns and laywomen in an Italian community, in prisoners and their guards in Alcatraz, and in patients with Down syndrome in Great Britain.

Nuns and Laywomen.   The BPs of nuns belonging to a secluded order were studied over a period of 30 years, during which they were compared with those of laywomen, many of whom were relatives of the nuns (Timio et al., 1988, 1997). The groups were well matched for age, BP, and salt intake and had similar family histories of EH. None of the participants smoked, used contraceptive pills, or had hormone replacement therapy after menopause. At the end of the study both groups had similar dietary salt intakes and body mass index (BMI) and their physical activity and consumption of alcohol were also similar.

Over the 30-year observation period, the BP in the laywomen rose on average by 30/12 mmHg, with most of the rise during the first 8–12 years (figure 4.8). Moreover, their cardiovascular mortality and morbidity were significantly greater than in the nuns (figure 4.9). In the absence of dietary differences or in their level of physical activity between the groups, the greater prevalence of EH in the laywomen was thought to be due to the stresses of family, village, and city life (Hansson et al., 1997). In contrast, the nuns lived a predictable well-ordered life, where their day-to-day stresses appeared to be offset by the social support within the group, and its cultural solidarity and common objectives.

Prisoners and Guards.   Rather similar differences were observed in a study by Alvarez and Stanley (1930) in a study of 6000 convicts and 400 prison guards at the Alcatraz penitentiary (see Henry, 1997a). It suggests that divine intervention probably

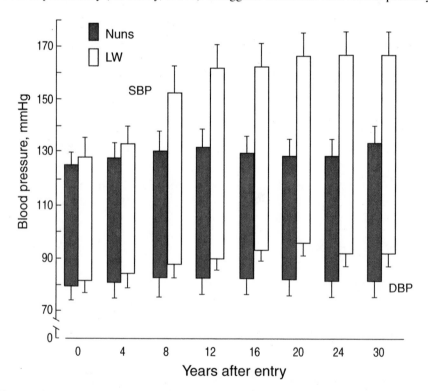

Figure 4.8. Systolic and diastolic BPs (SBP, DBP, mmHg) taken over 30 years in a case control study in nuns of a secluded order (dark rectangles) and laywomen (clear rectangles). Results are means ± SDs. Redrawn from Timio et al. (1988, 1997), with permission of *Blood Pressure* and Taylor and Francis.

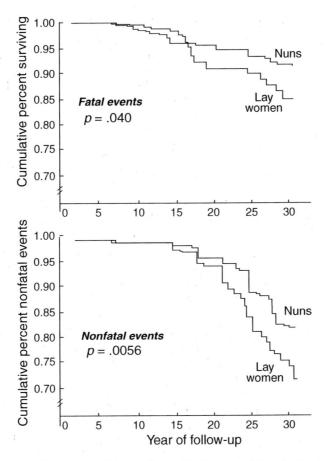

Figure 4.9. Life table analysis of data in figure 4.8. Top, cumulative decline in each group due to fatal events, which was greater in laywomen, $p = .04$. Bottom, cumulative changes due to nonfatal morbid events, which were more frequent in laywomen, $p = .0056$. From Timio et al. (1997), with permission of *Blood Pressure* and Taylor and Francis.

did not account for the low prevalence of EH in the nuns. At Alcatraz, the slope of the age-BP relationship was steeper in the guards than in the prisoners.[3] Life for the prisoners was stable and predictable, while the guards feared for their personal safety and were also anxious about losing their jobs at the time of the Great Depression.

Down Syndrome.   This common developmental abnormality is a genetic disorder due to trisomy of chromosome 21 (Gardner-Medwin, 1996). The patient has a characteristic facial appearance and a low IQ, but typically an affectionate and cheerful demeanor. Down patients appreciate music but have a very limited capacity for abstract thought. Their BP does not rise with age, whether they live at home or in institutions (figure 4.10; Morrison et al., 1996). In contrast, in patients with other types of mental handicap the age-BP relationship tends to be normal. Possibly their cognitive impairment reduces the perception of stress.

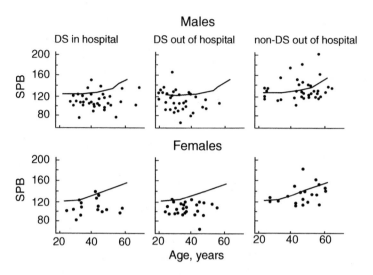

Figure 4.10. Left, age-SBP relationships in men and women with Down syndrome (DS) living in hospital (circles). Middle, Down patients living at home (circles). The solid lines are the UK reference populations for men and women. Right, p age-BP relationship in persons with other mental disorders (circles) are similar to those of reference groups. Data from Morrison et al. (1996).

Stresses of Shorter Duration

Shorter-duration stresses include those experienced by: (1) British soldiers during a western desert battle in World War II, (2) members of the Australian Antarctic expedition during the winter months, (3) prisoners living communally or alone, and (4) Americans after the terrorist attack on New York on September 11, 2001.

Battle-Related Stress.   A high proportion of members of a British armored brigade developed transient hypertension during the battle for Tobruk against Field Marshal Rommel's army (Graham, 1945). The soldiers were aged 20–38 years and when their BPs were first measured immediately after the battle, SBP/DBP of the whole group averaged 158/98 mmHg, with 30% of the soldiers having BPs ≥175/100 mmHg. Two months later, after a period of rest from battle, the group's BP had fallen on average by 20/10 mmHg without medication. The stress associated with the prolonged battle was thought to have caused the transient BP rise, which subsided within weeks after the danger had passed.

Winter in Antarctica.   During the Antarctic summer, most members of the expedition engage in daily hard physical work, which they enjoy. However, during the winter months they become completely housebound because of the harsh weather. Most do not like to be confined indoors: Colleagues get on each other's nerves, alcohol consumption rises, and they feel claustrophobic and easily stressed (Jennings, Deakin et al., 1989, 1991). The winter BPs are greater than in summer (figure 4.11).

Antarctica

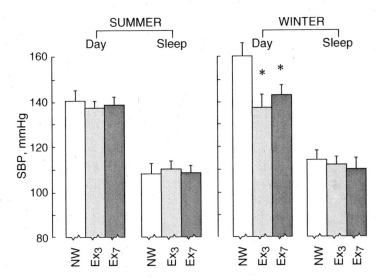

Figure 4.11. Resting ambulatory systolic BP (SBP, mmHg) during the day and while asleep from Australian Antarctic expedition members. Each period consisted of 3-week periods when subject performed normal work (NW), or standard bicycling of 40 min at 65% of W_{max} three and seven times per week (Ex$_3$, Ex$_7$). SBP during NW period was greater in winter than in summer ($p < .01$); bicycling restored BP to summer level (*$p < .01$). In summer, low BP was unaffected by cycling. Based on Jennings et al. (1989).

However, those engaging in regular submaximal exercise training during the winter maintain their BPs between training sessions at the summer levels (chapter 10).

Prison Habitat. D'Atri and Ostfeld (1975) observed that in male prisoners who had lived for several months in a communal dormitory, SBP was 16 mmHg higher than in those living in single-occupancy cells (131 vs. 115 mmHg), which was not due to dietary difference. The BP rise developed within days of transfer from cell to dormitory, while a fall in BP accompanied transfer in the reverse direction (D'Atri et al., 1981).

Terrorist Attack on New York. The long-term impact of the attack on the World Trade Center on September 11, 2001, on BP was assessed in some 400 subjects on a regular monitoring program from four centers in the United States (New York, Chicago, Washington, DC, and Mississippi). Their BPs were taken at home and had been telemonitored at a central clinic for 2 months before, which continued for 2 months after the attack (Gerin et al., 2005). The SBPs after the attack were on average 2–4 mmHg greater than before the attack, which was statistically significant. Seasonal variation was eliminated on the basis of corresponding measurements taken in a proportion of the subjects during the previous year. The BP response differed from the changes after a large earthquake, where in a single subject MAP increased immediately by ~30 mmHg, but subsided completely within the hour (Parati et al., 1991; Unger and Parati, 2005).

The persistence of the BP rise after the New York attack was attributed to the frequent media references to the event over the next few months, which generated on ongoing sense of present danger.

Exercise Training

Regular physical exercise is regarded as being beneficial for health (Arakawa, 1993; Jennings and Kingwell, 1994). A survey of Harvard College alumni concluded that the level of college sport activity performed many years earlier had no detectable effect on later health, but that the chief determinant of risk of developing hypertension was the amount of exercise performed at the time of the survey (Paffenbarger et al., 1983).

There is wide agreement that with regular aerobic exercise (e.g., running, bicycling), the resting BP between bouts is reduced. In contrast, BP rises or remains unchanged when training involves isometric exercise (e.g., weight lifting). A good way of

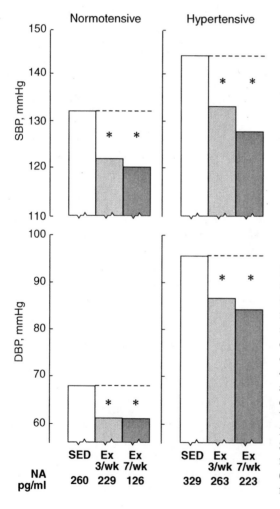

Figure 4.12. Average (+SEM) supine systolic and diastolic BPs (SBP, DBP, mmHg) in normotensive and hypertensive subjects; plasma noradrenaline concentration (NA, pg/mL) at foot of columns. BPs measured at end of 4 weeks' sedentary period (SED), after 4 weeks' standard bicycle exercise performed at 60–70% of W_{max} 3 and 7 times per week (Ex 3/wk, 7/wk). *$p < .05$, for ΔBP from SED. Data from normotensives from Jennings, Nelson, Nestel et al. (1986), and from hypertensives from Nelson et al. (1986).

producing a long-term reduction of BP in sedentary persons is by exercising three times per week on a bicycle ergometer for 30–40 minutes per session at 60–70% of maximum work capacity (W_{max}) (Jennings, Nelson et al., 1986; Nelson et al., 1986). After 4 weeks of the above regimen, resting SBP/DBP between bouts fell by 11/7 mmHg from the value before training. The changes were similar in normotensives and persons with EH (figure 4.12).[4] With less strenuous cycling or brisk walking, the fall in BP is smaller than with the standard regimen.

This also applies if the exercise is more strenuous and is perceived as stressful by the subject. At rates above about 75% of W_{max} performed 6–7 times per week, BP either rises between bouts from the pretraining level or remains unchanged (figure 4.13). The mechanisms of the effects of exercise and long-term changes in training are discussed in chapter 11.

Dietary Salt

Dahl (1961) was one of the first to suggest that high dietary salt intake was the major cause of EH. His straight line graph related salt intake to the prevalence of EH in different parts of the world (figure 4.14). His views have received much support and also much opposition (Gleibermann, 1973; Freis, 1976; Swales, 1995; Simpson, 2000). Denton (1982) has emphasized the role of the CNS in providing the drive for salt appetite. Dahl, like Platt, used "hypertension" as a qualitative variable with the ordinate scale in figure 4.14 extending over only a few mmHg (Swales, 1995), which overemphasizes the role of salt in EH. In addition, the BP responses to changes in dietary salt are rather variable in any given population (chapter 12). The polarization of opinion about the role of salt resulted in the Intersalt study to try to resolve the issue.

Intersalt

Intersalt was a large international study in which 10,079 subjects were recruited from 52 centers in 32 countries (Intersalt, 1988; Grobbee, 1994; Swales, 1995). In this study, 24-hour urine samples were used to estimate dietary salt intake. Each center recruited

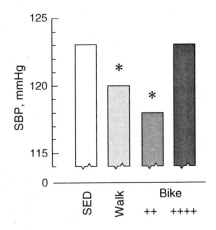

Figure 4.13. Effects on resting supine systolic BP (SBP, mmHg) of four types of exercise training in 14 healthy subject. Each period lasted 4 weeks: SED, sedentary; Walk, 60 minutes at 50% of W_{max} for 5 days/week; Bike+ +, 30 minutes cycling at 65% W_{max} for 3 days/week; Bike+ + + +, 15 minutes cycling at 85% W_{max} for 5 days per week. After Kingwell and Jennings (1993), with permission of the *Medical Journal of Australia.*

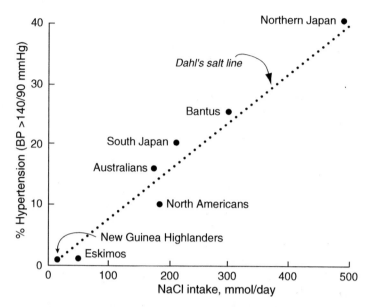

Figure 4.14. Dahl's relationship between salt intake (mmol/day) and the prevalence of hypertension in various populations, defined as the percentage of the population with BP ≥ 140/90 mmHg. Adapted from Dahl (1961).

200 subjects aged between 20 and 59 years, so that an age-BP relationship could be calculated. The slopes of the relationship in each center were related to the median salt intake.

The sodium intake was lowest in the Yanomamo Indians of Brazil and was greatest in the Tianjin region of northern China. The between-center comparisons suggested that in those on a habitually high salt intake, both SBP and DBP increased more than in those on low salt (figure 4.15). On average, a 50 mmol/day lowering of sodium intake resulted in ΔSBP/ΔDBP of −4.5/−2.3 mmHg, which would achieve significant reduction in cardiovascular risk.

The Intersalt investigators also estimated the effect of salt on the age-BP relationship within the "average" center, and the results were similar to the between-center estimates. The Intersalt study has provided a fair assessment of long-term differences in salt intake on BP over a large population spectrum and is in accord with the results of several clinical trials.

A Clinical Trial on Lowering Salt Intake

One trial conducted by the Australian National Health and Medical Research Council (1989) incorporated a design used in an earlier study by MacGregor et al. (1982), where the subject is unaware whether he or she is receiving normal or low amounts of salt. Lowering daily sodium intake by 60 mmol reduced SBP and DBP by 6.1/3.7 mmHg over the 8-week intervention phase. After statistical adjustments for differences in age and BMI, the estimated reduction in BP was 4.8/3.5 mmHg, similar to the

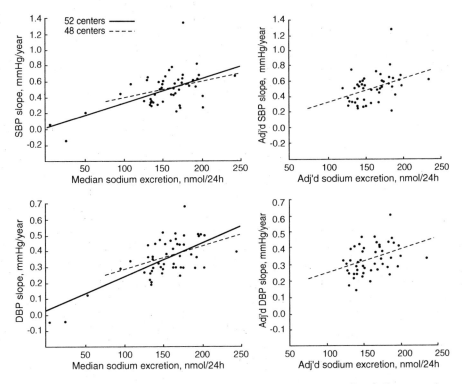

Figure 4.15. Intersalt findings, showing (left) relationship between median sodium excretion (mmol/24 hours) and slope of age-BP relationship (mmHg/year) from each center, adjusted for sex; solid line average regression equation based on 52 centers and dashed line equation from 48 centers after exclusion of lowest outliers. Right, relationship between salt intake and adjusted slopes, after allowing for variation in body mass index and alcohol intake. Data from Intersalt Research Group (1988), with permission of the *British Medical Journal*.

Intersalt estimates. Another important study has been the DASH (Dietary Approaches to Stop Hypertension) study (Sacks et al., 2001). This has demonstrated falls of BP of the same order.

Increasing Salt Intake

During short-term elevation of dietary sodium, the rises in BP are smaller than the falls associated with corresponding reduction in sodium intake. This was observed in 14 subjects whose sodium intake was raised from low to very high levels in large stepwise increments, with each level maintained for 3 days (table 4.2) (Luft, Rankin et al., 1979; Weinberger et al., 1981). The average rise in $\Delta SBP/\Delta DBP$ was only 1.3/0.8 mmHg per 100 mmol increase in sodium per day. Moreover, this is an over-estimate, because raising sodium intake increases loss of potassium. When this is replaced, the rise in BP is only about half the above figure. The small magnitude of these changes is partly due to the many homeostatic mechanisms that safeguard the constancy of body sodium.

Table 4.2. Response of Systolic and Diastolic Blood Pressure (SBP, DBP) to Sodium Loading in 14 Normal Adults

Sodium Intake (mEq/24 h)	SBP (mmHg)	DBP (mmHg)	SBP (mmHg) K Replaced	DBP (mmHg) K Replaced
10	111 ± 2	69 ± 3	114 ± 2	67 ± 5
300	116 ± 2	71 ± 3	115 ± 3	65 ± 5
800	121 ± 3	76 ± 3	122 ± 4	69 ± 5
1500	131 ± 4	85 ± 3	124 ± 4	72 ± 5

Note: Results are means $\pm$ SEM. Age range 18–40 years; 7 were Caucasian, 7 were African American. Subjects spent 7 days on lowest intake of sodium and 3 days on all other levels. The two columns on right indicate effect after replacement of potassium loss.

Source: Luft, Rankin et al. (1979), with permission of *Circulation*, American Heart Association, and Lippincott, Williams and Wilkins.

Unfortunately, there are no experimental studies in humans on long-term elevation of sodium intake. However, such an investigation has been performed by Denton et al. (1995) in 13 chimpanzees, in which salt intake was increased in three steps from 10 to 230 mmol sodium per day over 84 weeks. Rises in SBP/DBP of 33/10 mmHg were observed in eight monkeys, while in five animals there was little or no BP change. There are thus salt-sensitive and salt-resistant monkeys, as with humans. The BP measurements were obtained under ketamine-valium anesthesia, which inhibits barore-flexes and raises BP (Wong and Jenkins, 1975; Blake and Korner, 1981). This could accentuate the effect of salt. However, the control monkeys received the same treatment and, assuming that this was an effective control, the average rises in SBP/DBP of 7.5/2.3 mmHg for 50 mmol increase of sodiumper day are in the range of the Intersalt estimates and mirror the effects on BP of reduction in salt intake. The mechanisms of the effects of salt are discussed in chapter 12.

Obesity

In Australia, Europe, and the United States, more than 50% of hypertensives have a greater than recommended BMI (Chiang et al., 1969; Kannel et al., 1967; MacMahon et al., 1984; Tuck, 1994; Krieger and Landsberg, 1995). This contributes to the elevation of BP, while after weight reduction BP falls (MacMahon et al., 1985). The falls in BP appear to be similar whether the subject's sodium intake is normal or low, that is, 120 or 40 mmol/day (Tuck et al., 1981; Tuck, 1994).

One study examined the effects on BP of both weight reduction and exercise (Reid et al., 1994). Matched overweight subjects were randomly assigned to groups on exercise alone, weight loss alone, and weight loss plus exercise. A crossover experimental design was employed, so that the results in each subject of 12 weeks of treatment were compared with the effects of 12 weeks' normal sedentary activity on the baseline diet (figure 4.16). Weight loss alone and exercise alone lowered MAP by ~ 7 mmHg, while the combined intervention resulted in a fall of ~ 14 mmHg, suggesting additive effects on BP.

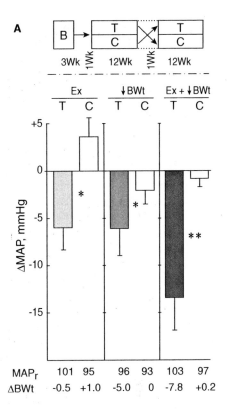

Figure 4.16. Results in three groups of subjects treated with exercise alone, body weight (BWt) reduction alone, and the combined effects of exercise plus BWt reduction. (A) General protocol: Baseline (B) after which half the group had 12 weeks of treatment (T) followed by 12 weeks of control (C, baseline activity); order was reversed in the other half of each group. Lower graphs: ΔMAP (mmHg) at the end of T (shaded) and C (clear). From left to right: (1) bicycle exercise alone (65% W_{max} for 40 minutes, 3×/week); (2) weight reduction alone; (3) exercise plus weight reduction. Numbers at bottom are resting MAP (MAP$_r$, mmHg) and ΔBWt (kg) during T and C. $*p < .05$; $** < .01$. Based on Reid et al. (1994).

As with salt, the effects of weight gain on BP are best studied under steady-state conditions, when the average changes of calorie-induced weight gains and losses alter MAP by ±5–8 mmHg for a ±5 kg change in body weight (chapter 14).

Other Diet-Induced Changes and Alcohol

A high-fiber diet, a vegetarian diet, and an increased intake of fish oils all produce small but definite falls in BP of 2–3 mmHg (Beilin, 1987, 1994, 1995; Burke et al., 1994; Margetts, 1986). Falls in BP of the same order also accompany increases in intake of calcium and magnesium (Cappucio, 1994).

In subjects drinking more than 2–3 standard alcoholic drinks per day, BPs are above those of nondrinkers (MacMahon, 1987). Controlled intervention studies in which alcohol intake has been raised for several weeks have observed that BP rises by 2–5 mmHg (Vandongen and Puddey, 1994). The rise is accentuated by occupational stress (chapter 11; Schnall et al., 1992).

The small magnitude of all the above changes and the likelihood that several of them act through a number of mechanisms makes analysis of their mode of action difficult. Furthermore, eating habits and a high intake of alcohol are often closely related to psychosocial stress.

Redevelopment of Hypertension After Stopping Treatment

Some 20–25 years ago, our group studied how quickly EH redevelops after stopping antihypertensive treatment following a long period of good control of BP, mostly with β-blockers and diuretics (Jennings et al., 1980, 1984; Jennings, Korner et al, 1991; Korner, 1982; Korner et al., 1991). We wondered whether some of the factors that initially raised BP in EH might disappear in the course of treatment.

Our first study was performed in 13 subjects with moderate EH, before and after treatment (figure 4.17). Before treatment, MAP and TPR were raised, including the nonautonomic component, which was assessed after pharmacological autonomic blockade and is an approximate indicator of structural changes. After one year's drug treatment and one week after stopping the drugs, MAP and TPR were in the range of healthy normotensive subjects, as was the nonautonomic component of TPR. We had thought that significant regression of the structural changes had occurred owing to treatment, but this turned out to be incorrect. The widening of the bed due to treatment is probably due to a diminished myogenic component of vascular tone, simply as a result of the reduction in BP (chapter 6). The most remarkable finding was the speed at which hypertension redeveloped after stopping the drugs in this and subsequent studies. Out of 49 subjects who received treatment for one year or more (mean 8.8 ± 1.6 years), hypertension redeveloped in 33 (67%) within 10 weeks of stopping

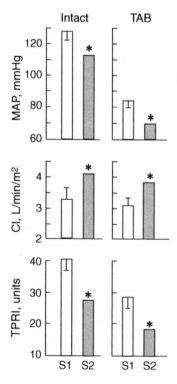

Figure 4.17. Results from hemodynamic studies in 13 subjects with moderate EH: Study 1 (S1) before drug treatment; Study 2 (S2) after 12 months on β-blockers and diuretics and 5–7 days after stopping drugs. From above, mean arterial pressure (MAP, mmHg), cardiac index (CI, L/min/m^2), total peripheral resistance index (TPRI, units), with intact ANS effectors (Intact) and after total autonomic blockade (TAB). Bar on rectangle is SE of difference between S1 and S2, *$p < .05$. Adapted from Jennings et al. (1980) and Korner (1982), with permission of *Clinical Science*, the Biochemical Society, and the Medical Research Society.

treatment; in another 9 (18%) within 20 weeks, and in only 7 (14%) did BP remain in the normal range for over 12 months.[5] This does suggest that in the present state of knowledge, drug treatment of EH should be a lifelong affair.

Clearly, β-blockers plus diuretics restore BP to normal without addressing the underlying cause of hypertension, and these drugs cause little regression of structural cardiovascular changes (Schiffrin et al., 1994). This appears to be achieved somewhat more successfully with ACE inhibitors or AT_1 receptor antagonists (Dahlöf and Hansson, 1992; Dahlöf et al., 1992; Schiffrin et al., 1994). However, it is not known whether any of the drugs in current use affect the rapidity with which EH redevelops after drug withdrawal.

Arterial Blood Pressure as a Pointer to the Causes of EH

SBP and DBP increase by similar amounts up to the age of about 60 years, when they are largely due to increased systemic vasoconstriction. After that, DBP reaches a plateau, while SBP continues to increase due to greater arterial pulse wave summation in the conduit arteries as the latter become stiffer. Isolated systolic hypertension sometimes develops in older persons in the absence of elevation of DBP.

Of the likely early determinants of EH, psychosocial stress elicits the largest rises in SBP/DBP of ~20/10 mmHg. High alcohol consumption accentuates the development of EH in certain types of occupational stress. Increasing salt intake by 50 mmol sodium per day raises BP on average by ~5/3 mmHg, while in obesity BPs the corresponding rise is ~7/6 mmHg for an 8 kg rise in body weight. As discussed in later chapters, the effects of salt on BP are enhanced by stress and other constrictor factors, while in obesity the increase in BP is relatively independent of the effects of salt or stress (chapters 12, 13). The presence of obesity predisposes to OSA-related hypertension.

Chronic stress of sufficient intensity raises BP in virtually everyone, but it is only in those susceptible to EH that the high BP becomes permanent with repeated exposure. The effect of stress on BP is accentuated by a high salt intake in salt-sensitive persons. The effect is most striking in Chinese, Japanese, and African Americans, who are more sensitive to salt than Caucasians.

When exposure to high levels of stress lasts over weeks or months, daytime BP rises in almost everyone but then returns to normal once the stress is over. Figure 4.7 helps to visualize the BP trajectory over the course of the day: In those developing EH, home BP in the early morning is close to normal; it then rises to the levels of persons with mild EH in the figure; this accords with observations in the Antarctic study in figure 4.11 (NW). As the defense pathway becomes more sensitized, daytime BP rises to higher levels and BP is also raised at night.

In figure 4.7, the maximal daytime BP minus that during sleep is 2–3 times greater in EH than in normotensives. The difference is due to raised SNA in EH and to the amplifier effect of the structural changes (chapters 5, 6). Although the difference is substantial, it suggests that the sensitization of the defense pathway is considerably smaller than the corresponding change in *Aplysia*. The reasons for this are considered in chapter 11. They relate to the highly developed inhibitory systems of the mammalian brain, which moderate the autonomic changes even when intrinsic responsiveness of the defense pathway is increased. No apparent sensitization occurs in patients with Down syndrome, in whom EH is virtually absent. The reasons for this are not known, but one possibility is genetically determined impairment of the perception of stress.

The truly long-term effects of stress in the development of EH are illustrated by the 30-year study of a cohort of Italian nuns and laywomen. Most of the rise in BP in the laywomen took place over the first 8–12 years; by then all those susceptible to EH will have developed high BP.[6] The above time is similar to the recent estimate of 5–15 years to develop EH by Julius et al. (2004), which is what it takes for those with high normal BPs to become frankly hypertensive.

The difference in age-BP curves between nuns and laywomen resembles the effects of changing from a rural to an urban environment, suggesting a similar difference in the levels of stress. Even greater differences in stress levels may account for the greater prevalence of EH in black Americans than in white Americans, which may be compounded by the former group's greater BP susceptibility to dietary salt. Figure 4.6 suggests that the threshold for developing EH is similar in African Americans and whites, which is consistent with the former's greater exposure to more intense environmental stimuli than to intrinsic genetic differences between the groups.

Regular submaximal aerobic exercise is a physiological antagonist to the autonomic effects of stress, which appears to be due to lowering constrictor tone between training sessions. As discussed in chapter 10, submaximal exercise elicits pleasurable feelings of the type that becomes addictive. In contrast, near-maximal exercise is perceived as stressful and is something to be endured, like occupational stress.

Submaximal regular exercise is often capable of maintaining BP within normal limits in persons with EH, particularly when combined with reduction in salt intake and reduction in body weight. However, in more severe grades of hypertension the reduction in BP is insufficient to reduce cardiovascular risk.

EH is one of the few diseases in which there is a pronounced long-term benefit from nonspecific treatment with antihypertensive drugs. This is simply because reduction in BP lowers future cardiovascular mortality and morbidity, even though the outlook in treated hypertensives is not as favorable as in those who never had EH (Bulpitt et al., 1986). The rapid redevelopment of hypertension when the antihypertensive drugs are withdrawn is an indicator that drugs like β-adrenoreceptor antagonists and diuretics do not address the causes of EH despite their effectiveness in lowering BP. These are addressed by the nonpharmacological lifestyle measures discussed in this chapter, suggesting that both methods of treatment have a place in management of persons with EH.

5

Output Patterns in Nonobese Hypertensives

In nonobese persons, the hemodynamic and neurohumoral output patterns provide useful clues about the nature of the more proximal operations of the control system, including possible interactions about some of the inputs considered in the previous chapter. In contrast, in obese individuals the substantial vasodilatation associated with hyperinsulinemia masks the constrictor factors that raise BP. Accordingly, the output patterns in obesity are considered separately (chapter 13).

The hemodynamic patterns in lean individuals with EH suggest early hypothalamic involvement, with autonomic changes accounting for much of the vasoconstriction in mild and moderate EH. Over the next few years, a number of nonautonomic factors assume increasing prominence. Initially blood volume is normal, but it declines as hypertension becomes more severe, which is a consequence of constrictor hypertension. There is also some elevation of glucocorticoid hormones as part of the defense response. Participation in some of the regulation of the renin-angiotensin system is suggested by the much greater variance in plasma renin activity (PRA) in a population of persons with EH.

Central and Regional Hemodynamics

For some 20–30 years from the mid-1940s, research on the hemodynamics of hypertension formed a substantial component of the overall research effort in human hypertension. This resulted in determining the changes in mean arterial pressure (MAP), cardiac output (CO), total peripheral resistance and regional vascular resistances (TPR, Vas Rs), and the corresponding conductances (TPCs, Cs). Over this period, considerable research was also undertaken into the factors that cause changes in the arterial pressure pulse in the course of hypertension.

MAP, CO, and TPR, and severity of EH

In mild untreated EH, the TPR index (TPRI, TPR/m² body surface area) remains normal, while the cardiac index (CI) is 15–20% greater than in normotensives (figure 5.1; Lund-Johansen, 1977). Continuing elevation of BP is mostly due to rising TPRI, while CI returns to normal at first and gradually declines. Right atrial pressure (RAP) tends to increase slightly (Safar, 1989; Safar and London, 1989). The findings in figure 5.1 are typical of the results of many other hemodynamic investigations.[1] They are also in accord with longitudinal studies in which the same subjects have been studied on at least two occasions (e.g., Lund-Johansen, 1980, 1994).

At first the high CO was thought to be due to elevation in blood volume, until it became clear that this was below normal in EH (Tarazi et al., 1968). Another theory was that a high metabolic rate caused elevation of CO, but this finding was not uniform (Amery et al., 1967; Levy et al., 1967; Julius and Conway, 1968; Sannerstedt, 1969; Murakami, 1973; Lund-Johansen, 1977). It may have reflected variation in adrenaline secretion rates at the time of the investigations.

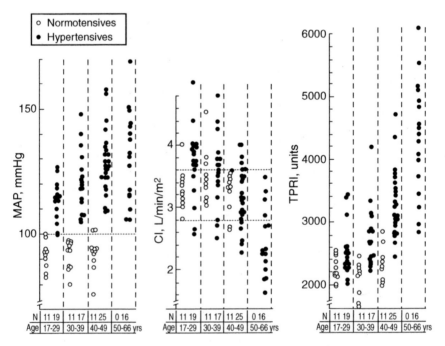

Figure 5.1. Individual results of mean arterial pressure (MAP, mmHg), cardiac index (CI, L/min/m²), and TPRI (total peripheral resistance index, units) in 77 men with EH (black circles) and 33 normotensives (open circles). Data arranged according to age, shown at foot of each column. N is the number of subjects. Modified from Lund-Johansen (1977), with permission of Blackwell.

Regional Properties and Hemodynamic Changes in EH

EH has significant effects on the renal, splanchnic, and muscle and skin beds, which all play a role in the normal regulation of BP. The circulation to the brain and heart is also affected by EH, but mostly in its later stages.

Blood Flow at Rest and during Maximum Activity

The resting regional blood flows in normal humans are summarized in table 5.1 (Mellander and Johansson, 1968). The kidney is the most richly perfused organ per 100 g of tissue, followed by myocardium, brain, gastrointestinal tract, and liver, while the lowest perfusion is in resting skeletal muscle (Mellander and Johansson, 1968; Folkow and Neil, 1971; Korner, 1974; Rowell, 1986, 1993).

The high resting renal blood flow (RBF) reflects its large metabolic activity, which accounts for 10% of the body's resting O_2 consumption. Resting renal Vas R is low, and the capacity for further dilation is modest. However, the renal bed is a major source of increased constrictor tone during rises in sympathetic neural activity (SNA) or other constrictor factors. The opposite obtains in resting skeletal muscle, in which both perfusion and metabolism are low. Hence, the capacity for further constriction is modest, while there is a large capacity for further dilation, for example, in exercise.

The properties of the main beds are summarized briefly below.

Table 5.1. Peripheral Blood Flow Data in Major Vascular Beds in Humans at Rest and during Maximum Activity

Organ	Rest			Maximum Activity			
	L/min	% of CO	mL/min/ 100 g	L/min	× Resting	mL/min/ 100 g	Weight kg
CNS	0.75	13.6	50	2.1	2.8 ×	140	1.5
Heart	0.21	3.5	70	1.2	5.7 ×	400	1.3
Skeletal muscle	0.75	13.6	2.5	18.0	24 ×	600	30
GI tract	0.7	12.7	35	5.5	7.9 ×	275	2
Liver A	0.5	9	29	3.0	6.0 ×	176	1.7
Skin	0.2	3.6	9.5	3.5	17.5 ×	167	2.1
Kidney	1.1	20	366	1.4	1.3 ×	466	0.3
Salivary gland	0.02	0.3	40	0.25	12.5 ×	500	0.05
Fat	0.8	14.4	6	3.0	5.9 ×	30	10–15
Other*	0.5	9	—	—	—	—	20
Total	5.5	100					

*Other tissues include bone, lung and bronchi, spleen, and lymphatic tissue.

Source: Mellander and Johansson, 1968.

Kidney

The functional unit of the kidney is the nephron. Humans have over 1 million nephrons, each consisting of a glomerulus, proximal convoluted tubule, Henle's loop, distal tubule, and collecting duct (Sands et al., 1992). In the outer and middle cortex, the loops of Henle are short. This is also the case in some juxtamedullary glomeruli, but in most of them the loops extend far into the medulla. They are accompanied by long vascular leashes, the vasa recta, which arise from the efferent arteriole and return to the interlobular veins.

The renal artery divides into interlobar arteries, which become the arcuate arteries (figure 5.2). The latter form the interlobular branches, which give rise to the afferent arterioles. Each afferent arteriole supplies a single glomerulus and is the source of the

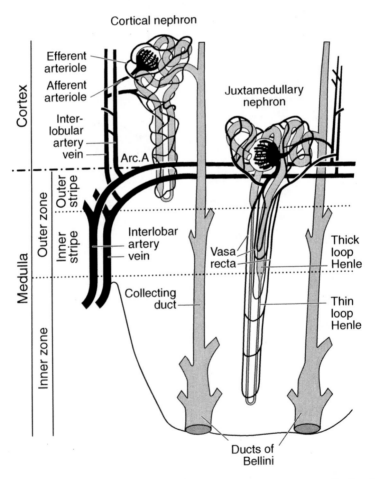

Figure 5.2. Arteries and arterioles in cortical and juxtamedullary nephrons. Further description in text. After Pitts (1963).

glomerular capillaries. Blood then passes through the efferent arteriole to the tubular capillaries.

Glomerular capillary BP is about 50 mmHg, while tubular capillary BP is 15–20 mmHg. In each glomerulus, the pressure for filtration is the net glomerular hydrostatic pressure minus net colloid osmotic pressure. The latter is greater in the efferent than in the afferent arteriole, which assists reabsorption of tubular fluid into the peritubular capillaries (Dworkin and Brenner, 1992; Cowley and Roman, 1997).

The interlobular arteries are long tapering vessels with a high resistance to blood flow. As a result, BP in the afferent arterioles of the outer cortex is lower than in those of the inner cortex (Aukland, 1989; Ulfendahl and Wolgast, 1992). Hence, during constrictor stimuli or falls in renal perfusion pressure reduction in nephron perfusion is greatest in the outer cortex. Normally, about 90% of the total RBF goes to cortical nephrons and about 10% to juxtamedullary nephrons (Ulfendahl and Wolgast, 1992).

The kidney's sympathetic innervation supplies the VSM cells of the afferent and efferent arterioles, and also the renin-producing cells in the distal segment of these arterioles. Innervation density is greater in the outer than in the inner cortex; furthermore, in each region the afferent arteriole is more densely innervated than the efferent arteriole (Denton et al., 2004; Eppel et al., 2004). The effects of increased SNA on renin-producing cells are mediated through β-ARs and cause a local increase in angiotensin II (Ang II) formation. This causes a greater degree of constriction of the efferent than the afferent arterioles, which raises filtration fraction (glomerular filtration rate/renal plasma flow [GFR/RPF]).

Renin production alters reciprocally as local renal artery BP changes. Vasodilators also increase renin release. The latter changes during alterations in tubular sodium load, which acts through a local sodium chloride sensor in the wall of the thick segment of the ascending loop of Henle, which is called the macula densa. This is part of the juxtaglomerular apparatus (JGA) at the vascular pole of each glomerulus; it extends between the afferent and efferent arterioles, making contact with both vessels and with the mesangium. A change in NaCl delivery at the macula densa induces an inverse change in renin secretion by the juxtaglomerular cells (Vander, 1967; Schnermann and Briggs, 1992).

Effect of EH.   Renal Vas R is already raised and RBF reduced in mild EH, and the changes become more pronounced with greater severity of EH (figure 5.3; Goldring et al., 1941; Goldring and Chasis, 1944; Talbott et al., 1943; Hilden, 1948; Corcoran et al., 1948; Bolomey et al., 1949; Cottier, 1960; Brod et al., 1962; Hollenberg et al., 1978; de Leeuw et al., 1983; Ljungman and Granerus, 1995). In the early stages of EH, the constriction is mediated through α-ARs (Hollenberg et al., 1981; de Leeuw et al., 1985).

Aging causes similar renal changes, but for a given age the constriction is greater in EH (Bauer et al., 1982; Messerli, Sundgaard-Riise, Ventura et al., 1983; London et al., 1984). The decline in GFR begins when EH is moderately severe. Before then it has been maintained by the raised filtration fraction. Another change associated with severe EH is the decline in para-amino hippurate extraction ratio (E_{PAH}) by the kidney (figure 5.3), which is an indicator of enhanced heterogeneity of nephron perfusion (Pappenheimer and Kinter, 1956; Kinter and Pappenheimer, 1956; Stokes and

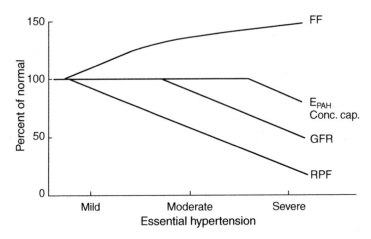

Figure 5.3. Average changes in patients with mild, moderate, and severe EH, in renal plasma flow (RPF), glomerular filtration rate (GFR), filtration fraction (FF), renal extraction ratio of PAH (E_{PAH}), and urinary concentrating capacity (Conc. cap.); results expressed as percentage of matched healthy normotensives. Based on data from several series. From Ljungman and Granerus (1995), with permission of Raven Press and Lippincott, Williams and Wilkins.

Korner, 1964; Birkenhäger and Schalekamp, 1976; de Leeuw et al., 1978; Reubi et al., 1978; Ljungman et al., 1980; Katzman et al., 1990; Ljungman and Granerus, 1995).

Glomerular pressure is often raised in EH, as estimated from the renal vein wedge pressure (Lowenstein et al., 1967, 1970). This is a sign of renal damage (Anderson and Brenner, 1995), which relates to increased renal perfusion heterogeneity.

Splanchnic Circulation

The splanchnic circulation includes the vessels supplying the gastrointestinal tract, liver, pancreas, and spleen. The veins from stomach, intestine, spleen, and pancreas drain into the portal vein, which provides the liver with two thirds of its blood flow and one third of its O_2 supply (Donald, 1981; Lundgren, 1986). The hyperemia during digestion is mediated through release of local intestinal hormones (gastrin, histamine, cholecystokinin). Intestinal resistance vessels are richly innervated and are very sensitive to hypoxia and hypercapnia (Korner et al., 1967; Korner, 1974).

The intestinal veins are the most distensible veins of a major organ. During arteriolar dilation, they become passively distended and accommodate a substantial volume of blood. The opposite happens during arteriolar constriction, when the veins empty through passive recoil, often reinforced by sympathetic venomotor activity (Folkow and Neil, 1971; Rothe, 1983; Rowell, 1986; Monos et al., 1995).

Effects of EH.   Splanchnic Vas R is increased in mild EH, increasing further as EH becomes more severe (Culbertson et al., 1951; Brod, 1960; Messerli et al., 1975, 1978). The high sensitivity of intestinal resistance vessels to tissue hypoxia and hypercapnia tends to mask SNA-mediated constrictor effects (Korner et al., 1967, 1990). The rise in splanchnic SNA is probably of the same magnitude as in the renal sympathetic nerves.

Skeletal Muscle and Skin Beds

The muscle bed's capacity for metabolic dilation is large (Rowell, 1986). Neural vasoconstriction is through stimulation of α-ARs, while stimulation of β_2-ARs produces vasodilation. In acute stress, the dilator effect is due to a small increase in plasma adrenaline concentration, which masks the neural vasoconstriction that generally occurs simultaneously (figure 5.4; Chalmers et al., 1966; Uther et al., 1970; Bolli et al., 1981; chapters 9, 10, this volume). At higher concentrations, the affinity of adrenaline is greater for α- than for β-ARs, thus reinforcing neural constrictor effects.

The skin circulation plays little role in baroreflex control but is important in thermoregulation (Delius et al., 1972b; Korner, 1974; Rowell, 1986; Victor and Mark, 1995). The richly innervated arteriovenous anastomoses are plentiful in the nail beds of fingers and toes and sparse in central body skin. They constrict in the cold and dilate when it is warm. The subcutaneous venous plexuses are very distensible and, like the gastrointestinal veins, can accommodate a large fraction of the blood volume.

Effect of EH.   In mild hypertension, resting blood flows in forearm and leg reflect mainly the vasodilation in muscle (Abramson and Fierst, 1942; Amery et al., 1969; Bolli et al., 1981; Hulthen et al., 1982). In the presence of β-AR antagonists, the underlying α-AR-mediated vasoconstriction becomes unmasked (Bolli et al., 1981; Kiowski et al., 1981).

In severe EH, resting muscle Vas R becomes raised (Amery et al., 1967; Bolli et al., 1981). Much of this is due to the amplifier action of R_1 vessel structural changes and reduction in availability of NO (chapter 6). However, during stress muscle vasodilation also occurs in severe EH, owing to phasic secretion of adrenaline (see below).

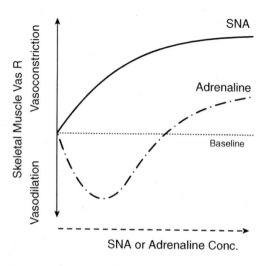

Figure 5.4. Relationship between sympathetic activity (SNA) and vascular resistance (Vas R) in skeletal muscle is monotonic, with Vas R rising as SNA increases. In contrast, relationship between plasma adrenaline concentration (Conc) is biphasic, with a fall in Vas R during small concentration rises and an increase in Vas R at high concentrations. Based on Uther et al. (1970).

Skin bed Vas R increases at all levels of severity of EH. The size of the bed is often reduced, which is best seen in the nailfold capillaries and conjunctiva (Lack, 1949; Harper et al., 1978; Sullivan et al., 1983; Shore and Tooke, 1994; Antonios et al., 1999a, 1999b). It is a consequence of sustained vasoconstriction reinforced by the development of structural changes.[2]

Effect of Regional Patterns on Central Hemodynamics

Table 5.2 indicates average resting CO and regional blood flows, conductances, and Vas Rs in mild and moderate/severe EH, expressed as percentages of the values in normotensive controls (references in reviews by Brod, 1960; Brod et al., 1962; Korner and Fletcher, 1977; Korner, 1982; Conway, 1984; Lund-Johansen, 1980, 1994). Jan Brod, then in Prague, was the first to recognize that the regional hemodynamic pattern in EH resembles the defense response (Brod, 1960; 1963).

When relating vascular tone in individual beds to the overall effects, it is most convenient to use conductances (C = flow/pressure), since TPC is the sum of the

Table 5.2. Resting Cardiac Output (CO) and Blood Flows in Kidney (RBF), Gastrointestinal (GI), Skeletal Muscle (SkMBF), and Other Beds, and Corresponding Vascular Conductances (C) and Vascular Resistances (Vas R) in Normotensive Controls, and Mild and Moderate to Severe EH

MAP	Normal BP 100 mmHg	Mild EH 115 mmHg	Mod/Severe EH 130 mmHg
Blood Flows			
CO	100	115	96
RBF	100	80	55
GIF	100	97	84
SkMBF	100	160	113
Other	100	121	111
Conductance			
TPC	100	100	74
Ren C	100	70	42
GI C	100	84	64
SkM C	100	139	87
Other	100	105	85
Vascular Resistance			
TPR	100	100	135
Ren R	100	143	238
GI R	100	119	154
SkM R	100	72	114
Other R	100	114	117

Note: Results expressed as percentage of normotensive controls. In appropriate units, TPC = Ren C + GI C + SkM C + Other C, while TPR = 1/Ren R + 1/GI R + 1/SKM R + 1/Other R.

regional Cs; the relationship between TPR and regional Vas Rs is not as easy to take in (see formulas in table 5.2).

In mild EH, TPC is the same as in normotensive controls, because the falls in renal and splanchnic Cs (i.e., vasoconstriction) is offset by the skeletal muscle vasodilation.[3] Hence, the 15% elevation in BP is entirely due to elevation in CO.

In more severe EH, there is net resting vasoconstriction as indicated by the fall in TPC and a normal CO (table 5.2). Resting renal, gastrointestinal, muscle, and skin beds have all constricted. However, in the study by Brod et al. (1960) there was pronounced skeletal muscle vasodilation, despite the presence of relatively severe EH (figure 5.5). Subsequent work has indicated that while resting plasma adrenaline is normal, it increases phasically during mild stress, which is responsible for the vasodilator response (see below). The stress is mild enough to have no effect in healthy normotensives.

Pulsatile Arterial Pressures, TPR, and Distensibility

The MAP helps in the assessment of the types of circulatory changes just considered. However, during aging SBP rises far more than DBP (figure 4.2). We know that in isolated systolic hypertension the risk for developing stroke and heart failure is substantial; hence the importance of determining what causes elevation of arterial pulse pressure in aging and hypertension.

The first to measure arterial BP was Stephen Hales (1733), who regarded the large arteries near the heart as having a cushioning function that allowed the transformation of the pulsatile blood flow in the aorta to steady flow in the capillaries (Taylor, 1966b). The cushioning was likened to a "Windkessel," which fulfilled the above function in the fire engines of the period.

For the next 150 years, no instruments were available for measuring phasic BP and blood flow adequately. It was only in the first half of the 20th century that

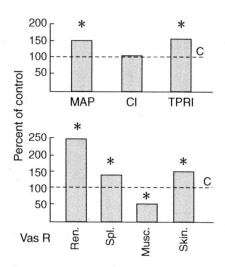

Figure 5.5. Top, resting mean arterial pressure (MAP), cardiac index (CI), and total peripheral resistance index (TPRI) in 15 subjects with moderate to severe EH, expressed as percentages of means of 12 age-matched normotensives. Bottom, resting renal, splanchnic, forearm muscle, and forearm skin Vas Rs in same group. Adapted from Brod (1960).

high-frequency optical manometers and strain gauges were developed (Frank, 1905; Wiggers, 1928; Hamilton, 1944; Remington, 1963). By the 1930s and 1940s, Kolin and Wetterer had developed the electromagnetic blood flowmeter, and ultrasonic flow probes were later added to the measuring equipment, allowing pulsatile hemo-dynamics to be placed on a firm theoretical footing (McDonald and Taylor, 1959; McDonald, 1960).

As is evident in figure 1.2, there are considerable differences between central and peripheral arterial pressure pulses (McDonald, 1960). In the ascending aorta, the arterial pulse is broad, and BP during systole reaches a later peak than the velocity of blood flow; the incisura marks the end of ventricular systole, and is followed by a well-defined diastolic wave.[4] However, in the peripheral arteries (e.g., femoral and saphenous) the systolic pressure peak is greater than in the central aorta: The incisura is absent, but there is a wave in diastole (figure 1.2).

In the ascending aorta, over 90% of flow (and 100% of the forward flow) is in sys-tole, while in diastole flow is mostly zero, except for a backflow spike as the aortic valve closes. In the peripheral arteries, the peak blood flow velocity is less than in the upper aorta, but a high proportion of the blood flow during diastole is in a forward direction.

Pulse Wave Velocity and Wave Reflection

In 1850, the Weber brothers showed that the arterial pulse propagated as a wave that travels much more rapidly than the blood (Taylor, 1966b). Its velocity is given by the Moens-Korteweg equation (McDonald, 1960; O'Rourke, 1982a).

$$\text{PWV} = \sqrt{E} \times w/2r_i\rho,$$

where PWV is pulse wave velocity, E is Young's modulus, w and r_i are wall thickness and internal radius, and ρ is density. In general, if the pulse wave velocity is more rapid, the wall is less distensible.

Otto Frank recognized the compound nature of the arterial pulse wave, which he thought was made up of a wave generated by ventricular ejection traveling away from the heart, and waves reflected from the periphery traveling toward the heart. Hamilton and Remington thought that the arterioles were the main reflecting sites and lumped them into a single reflecting site in the lower part of the body, with the incident (centrifugal) and reflected (centripetal) waves bouncing back and forth between the latter site and the aortic valve (Hamilton and Dow, 1939; Hamilton, 1944; Remington, 1963). This was known as the standing wave theory.

The general idea is still accepted, but there have been subsequent modifications (Taylor, 1965, 1966b; Mills et al., 1970; O'Rourke, 1982b; Latham et al., 1987). In O'Rourke's modification of the Hamilton-Remington model, the arterial system is an asymmetric T-tube, where one reflecting site is at the upper part and another in the lower part of the body (figure 4.3). At each site, the reflected waves summate with the incident wave from the heart at different times of the cardiac cycle, as discussed in chapter 4.

In the above model, Vas R and distensibility can be altered independently (O'Rourke, 1982b). When Vas R increases and distensibility stays normal, the rises in SBP and DBPs are similar, with little change in pulse pressure (figure 5.6, middle). When Vas R

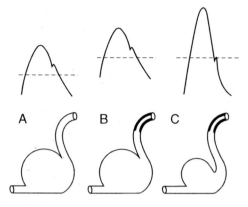

Figure 5.6. Arterial pulse waves in three models of the arterial system: (A) normal Vas R and distensibility; (B) high Vas R and normal distensibility; (C) high Vas R and reduced distensibility. From O'Rourke (1982a), with permission of Churchill-Livingstone-Elsevier.

remains high and distensibility is reduced, MAP rises as before, but the rise is largely in SBP; DBP is little changed so that there is simulation of isolated systolic hypertension (figure 5.6C). In chronic EH, DBP is mostly raised significantly, but the increases in SBP and pulse pressure are greater when distensibility is low.

Blood Volume and Viscosity in EH

The early findings on blood volume in hypertension were variable, mainly because all etiological types were lumped together.

In mild EH, plasma and blood volumes are either normal or slightly reduced (Tarazi et al., 1968; Julius et al., 1972; Dustan et al., 1973; Parving and Gyntelberg, 1973; Safar et al., 1995). As EH increases in severity, the total plasma and blood volumes decline to about 20% below normal (figure 5.7). This contrasts with the rise in central blood volume, which occurs at all levels of EH (Julius and Esler, 1976; Safar et al., 1995).

Mechanism of Redistribution and Reduction of Blood Volume

August Krogh (1912) first recognized the role of regional venous distensibility in redistributing blood volume between the thoracic and extrathoracic venous compartments. Arteriolar constriction in a bed in which the veins are very distensible causes them to empty passively, shifting blood to the central compartment and raising central venous pressure (Rowell, 1986). The opposite changes occur during arteriolar dilation when its venous volume increases, drawing on blood from the central compartment. On the other hand, in a bed with nondistensible veins, neither constriction nor vasodilation affects its venous blood volume. In humans with EH, the distensible gastrointestinal and skin veins are the chief sources for shifting blood volume to and from the central compartment (Rowell, 1986; Antonios et al., 1999a, 1999b).

This mechanism has been rediscovered on several occasions (Barcroft and Samaan, 1935; Brooksby and Donald, 1971; Caldini et al., 1972). The experiments of Brooksby and Donald are of particular interest: Splanchnic sympathetic nerve stimulation caused passive emptying of intestinal veins, but also caused SNA-mediated venoconstriction.

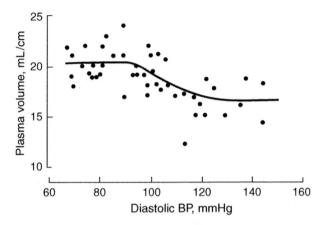

Figure 5.7. Relationship between diastolic BP (mmHg) and plasma volume (mL/cm body height) from a population of healthy normotensives and subjects with EH. Plasma volume declines from about 100 mmHg, reaching a plateau at diastolic BP ≥ 120 mmHg. From Tarazi et al. (1968), with permission of the *New England Journal of Medicine* and Massachusetts Medical Society.

Mechanism of Reduction in Blood Volume in EH

The Krogh mechanism explains redistribution of blood volume but does not indicate why total blood volume is reduced. It is well known that in EH exchangeable sodium and extracellular fluid volumes tend to be reduced (Dustan, 1973; Lever et al., 1981; Beretta-Piccoli et al., 1983; Harrap et al., 2000). It raises the question as to the effects of the tonic vasoconstriction on the microcirculation and extravascular compartment.

Somewhat serendipitously, some answers had been provided many years earlier, when I studied the effects of vasoconstriction on blood-tissue exchange and protein turnover between plasma and thoracic duct lymph (Korner and Courtice, 1954). It was thought that vasoconstriction might alter capillary permeability (Courtice and Yoffey, 1970). However, this is difficult to determine at normal low resting rates of lymph flow (Korner et al., 1954). Accordingly, anesthetized cats were infused with varying rates of Ringer-Locke solution in order to increase lymph flow and shorten the time for plasma-lymph protein equilibrium. One group of cats was infused with Ringer-Locke solution for 5 hours, at low, moderate, or high infusion rates. Another group received the electrolyte solution plus noradrenaline (NA; 0.3 μg/kg/min) to induce vasoconstriction.

The NA raised MAP and accentuated the rise in central venous BP (figure 5.8).[5] In both groups, lymph flow was similar at each infusion rate, as was the amount of total protein and labeled albumin recovered in lymph (table 5.3).

In animals receiving electrolyte solution alone at low and moderate rates, the specific activities of labeled albumin in plasma and lymph did not come into equilibrium over the 5-hour infusion, but this did occur at the highest rate of infusion (figure 5.9, left). In contrast, in NA-treated animals equilibrium was attained within 1–2 hours at all three infusion rates (figure 5.9, right).

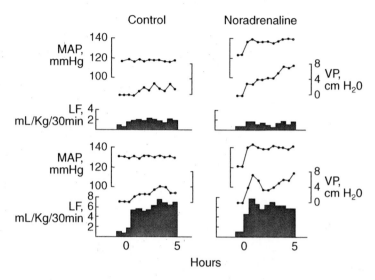

Figure 5.8. Results obtained in anesthetized cats infused with (left) Ringer-Locke solution alone, and (right) Ringer-Locke solution plus noradrenaline (0.3 μg/kg/min). In the top panels, the net rate (infusion-urine output) of IV infusion was low (30 mL/kg/5 hours), while in the lower panels the net rate was high, at a rate of 150 mL/kg/5 hours. Variables: mean arterial pressure (MAP, mmHg), inferior vena caval pressure (VP, cm H_2O), and thoracic duct lymph flow (LF, mL/kg/5 hours). Data from Korner and Courtice (1954).

The equilibrium time depends on the rate of protein leakage from plasma and the amount of protein in the interstitial fluid with which the plasma protein must mix (Wasserman and Mayerson, 1952). The control and NA-treated animals had similar leakage rates of plasma protein and albumin (table 5.3). Hence, the more rapid equilibrium during vasoconstriction suggests that the interstitial protein pool is smaller than in the nonconstricted controls.

Table 5.3. Loss of Total Protein and T-1824-Labeled Albumin from Plasma in Cats Infused with Ringer-Locke Solution Alone, or with Ringer-Locke Solution Plus Noradrenaline (NA Infusion)

Variable	Control	NA Infusion
Total protein loss mg/kg/5 hours	610 ± 21	500 ± 10*
Total protein loss % initial value	25 ± 3.5%	24 ± 1.1%
Albumin loss % initial value	50 ± 3.1%	59 ± 1.8%

Note: Rate of electrolyte infusion 120 mL/kg/5 hours IV; NA infusion 0.3 μg/kg/min IV; *$p < .05$ for difference between groups; percentage loss of albumin over 5 hours greater than loss of total protein.

Source: Korner and Courtice (1954).

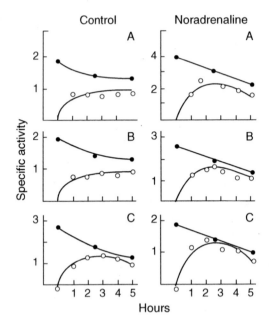

Figure 5.9. Specific activity (T-1824-labeled albumin)/(total albumin concentration) in plasma (black circles) and lymph (open circles) in control cats receiving Ringer-Locke alone (left), and cats receiving Ringer-Locke plus noradrenaline (0.3 μg/kg/min) (right). (A) minimal rate of infusion; (B) net rate of 30 mL/kg/5 hours IV; (C), net rate of 150 mL/kg/5 hours IV. Discussion in text. Data from Korner and Courtice (1954).

The Smaller Protein Pool Is an Indicator of Rarefaction

The lymph capillaries originate in the extravascular space close to the blood capillaries. During vasoconstriction, more blood flows through arteriovenous anastomoses and less through the exchange capillaries (Zweifach, 1983). Some arterioles and capillaries become closed, reducing the size of the capillary filtration area and of the interstitial protein pool. However, in the patent arterioles and capillaries there are rises in blood flow and capillary pressures, which increases the leakage of plasma albumin. More rapid leakage into a smaller pool accounts for the rapid vasoconstriction-induced equilibration.

In EH, the corresponding closure of some of the arterioles and capillaries could be transient or permanent, depending on changes in blood viscosity or on availability of NO, which affects aggregation of blood cells and platelets (chapter 6).

In the kidney, vasoconstrictor-induced rarefaction reduces the proportion of functioning nephrons. The venous and extracellular compartments are small, and rarefaction has a smaller effect on vascular capacity and total blood volume than the corresponding constriction of the gastrointestinal and skin beds.

The above mechanisms account for the reduction in total blood volume in EH. In moderate and severe EH, the constriction appears to be of the same order as in the lymph experiments. It is mediated through the raised SNA and through structural and functional R_1 vessel changes. The neurally induced reduction in venous capacity is accompanied by greater excretion of water and salt. This is helped by the raised renal vein pressures and by the renal action of atrial natriuretic peptide (ANP; Sudhir et al., 1988).

Vasoconstriction Does Not Increase Capillary Permeability

Parving and Gyntelberg (1973) suggested that capillary permeability increased in EH. This was based on the greater rate of disappearance of labeled albumin from plasma in persons with EH than in normotensives (7.2% vs. 5.6% per hour).

This is not in accord with the findings in the lymph experiments. At high electrolyte infusion rates the interstitial protein is rapidly washed out of the extravascular space, so that lymph protein concentration approaches that of the capillary filtrate (Korner, Morris and Courtice, 1954). In the NA-treated cats, this concentration averaged 0.3 g protein/100 mL plasma, which is close to other estimates of capillary filtrate composition (Crone, 1963; Landis and Pappenheimer, 1963; Michel, 1984). It is well below the average concentration of 0.9 g protein/100 mL in the control cats, in which the interstitial protein pool is greater and the rate of protein washout slower. It suggests that vasoconstriction does not alter capillary permeability.

Viscosity Changes in EH

Blood viscosity is often increased in EH. The reasons are uncertain: Factors that suggest increased viscosity in EH are the tendency toward higher hematocrits and changes in plasma protein composition (Letcher et al., 1981; Chabanel and Chien, 1995).

One speculation is that the changes in plasma proteins are related to greater protein synthesis due to the high turnover associated with the vasoconstriction-induced microcirculatory changes just considered. Another factor is greater catecholamine (CA) turnover in the splanchnic sympathetic outflow, which raises hepatic synthesis of plasma proteins (Chabanel and Chien, 1995). It seems more likely that raised viscosity is a consequence of these changes in EH. The altered plasma proteins could affect platelet aggregation and increase the chances of permanent microcirculatory rarefaction.

Autonomic Outflow Patterns

In EH, there are changes in resting vagal activity and cardiac SNA and in the activity of main sympathetic constrictor outflows. The sympathetic changes explain the initiation of EH, and SNA remains high for many years.

Autonomic Effects on Heart Rate

Up to about 60 years of age, resting heart rate is about 10–25% greater in persons with EH than in normotensives, but in older people the rates are often similar (Julius et al., 1971, 1975; Korner, Shaw, Uther et al., 1973; Lund-Johansen, 1980, 1994; Korner, 1982, 1983). The tachycardia is due to an increase in cardiac SNA and lower vagal activity in EH, while the "intrinsic" heart rate (i.e., during cardiac autonomic blockade) is the same in both groups (Jose and Taylor, 1969; Korner, Shaw, Uther et al., 1973).

The vagal and cardiac sympathetic effects on heart rate have been estimated from the changes elicited by successively blocking muscarinic receptors and β-ARs.

However, the estimates differ, depending on the order of administration of the antagonists (figure 5.10). This is because the circulatory changes associated with each drug are accompanied by changes in arterial, cardiac, and pulmonary BPs, by which the reflex heart rate changes are evoked through the unblocked pathway. It illustrates

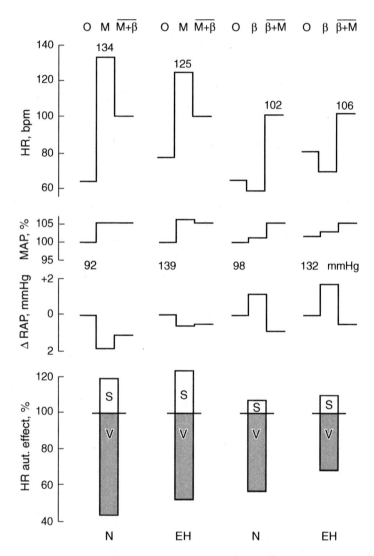

Figure 5.10. Changes in heart rate (HR, bpm), mean arterial pressure (MAP, % of baseline), right atrial pressure (ΔRAP, mmHg), sympathetic and vagal effect on heart rate (S, V; % of baseline) in subjects with EH (EH) and normotensives (N). In left two panels, atropine (M_2 muscarinic receptor antagonist) given first; followed by propranolol (β-AR antagonist); in the right two panels, propranol given first, followed by atropine. Numbers on top of HR graph, peak steady-state values; numbers on MAP graph, baseline MAPs. O, baseline; β, propranolol; M, atropine. After Korner and Fletcher (1977).

one of the problems of indirect assessment of autonomic function. To arrive at something close to the "true" autonomic effects on heart rate, Korner, West, and Shaw (1973) alternated the order of giving each antagonist to each subject in two separate experiments and averaged the estimates.

After muscarinic blockade, the average rise in heart rate was 41.5 bpm in EH and 52.5 bpm in normotensives, suggesting a lower resting vagal tone in EH. As discussed in chapter 9, this occurs in every type of hypertension and is a consequence of elevation of cardiopulmonary load.

After β-AR blockade, heart rate slowed by 18.5 bpm in EH and by 14.5 bpm in normotensives, suggesting an increase in cardiac SNA in EH.[6] The elevation of cardiac SNA is part of the defense response.

Sympathoadrenal Function in EH

SNA in humans is assessed by (1) microneurography, where a microelectrode is used to record SNA from a postganglionic sympathetic nerve; and (2) the NA "spillover" method, which is an index of SNA in a given sympathetic outflow related to the NA turnover rate.

Microneurography

Microneurography has been used in recording SNA in sympathetic nerves to skeletal muscle and skin. The nerves to skeletal muscle are mostly vasoconstrictor fibers to the resistance vessels: they discharge in pulse-synchronous bursts and respond to changes in BP and respiration (Delius et al., 1972a; Wallin and Fagius, 1988; Eckberg and Sleight, 1992; Victor and Mark, 1995; Mancia, 1997; Grassi, 1998). The skin sympathetic fibers supply blood vessels, sweat glands, hair follicles, and fat (Jänig, 1985). Skin SNA is relatively insensitive to BP changes, but participates in thermoregulation (Delius et al., 1972b; Iriki et al., 1979).

The first measurements in subjects with EH found that their SNA was similar to that in normotensives (Wallin and Sundlöf, 1979; Wallin and Fagius, 1988). However, subsequent studies in subjects with mild EH have uniformly observed elevation in muscle SNA compared to the levels in well-matched groups of normotensives (figure 5.11); SNA increases further as EH becomes more severe (Anderson et al., 1988; Yamada et al., 1989; Floras and Hara, 1993; Victor and Mark, 1995; Grassi, 1998; Grassi et al., 1998). The reason for the discrepancy is unclear: It may be due to better matching of groups in the later studies, or even technical improvements (Victor and Mark, 1995).

Catecholamine-Based Biochemical Indices

The tissues in which CA biosynthesis occurs include (1) peripheral sympathetic nerves, (2) chromaffin cells of the adrenal medulla, and (3) central CA neurons (Bowman and Rand, 1980; Cooper et al., 1991). The transmitter released at the endings depends on which biosynthetic enzymes are present in the particular cell (figure 5.12). For example, NA neurons lack the enzyme phenylethanolamine transferase, which is necessary for adrenaline synthesis from NA.

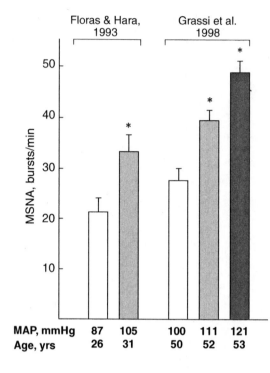

Figure 5.11. Resting muscle sympathetic nerve activity (MSNA, burst/min) in normotensives (open rectangle) and those with mild and moderate EH (light and dark gray). Left, data from young subjects; right, data from older subjects. *$p < .05$ for Δ between EH and normotensives. Numbers, average mean arterial pressures (MAP, mmHg) and age (years). After Floras and Hara (1993) and Grassi, Cattaneo, Seravalle et al. (1998).

Metabolic inactivation of CAs is through one or more of the following: (1) *oxidative deamination* by monoamino oxidase, which is the sole metabolizing enzyme in CA neurons; its metabolites are markers of intraneuronal metabolism, such as dihydroxyphenylglycol; (2) *O-methylation* with catecholamine methyltransferase; its metabolites are markers of extraneuronal metabolism; (3) *conjugation* by sulfotransferases or glucuronidases; and (4) *dehydrogenation* to homovanillic acid and vanillylmandelic acid (VMA) by alcohol dehydrogenase; VMA is the main NA metabolite in urine (figure 5.12), where it is an index of peripheral NA turnover from postganglionic sympathetic nerves (Cooper et al., 1991; Boulton and Eisenhofer, 1998).

Noradrenaline

Plasma NA concentration is still useful as an index for assessing SNA. However, it depends on both NA entry from the terminals and the clearance rate into tissues and urine. The latter is often low in the sick and elderly, which may complicate interpretation of results.

Any ambiguity is avoided by the NA spillover method, which measures entry of NA from sympathetic terminals into plasma (Esler et al., 1979, 1990; Esler, 1982, 1995). Tritiated NA (^{3}H-L-NA) is infused at a constant rate until a steady plateau

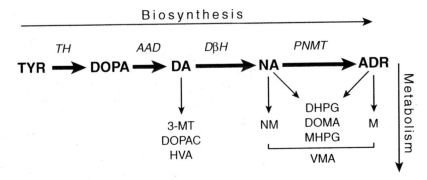

Figure 5.12. Steps in catecholamine biosynthesis from tyrosine (bold). Biosynthetic enzymes in italics; main metabolic products are below line for synthesis. Tyr, tyrosine; TH, tyrosine hydroxylase; DOPA, 3,4,dihydroxyphenylalanine; AAD, aromatic acid decarboxylase; DA, dopamine; DβH, dopamine-β-hydroxylase; NA, noradrenaline; PNMT, phenylethanolamine methyltransferase; ADR, adrenaline. Metabolic products for dopamine: 3-MT, 3-methoxytyramine; DOPAC, dihydroxyphenylacetic acid; HVA, homovanillic acid. Metabolites of NA and ADR shown by downward arrows: NM, normetanephrine; DHPG, dihydroxyphenylethylene-glycol; DOMA, dihydroxymandelic acid; MHPG, 3-methoxy-4-hydroxyphenyl-glycol; VMA, vanillyl mandelic acid. Adapted from Esler et al. (1990), with permission of *Physiological Reviews* and the American Physiological Society.

concentration is reached in the arterial blood, when NA spillover, clearance, and extraction ratios are calculated from the following formulas:

$$\text{Total NA spillover} = {}^{3}\text{H-NA infusion rate/plasma NA SpA}$$
$$\text{Regional NA spillover} = [(NA_a - NA_v) + NA_a \times E] \times PF$$
$$\text{Total NA clearance} = {}^{3}\text{H-NA infusion rate/plasma }{}^{3}\text{H-NA}$$
$$\text{concentration}$$
$$E = (NA_a - NA_v)/NA_a$$
$$\text{Plasma NA SpA} = {}^{3}\text{H-NA concentration/total plasma NA}$$

Where NA = noradrenaline; ^{3}H-NA = tritiated noradrenaline; plasma NA SpA = plasma noradrenaline-specific activity; NA_a, NA_v = noradrenaline concentration in arterial and venous blood; E = extraction ratio; PF = plasma flow. The main assumption is that the fraction of NA reaching plasma bears a constant relationship to the total transmitter released from a particular outflow. This has been validated in some beds (Esler, 1982, 1995; Blombery and Heinzow, 1983; Esler et al., 1990; Hjemdahl and Friberg, 1996). Some uncertainties arise about whether the low perfusion in resting skeletal muscle or the intrinsic heterogeneity of the "hepatomesenteric" sympathetic outflows could compromise the results. I have assumed that NA spillover provides reliable estimates of average (total) SNA and renal and cardiac SNA, while microneurography is the most reliable method for assessing muscle SNA.

Effect of EH.   Plasma NA concentration is raised in EH, but the effect is small (figure 5.13, top; Goldstein, 1983; Esler et al., 1987; Grassi, 1998). In contrast, average

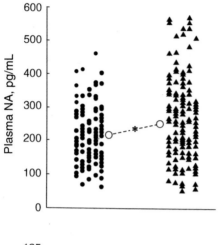

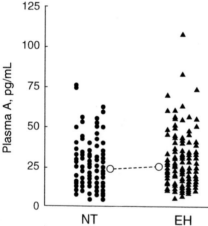

Figure 5.13. Data from 131 normotensives (NT) and 172 untreated essential hypertensives (EH). Top, plasma NA (pg/mL); bottom, plasma adrenaline (A, pg/mL) concentration. Open circles, average NA and A values in each group; asterisk denotes $p < .05$ for difference between groups. Average MAP $\pm$ SEM in normotensives 91 $\pm$ 0.6 mmHg; in hypertensives 111 $\pm$ 0.7 mmHg. From Grassi (1998), with permission of the *Journal of Hypertension* and Lippincott, Williams and Wilkins.

($\equiv$ total), renal, and cardiac NA spillovers between the ages of 20 and 60 years are greater in EH (figure 5.14; Esler et al., 1989; Esler, 1995). However, in the small number of older persons, spillover has been similar to that of normotensives.

The early increase in spillover suggests that the raised SNA accounts for the early elevation of BP. The elevation remains constant between 40 and 60 years of age or may decline slightly, which does not explain the substantial rises in BP and TPR between those ages in EH (figure 5.1; table 5.2). It suggests that nonneural as well as neural factors must contribute to the elevation in BP over this period (chapter 6). The apparent normalization in NA spillover in older persons must be interpreted with caution. The number of subjects was small and they may have been healthier than the average older person with EH. Other suggestions for the fall in spillover include a baroreflex response to high cardiopulmonary load (chapter 9); a central inhibitory action of ANP (Gutkowska et al., 1997); or an increased production of oxygen radicals resulting in reduction synthesis of CAs in CA neurons (Girouard et al., 2003). In older patients with EH and cardiac failure, NA spillover is raised (Hasking et al., 1986).

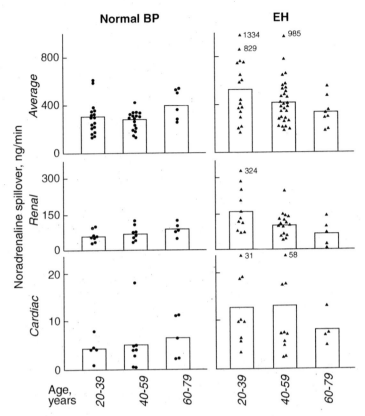

Figure 5.14. Noradrenaline spillover rates (ng/min) including average (i.e., total), renal, and cardiac spillover in groups of different age (see bottom of each column). Subjects with normal BPs (left) and with essential hypertension (EH; right). Up to 59 years of age, spillover is significantly greater in EH group. Based on Esler (1995), with permission of Raven Press and Lippincott, Williams and Wilkins.

It has been suggested that a fault in the NA reuptake pump may accentuate the enhanced NA spillover (Esler et al., 1981; Schlaich et al., 2004). This too should be interpreted cautiously, since current methods for in vivo assessment are indirect. In vitro studies in SHR suggest that the NA reuptake pump functions normally at the terminals of the vasculature (Dyke et al., 1989).

Adrenaline

Acute stress elicits skeletal muscle vasodilation, which is caused by increased secretion of adrenaline, which subsides as soon as the stress is over (figure 5.15). The small increase in its concentration stimulates β-ARs (Hjemdahl et al., 1984). This has also been observed in animals during acute hypoxic stress (Fukuda and Kobayashi, 1961; Chalmers et al., 1966; Korner et al., 1967). Pretreatment with β-blockers in these

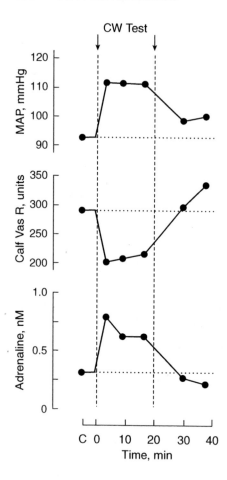

Figure 5.15. Stress induced by color-word conflict test (CW Test) on mean arterial pressure (MAP, mmHg), calf vascular resistance (Vas R, units), and plasma adrenaline (nM). Adapted from Hjemdahl et al. (1984).

experiments unmasks the simultaneous increase in neural α-AR-mediated vasoconstriction during the stress.

In EH, plasma adrenaline concentrations are closely similar to those of normotensives (figure 5.13; Grassi, 1998; Rumantir et al., 2000), although in some earlier studies plasma concentrations were raised in mild EH (De Champlain et al., 1979; Franco-Morselli et al., 1979). How then to account for the skeletal muscle vasodilation that occurs under resting conditions in EH, as in figure 5.5? On the face of it, adrenaline secretion is responsible for this effect, since β-AR antagonists uniformly unmask coexisting neural vasoconstriction (Bolli et al., 1981; Kiowski et al., 1981).

A hypothesis that explains these findings is that plasma adrenaline concentration is normal at rest but increases phasically during slight accentuation of stress. Assuming that the defense pathway responsiveness is accentuated in EH, the stimulus provided by the invasive laboratory procedures elicits a defense response, including phasic elevation of plasma adrenaline in persons with EH, while the same procedures have no effect in normal subjects (chapters 9, 10).

Table 5.4. Cardiac Adrenaline and Noradrenaline (NA) Kinetics in Subjects with Normal BP and with EH

Variable	Normal BP	EH
Art. adrenaline, pg/mL	72 ± 8.2	72 ± 13.3
CS adrenaline, pg/mL	36 ± 4.4	50 ± 8.9
Cardiac adrenaline spillover, ng/min	0.27 ± 0.31	1.46 ± 0.47*
Cardiac NA spillover ng/min	15.4 ± 2.2	24.9 ± 4.7*
n (M/F)	13 (10 M,3F)	27 (27M,0F)
BMI, kg/m²	24.6	28.7*
SBP/DBP, mmHg	143 ± 2.8/72 ± 1.3	166 ± 4.1/88 ± 2.7

Note: Values are means ± SEMs; *$p < .05$ for $\Delta_{\text{hypert-normot}}$; Art. arterial; CS, coronary sinus; NA, noradrenaline; BMI, body mass index; SBP, systolic blood pressure; DBP, diastolic blood pressure; n, number; M, male; F, female.

Source: Rumantir et al. (2000), with permission of *Journal of Hypertension* and Lippincott, Williams and Wilkins.

The above is in accord with findings by Rumantir et al. (2000): Despite the absence of change in plasma adrenaline, there was significant adrenaline spillover into coronary sinus blood in persons with EH, which was not observed in age-matched normotensives (table 5.4). Assuming that in persons with EH mild stress elicits an increase in plasma adrenaline concentration, this is rapidly taken up by the NA reuptake pump when the stress is over. Some of the adrenaline is metabolized gradually in the terminals and some is released during neural activity but in too low concentrations to have systemic effect.

Prejunctional Modulation at Sympathetic Nerve Terminals

In the heart, neural release of NA from sympathetic terminals stimulates prejunctional α_2-ARs, which inhibits transmitter released by subsequent nerve impulses (Rand et al., 1973; Langer et al., 1977; Starke, 1977; Medgett et al., 1978; Rand et al., 1980; Langer, 1981; Angus et al., 1990; Langer and Arbilla, 1990). This is termed autoinhibitory feedback (figure 5.16, top) Some have regarded this feedback as modulating cardiac SNA on a beat-to-beat basis (Rand et al., 1980; Langer and Arbilla, 1990). However, our group found that this only occurs at very high levels of cardiac SNA (Angus and Korner, 1980; Angus et al., 1984, 1990). It suggests that the release site is some distance from the prejunctional receptor (figure 5.16, bottom).

In contrast, during sympathetic excitation of R_1 vessel VSM cells, the autoinhibitory feedback comes into play in the physiological range of SNA (Angus et al., 1990). Presumably, at these terminals the prejunctional receptors are close to the NA release site.

Adrenaline-mediated stimulation of prejunctional β-ARs causes an increase in NA release during subsequent nerve impulses. This mechanism was at one time proposed as the major determinant of the elevation of BP in EH (Majewski and Rand, 1981a; Majewski, Rand, and Tung, 1981; Majewski, Tung, and Rand, 1981). However, there is ample evidence of CNS mechanisms that elevate SNA in EH (chapter 8). Bearing in

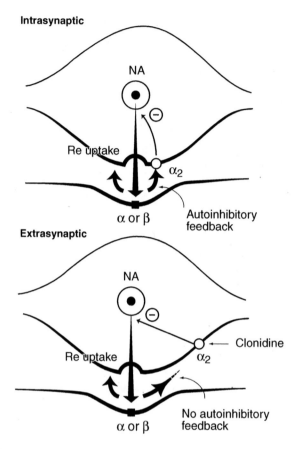

Figure 5.16. Schema of sympathetic nerve terminal: postjunctional changes in heart rate and VSM cells is through noradrenaline (NA) stimulating, respectively, β-ARs or α-ARs. Top, simulation of prejunctional α_2-AR, which is intrasynaptic close to site of NA release, autoinhibitory feedback $(-)$ results, with less NA released during subsequent nerve impulse. Bottom, if prejunctional α_2-AR is extrasynaptic, NA concentration is too low to stimulate the receptor, which can still be stimulated by circulating agonists such as clonidine. Based on Angus et al. (1990), with permission of *Annals of the New York Academy of Sciences.*

mind that plasma adrenaline is raised only phasically in EH, it is unlikely that it plays a major role in the pathogenesis of EH.

Plasma Renin Activity

The enzyme renin cleaves angiotensinogen to form the decapeptide Ang I, which is converted to the octapeptide Ang II by ACE (Jackson and Garrison, 1996). Further cleavage gives rise to smaller peptides, including angiotensin III and angiotensin-(1–7).[7] The kidney is the major source of PRA; the changes in PRA are usually associated with parallel changes in plasma Ang II concentration. However, renin is present in many other tissues including the heart, vasculature, and CNS. These tissues have local renin-angiotensin systems, with important physiological actions, some of which are discussed in later chapters (Allen et al., 2000; Husain and Graham, 2000).

PRA in EH.   PRA is lower in EH than in normal subjects on a similar diet, but the variance (i.e., SD^2) of the distribution is significantly greater than in normotensives (figure 5.17; Padfield et al., 1975; Thurston et al., 1978; Thomas et al., 1996). The greater variance in EH suggests that additional factors are involved in its regulation.

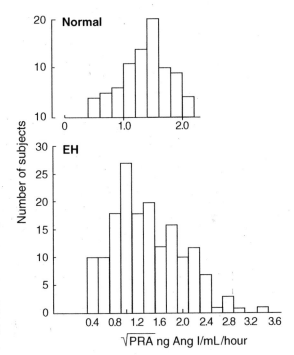

Figure 5.17. Frequency distribution of square root of plasma renin activity (PRA) in 176 subjects with essential hypertension (EH) and 83 matched normotensives. From Thurston et al. (1978), with permission of *Quarterly Journal of Medicine* and Oxford University Press.

The proportion of subjects with high PRAs (≥ 4 ng Ang I/mL/hour) is greater in EH than in normal subjects. This may be due to the greater rise in renal SNA and associated greater perfusion heterogeneity (Esler et al., 1975; Julius and Esler, 1975; Sands et al., 1992). However, in the majority of those with EH, PRAs are below values in normotensives (figure 5.17). One factor may be the greater central blood volumes in low-renin subjects (Esler et al., 1976). It has been suggested that depressed renin secretion could be mediated through the baroreflex pathways (Dampney et al., 1979). However, this seems unlikely in view of the elevation of constrictor SNA: A more plausible explanation is that renin secretion may be depressed by the action of the high renal BP on the peripheral renal barostat (see chapter 15).

In the high-renin group, plasma Ang II concentrations are usually also raised (Caravaggi et al., 1976). Ang II could accentuate transmitter release per sympathetic nerve impulse through stimulation of prejunctional AT_1 receptors (Zimmerman, 1978; Antonaccio and Kerwin, 1980, 1981). A corollary is that long-term administration of ACE inhibitors reduces neural SNA (Adams et al., 1990).

Steroid Hormones

Aldosterone is the main adrenal mineralocorticoid hormone and is formed in cells of the zona glomerulosa in the outer part of the adrenal cortex (Biglieri et al., 1995). Its secretion is regulated through the renin-angiotensin system and plasma K^+.

Other mineralocorticoids (e.g., 18-hydroxydeoxycorticosterone, 18-OH-DOC) are synthesized in cells of the zona fasciculata.

Cortisol is the main glucocorticoid hormone in humans, with corticosterone the corresponding hormone in rats. The secretion of cortisol is formed in the zona fasciculata and regulated by adrenal corticotrophic hormone (ACTH) from the anterior pituitary. In turn, ACTH is under the control of corticotrophin-releasing hormone (CRH) and arginine vasopressin (AVP; Berecek, 1992; Orth et al., 1992). The innermost adrenal cortical layer is the zona reticularis, which is the source of adrenal androgens and oestrogens.

Steroids in EH

It has been suggested that EH is a variant form of steroid hypertension, with features of primary aldosteronism or Cushing's syndrome. However, stress-related elevation of glucocorticoid secretion is also part of the defense response.

Plasma cortisol has a circadian rhythm, with the maximum concentration in the morning. At that time, resting plasma cortisol is about 20% greater in EH than in normotensives (figure 5.18; Filipovsky et al., 1996). Phasic increases in psychosocial stress raise cortisol secretion (Björntorp et al., 2000).

Whitworth et al. (1989) estimated the contribution of cortisol to the elevation of BP in EH by suppressing ACTH secretion with a daily low dose of dexamethasone for 4 weeks. This produced a BP fall of about 6 mmHg in those with EH, but had no effect in normal subjects (table 5.5).

Is EH a Form of Steroid Hypertension?

Soon after discovering primary aldosteronism, Conn suggested that at least 20% of persons diagnosed as having EH had a variant form of primary aldosteronism (Conn, 1964; Lim et al., 2001; Stowasser, 2001). There are patients regarded as having EH,

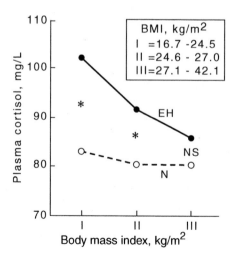

Figure 5.18. Relationship between body mass index (BMI, kg/m^2) and plasma cortisol (mg/L) in normotensive males (N, dashed line) and those with essential hypertension (EH, solid line). *$p < .01$, for difference between groups; NS, not significant. From Filipovsky et al. (1996), with permission of *Journal of Hypertension* and Lippincott, Williams and Wilkins.

Table 5.5. Effect on Mean Arterial Pressure (MAP) of 4 Weeks'
Treatment with 0.5 mg/Night Dexamethasone in 8 Normal
Subjects and 6 Subjects with EH

MAP, mmHg	Control	3, 4 Week R_x
Normal BP	80	79
EH	112	106*

Note: Control, value before treatment; 3, 4 week, average of values after 3 and 4
weeks of treatment (R_x) within subjects. *$p < .05$, for difference within subjects.

Source: Whitworth et al. (1989).

in whom there is moderate elevation of aldosterone (Helber et al., 1980; Henry and
Grim, 1990). In other patients thought to have EH, plasma 18-OH-DOC was raised
and accounted for much of the BP rise (Melby et al., 1972; Brownie, 1995).
However, in most patients with EH, plasma aldosterone is normal for a given salt
intake (Espiner and Nicholls, 1993; Padfield and Edwards, 1993; Swales, 1993).

Some patients with raised mineralocorticoids have been misdiagnosed as having
EH, and some patients with hard-to-treat EH benefit from the administration of
spironolactone. However, a recent careful assessment of the prevalence of primary
aldosteronism in persons thought to have mild to moderate EH is 3.2%, which is far
smaller than suggested by Conn (Williams et al., 2006). One distinction is that in
mineralocorticoid hypertension, blood and plasma volumes are high (chapter 15),
while in EH these volumes are low.

EH has also been regarded as a variant form of Cushing's syndrome in which a
pituitary adenoma is the source of raised ACTH and cortisol secretion (Whitworth,
1994; Whitworth et al., 2000). However, patients with Cushing's syndrome usually
present with severe hypertension, abdominal striae, hirsutism, acne, ecchymoses,[8]
and skeletal muscle wasting, while sympathoadrenal activity is usually normal.

EH Is a Largely Constrictor Type of High BP

Lean individuals with mild EH have a resting hemodynamic pattern resembling the
defense response. There is vasoconstriction in renal, gastrointestinal, and skin beds
and vasodilation in skeletal muscle, which offsets the vasoconstrictor responses in
the other beds (figure 5.19). This explains why TPC and TPR are normal in mild EH
and why the elevation of CO accounts for the high BP.

The high CO is due to the increased cardiac SNA and raised cardiac stroke volume. The latter is a consequence of the raised central blood volume that results from
the shift of blood from gastrointestinal and skin veins to the central cardiopulmonary
compartment. The shift is a consequence of SNA-mediated precapillary arteriolar
constriction and postcapillary venomotor changes.

The regional hemodynamic pattern in mild EH is largely due to the sympathoadrenal changes. In humans, the rise in regional Vas R is greater in the renal than in the
gastrointestinal bed, which is probably due to the latter's greater susceptibility to the

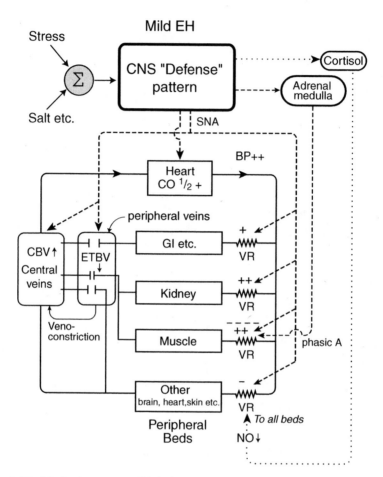

Figure 5.19. Mechanisms responsible in lean persons for hemodynamic pattern of mild EH. Sympathetic neural activity (SNA) is raised in kidney, gastrointestinal, and skeletal muscle beds. Adrenaline (A) masks the neural constriction in skeletal muscle. Net changes in vascular resistance (VR) on each bed denoted by sum of pluses and minuses. Renal and gastrointestinal vasoconstriction is offset by muscle vasodilation, so that TPC is unchanged, but CO is raised. Precapillary constriction and venomotor changes shift blood from distensible GI and skin veins to central compartment. Plasma cortisol also rises, inhibiting nitric oxide synthase (NOS) and reducing availability of NO. It is assumed that structural changes are small in mild EH. CBV, central blood volume; ETBV, extrathoracic blood volume.

tissue hypoxia (Korner et al., 1967; chapter 9, this volume). This is suggested from results in animals, in which the defense response elicited rises of similar magnitude in renal and splanchnic SNA (Iriki et al., 1977b; Iriki and Korner, 1979).

Reduction of vagal activity is a "whole organism" baroreflex response to elevation in cardiopulmonary load (chapter 9). The same mechanism may attenuate renal renin production in the majority of persons with mild and moderate EH.

In EH resting SNA is raised in all major sympathetic outflows involved in the regulation of BP. The hypothesis is that after prolonged exposure to chronic stress the defense pathways have become sensitized, so that SNA is raised by very low stimuli. Normally, plasma adrenaline secretion is not raised in EH, suggesting that its response threshold is greater than that for SNA. However, it increases phasically in response to mild stresses that have no effects in normal subjects (see chapters 9 and 11).

The raised plasma cortisol accounts for a small part of the BP rise in mild EH, which is probably due to its inhibitory action on the enzyme nitric oxide synthase (NOS). This explains the reduced availability of NO at an early stage of EH, as a result of which there is some increase in constrictor tone (chapter 6). This is the harbinger of regulatory problems in the peripheral circulation in chronic EH.

As the severity of EH increases, TPR and regional Vas Rs continue to rise while SNA and the concentrations of the major pressor hormones remain unchanged. By exclusion, the enhanced vasoconstriction must be due to nonneural factors. They include the amplifier action of the R_1 vessel structural changes, an increase in stiffness of the conduit arteries (figure 5.6) and several functional changes, as discussed in chapter 6.

In moderate and severe EH, the elevation of central blood volume is accompanied by a reduction in total blood volume of up to 20%. The reduction in venous capacity in gastrointestinal and skin beds shifts blood to the central compartment, while other homeostatic mechanisms increase sodium and water excretion by amounts equivalent to the reduction in venous capacity. As EH increases in severity, the vasoconstriction reduces the microcirculatory exchange area, producing rarefaction. It is functional at first, but in time permanent closure of some of the small arterioles and capillaries develops. Rarefaction affects all vascular beds and accounts for the deterioration in organ function in EH.

In conclusion, neural autonomic mechanisms initiate EH, while its progression depends largely on additional nonneural factors. Their role is considered in the next two chapters.

PART IV

INTRINSIC CARDIOVASCULAR PROPERTIES IN HYPERTENSION

6

The Peripheral Vascular Integrator

A brief account of the main cell types in the vascular wall and their sympathetic innervation is followed by discussion of myogenic and metabolic regulation and how they are affected by EH. In the intact organism, the vascular tone of a given bed depends on interactions between local and neurohumoral factors. The vascular endothelium is the source of additional modulators of vascular tone, including nitric oxide (NO) and other autacoids. These too are affected by EH and, in conjunction with the structural changes in resistance vessels and conduit arteries, make a substantial contribution to the progressive rise in BP and the long-term deterioration of vital organ function.

Some Features of the Normal Vasculature

The aorta and conduit arteries have strong walls that contain much elastin and collagen as well as vascular smooth muscle (VSM) cells (Burton, 1962; Folkow and Neil, 1971; Milnor, 1982; O'Rourke, 1982a; Rhodin, 1980). The collagen and elastin largely determine wall distensibility and other mechanical properties. The innermost layer of the wall is the intima, which is covered by a continuous layer of endothelial cells separating the wall from the bloodstream. Next come the internal elastic lamina and the media with its VSM cells. The adventitia is the outermost layer and is traversed by the sympathetic nerves to the VSM cells. The small arteries and arterioles are the resistance arteries: Their wall to lumen ratio is greater than in the conduit arteries due to a greater proportion of VSM cells in their media. The capillaries consist of a single layer of endothelial cells, with varying permeability characteristics in different beds. The veins are highly distensible vessels with a large lumen and thin media and accommodate about 70% of the blood volume.

Much of the bed's capacity to integrate the responses to neurohumoral and local stimuli depends on the organization of the resistance vessel network (figure 2.6). This consists of the R_1 vessels, comprising small arteries and large arterioles (A_1, A_2 branches), which are mainly responsive to neural and hormonal stimuli, and the smaller R_2 arterioles, including the A_3, A_4, and higher order arterioles, which are more responsive to local metabolites and changes in transmural BP than the R_1 vessels.

VSM Cells and Contractile Machinery

These cells are narrow and long and contain myosin and actin filaments. One end of the actin filaments is attached to the *dense bodies*, which are homologues of the Z-bands of striated muscle (figure 6.1) (Mulvany, 1984). Adjacent dense bodies are joined by intermediate filaments, and the cells have an extensive sarcoplasmic reticulum (SR) for storing calcium. The actin and myosin filaments are arranged in parallel between dense bodies. They communicate with adjoining cells through gap junctions, which coordinate vascular contraction through the precapillary vasculature.

VSM cells of R_1 and R_2 vessels differ in their responsiveness to neurohumoral and local stimuli (Sun et al., 1992). They subserve a number of functions in addition to contraction, including participation in repair processes, growth, and proliferation. The large number of ionic channels in their cell membranes may help activate discrete functional pathways related to the above tasks (Beech, 2005).

Entry of calcium ions (Ca^{2+}), sodium (Na^+) and magnesium (Mg^{2+}) ions, and efflux of potassium ions (K^+) is important for the VSM cell's normal contractile function (Darnell et al., 1990; Hille, 1992; Bobik et al., 1994; Khalil and Breemen, 1995). The initiation of excitation-contraction coupling in VSM cells is usually associated with the opening of L-type voltage gated Ca^{2+} channels. T-type Ca^{2+} channels contribute to pacemaker functions, maturation processes, and proliferation. Stretch-sensitive Ca^{2+} channels play a role in the myogenic response.

VSM potassium channels include: (1) Ca^{2+} and voltage-sensitive K^+ channels (Kc_a); (2) delayed rectifier K^+ channels (K_{DR}); and (3) ATP-sensitive K^+ channels (K_{ATP}). The K_{Ca} channel helps set the level of the membrane potential and may also limit the contractile responses to vasoconstrictor stimuli (Brayden and Nelson, 1992). Opening K_{ATP} channels (e.g., through metabolic factors) hyperpolarizes the cell membrane and promotes the closure of Ca^{2+} channels and VSM relaxation.

VSM Contraction

Force is generated through crossbridge formation when myosin attaches to actin and ATP is hydrolyzed (Somlyo and Somlyo, 1986; Elliott and Elliott, 1997). VSM has fewer myosin filaments per actin filament than striated muscle but is able to develop similar tension at a lower energy cost (Stull et al., 1991; Murphy, 1994).

The contractile apparatus is activated through the electromechanical and pharmacomechanical pathways (figure 6.2; Somlyo and Somlyo, 1994). Cytosolic Ca^{2+} increases through inflow of calcium from both extracellular sources and the SR stores.

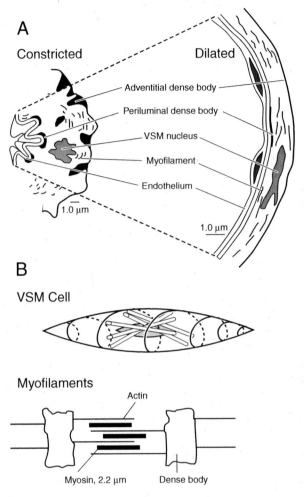

Figure 6.1. (A) Sketch of resistance vessel during dilatation and constriction. (B) Contractile units are stacked into narrow VSM cell so that striations are hard to see, despite parallel arrangement of filaments shown in lower graph. Note attachment of actin to dense bodies. (A) After Sleek and Duling (1986); (B) after Mulvany (1984).

The activation of the electromechanical pathway requires membrane depolarization, which opens voltage-gated Ca^{2+} channels (Shaw and McGrath, 1996). The pharmacomechanical pathway is activated by agonists that increase $[Ca^{2+}]_i$ by stimulating membrane receptors (Somlyo and Somlyo, 1994; Aaronson and Smirnov, 1996; Shaw and McGrath, 1996). A Ca^+-calmodulin complex (Cam) binds to myosin light chain kinase. The 20 kDa myosin light chain (MLC_{20}), when phosphorylated at serine-19, is part of the cross bridge between myosin and actin. Some agonists sensitize the contractile machinery, so that force and cross-bridge phosphorylation can increase without a rise in $[Ca^{2+}]_i$. One mechanism is through inhibition of smooth muscle light

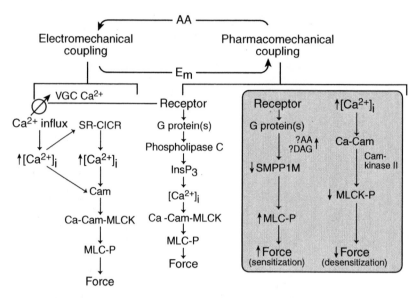

Figure 6.2. Electromechanical and pharmacomechanical pathways for contraction in VSM. Left, in the electromechanical pathway $[Ca^{2+}]_i$ there is (1) calcium influx through voltage-gated calcium channels (VGC); and (2) calcium-induced calcium release from sarcoplasmic reticulum (SR-CICR). Calcium-calmodulin complex (Cam) binds to myosin light chain kinase (MLCK). After phosphorylation of MLC (MLC-P), force is generated through myosin-actin interaction. Middle, agonist activates pharmacomechanical pathways by stimulating receptors coupled to G-proteins; second messengers (e.g., phospholipase C); inositol 1,4,5-triphosphate ($InsP_3$) cause a rise in $[Ca^{2+}]_i$. Shaded, force alters without change in $[Ca^{2+}]_i$ because of phosphorylation or dephosphorylation of MLC and MLCK by light chain phosphatase, SMPP1M. AA, arachidonic acid; DAG, diacylglycerol; E_m, membrane potential. From Somlyo and Somlyo (1994), with permission of *Nature* and Macmillan Publishers, Ltd.

chain phosphatase (SMPP1M), which raises the proportion of MLC that is phosphorylated (MLC-P; figure 6.2, shaded right; Stull et al., 1991; Somlyo and Somlyo, 1994).

Endothelial Cells

NO is produced by the endothelial cell, and its functions include modulation of VSM tone and minimizing platelet aggregation and capillary permeability (Angus and Cocks, 1989; Moncada et al., 1991; Dusting, 1995). Its effect on VSM tone was discovered by Furchgott and Zawadski (1980), who found that after removal of endothelium the dilator action of acetylcholine (ACh) was transformed into a constrictor response. The ACh stimulates muscarinic receptors on endothelium, which increases production of an endothelium-dependent relaxing factor (EDRF). EDRF is now known to be the NO molecule (Moncada et al., 1991). NO diffuses to VSM cells, increasing the concentration of cyclic guanylyl monophosphate (cGMP), which lowers $[Ca^{2+}]_i$ and causes VSM to relax (Ignarro and Kadowitz, 1985).

The synthesis of NO radicals by endothelial cells derives from L-arginine $\rightarrow$ L-citrulline + NO•, through the action of the enzyme NO synthase (NOS). Endothelial NOS (eNOS) accounts for basal NO production. NO has a half-life of about 40 seconds (Angus and Cocks, 1987), so that it has to be continuously synthetized to maintain the relatively low basal tone of many vascular beds (Kelm et al., 1995; Tschudi et al., 1996). NO is inactivated by superoxide ions (O_2^-), which are mopped up by superoxide dismutase. Another form of NOS is inducible NOS, which forms in macrophages and endothelial cells due to stimulation by cytokines. A third form is neural NOS, which is produced in some neurons and in skeletal muscle.

Endothelial NO increases in response to two types of stimuli. First, in response to stimulation of specific endothelial membrane receptors by a number of agonists, including ACh, noradrenaline (NA), angiotensin II (Ang II), bradykinin, and so on (Pearson and Vanhoutte, 1993; Cocks, 1997). Second, its production increases in response to elevation of blood flow velocity (shear stress), which stimulates integrins and other receptors on the endothelial surface (Davies and Barbee, 1994; Davies, 1995).

The increased cortisol secretion in EH partially reduces NO biosynthesis by inhibiting NOS. This can also be done experimentally by the administration of various analogues of L-arginine, such as L-NAME (N^G-nitro-L-arginine methyl ester; Moncada et al., 1991).[1] NOS inhibitors attenuate or abolish NO-mediated vasodilation, but have no effect on the dilation produced by exogenous nitrates, such as sodium nitroprusside and glyceryl trinitrate, which also increase cGMP in VSM cells (Ignarro and Kadowitz, 1985). Other endothelial autacoids with a vasodilator action are prostacyclin (PGI_2) and several endothelium-derived hyperpolarizing factors (EDHFs; Pearson and Vanhoutte, 1993; Edwards et al., 1998; Faraci and Heistad, 1998).

Hemoglobin in red blood cells is another physiological source of NO affecting VSM tone (Jia et al., 1996; Perutz, 1996; Stamler et al., 1997). In the lungs, HbO_2 is S-nitrosylated with locally produced NO• and S and reacts with glutathione to form S-nitroso (SNO)-glutathione in red cells, which binds tightly to HbO_2. In the tissues, the rate of dissociation of S-nitroso compounds from HbO_2 is enhanced at low tissue pO_2, since NO binds less strongly to reduced hemoglobin.

Endothelial NO inhibits platelet aggregation and prevents adhesion of leucocytes to the walls of capillaries and venules (Kurose et al., 1993). After administration of L-NAME and inhibition of NOS, more leucocytes migrate from the capillaries to tissues because of weakening of the adhesion proteins between adjoining cells, which also increases leakage of plasma proteins into the tissues.

Endothelium also produces vasoconstrictor autacoids, including endothelin-1 (ET-1) and thromboxanes (Yanagisawa et al., 1988; Pearson and Vanhoutte, 1993; Lüscher, 1994; Vanhoutte, 1996; Faraci and Heistad, 1998). ET-1 is a potent vasoconstrictor and a growth promoter (Dzau and Gibbons, 1987; Bobik and Campbell, 1993). It stimulates ET_A and ET_B receptors on VSM cells. In addition, ET_B receptors on adjoining endothelial cells are stimulated to increase NO production.

Sympathetic Innervation

The sympathetic constrictor nerves supply all blood vessels except the capillaries. They release transmitter from the terminal varicosities near the outer part of the media.

In the conduit arteries the gap between the varicosities and VSM cells is relatively wide (Burnstock and Costa, 1975; Burnstock, 1986). However, in the resistance vessels there are close synaptic junctions between varicosities and VSM cells, similar to synapses in CNS (Luff et al., 1987; Luff and McLachlan, 1988, 1989; Sjöblom-Widfeldt, 1990). Typically, two or more cotransmitters are released from a terminal with transmitters often differing between regions (Morris, 1995; Ralevic and Burnstock, 1995; Kelly and Garland, 1996).

Stimulation of sympathetic constrictor nerves to the resistance vessels increases force of contraction and evokes excitatory junction potentials (EJPs; Burnstock and Holman, 1963; Hirst and Edwards, 1989; Hirst and Neild, 1980). The current view is that about 90% of the force of contraction is due to stimulation of α_1-adrenoceptors (ARs) by neurally released NA, while the remaining force is due to stimulation of P_{2x} purinergic receptors by coreleased ATP, which also elicits EJPs (Angus et al., 1988; Sjöblom-Widfeldt, 1990). Neuropeptide Y (NPY) acts on Y_1 receptors but is a weak constrictor in vivo; it potentiates the action of "strong" agonists such as NA, phenylephrine, Ang II, and AVP (Potter, 1988; Prieto et al, 1997).

Myogenic Regulation and Related Factors

The myogenic response is evoked in the resistance vessels by changes in local transmural BPs, that is, by the degree of stretch.

The Myogenic Response

Bayliss (1902) first described the myogenic response and regarded it as an intrinsic response to stretch that helped to maintain blood flow constant during fluctuations in BP. In a perfused sympathectomized limb, a step increase in perfusion pressure raises blood flow transiently, but restoration of the flow occurs within 30–60 seconds owing to stretch-induced increase in vascular resistance (Vas R; figure 6.3). This autoregulatory response can be evoked over a range of BPs on either side of resting. Below the autoregulatory range, vessel caliber decreases passively, while at high BPs beyond the range the vasculature is often damaged, resulting in increased permeability of the blood-brain barrier.

For many years there was controversy about whether the myogenic response was solely due to stretch or whether flow-induced changes in tissue metabolite concentrations also played a role (Anrep, 1912). We now know that in appropriate preparations both can alter vascular tone independently of one another (see Folkow, 1949, 1964).

However, in the intact organism it may be difficult to separate the effects of stretch from other factors. Stretch is determined by the level of BP, which in turn depends on changes in SNA, pressor hormones, or locally produced molecules. Thus stretch, like BP, is multifactorial. As to the intrinsic nature of the myogenic response, tone evoked by distension often develops in isolated vessels, but sometimes it requires an agonist such as NA.

Raising transmural BP in an isolated vessel in the absence of tone causes vessel diameter to increase passively (Kuo et al., 1988). However, when resting tone is present,

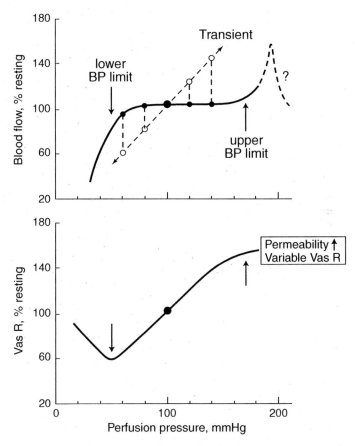

Figure 6.3. Top, relationship between perfusion pressure (mmHg) and blood flow (% resting) after step changes in BP. Each step elicits a transient blood flow change (dashed line, open circles), but resting level is restored at the raised pressure through myogenic increase in tone, as shown in bottom graph (thick line, small black circles). Bottom, perfusion pressure–vascular resistance (Vas R) relationship is monotonic over autoregulatory range between arrows. Resting values (large black circle).

raising transmural BP increases active tension and produces an increase in active tension and narrowing of the vessel lumen.

In an isolated perfused organ, raising BP largely increases tone in R_2 arterioles, while that of R_1 vessels remains unchanged (Bjoernberg et al., 1988; De Wit et al., 1998). This is because blood flow velocity also increases, raising NO production and inhibiting the myogenic response (Ekelund et al., 1992).

The myogenic response is normally absent in the renal papillary bed, in which blood flow increases linearly with perfusion BP (figure 6.4; Thurau, 1964; Fenoy et al., 1995; Cowley and Roman, 1997). Here too the increased NO production suppresses the myogenic response, which becomes manifest in the presence of NOS inhibitors (Fenoy et al., 1995).

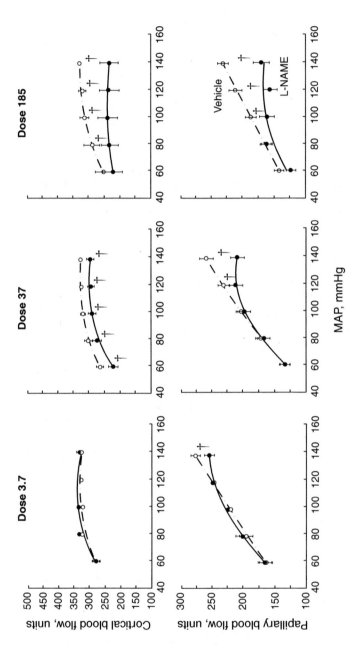

Figure 6.4. Relationship between mean arterial pressure (MAP, mmHg) and renal cortical blood flow (top) and renal papillary blood flow (bottom). Open circles, dashed line, vehicle treated controls for each group; closed circles, solid line, animals infused with L-NAME at, respectively, 3.7, 37, and 185 nmol/kg/min (top of graph). Myogenic response occurs in these R_1 vessels after inhibition of NO synthesis. † for Δ. $p < .05$. From Fenoy et al. (1995), with permission of *Hypertension*, American Heart Association, and Lippincott, Williams and Wilkins.

Mechanism of the Myogenic Response

Spontaneous arteriolar vasomotion occurs in a proportion of arterioles in which there are pacemaker cells that increase their rhythm in response to stretch (Folkow, 1964; Osol and Halpern, 1988; Johansson, 1989). However, the response can also be evoked without spontaneous vasomotion, since stretch induces an increase in cytosolic Ca^{2+} (Johansson and Somlyo, 1980; Bevan and Laher, 1991; Brayden and Nelson, 1992; Khalil and Breemen, 1995; Aaronson and Smirnov, 1996; Wesselman et al., 1997). Once the lumen starts to narrow during contraction, the tension required to maintain the raised BP diminishes progressively in accordance with Laplace's law ($T = BP \times r_i$; Johnson, 1964b, 1980). Coordination of VSM contraction in the branching microcirculatory network depends on the function of the gap junctions (Tsai et al., 1995). Calcium antagonists abolish the myogenic response (Ono et al., 1974; Ogawa and Ono, 1987; Nordlander, 1989).

The evoked vascular response to agonists depends on whether the conditions of studying the isolated vessel are isobaric (constant pressure) or isometric (constant circumference; VanBavel and Mulvany, 1994). Under isobaric conditions, increasing concentrations of agonist produce gradual narrowing of the vessel lumen, which is what happens in vivo. In contrast, under isometric conditions a small increase in agonist concentration above threshold evokes an abrupt increase in tension to near maximum, which suggests a strong interaction between electromechanical and pharmacomechanical pathways (Davis and Hill, 1999).

Myogenic Responses in Chronic Hypertension

In figure 6.5 the autoregulatory range of the spontaneously hypertensive rat (SHR) is reset about its raised resting BP, to the right of that of WKY (Harper and Bohlen, 1984). However, the two curves become virtually superimposable when each strain's BP is expressed as a percentage of its own resting value. Similar resetting of the autoregulatory range occurs in humans (Strandgaard, 1976; Johansson, 1984; Johansson, 1992; Strandgaard and Poulson, 1994; Strandgaard and Paulson, 1995). Clearly, the myogenic response remains robust in EH.

Do Myogenic Mechanisms Enhance the Action of Agonists in Hypertension?

It has been suggested that in hypertension the initial rise in BP increases the myogenic component of Vas R, potentiating the constrictor action of the agonist (Meininger et al., 1984, 1985; Meininger and Trzeciakowski, 1988). It suggests an interaction between electromechanical and pharmacomechanical pathways similar to that in the isometric preparation (Cowley, 1992; VanBavel and Mulvany, 1994; De Wit et al., 1998).

The hypothesis has received support from experiments in isolated R_1 vessels studied isobarically (Nilsson, Ljung et al., 1985; Speden and Warren, 1986; Lombard et al., 1990; Meininger and Faber, 1991; VanBavel and Mulvany, 1994). For example, renal R_1 arterioles were about 100 times more sensitive to NA when perfused at a pressure of 140 mmHg than at 60 mmHg (figure 6.6). However, raising BP in an isolated

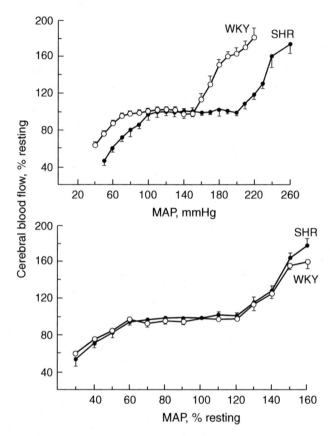

Figure 6.5. Autoregulatory curves in cerebral vasculature of SHR and WKY. Top, relationship between MAP (mmHg) and cerebral blood flow (% of resting). Bottom, same data, but MAP expressed as a percentage of each group's resting value. From Harper and Bohlen (1984), with permission of *Hypertension*, American Heart Association, and Lippincott, Williams and Wilkins.

vessel increases its length and width considerably (figure 6.7; Lew and Angus, 1992). The resulting depolarization of the cell membrane increases its sensitivity, which suggests that the data in figure 6.6 are preparation artifacts. Under in vivo conditions the dimension changes are much smaller because of the tethering of the vessels to the surrounding tissues.

The above hypothesis was also examined in vivo during acute induction of 2K-1C hypertension, when elevation of Ang II raises BP, TPR, and regional Vas R (Meininger et al., 1984, 1985, 1986; Meininger and Trzeciakowski, 1988). The aim was to partition the rise in Vas R in hindquarter and gastrointestinal beds into myogenic and Ang II-mediated components. This was done by comparing the normal Vas R changes in each bed with those occurring when holding perfusion pressure at the BP preceding induction of hypertension; this was achieved by inflating a perivascular cuff around the artery supplying the particular bed.

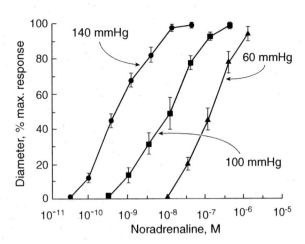

Figure 6.6. Relationship between noradrenaline concentration (M) and diameter (% of maximum constriction) in isolated renal small artery studied under isobaric conditions at pressures 60, 100, and 140 mmHg. From Lombard et al. (1990), with permission of *American Journal of Physiology* and American Physiological Society.

During cuff-induced "protection" from the high BP, the rise in Vas R was less than one quarter of the normal unprotected response (figure 6.8). It was concluded that most of the rise in Vas R was myogenically mediated and not due to the direct action of the agonist. However during hypertension, intestinal blood flow in the protected bed was below that in the unprotected bed.

The major flaw in the hypothesis is the idea of partitioning ΔVas R into myogenic and agonist components. In early 2K-1C hypertension, the rises in Vas R (or TPR) and BP are totally linked to the action of the agonist. If the action of the agonist is

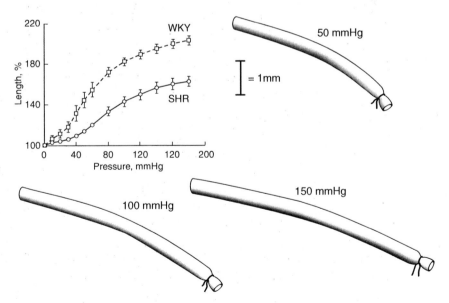

Figure 6.7. Cannulated small mesenteric arteries of WKY at pressures of 50, 100, and 150 mmHg. Note increases in diameter and length with rises in perfusion pressure. (Insert) Length-pressure curves in adult WKY and SHR indicate lower distensibility in SHR. Adapted from Lew and Angus (1992).

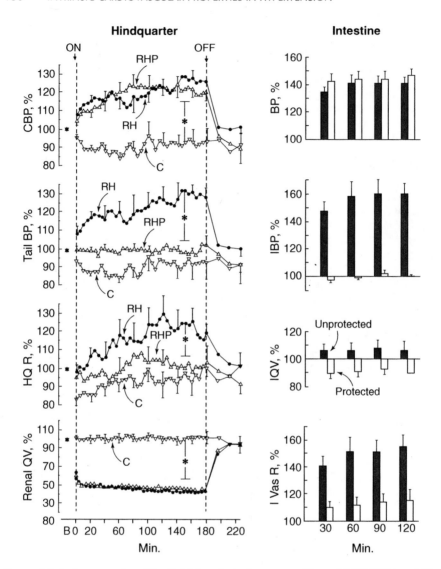

Figure 6.8. Left, mean values (% of initial resting) of mean carotid arterial BP (CBP), tail BP, hindquarter vascular resistance (HQ R), and renal blood flow velocity (Renal QV, Doppler) during acutely induced 2K-1C renal hypertension (RH) or control (C). In some rats, tail BP maintained at preclip resting level (Protected, RHP) using a cuff around lower aorta. Right, intestinal bed during hypertension, including systemic BP, intestinal BP (IBP), intestinal blood flow velocity (IQV), and vascular resistance (IVasR) in unprotected bed (black rectangles) and protected bed (open rectangle). Adapted from Meininger et al. (1984, 1985).

prevented or abolished by ACE inhibitors or AT_1 antagonists soon after clipping, there is no rise in either BP or Vas R (Barger, 1979; Laragh and Sealey, 1995). Cuff inflation provides a method for manipulating myogenic tension that is independent of the action of the agonist and can mask it completely. The small residual increase in Vas R in the protected bed is probably due to inability to match blood flows at the two perfusion pressures. It does not appear to have much to do with the action of the agonist.

Chapter 4 discussed the results of a study that illustrates how myogenic tone alters simply in response to BP changes. Figure 4.17 gives results from patients with EH studied before and soon after 1 year's treatment with β-blockers and diuretics; on each occasion the effects of acute autonomic blockade were also examined (Jennings et al., 1980). The changes in TPR were approximately the same as the changes in BP, both within each study and between studies (table 6.1). Before treatment (S1) autonomic blockade reduced BP by 35%, with a similar change in TPR; after 1 year the BP was about 30% below the initial baseline value, as was TPR. During the first and second studies, the relative magnitude of autonomic:nonautonomic components of TPR were thus approximately the same. It suggests that the treatment had lowered BP and relaxed the vasculature as a consequence of the reduction in BP. The relaxation accounted for the high CO in the second study both with intact effectors and after total autonomic blockade (TAB). In both studies, the ratio of the autonomic:nonautonomic components of TPR was similar, about 30:70, which suggests that treatment affected BP and TPR nonspecifically. This is further supported by the rapid redevelopment of hypertension within weeks after stopping treatment, as links with the original neural mechanisms in EH again become manifest (Korner, 1982).

Because changes in BP alter myogenic tone so readily, the difference between TPR with effectors intact and during TAB, that is, $TAB_{(intact-TAB)}$, may not be closely related to the actual magnitude of the autonomic effector activity. This is suggested from results obtained on the effects of TAB on hindquarter (HQ) Vas R in rabbits with cellophane wrap hypertension and sham-operated animals (figure 6.9; West et al., 1975; Angus et al., 1976). The fall in BP elicited by TAB in wrapped rabbits was 2.5 times that of sham-operated animals, although ΔMAP was the same in both. In wrap hypertension, the high BP is due to elevation of Ang II, amplification of constrictor factors by the structural changes, and possibly a small increase in SNA (chapter 15). Clearly, the magnitude of the autonomic component of HQ Vas R is not 2.5 times

Table 6.1. Partitioning of MAP and TPR in Figure 4.17 into Autonomic and Nonautonomic Components

	Intact ANS	TAB	Autonomic C (%)	Nonautonomic C (%)
MAP				
S1	128 mmHg	84 mmHg	34	66
S2	92 mmHg	69 mmHg	25	75
TPR				
S1	40 units	28 units	30	70
S2	27 units	18 units	33	67

Note: The 13 subjects were studied before and after one year's antihypertensive treatment with β-blockers and diuretics. S1, study 1 before treatment; S2, study 2 after 12 months' treatment with β-blockers and diuretics and 5–7 days after withdrawal of all drugs.

Source: Jennings et al. (1980).

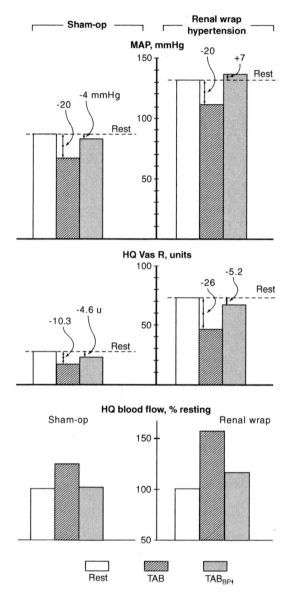

Figure 6.9. Hindquarter hemodynamics of sham-operated and renal cellophane wrap rabbits under resting conditions and during total autonomic block. From above: mean arterial pressure (MAP, mmHg), hindquarter vascular resistance (HQ Vas R, units), HQ blood flow (% of resting). Left, resting (open rectangle); middle, total autonomic block (TAB, hatching); TAB after restoring MAP to initial resting (TAB$_{BP\uparrow}$, gray). Fall in Vas R and rise in blood flow in middle graph greater in wrapped than sham-operated rabbits ($p < .01$). Based on data in West et al. (1975) and Angus et al. (1976).

normal, but reflects the size of the structural amplifier. Accordingly, when the BP was restored to resting by infusing dextran. HQ Vas R$_{(resting-TAB)}$ was the same in both groups and blood flows too were close to normal.

Thus, when the rise in BP in hypertension is closely related to the action of an agonist, it is unrealistic to partition vessel tone into agonist-related and myogenic components. The response is best regarded as due to the agonist. The hemodynamic effects on vessel tone are closely related to the effects of the agonist on BP in vivo.

Disruption of the Blood-Brain Barrier

A large and abrupt rise in BP often disrupts the blood-brain barrier transiently. Byrom (1954) thought that this was due to myogenically induced arteriolar vasospasm, causing local ischemia followed by cerebral edema. Another theory is that if the rise in BP exceeds the muscle's "yield point," the sudden dilation of the vessels after a period of constriction disrupts the capillaries and venules (Haggendal and Johansson, 1971; Johansson, 1984, 1992; Strandgaard and Poulson, 1994). Support for this view has come from a study of the effects of stimulation of the sympathetic nerves on the cerebral blood vessels, which restores VSM tone and reduces the degree of edema (Bill and Linder, 1976).

A third mechanism is based on the finding that leaks around the small venules are the first sign of blood-brain barrier disruption in stroke-prone SHR (SHR.SP; Kurose et al., 1993). This is due to impaired endothelial cell function, with low NO and high concentrations of superoxide ions reducing adhesion between adjoining endothelial cells. It accounts for leakage of plasma proteins and greater platelet aggregation. In humans with severe EH, indications of small areas of focal brain edema are common.

The important point is that at high BPs autoregulation fails. Enhanced blood-brain barrier permeability to the sodium ion may then accentuate the hypertension (chapter 12).

Role of Myogenic Tone in Local Vascular Regulation

Myogenic tone is active VSM contraction, generated in response to stretch and associated membrane depolarization. In isolated arterioles, baseline stretch has to be sufficient to allow the contractile machinery to respond to further BP changes. Such conditions are created by pulse pressure changes with every heartbeat, which is important for the VSM pacemaker cells. Any change in BP alters active VSM tone, which makes it the ideal short-term regulator of regional blood flow.

Long-term alterations in BP are largely mediated through changes in sympathoadrenal activity, hormones, metabolic changes, and local molecules in the vascular wall. All of them alter Vas R and affect systemic BP. Changes in myogenic tone are a consequence of changes in BP rather than an initiator of its elevation. Most long-term BP changes are mediated through specific agonists or chronic remodeling of the vasculature, which makes it virtually impossible to define a separate myogenic component of Vas R that is independent of the above mechanisms.

It is doubtful whether the large interaction between stretch and agonists observed in figure 6.6 ever occurs in vivo. It certainly plays no independent role in the rises in Vas R in renovascular hypertension. In the treatment of hypertension, long-term lowering of BP reduces vascular tone through the myogenic mechanism, even when the treatment does not specifically address the causes of EH.

Metabolic Regulation

The peripheral vasodilation of the resistance vessels that occurs during metabolic activity is due to tissue hypoxia and various products of tissue metabolism (Roy and

Brown, 1879; Gaskell, 1880; Berne, 1964; Johnson, 1964b; Korner, 1974; Sparks, 1980; Folkow et al., 1989; Pearson and Vanhoutte, 1993; Rowell, 1993). When exercise is severe, the dilation of the conduit arteries is also of great importance. NO and other dilator autacoids are important in the above responses and in their absence in hypertension, metabolic regulation becomes impaired.

Metabolic Regulation Is Multifactorial

Here the main focus is on metabolic regulation in skeletal and cardiac muscle. These serve as models for regulation in other organs, in which additional factors usually come into play, related to the organ's specialized function.

At the start of aerobic exercise, muscle and blood flow and conductance increase as tissue pO_2 declines (Saltin, 1985). The precapillary sphincters and R_2 arterioles are the first vessels to dilate, followed by the R_1 vessels (Duling and Berne, 1970; Mellander and Bjoernberg, 1992). At high rates of work, the dilation extends to the conduit arteries, hence the term *ascending vasodilation* (Schretzenmayr, 1933; Hilton, 1959; Lie et al., 1970; Rodbard, 1975).

The dilation is mediated by hypoxia, adenosine, ATP, H^+, K^+, tissue osmolality, and local elevation in temperature (Korner, 1974; Sparks, 1980; Loutzenhiser and Parker, 1994; Mubagwa et al., 1996; Ishibashi et al., 1998). NO, PGI_2, and other dilator prostaglandins may enhance the rise in blood flow. At low tissue pO_2 there is dissociation of SNO bound to HbO_2, and this diffuses into VSM cells where it increases activity of cGMP.

Ishibashi et al. (1998) elucidated the role of local hypoxia, adenosine, and endothelial NO in the coronary vasodilation of exercising dogs by means of selective inhibitors and antagonists. The opening of K^+_{ATP} channels by tissue hypoxia causes relaxation of VSM, while stimulation by adenosine of A_2 adenosine receptors produces the same effect. Increased production of endothelial NO occurs largely in response to the rise in blood flow and increases cGMP in VSM cells.

Blocking only the K_{ATP} channels or the A_2 receptors has no effect on the circulatory response, because of compensation through the unblocked pathways, but blocking both the above mechanisms attenuates the rise in coronary conductance by about half (figure 6.10). When NO production is also suppressed, the dilator response is attenuated further and the heart's mechanical performance deteriorates. The small residual vasodilation may be due to an increase in H^+.

Additional factors that play a role in metabolic vasodilation include ATP from muscle or the regional sympathetic nerves (Burnstock and Holman, 1963; Ralevic and Burnstock, 1995). In skeletal muscle, the ACh released from motor nerves may raise production of EDHFs, which open ouabain-sensitive K^+ channels in VSM cells (Edwards et al., 1998).

Other Dilator Factors: Prostaglandins and Peptides

In the renal bed, additional modulators of VSM tone are prostaglandins E_2, $F_{2\alpha}$, and D_2, formed in the renal papilla. Arachidonic acid is also metabolized by cytochrome P-450 enzymes to epoxyeicosatrienoic acids and 20-hydroxyeicosatetraenoic acid,

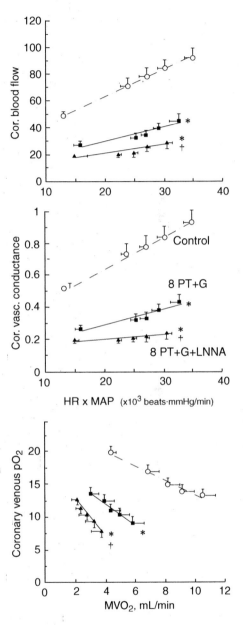

Figure 6.10. Relationship in conscious dogs between heart rate (HR) × MAP product (beats × mmHg/min × 10^3; an index of LV work) and coronary blood flow (mL/min/kg, top) and vascular conductance (middle). Lowest panel, relationship between myocardial oxygen consumption (MVO_2) and coronary venous pO_2 (mmHg). Control (no treatment), open circles; adenosine receptor blockade with 8-phenyl theophylline (PT) plus K_{ATP} channel blockade with glibenclamide (G), closed squares; blockade with PT + G + N^w-nitro-L-arginine (LNNA), a NOS inhibitor, closed triangles. *$p < .05$ for difference from intact animals; †$p < .05$ from partial block preparation. From Ishibashi et al. (1998), with permission of *Circulation Research*, American Heart Association, and Lippincott, Williams and Wilkins.

which, respectively, constrict and dilate the vasculature (Campbell et al., 1996; Cowley and Roman, 1997; Roman and Alonso-Galicia, 1999).

Reactive Hyperemia

After a period of occlusion of the arterial blood supply to a vascular bed, its removal gives rise to an increase in blood flow to a maximum, followed by an exponential return to the preocclusion level. The peak response and the area under the curve are proportional to the duration of occlusion. It suggests that during occlusion normal resting metabolism continues and that the postocclusion changes are due to accumulation of metabolites and other dilator factors. In EH, the peak forearm reactive hyperemia response is attenuated by 20–50%, largely due to diminished availability of NO (Kelm et al., 1996).

Reactive hyperemia in skin is mediated through dilator substances from sensory nerves, including substance P and calcitonin gene-related peptide (Gibbins et al., 1985; McEwan et al., 1988). Brachial plexus avulsion attenuates the response (Duff and Shepherd, 1953). Often cyclooxygenase products (PGE_2, PGI_2) release the peptides from the nerve endings (Larkin and Williams, 1993). Hence, intradermal injection of either a local anesthetic or indomethacin eliminate the reactive hyperemia.

Ascending Vasodilation and "Steal" Syndromes

The mechanisms involved in ascending vasodilation include (1) centripetal cell-to-cell dilation, which starts at the distal arterioles and depends on the integrity of gap junctions (Frame and Sarelius, 1993, 1995; Segal, 1994); (2) dilation of resistance and conduit arteries through blood flow-related rises in NO production; and (3) increased production of dilator autacoids such as EDHF and PGI_2.

Large artery diameter increases by 30–40% in response to a three-fivefold increase in blood flow due to increased NO production (Melkumyants et al., 1989; Khayutin et al., 1995). This maximizes blood flow throughout the active bed. Elevation of NO in the smaller resistance vessels and capillaries makes microcirculatory blood flow distribution more uniform (Griffith et al., 1987, 1990).

When production of NO is impaired in long-standing hypertension, the dilator capacity of large arteries is diminished. At high levels of exercise, the resistance of the large arteries to blood flow may be too great to satisfy the metabolic requirements of the active tissues. When this happens, the latter "steal" blood flow from the less active regions (figure 6.11). Reivich et al. (1961) first described a steal syndrome in a patient with complete unilateral obstruction of the first part of one subclavian artery. On exercising the forearm muscles on the affected side, vertebral artery blood flow became temporarily reversed and supplied blood to the active limb muscles instead of to the brain. This gave rise to neurological signs of vertebrobasilar insufficiency, which disappeared when exercise stopped. Steal syndromes readily produce focal damage in the myocardium, kidney, and brain.

Nitric Oxide and Other Endothelial Autacoids in Hypertension

NO-mediated vasodilation is impaired in many types of hypertension (Moncada et al., 1991; Panza, Casino, Badar et al., 1993; Panza, Casino, Kilcoyne et al., 1993). This is an early event in EH due to the rise in plasma cortisol. High BP per se attenuates NO

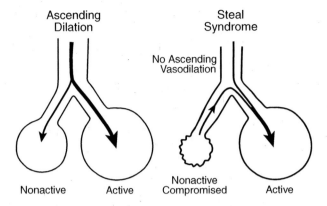

Figure 6.11. Left, in a very active organ, dilation of the conduit artery maximizes its blood flow without compromising that of nearby less active regions. Right, absence of ascending dilation gives rise to steal syndrome: Active region draws on the blood supply of less active regions, which may cause damage.

production, while antihypertensive drug treatment restores it toward normal (Vanhoutte, 1993, 1996; Lüscher, 1994).

Impairment of Endothelium-Dependent NO Vasodilation in Vivo

In the human forearm, NO-mediated vasodilation induced by ACh or bradykinin is attenuated in EH (figure 6.12; Vallance et al., 1989; Panza, Casino, Kilcoyne, and Quyyumi, 1993; Taddei et al., 1993; Kelm et al., 1995). Muscle vessels rather than those in skin are mainly affected. Enhanced production of cyclooxygenase constrictor autacoids may also diminish dilator responses in EH.

Role of Agonists and Blood Flow

Under in vivo conditions, endothelial NO production is increased by stimulation of endothelial receptors by agonists and by a blood flow velocity-related increase in shear stress. The effect of hypertension on the two factors is most readily separated under controlled conditions in vitro (Angus and Cocks, 1989; Angus and Lew, 1992; van Zwieten et al., 1995; Vanhoutte, 1996).

Agonists

Preconstricted aortic rings of SHR relax in response to stimulation by low concentrations of ACh, but at higher concentrations the tension rises again due to the action of constrictor prostanoids (Vanhoutte, 1996). When the latter effect is abolished by pretreatment with indomethacin, the dilator response is the same as in WKY. It suggests that receptor-mediated NO production is not impaired. This was also observed in intestinal R_1 vessels of SHR (figure 6.13, top; Angus and Lew, 1992; Angus et al., 1992).

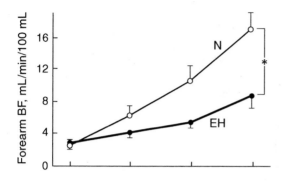

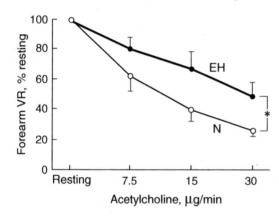

Figure 6.12. Relationship between infusion rate of acetylcholine (μg/min) and (top) forearm blood flow (BF, mL/min/100 g) and (bottom) forearm vascular resistance (VR, % resting) in persons with EH (black circles) and normotensives (N; open circles). From Panza et al. (1993), with permission of *Circulation*, American Heart Association, and Lippincott, Williams and Wilkins.

Increases in vascular wall thromboxanes and endoperoxides are responsible for the greater destruction of NO in the vascular wall compared to that in WKY (Küng and Lüscher, 1995). This has been demonstrated in endothelial cultures in which adding superoxide dismutase mops up the constrictor autacoids and restores NO concentration (figure 6.13, bottom; Grunfeld et al., 1995; Tschudi et al., 1996). Consentino et al. (1994) have suggested that the agonists raise endothelial $[Ca^{2+}]_i$, which raises production of $NO^\bullet$ and arachidonic acid metabolites in parallel; the latter are responsible for the raised superoxide concentration.

Effect of Flow Velocity (Shear)

In isolated gracilis arterioles, vasodilation is induced by an increase in flow in the perfused vessel mediated through raised production of NO and PGI_2 (figure 6.14; Koller et al., 1993; Koller and Huang, 1994). In SHR, the virtual absence of NO production accounts for the attenuated dilator response.

Other Modulators of NO Production

Recall from chapter 5 that NO production is suppressed by elevation in plasma glucocorticoids (Kelly et al., 1998, 2001; Mangos et al., 2000; Lou, 2001). Reduction in

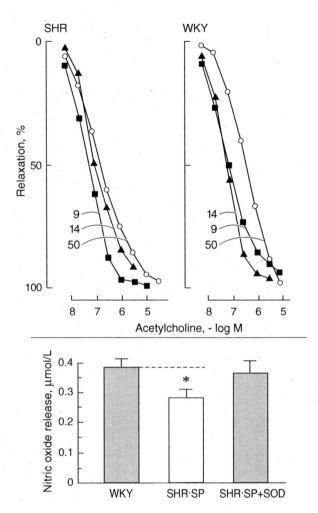

Figure 6.13. Top, relaxation responses in mesenteric resistance arteries (150–250 μm i.d.) pre-contracted with methoxamine, in 9-, 14-, and 50-week-old SHR and WKY studied in isometric myograph. From Angus et al. (1992). Bottom, NO concentration (μmol/L) in isolated rat mesenteric artery after giving calcium ionophore A23187. Responses in WKY (left), SHR.SP (middle), and SHR.SP after addition of superoxide dismutase (SHR.SP + SOD, right). In the absence of SOD, NO release in SHR.SP is lower than in WKY. From Tschudi et al. (1996).

NO production also occurs after the menopause and is restored by giving estrogens (Sudhir et al., 1996; Sudhir, Jennings, et al., 1997). Exercise training has the opposite effect (Wang et al., 1993; Kingwell, Sherrard et al., 1997).

Hypertension Due to NOS Inhibition

Giving a NOS inhibitor acutely raises BP by 20–40 mmHg depending on the dose (Vallance et al., 1989; Chu et al., 1991). Long-term NOS inhibition causes sustained

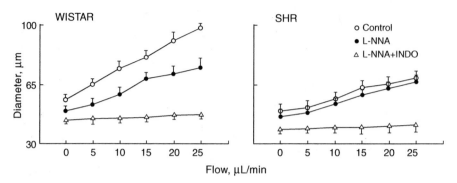

Figure 6.14. Relationship between flow rates (μL/min) and diameter in isolated perfused arterioles of Wistar rats and SHR. Controls, saline, open circle; L-NNA, black circles; L-NNA + indomethacin, open triangles. LNNA, N^w-nitro-L-arginine. From Koller and Huang (1994), with permission of *Circulation Research*, American Heart Association, and Lippincott, Williams and Wilkins.

hypertension in rats, rabbits, and mice (Gardiner et al., 1992, 1993; Ward and Angus, 1993). This also occurs in transgenic mice with disruption of the eNOS (Huang et al., 1995; Gödecke et al., 1997).

The hypertension is due to widespread vasoconstriction, which is most pronounced in the hindquarter (Gardiner et al., 1993).[2] When NOS inhibition stops after 2 weeks, BP recovers rapidly. However, after more prolonged NOS inhibition, recovery is only partial (Manning et al., 1993; Morton et al., 1993).

Mechanisms of Hypertension

The hypertension is prevented by infusing L-arginine together with the NOS inhibitor, indicating that it is due to suppression of biosynthesis (figure 6.15A, B) (Manning et al., 1993; Hu et al., 1994). If the L-arginine infusion is delayed for several days, it attenuates rather than prevents the hypertension (figure 6.15C).

Renal involvement appears to be responsible for the residual elevation of BP, suggested by the two-fourfold rise in PRA and elevation of constrictor prostanoids and thromboxanes (Morton et al., 1993; Pollock et al., 1993; Hu et al., 1994; Küng et al., 1995). ACE inhibitors or AT_1 antagonists greatly attenuate the hypertension.

In chronic L-NAME hypertension, focal lesions in renal, arcuate, and interlobular arteries are extensive, with deposits of sudanophilic lipid droplets (Bouriquet et al., 1996). The animals have widespread glomerular injury and albuminuria, some of which is caused by endothelin.

Surprisingly, structural changes in R_1 vessels are generally absent (Dunn and Gardiner, 1995). In the basilar artery, the wall is thickened through adventitial fibrosis, while medial VSM cell numbers are reduced (Arribas et al., 1997). Clearly, the NO molecule normally maintains VSM cell integrity during hypertrophy and remodeling.

In transgenic mice in which the NOS gene has been knocked out, the hypertension is of the same magnitude as in drug-induced NOS inhibition, but there is less pathology (Huang et al., 1995; Gödecke et al., 1997). PGI_2 levels are raised, which compensates

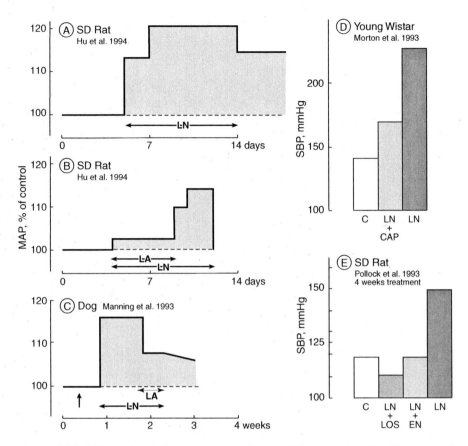

Figure 6.15. Effects of various maneuvers on L-NAME hypertension. (A) Nine days of L-NAME (LN) in adult Sprague-Dawley (SD) rats (Hu et al., 1994). (B) L-arginine (LA) given for 5 days together with LN (Hu et al., 1994). (C) After delay in starting LA infusion, attenuation of hypertension is less effective (Manning et al., 1993). (D) Systolic BPs over 6–7 weeks in young Wistar rats: groups include controls (C, no treatment); LN, treatment; LN plus captopril (LN + CAP; Morton et al., 1993). (E) Systolic BP (SBP) after 4 weeks in adult SD rats: LN, LN + losartan (LOS); LN + enalapril (EN; Pollock et al., 1993).

for some of the effects of NO on the vascular wall (Sun et al., 1999). Presumably it is easier to recruit alternative pathways during development than in adulthood.

Endothelin

Endothelin is a local paracrine autacoid and may contribute to the development of structural changes. However, in EH, SHR, and other types of hypertension, plasma levels are normal. In DOCA-salt- and cyclosporin-induced hypertension, its renal vascular effects contribute to the elevation of BP (Lariviere et al., 1993; Takeda, Miyamori, Wu et al., 1995).

Hemangioendothelioma is an endothelin-producing tumor that causes a rare type of hypertension. Plasma endothelin is markedly raised and the high BP is cured by removal of the tumor (Lüscher et al., 1993; Vanhoutte, 1993).

Role of Structural Changes in Chronic Hypertension

A characteristic feature of EH and other types of chronic hypertension is the development of structural changes in R_1 vessels, conduit arteries, and veins. R_1 vessel changes contribute significantly to the rise in TPR and BP and promote microcirculatory rarefaction. The decrease in distensibility in conduit arteries accentuates the rises in systolic BP and pulse pressure.

Vascular Resistance Properties and Other Features

Folkow was the first to note that the minimum Vas R (R_{min}) was greater in persons with EH than in normotensives in the fully dilated human forearm in which VSM tone was completely abolished (Folkow, 1956; Folkow et al., 1958). He deduced that this must be due to greater narrowing of the arteriolar lumen in EH, possibly as a consequence of inward growth during medial hypertrophy. His analysis suggested that the structural changes were hemodynamically important: (1) R_{min} was closely related to resting MAP in a population of hypertensives and normotensives (figure 6.16, top); and (2) vascular responsiveness to pressor agents was greater in hypertensives than in normotensives (figure 6.16, bottom; Sivertsson and Olander, 1968; Sivertsson, 1970). These findings were soon confirmed by other investigators and in other types of hypertension (e.g., Doyle et al., 1959; Conway, 1963, 1984; Folkow, 1982; Korner, 1982; Mark, 1984; Egan et al., 1988). The work led to much research on the nature and implications of vascular remodeling in EH.

Morphology of R_1 and R_2 Vessels

In chronic hypertension, the internal radius (r_i) in R_1 vessels is narrower and the ratio of wall thickness (w)/r_i is greater than in the corresponding vessels in normotensives (Furuyama, 1962; Suwa and Takahashi, 1971; Schmid-Schoenbein et al., 1986; Heagerty et al., 1993; Mulvany, 1993, 1994; Mulvany et al., 1996; Thybo et al., 1994; Kett et al., 1995; Rizzoni et al., 1996). The reduction in conduit artery distensibility is an obvious source of elevation of central aortic BP (figure 5.6; Safar et al., 1983, 1995; Weber et al., 1996; O'Rourke, 2002). However, in the smaller R_2 vessels, vascular geometry remains normal. One exception is the renal afferent arteriole, which develops changes similar to those of R_1 vessels (Gattone et al., 1983; Skov et al., 1992; Anderson and Brenner, 1995; Kett et al., 1995; Notoya et al., 1996).

Folkow thought that the R_1 vessel changes were due to medial VSM cell hypertrophy or hyperplasia (Folkow et al., 1958; Folkow, 1978). However, Short discovered not long afterward that the medial mass in the R_1 vessel was often unchanged in patients with severe EH, although r_i was still narrower and the w/r_i ratio greater

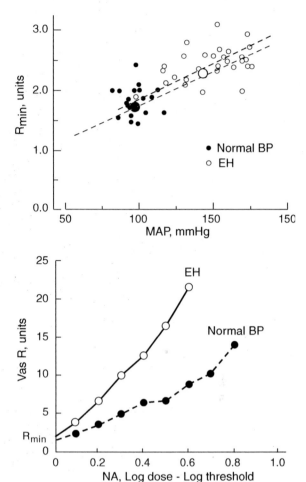

Figure 6.16. Top, relationship between resting mean arterial pressure (MAP, mmHg) and minimum Vas R (R_{min}, units) after abolishing local vascular tone (subjects with EH, open circles; normotensives, closed circles). Large circles, mean values of each group. Bottom, effect of graded doses of noradrenaline (NA) on forearm Vas R (multiples of basal Vas R) in EH and normotensives. Note steeper slope in hypertensives. After Folkow (1956) and Folkow et al. (1958).

(Short and Thompson, 1959; Short, 1966). Later these changes were termed eutrophic remodeling to distinguish them from remodeling associated with frank hypertrophy (figure 6.17; Mulvany et al., 1996).

Wall Stress

In acute elevation of BP, average circumferential tension and stress increase in proportion to the rises in BP (table 6.2). However, in chronic hypertension the increase in w/r_i ratio restores average circumferential stress to normal; inner wall stress remains slightly raised and outer wall stress is slightly subnormal. *Residual stress* is stress at zero load, which depends on the nature of the attachments of the cytoskeleton to surrounding structures (Fung, 1990).

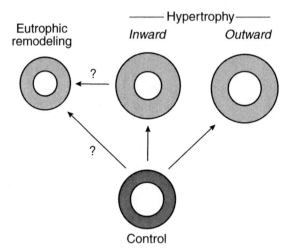

Figure 6.17. R_1 vessel cross-section in hypertension. Control, dimensions at bottom. Top middle and right, medial hypertrophy due to both inward and outward growth. Top left, eutrophic remodeling, where r_i is narrower and w/r_i ratio greater than control, but wall volume is unchanged. Modified from Mulvany et al. (1996).

Resistance Properties: R_{min}, R_{max}, and Slope (S)

The resistance properties in different types of experimental hypertension have been studied in isolated vascular beds under controlled conditions (Folkow et al., 1970; Lundgren, 1974; Göthberg et al., 1976; Göthberg, 1982; Folkow and Karlström, 1987; Mueller, 1983; Baumbach and Heistad, 1988; Smeda et al., 1988; Adams et al., 1989, 1990; Korner et al., 1993; Simpson et al., 1994; Korner and Bobik, 1995). In all of them, a given constrictor stimulus evoked greater rises in Vas R.

This is illustrated by comparing the effects of methoxamine on the isolated HQ bed of adult SHR and WKY (figure 6.18). Vas R is greater in SHR than in WKY over the

Table 6.2. Formulas for Radial Stress, Circumferential Stress, and Shear Stress in a Cylindrical Vessel

Stress	Formula
Radial stress	$RS_{inn} = P$
	$RS_{out} = 0$
Circumferential stress	$CS_{ave} = P \times r_i/w$
	$CS_{inn} = P \times (r_o^2 + r_i^2)/(r_o^2 - r_i^2)$
	$CS_{out} = P \times 2r_o^2/(r_o^2 - r_i^2)$
Shear stress	$\tau = \eta \times Q/\pi \times r_i^3$

Note: P, intravascular blood pressure; w, wall thickness; r_i, r_o, inner and outer radius; CS_{inn}, RS_{out}, radial stress on inner and outer parts of the wall; CS_{ave}, CS_{inn}, CS_{out}, circumferential stress: average, inner, and outer edge of wall; τ, shear stress; Q, blood flow/min; η = viscosity.

Source: Milnor (1982), with permission of Lippincott, Williams and Wilkins.

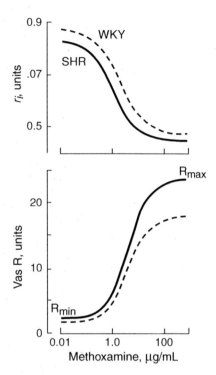

Figure 6.18. Bottom graph, relationship between log methoxamine concentration (μg/mL perfusate) and Vas R (units) in isolated hindquarter of 50-week-old SHR and WKY. Top, relationship between log methoxamine concentration to internal radius (r_i, units), calculated as $(1/Vas\ R)^{0.25}$. Vas R responses are enhanced in SHR, but narrowing of r_i is approximately constant. From Korner, Bobik and Angus (1992), with permission of *Kidney International* and Nature Publishing Group.

full range of vascular tone, from full dilation (R_{min}) to maximum constriction (R_{max}), while the SHR's slope S is steeper, with a ratio $S_{SHR}:S_{WKY}$ of ~1.5. This ratio provides a measure of the average enhancement of the Vas R response. The amplification in SHR is similar to that in moderate EH (Folkow, 1995a; Korner and Angus, 1992).

The Vas R data at the top of figure 6.18 has been replotted in r_i units ($r_i = 1/$ Vas $R^{0.25}$), in accordance with Poiseuille's law. The graph suggests that the bed in SHR is narrower by an approximately constant amount over the full range of vascular tone.

Isolated R_l vessels have been studied in the Mulvany-Halpern isometric myograph (Mulvany et al., 1978; Mulvany and Aalkjaer, 1990; Mulvany, 1994). The maximum force during contraction at optimum length is greater in SHR than in WKY, approximately in proportion to the difference in w/r_i ratio.

In vivo assessment of active force in mesenteric arterioles during local administration of pressor agents indicates that force is greater in young SHR than in young WKY, similar to findings in the isometric myograph. In adult SHR and WKY the difference is smaller, owing to the greater stiffness of SHR vessels (Bohlen and Lash, 1994).

In Vivo Studies

In awake rabbits with chronic cellophane wrap-hypertension subjected to TAB, the enhancement of the HQ Vas R responses was the same for NA, Ang II, and AVP (West et al., 1975; Angus et al., 1976).[3] It suggests that the structural Vas R amplifier has a nonspecific action, which is simply due to alteration in geometry (Folkow, 1956;

Korner and Angus, 1992).[4] However, Hamilton and Reid (1983) reported that the rises in MAP in wrap hypertension were greater with α-AR agonists than with Ang II, which suggests that regulation of receptors might affect the response.

To resolve this issue, Wright et al. (1987) studied the HQ bed vascular responses to constrictor and dilator agonists in wrapped and sham-operated rabbits subjected to TAB. Changes in Vas R rather than in MAP were studied, since they are better indicators of vascular constriction.[5]

The dose-response curves to the constrictor and dilator drugs were combined into a single sigmoid curve (figure 6.19). As before, R_{min}, R_{max}, and S were all greater in hypertensive rabbits than in controls. The slope ratios were similar for each of the drugs used (S_{hyp}:S_{norm}) and averaged ~2:1.[6]

The reason for blocking the ANS was to avoid reflex effects during the drug-induced BP changes. However, this still leaves open the question whether in the

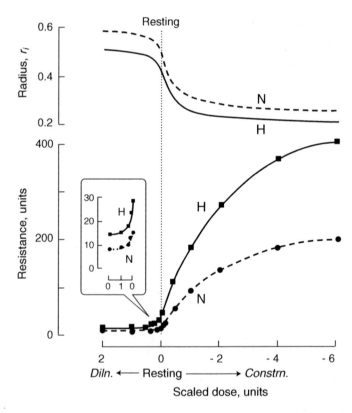

Figure 6.19. Dose-hindquarter response curves in conscious autonomically blocked rabbits with cellophane wrap hypertension (H) and normotensive controls (N). Bottom, relationship between scaled doses of dilator and constrictor agonists and Vas R (units). Top, relationship between doses and average hindquarter r_i, calculated as $(1/Vas R)^{0.25}$. Vertical dotted line, resting value; insert is dilator responses on an enlarged scale. Based on Korner and Angus (1992) and Wright et al. (1987).

intact organism with functioning baroreflexes such enhanced rises in TPR and BP would occur, as implied in Folkow's graph in figure 6.16 (top).

To answer this, Wright et al. (1999, 2002) examined the TPC and TPR responses to dilator and constrictor drugs in rabbits with intact effectors and compared them with the responses in the same animals during combined neurohumoral blockade (NHB; figure 6.20; Wright et al., 1999, 2002).[7]

In both intact and blocked animals, resting vascular tone was greater in hypertension rabbits than in control rabbits (table 6.3). Table 6.4 indicates that the slope ratio $S_{wrap}:S_{sham}$ was approximately 0.5 for TPC, 2.0 for TPR, and 1.9 for MAP, with the ratios similar in intact and blocked rabbits. This suggests that baroreflexes exerted

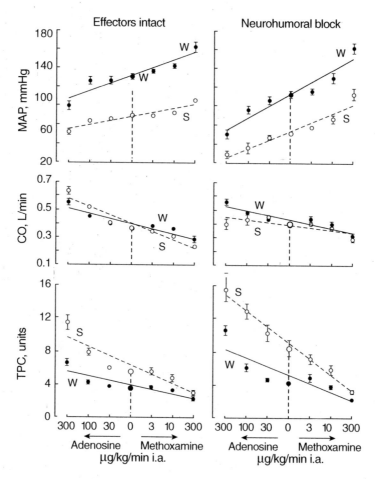

Figure 6.20. Effects of graded doses of methoxamine and adenosine on mean arterial pressure (MAP, mmHg), cardiac output (CO, L/min), and total peripheral conductance (TPC, units) in cellophane wrapped (W) and sham-operated (S) rabbits with effectors intact and during neurohumoral block. Circles, resting values (no drugs). From Wright et al. (2002), with permission of *Journal of Hypertension* and Lippincott, Williams and Wilkins.

Table 6.3. Resting Hemodynamic Variables in Renal Cellophane Wrapped (Wrap) and Sham-Operated Rabbits with Intact Effectors and during Neurohumoral Block (NHB)

	Resting Values	Wrap	Sham	Δ(W–S)
Intact	MAP, mmHg	114	68	46*
	CO, L/min	0.35	0.32	0.03
	TPC, units	3.08	4.66	−1.58*
	TPR, units	337	216	121*
NHB	MAP, mmHg	87	46	41*
	CO, L/min	0.38	0.41	−0.03
	TPC, units	4.50	9.07	−4.57*
	TPR, units	236	118	118*

Note: MAP, mean arterial pressure; CO, cardiac output (transonic Doppler flowmeter); TPC, total peripheral conductance, mL/min/mmHg; TPR, mmHg/L/min. W, wrap; S, sham. *$p < .05$.

Source: Wright et al. (2002), with permission of *Journal of Hypertension*, and Lippincott, Williams and Wilkins.

similar effects during administration of vasoactive drugs in wrapped and sham-operated rabbits.

However, the slope ratios for ΔMAP were different in intact and blocked rabbits, because of differences in CO responses in the wrapped and sham groups (figure 6.20; table 6.4). Nevertheless, the responses of both TPR and MAP were enhanced in hypertension. As the model simulation suggests, this was largely due to the structural changes.

The structural enhancement of TPR equals

$$\Delta TPR = (S_{hyp}:S_{norm}) \times (\Sigma\Delta[NH + Local\ factors]) + Rarefaction,$$

where $(S_{hyp}:S_{norm})$ is the amplification factor given by the slope ratios, NH are the neurohumoral stimuli, and local factors are alterations in dilator and constrictor autacoids.

Table 6.4. Average Slope (S) of Sigmoid log Concentration–Response Curve in Cellophane-Wrapped Hypertensive (Wrap) and Sham-Operated Rabbits (Sham) with Effectors Intact (Intact) and during Neurohumoral Block (NHB)

	Slope*	Wrap	Sham	Ratio $S_{WRAP}:S_{SHAM}$
Intact	S_{TPC}	0.465	0.984	0.47
	S_{TPR}	2.15	1.02	2.11
	S_{MAP}	8.35	4.41	1.89
NHB	S_{TPC}	1.03	1.90	0.54
	S_{TPR}	1.23	0.70	1.75
	S_{MAP}	12.77	9.56	1.34

Note: The responses were the changes in TPC, TPR, and MAP and the slopes determined in both adenosine–methoxamine and acetylcholine–angiotensin II sequences. *p for Δ (wrap–sham) $< .01$ for all variables.

Source: Wright et al. (2002).

Rarefaction is assumed to account for an additional increase of 30% (Greene et al., 1989; Korner and Angus, 1992).[8]

Table 6.5 summarizes the differences in the above factors in wrapped and sham-operated rabbits. During neurohumoral blockade, there are more constrictor autacoids, less NO, and more rarefaction in the hypertensive rabbits than in controls. With intact effectors, the raised plasma Ang II and slight increase in SNA provide additional constrictor drive (Chalmers et al., 1974; Korner et al., 1975; Brody et al., 1991). About 75% of the rise in TPR was due to nonautonomic factors.

Some Dissenting Findings

A number of investigators have not observed that Vas R or TPR responses to agonists are enhanced in hypertension (Lais and Brody, 1978; Fink and Brody, 1979; Touw et al., 1980; Toal and Leenen, 1985; Leenen et al., 1994). This led to an animated debate (Izzard et al., 1999, 2002; Folkow, 2000; Wright et al., 2002b; Lee and Bund, 2002; Bund and Lee, 2003). As is the way of such debates, in the short term they generate more heat than light.

Models of the resistance vasculature support the view that the enhanced Vas R responses are largely due to alterations in R_1 vessel geometry (see below). The enhancement would diminish if there was marked impairment of VSM contractile function, or the vessels were very stiff. Neither appears to be the case (Mulvany et al.,

Table 6.5. Factors Contributing to the Differences in Resting TPR between Renal Cellophane-Wrapped and Sham-Operated Rabbits, Expressed in Arbitrary Constrictor (+) and Dilator (units)

Factor	Intact		NHB	
	Wrap	Sham	Wrap	Sham
Constrictor Stimulus				
Sympatho	+?	+	0	0
Ang II	++	+	0	0
Local aut	++	0	++	0
Dilator Stimulus				
Metabolic	−	−−	−	−−
NO/EDHF	−	−−−	−	−−−
Σ(wrap–sham)	5.5+		4+	
Rarefaction	+++	0	++	0
R_1 vessel TPR amplifier	$S_{wrap}/S_{sham} = 2.0$		$S_{wrap}/S_{sham} = 2.0$	
$\Delta TPR_{wrap-sham}$ + units	$2.0 \times 5.5 + 3 = 14$		$2 \times 4 + 3 = 11$	

Notes: $\Delta TPR_{wrap-sham}$ = R_1 amplifier $\times$ $\Sigma(\Delta N–H$ + local stimuli) + rarefaction. Sympatho, sympatho–adrenal; Local constrictor autacoids; metabolic, differences due to impaired ascending dilation in active organs; EDHF, endothelium-dependent hyperpolarizing factor; Rarefaction, reduction in microcirculatory density; R_1 amplifier assessed from slope ratio S_{wrap}/S_{sham}; $\Delta TPR_{wrap-sham}$, resting ΔTPR between groups.

Source: After Wright et al. (2002), with permission of *Journal of Hypertension*, and Lippincott, Williams and Wilkins.

1978; Adams et al., 1989; Dyke et al., 1989; Mulvany and Aalkjaer, 1990). Failure to repeat the results in intact animals are probably generally due to technical differences, for example, using bolus injections of vasoactive drugs rather than steady-state infusions, which leads to mismatches between cardiac and peripheral circulatory performance. Another factor may be that during TAB venous filling may be inadequate.

However, the enhanced vascular responsiveness in hypertension has been observed by a large number of investigators. Structure is the most important factor in the enhanced resistance responses to neurohumoral stimuli, but, as indicated in table 6.5, several local functional effects associated with hypertension are also important.

Model Simulation

Several models have been developed over the years to simulate the effects of vascular geometry on Vas R, most of them with similar features (Folkow, 1956; Folkow et al., 1958; Egan et al., 1988; Korner and Angus, 1992). The Korner-Angus model combines the effects of dilator and constrictor drugs into a single logistic dose-response curve, as in the experiments just considered. The bed is lumped into a single vessel. It is assumed that Poiseuille's law applies, that changes in contractile force start at the outer media, and that contractile VSM function per unit mass is normal; further, that the w/r_i-related enhancement of contraction depends on the thickness of the entire wall. Distensibility has been assessed by an elongation ratio E, comparing the extensile properties of hypertensive vessels relative to normotensive vessels.[9]

Inward hypertrophy is simulated by increasing w/r_i and reducing r_i and holding r_o constant, which raises R_{min}, R_{max}, and S (figure 6.21, left). In curve A, narrowing r_i by 9% and increasing w/r_i by 50% (E constant) causes a 2.4-fold increase in S. When the magnitude of the changes in r_i and w/r_i is increased further in curve B, S, and R_{max} become unrealistically large, unless distensibility is reduced. Simulation of outward hypertrophy in figure 6.21 (right) again causes rises in R_{max} and in S, but R_{min} declines below initial control.

One advantage of the model is that one can determine the effects on resistance properties of altering one component of wall geometry at a time. As indicated in the multiple regression equation in table 6.6, slope is inversely related to r_i^4, directly related to $(w/r_i)^2$, and decreases linearly when distensibility is reduced. Narrowing of r_i causes the greatest increase in S, but the effect of raising w/r_i is also substantial: For a given rise in w/r_i, the increase in S is greater the narrower r_i. A corollary is that widening r_i during vasodilation attenuates the rise in S: This is the situation in obesity where the structural amplifier is less powerful (chapter 13).

Eutrophic Remodelling of R1 Vessels

Inward growth is an economical way of enhancing constriction because less VSM mass is necessary to increase w/r_i than with outward growth. In figure 6.22, narrowing of r_i by 15% and increasing w/r_i by 50% and 30% require wall volume to increase, respectively, by only 5% and 2% of Δ wall volume associated with outward growth. Most histologists would report a 2% increase as eutrophic remodeling, although it still represents some vascular growth (Korner and Angus, 1992).

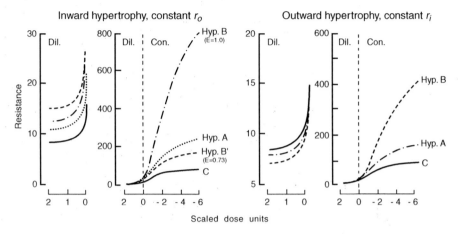

Figure 6.21. Model simulation of inward hypertrophy, r_o held constant and increase in w/r_i narrows r_i. Full dose-Vas R curve toward center; left graph: dilator response on expanded scale. C, control: baseline $r_i = 0.507$ units, $w/r_i = 0.2$; $E = 1.0$. In Hyp. A, baseline $r_i = 0.464$ units, $w/r_i = 0.3$, $E = 1.0$; in Hyp. B, baseline $r_i = 0.434$ units, $w/r_i = 0.4$, $E = 1.0$; in Hyp. B', baseline $r_i = 0.434$, $w/r_i = 0.4$, $E = 0.73$ (decreased distensibility). Right, simulated outward hypertrophy with r_i constant; on right shows full dose–Vas R curve; middle, dilator response on expanded scale; C, control; Hyp. A: $r_i = 0.507$, $w/r_i = 0.3$, $E = 1.0$; Hyp. B, $r_i = 0.507$, $w/r_i = 0.4$, $E = 1.0$. Dil., dilation; Con., constriction. From Korner and Angus (1992), with permission of *Journal of Vascular Research* and S. Karger, Basel.

Recall that eutrophic remodeling was first decribed in patients with long-standing severe EH (Short and Thompson, 1959). Later, the same phenomenon was observed in cerebral vessels of 6–10-month-old SHR.SP rats (Baumbach and Heistad, 1989, 1991). However, in younger SHR.SP the increase in medial mass was greater (Baumbach, personal communication), suggesting that eutrophic changes develop from earlier hypertrophic changes.

The following seems a reasonable hypothesis to explain eutrophic remodeling. Initial growth of the VSM mass in hypertension narrows r_i and increases r_o. In the inner part of the vessel, circumferential wall stress remains slightly raised despite

Table 6.6. Multiple Regression Equations Relating S, R_{min}, and R_{max} to r_i, w/r_i, and E from 28 Simulations

Equation	MC	$F_{1.24}$	SE_{inter}	SE_{b1}	SE_{b2}	SE_{b2}
1) Log S = $1.734 + 1.89\,w/r_i - 3.60\,r_i + 1.15\,E$	0.96	99.2	± 0.21	± 0.18	± 0.38	± 0.11
2) $R_{min} = 67.8 - 9.47\,w/r_i - 99.9\,r_i - 6.97\,E$	0.99	533.4	± 1.44	± 1.24	± 2.63	± 0.75
3) $\mathrm{LogR}_{max} = 1.53 + 2.39\,w/r_i - 3.02\,r_i + 1.53\,E$	0.94	65.6	± 0.31	± 0.26	± 0.56	± 0.16

Note: The sums of squares (SS) accounted for by regression equal the square of multiple correlation coefficient (MC); the fraction of SS due to regression (from equation 1 down) was 92%, 98%, 88%; $F_{1.24} = F$ value for 1 and 24 degrees of freedom; SE_{int} = standard errors (SEs) of intercept; SE_{b1}, SE_{b2}, SE_{b3} are SEs of partial regression coefficients.

Source: Korner and Angus (1992, 1995), with permission of *Journal of Vascular Research* and S. Karger, Basel.

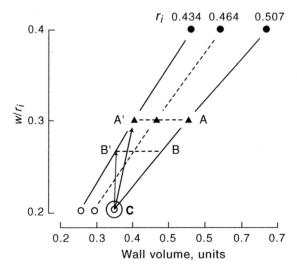

Figure 6.22. Relationship between w/r_i ratio and wall volume (units), at three values of r_i in model. C, control value; A' and A, and B' and B are two sets of w/r_i values at different r_i. For a given increase in w/r_i the narrower r_i, the smaller the increase in wall volume; see comparisons A' versus A, or B' versus B, by reading difference from C on abscissa. From Korner and Angus (1992), with permission of *Journal of Vascular Research* and S. Karger, Basel.

normalization of average wall stress, providing an ongoing stimulus for maintaining the increase in VSM mass. In contrast, stress near the outer part of the vessel wall is subnormal, NO is low, and concentrations of constrictor autacoids are high. Over months in rats (and years in humans) these changes produce some apoptosis of VSM cells in the outer part of the wall. In time, adventitial fibrosis results in a decrease in r_o and causes further narrowing of r_i.

Rarefaction: Reduction in Microvascular Density

Transient rarefaction is a consequence of vasoconstriction (see chapter 5 and figure 5.9; Hutchins and Darnell, 1974; Chen et al., 1981; Prewitt et al., 1982, 1984; Roy and Mayrovitz, 1982; Baumbach and Heistad, 1988; Bohlen, 1989; Struijker-Boudier et al., 1992; Shore and Tooke, 1994; Hutchins et al., 1996). Normally there is variation in size of both R_1 and R_2 vessels in a given bed (Kostromina et al., 1991; Aukland, 1989; Sands et al., 1992; Kopp and DiBona, 1992). The microvascular heterogeneity is accentuated by structurally enhanced vasoconstriction and closure of some R_2 vessels and capillaries, resulting in rarefaction. Some rise in Vas R occurs due to greater energy losses through the patent R_1 and R_2 vessels (Borders and Granger, 1986).[10]

In the course of normal acute-reflex vasoconstriction, rarefaction is mostly transient, waxing and waning in the course of the day. In persons with mild to moderate EH, the periods of rarefaction are longer than in normotensives. Much of the rarefaction is functional, but the chances of permanent closure increase as changes in autacoids cause platelet aggregation and intravascular thrombosis.

Steal Syndromes Give Rise to Rarefaction

Low NO gives rise to steal syndromes through impaired ascending vasodilation. The triad of structural changes, reduction in dilator autacoids, and frequent steal syndromes enhance the probability of permanent rarefaction. One manifestation of this is impairment of cerebral cortical perfusion in moderate to severe EH (Fujii et al., 1990). In one study in symptomless persons with moderate EH, cortical blood flow was 20% below that of normotensives, regional O_2 consumption was reduced, and the respiratory quotient was 0.7, indicating that energy came from substrates other than glucose (Lambert et al., 1994, 1996; Dickinson, 1995).

Conduit Arteries and Veins

Sustained hypertension causes reduction in conduit artery distensibility. The changes are greater and develop more rapidly than the effects of normal aging (Lakatta, 1987, 1993; Folkow and Svanborg, 1993).

In the aorta the intima is normal, while VSM cell hypertrophy causes thickening of the media, in proportion to the rises in MAP and pulse pressure (Black et al., 1988, 1989; Sudhir and Angus, 1990). Collagen formation increases and the elastic lamellae become thickened, particularly in the inner parts of the wall where circumferential stress is maximal (Wolinsky, 1970; Keeley et al., 1991; Berry et al., 1993; Weber et al., 1996). As distensibility decreases, the raised pulse pressure provides an independent myogenic source of microcirculatory vascular tension.

Veins

Large-vein distensibility is reduced in EH, SHR, and renovascular hypertension (Walsh et al., 1969; Takeshita and Mark, 1979; Sudhir, Angus et al., 1990; Sudhir, Smolich et al., 1990; Shore and Tooke, 1994). This is due to the slight elevation of venous pressure that results from the blood volume shifts to the central venous compartment. It contrasts with the variable changes in small-vein properties (Bohlen, 1989; Noble et al., 1990; Zweifach, 1983).

Cellular Mechanisms and Physiological Signals

The initial hemodynamic changes in EH alter circumferential and shear stresses in the vascular wall (figure 6.23). Some of these affect VSM growth, while neurohumoral factors also have direct effects on these processes. Such direct effects are suggested by finding differences in R_1 vessel geometry for the same rises in BP in different etiological types of hypertension (table 6.7; Rizzoni et al., 1996). In each type of hypertension, the particular physical, neuroendocrine, and paracrine signals may give rise to somewhat different profiles of growth factors, which account for some of the differences in VSM proteins (Berk and Alexander, 1989). The various signals also stimulate fibroblasts and other nonmuscle cells, which determine increases in collagen, elastin, and other matrix constituents. The local renin angiotensin system, PDGFs, FGFs, and ET-1 are all involved in VSM hypertrophy or hyperplasia (Albaladejo et al., 1994; Keeley et al., 1991; Simon et al., 1993). In addition, the sympathetic transmitters NA and NPY potentiate PDGF-mediated proliferation of VSM cells in culture (Bobik et al., 1990; Zukowska-Grojec et al., 1996; Zukowska-Grojec, 1998).

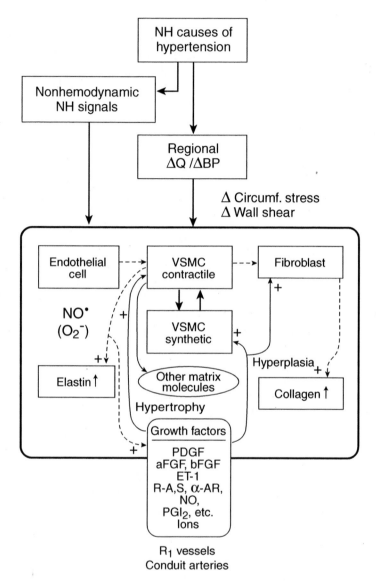

Figure 6.23. Neurohumoral (NH) causes of hypertension act on R_1 vessels and conduit arteries. Effect mediated through mechanical signals (Δ circumferential, shear stresses) and through direct nonhemodynamic signals. Most VSM cells (VSMC) are in contractile phenotype and can undergo hypertrophy, as do cardiac myocytes; during hyperplasia, many change transiently to synthetic phenotype. Growth factors expression differs in various types of hypertension. NO and superoxide ions affect hypertrophy, hyperplasia, and collagen formation.

Table 6.7. Wall Geometry in Subcutaneous R_1 Vessels in Patients with Different Types of Hypertension

	NT Control	EH	Pheochr	Prim Aldo	Ren Hypert
MAP, mmHg	94.2	125.5	118.5	125.1	127.8
Age, yrs	49	51	48	48	52
r_i, μm	149.5	120	120.5	111.5	116.5
r_o, μm	179.6	158.7	156.7	150.3	161.6
w, μm	30	38.7	36.2	38.8	45.1
w/r_i	0.20	0.32	0.30	0.35	0.39
Media, μm^2	14387	15931	15651	17076	22022
r_i, %	100	80.2	80.6	74.6	77.9
r_o, %	100	88.3	87.2	83.7	90
w/r_i, %	100	160	150	175	195
Media, %	100	111	109	119	154

Note: NT Control, normotensive control; EH, essential hypertension; Pheochr., pheochromocytoma; Prim Aldo, primary aldosteronism; Ren Hypert, renovascular hypertension; MAP, mean arterial pressure; r_i, r_o, w, inner and outer radius and wall thickness; Media, medial wall area (assumed to be proportional to wall volume).

Source: Rizzoni et al. (1996), with permission of Hypertension, American Heart Association, and Lippincott, Williams and Wilkins.

Table 6.8 lists molecules which are secreted by VSM cells that affect growth and matrix composition (Darnell et al., 1990; Dzau et al., 1994; Cooper, 1997). The mechanical stresses and strains alter the orientation and number of the connecting filaments and may cause migration of fibroblasts (Harris et al., 1981; Fung, 1990).

The VSM cell has at least two phenotypes: (1) the normal contractile phenotype, and (2) the synthetic phenotype, in which the cell proliferates and manufactures cellular proteins and growth factors. When a contractile cell is placed into culture, the switch to the synthetic phenotype is almost automatic. However, under in vivo conditions such a switch is a more gradual process (Chamley-Campbell et al., 1979; Berk et al., 1989; Scott-Burden et al., 1989; Schwartz et al., 1990; Bobik and Campbell, 1993; De Mey and Schiffers, 1993; Owens, 1995).[11] This may be the reason for the relatively slow development of structural changes in adults.

Some of the interactions between mechanical deformation and local growth promoters are indicated in figure 6.24. In cultured VSM cells plated on a silicone elastomer, Ang II induces a small degree of cell proliferation (Sudhir et al., 1993). With mechanical strain the response is somewhat greater, while when both are applied together, the response is markedly potentiated due to more secretion of PDGF by the cell. Interactions between other neuroendocrine signals and wall stresses and strains alter the pattern of expression of various growth factors (Owens, 1989; Dzau et al., 1994).

Increases in sodium ion and local renin-angiotensin system activity raise collagen production and reduce distensibility of conduit arteries (Safar et al., 1983; Cox and Bagshaw, 1988; Avolio, 1995; Benetos et al., 1995). Distensibility is partially restored by treatment with ACE inhibitors and diuretics.

Table 6.8. Some Examples of Local VSM Cell Growth Promoters and Inhibitors and Inducers and Mediators of Matrix Modulation

VSM Growth Promoters	VSM Inhibitors	Matrix Modulators*	Mediators of Modulation
aFGF, bFGF	Heparan sulf.	FGF family	Plasminogen activator
PDGF, AA, AB, BB	NO	PDGF family	Collagenases
TGF-β family	TGF-β family	TGF-β family	Stromalysin
HB-EGF	PGI_2	IL-1	Elastases
EGF	ANP ($\equiv$ANF)	EGF	Endoglycosidases
IGF-I	Fibronectin		Metalloproteinases
IL-1, IL-6	Interferon γ	Ang II	
Thrombin		AVP	
Prostanoid		Prostanoids	
LDL		Glucocorticoids	
Ang II			
Thromboxane			
Leukotrienes			

*Matrix modulation is linked to growth/apoptosis in VSM cells; it includes synthesis and degradation of glycosaminogly-cans, hyaluronic acid, collagen, elastin, etc. Proteolysis and matrix degradation are mediated by endogenous proteinases, e.g., tissue plasminogen activator, plasmin, elastase, etc. Endothelial cells also express molecules that regulate adhesion to extracellular matrix and cell-to-cell junctions.

Source: Adapted from Dzau and Gibbons (1993); Dzau et al. (1994), with permission of Journal of Cardiovascular Pharmacology and Lippincott, Williams and Wilkins.

Physiological Signals

Blood Pressure.   In a longitudinal study of R_1 vessel changes, severe stenosis of one iliac artery was induced in young SHR and WKY, and the structural changes in a particular R_1 vessel were examined at 12 and 24 weeks of age in the intact and stenotic limbs (figure 6.25). At these times the medial thickness, medial area, and media:lumen ratio of the intact limbs were all greater in SHR than in WKY.

MAP rose between 12 and 24 weeks by ∼20 mmHg in SHR and all the structural variables increased. In WKY the rise in MAP was slightly greater, but the structure of the intact limb barely altered.

At 12 weeks, the MAP in the stenotic limb of SHR was about 40 mmHg below that of the intact limb and VSM mass was smaller (figure 6.25).[12] Between 12 and 24 weeks, VSM mass increased in the stenotic limb, in which MAP had also risen. In 12-week-old WKY, the MAP in the stenotic limb was lower than in the intact limb, as was VSM mass. However, there was little further change in wall structure between 12 and 24 weeks in either intact or stenotic limb, despite the substantial rises in MAP.

These experiments indicate clearly that BP is not the sole determinant of the structural changes. Other likely factors are blood flow, direct neuroendocrine and paracrine changes, and genetic susceptibility.

Blood Flow.   Experimental stenosis sufficient to lower blood flow in a conduit artery causes long-term narrowing of their lumen. The low shear stress associated with the blood flow reduction reduces production of NO and other dilator autacoids, as a result of which vessel tone increases (Langille and O'Donnell, 1986; Langille et al., 1989;

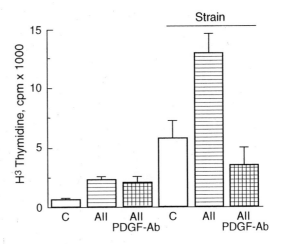

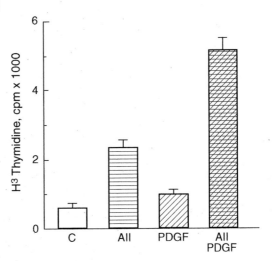

Figure 6.24. Top, in cells plated on a silicone elastomer, angiotensin II (AII) and mechanical strain each produce a small rise in VSM cell proliferation (thymidine incorporation) above control (C), which is potentiated when both are applied together. The response is abolished by antibody to PDGF (PDGF-Ab), which given alone does not affect the AII response in the absence of mechanical strain. Bottom, potentiation of the effect of AII by mechanical strain is simulated by coadministration of AII plus PDGF. From Sudhir et al. (1993), with permission of *Journal of Clinical Investigation*.

Langille, 1996). Similar changes have been observed in poorly perfused arterioles (Smiesko and Johnson, 1993).

The opposite occurs during long-term rises in conduit artery blood flow, as in patients with radial arteriovenous shunts (Girerd et al., 1996). Typically, arterial diameter widens by 40% for a sixfold increase in shunt flow. The dilation raises circumferential stress in accordance with Laplace's law, but there is no increase in wall thickness owing to the counterregulatory signals related to high blood flow velocity.

Circumferential and Shear Stress and Their Interaction. These were examined during a 3-month period of "arterialization" of vein grafts in dogs (Dobrin et al., 1989; Dobrin, 1995). Reducing blood flow velocity increased intimal thickness but had no effect on the media. Media thickness increased in response to raised circumferential stress and to greater deformation by a raised pulse pressure. Enhanced pulse pressure

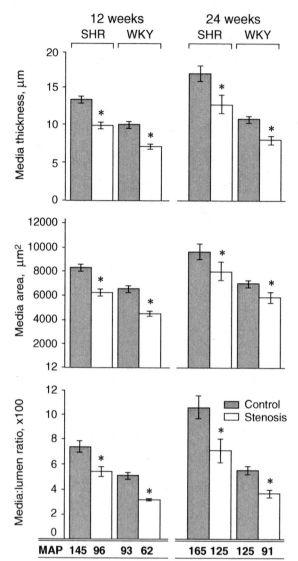

Figure 6.25. Changes in medial wall thickness (μm), medial area (μm^2), and $100 \times$ (media:lumen ratio) in designated R_1 vessel of 12- and 24-week-old SHR and WKY in normal hindlimb (shaded bar) and in hindlimb with marked stenosis of iliac artery (clear bar). Numbers at bottom refer to MAP (mm-Hg) in intact and stenotic limb. *$p < .05$ for Δ(control-stenotic limbs). Further discussion in text. After Bund et al. (1991).

in EH provides a relatively independent input to conduit arteries and R_1 vessels (O'Rourke, 1982a; Christensen, 1991).

Effect of Treatment.   Most antihypertensive drugs are very effective in lowering BP but are less effective in reducing structural changes. In mild EH, treatment with β-blockers for one year has no effect on medial thickness, while treatment with ACE inhibitors and Ca^{2+} antagonists reduces medial volume significantly but only partially (Schiffrin et al., 1994; Heagerty et al., 1988; Aalkjaer et al., 1989).

However, antihypertensive treatment restores production of dilator autacoids and diminishes formation of constrictor autacoids (Vanhoutte, 1993, 1996; Lüscher, 1994; Küng et al., 1995).

A Steroid Amplifier.   Vascular responsiveness to NA and Ang II increases following administration of glucocorticoids and mineralocorticoids in doses that cause steroid hypertension (Sudhir et al., 1989; Pirpiris et al., 1992). Both steroids cause the same enhancement, which is probably due to their direct actions on the contractile machinery. The increase in contractility is prevented by applying the synthetic steroid RU486 (mifepristone) to VSM cells. The drug has antiglucocorticoid and antiprogesterone activities and binds to the DNA steroid response sequences (Grunfeld et al., 1995). This interferes with expression of genes that regulate contraction (Clark et al., 1992; McNally et al., 2000).

The enhancement of Vas R by the steroid amplifier is similar to that produced by structural changes. However, it seems unlikely that in EH the much smaller rise in cortisol raises R_1 vessel contractility.

Integrative Vascular Regulation and Its Impairment in EH

Vascular smooth muscle of the resistance vessels is the peripheral integrator of the effects on Vas R of neurohumoral and local stimuli, which is due to the differential responsiveness of the R_1 and R_2 vessels. Peripheral vascular regulatory mechanisms include: (1) the myogenic response; (2) molecules involved in metabolic regulation; and (3) endothelial NO and various dilator and constrictor autacoids. The first two mechanisms function normally in EH from the viewpoint of VSM contractile function, but distortions may arise owing to reduced availability of NO. Structural changes in R_1 vessels enhance the effects of vasoactive stimuli on VSM tone, while the reduction in distensibility of the conduit arteries gradually raises arterial pulse pressure.

Myogenic autoregulation is a short-term mechanism for maintaining organ blood flow constant, mainly by altering R_2 vessel tone, during transient changes in BP. Autoregulation tends to be accentuated in hypertension because of reduced production of NO during rises in blood flow.

Myogenic tone is directly related to BP, which in turn depends on the circulatory actions of neurohumoral factors and local autacoids. This makes it undesirable to partition changes in Vas R into myogenic and agonist components.

Simply reducing BP lowers myogenic tone of the resistance vessels. This is why such a variety of antihypertensive drugs are beneficial, without addressing the basic causes of EH, as discussed in chapter 4. There are few diseases for which nonspecific therapy has been so successful.

During metabolic activity, blood flow is raised through the actions of tissue hypoxia, nitrothiol compounds, various metabolites, and neurotransmitters. Their actions are reinforced by increased production of NO, which may extend vasodilation into the conduit arteries. Ascending dilation maximizes blood flow in active tissues without compromising the blood supply of the less active ones. Increased NO production optimizes distribution of capillary blood flow, which benefits blood-tissue exchanges.

In EH, local NO availability is impaired, while production of constrictor autacoids tends to increase. Lack of NO particularly affects metabolically active organs (e.g., brain, kidney, myocardium, and skeletal muscle). Impairment of NO is particularly important for renal circulatory function (chapters 12, 15).

R_1 vessel structural changes develop in response to the actions of physical, neuroendocrine, and paracrine signals on VSM cells, fibroblasts, and other cells in the vascular wall. The result is medial VSM hypertrophy and increases in collagen, which increase as hypertension becomes more severe. The structural amplifier enhances the effects of neurohumoral and local inputs. Amplification is greater the narrower r_i and the greater the w/r_i ratio; amplification is reduced in stiffer R_1 vessels.

The initially hypertrophic changes give rise to eutrophic remodeling owing to changes in adventitial autacoids, which promote outer medial VSM apoptosis and increasing adventitial fibrosis. In eutrophic remodeling, structural amplification factor is largely maintained despite the smaller increase in VSM mass.

SNA is raised in EH through much of the day in renal, gastrointestinal, muscle, and skin beds. Only in the skeletal muscle bed is resting neural vasoconstriction masked during the phasic rises of adrenaline secretion. SNA remains high for many years because the relevant CNS has become sensitized. It may return to normal in older hypertensives. Cortisol secretion is slightly increased as part of the defense response, but probably not sufficiently to enhance VSM contractility. Its main effect on vascular tone is through inhibition of NO biosynthesis. Ang II may constrict the vasculature in high-renin subjects with EH.

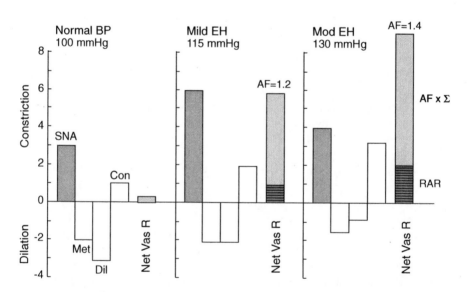

Figure 6.26. Main determinants of net Vas R in the renal bed in normotensives and in those with mild and moderate EH. Net Vas R is the sum of neurohumoral and local factors, including constrictor SNA, metabolites (Met), dilator autacoids (Dil), constrictor autacoids (Con), and rarefaction. The last column is Net Vas R × structural amplification factor (AF, shaded bar) plus a rarefaction component (RAR, horizontal lines).

Structural changes develop gradually as EH progresses. They enhance the level of vasoconstriction and increase the degree of rarefaction in all vascular beds, which increases elevation of BP. Rarefaction causes deterioration of organ function, which is accentuated by the steal syndromes that are associated with impaired ascending vasodilation.

As suggested in figure 6.26, the increase in renal Vas R (and TPR) starts with elevation of SNA. Vascular tone increases as local dilator factors diminish and constrictor factors rise. The functional changes are enhanced by the action of the structural amplifier and development of increasing rarefaction. By the time EH is moderately severe, nonautonomic factors account for the major part of the elevation of Vas R.

The structural changes are difficult to reverse with currently available antihypertensive drugs. However, many drugs (e.g., ACE inhibitors, AT_1 antagonists, and Ca^{2+} antagonists) partially reverse the changes in local autacoids. Because of the structural amplifier, removal of any sources of constrictor tone enhances reduction in TPR as long as BP remains low, which mostly requires pharmacotherapy.

7

Cardiac Performance

In hypertension, the heart pumps against a raised arterial BP while having to meet the body's requirements for O_2 and nutrients over a large range of metabolic activity. It maintains pump performance for many years through raised cardiac sympathetic nerve activity (SNA), greater preload, and development of left ventricular hypertrophy (LVH). However, in untreated hypertensives what eventually gives rise to deterioration of performance is, first, rarefaction of the coronary micro-circulation associated with the structural R_1 vessel changes, and second, excess enlargement of LV myocytes. This is why LV failure is common in poorly treated patients with severe EH, who are also at greater risk of life-threatening arrhythmias and sudden death.

Background Physiology

Myocardial performance depends on the heart's contractile properties, size, valvular function, and well-coordinated excitation, contraction, and relaxation of the ventricles.

Functional Anatomy

All myocardial fibers are attached to the atrioventricular (A-V) ring. The ventricles are enveloped by sheets of myocardium, with the superficial and deep spiral layers separated by a circular layer. The circular layer is most prominent in the LV, while the spiral muscles predominate in the right ventricle (RV; Rushmer, 1961; Streeter, 1979).

170

The blood supply is through the right and left coronary arteries (Gregg, 1950; Marcus, 1983). The left artery divides into left circumflex and anterior descending branches; the right coronary artery gives off branches to each ventricle from its position in the A-V groove.

The sympathetic nerves supply the sinoatrial (S-A) and A-V pacemakers and the atrial and ventricular myocardium. Sympathetic stimulation increases heart rate and force of myocardial contraction. The resulting metabolic vasodilation masks the direct α-AR-mediated coronary vasoconstriction (Feigl, 1983). The vagal motor nerves supply the S-A and A-V nodes, and their stimulation slows the heart and A-V conduction.

Cardiac Cycle

Cardiac excitation begins at the S-A node and is followed by sequential excitation of the atria, A-V node, Purkinje fibers, and ventricular myocardium, and atrial and ventricular contraction. At the start of diastole the opening of the A-V valves is associated with rapid inflow of blood into the ventricle, which gradually slows until atrial contraction provides a further boost near the end of diastole (figure 7.1). The transmitral blood flow velocity is greater in early ventricular diastole (E) than during atrial contraction (A), so that the E/A velocity ratio is high. The ratio declines during aging and in many types of LVH.

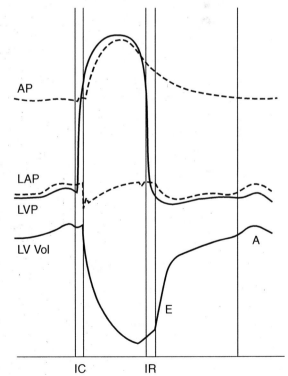

Figure 7.1 LV pressure and volume changes during cardiac cycle, showing aortic pressure (AP), left atrial pressure (LAP), left ventricular pressure (LVP), and left ventricular volume (LV Vol). IC and IR are phases of isovolumetric contraction and relaxation; E is the rapid LV volume change after opening of mitral valve; A is atrial booster action before opening of the aortic valve. After Rushmer (1961) with permission of *Physiological Reviews* and American Physiological Society.

The phase of LV isovolumetric contraction is the period between closure of the mitral valve and opening of the aortic valve, when all the LV myocardium has become activated. When the aortic valve opens, the stroke volume is ejected through radial compression of the LV by the deep constrictor muscles. In the RV, the action of the prominent spiral muscles causes descent of the base toward the apex during systole (Brecher and Galletti, 1963). Once the aortic and pulmonary valves have closed, ventricular pressures fall rapidly during the phase of isovolumetric relaxation.

Wall Stress

During isovolumetric contraction, the LV pressure (LVP) is related to the tension in the LV wall in accord with the Laplace relationship. A prolate ellipsoidal shape is maintained at low and moderate filling pressures when there are differences between circumferential and longitudinal wall stresses (Falsetti et al., 1971; Mirsky, 1979; Streeter, 1979; Milnor, 1982; Fung, 1993). At high filling pressures, the ventricle assumes a spherical shape, where circumferential and longitudinal stresses are the same, that is,

$$CS = (LVP \times r_i^2/w)/(2r_i + w),$$

where CS is circumferential wall stress, r_i is internal radius, and w is wall thickness.

In the normal heart, circumferential wall stress increases rapidly to a maximum during isovolumetric contraction (figure 7.2, left). As systole proceeds, r_i decreases so that

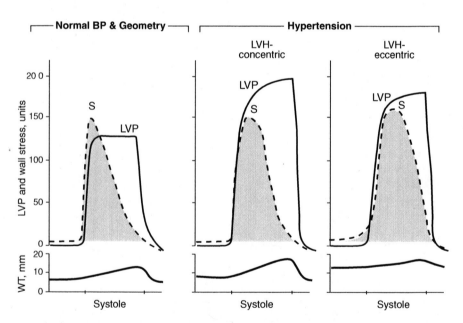

Figure 7.2. Changes during systole in LV pressure (LVP), circumferential stress (S), and wall thickness (WT, mm). Left, normal LV, BP LV geometry; middle, concentric LVH; right, eccentric LVH plus decompensation. Further discussion in text. Based on Grossman et al. (1975) and Mirsky (1979).

LVP is maintained by less wall stress (Grossman et al., 1975; Sasayama et al., 1977; Mirsky, 1979; Milnor, 1982). In concentric LVH, LVP and tension during isovolumetric systole are greater than in the normal heart, but average circumferential stress is normal owing to the thickened wall. At the start of ejection, r_i is below normal and w/r_i is raised, so that the higher LVP during the latter part of systole is maintained by a normal level of wall stress (figure 7.2, middle). When the LV is dilated (i.e., in eccentric LVH), there is an increase in end-diastolic wall stress. During isovolumetric systole, LVP is lower than in concentric LVH and stress is greater as ejection proceeds (figure 7.2, right).

Myocardial Contraction

Cardiac and skeletal muscle have a similar striated appearance, but very different functional properties. All myocardial cells are activated at every beat through intrinsic pacemaker mechanisms, while in skeletal muscle the number of fibers activated depends on the activity of the motor nerves.

Cardiac Sarcomere Structure

The myofibrils contain thin actin filaments and thick myosin filaments, arranged so that each thick filament is surrounded by a hexagonal array of thin filaments (Braunwald et al., 1967; Darnell et al., 1990). The actin molecule is a globular monomer called G-actin that polymerizes to filamentous F-actin, the polarity (positive and negative ends) of which determine the direction of assembly. Several hundred myosin molecules are arranged in bipolar fashion into a thick filament, with the tail of each anchored at the M line in the center (figure 7.3). The head protrudes toward an actin filament and binds to it during cross-bridge formation (Margossian et al., 1992; Murphy, 1996).

The thick filaments define the A band and extend symmetrically about the sarcomere center, where the H zone is the region without thin filaments. The I band (no thick filaments) extends over two halves of adjoining sarcomeres, with the Z disk in its middle, to which the positive end of each actin filament is attached.

Titin is a giant molecule extending from the Z disk to the M band (figure 7.3; Cooper, 1997; Labeit et al., 1997). Cardiac titin is shorter than skeletal muscle titin, which makes it into a stiffer spring, and is responsible for the lower compliance compared to skeletal muscle (Trombitas et al., 1995; Labeit et al., 1997). Additional cytoskeletal proteins maintain myocyte structure and connect with adjoining cells and extracellular matrix (Ganote and Armstrong, 1993; Cooper, 1997).

Contraction and Relaxation

In a test tube, actin and myosin filaments form a dense flocculate in the presence of the right concentrations of ATP, Ca^{2+}, Mg^{2+}, and other ions, simulating contracture of the muscle (Winegrad, 1982). In the relaxed state, the tropomyosin-troponin complex inhibits the binding of actin to myosin that normally occurs during contraction. As cytosolic Ca^{2+} rises to $\sim 10^{-6}$ M, there are changes in the steric relationship between tropomyosin and the three subunits of troponin (Tn-T, Tn-I, and Tn-C;

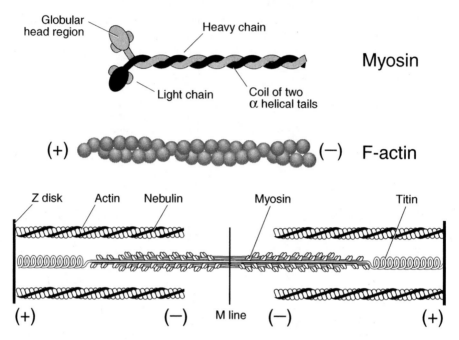

Figure 7.3. Top, myosin molecule has a heavy chain tail coiled into two α-helices; each has a globular head to which two light chains are attached. Middle, G-actin molecules polymerize into fibrillar F-actin with $(+)$ and $(-)$ polarity. Bottom, several hundred myosin molecules make up a thick filament. Their tails are attached to the M band in sarcomere center and their heads point toward the actin fibrils. The giant titin molecule is attached to the M band and Z disk. Note attachments of $(+)$ and $(-)$ ends of F-actin. From Cooper (1997) with permission of Sinauer Associates.

Darnell et al., 1990; Langer, 1992). The key disinhibitory reaction is the binding of some of the Ca^{2+} ions (known as activator calcium) to the low-affinity sites of Tn-C (Warber and Potter, 1986; Langer, 1992). This brings about a conformational change in the tropomyosin helix that permits the binding of actin to the myosin head (Warber and Potter, 1986). The extent of the rise in cytosolic Ca^{2+} concentration determines the number of cross bridges and their rate of cycling (Winegrad, 1982; Elliott and Elliott, 1997). Each cross bridge attaches and detaches itself a number of times during a single contraction (Finer et al., 1994; Howard, 1994).

   Ca^{2+} ions enter from both outside the cell and from the sarcoplasmic reticulum (SR) (Winegrad, 1982; Darnell et al., 1990; Langer, 1992; Katz, 1993). The entry from outside enhances Ca^{2+} entry through the SR release channel (calcium-dependent calcium release), which is located in "foot" structures of the transverse tubular SR and is the site of the ryanodine receptor (Fabiato, 1983). Rapid relaxation at the start of diastole is necessary for good mechanical function and requires rapid removal of Ca^{2+} from Tn-C and cytosol. The ion is returned to the SR through a Ca^{2+} pump-ATPase, which is regulated by the SR protein phospholamban. In the unphosphorylated state, phospholamban inhibits the pump, which operates after the protein has become phosphorylated. Blocking the SR Ca^{2+} pump impairs relaxation.

Mitochondria and Provision of Energy

Cardiac metabolism is largely aerobic and requires continuous provision of O_2 to the mitchondria, which is helped by the high concentration of myoglobin in heart muscle. Since the energy stores are minimal, ATP has to be produced constantly to meet moment-to-moment demands for energy for contraction. This occurs through oxidation of fatty acids, glucose, lactate, and pyruvate in the mitochondria (Mitchell, 1961; Alberts et al., 1989; Elliott and Elliott, 1997).[1] The ATP formed provides the energy for the binding of actin to myosin and the related cross-bridge cycling.

Determinants of Mechanical Force in Isolated Heart Muscle

The force developed by the heart depends on initial loading conditions, velocity of contraction, and stimulation by agonists.

Length–Tension Relationship

When initial length prior to contraction is altered, the active tension developed depends on the extent of overlap between thick and thin myofilaments (figure 7.4; Huxley, 1957; Winegrad, 1982). At physiological lengths, passive tension is considerably greater in the myocardium than in skeletal muscle. It is maximal at initial sarcomere lengths of 2.1–2.2 μm and falls on either side of this value (Sonnenblick et al., 1964). As fiber length increases, the troponin complex becomes more sensitive to Ca^{2+}, and more Ca^{2+} enters the cytosol (Allen and Kentish, 1985). There is also a "population factor" in the ascending limb in vivo, because the LV sarcomere lengths vary in different parts of the wall at low and moderate filling pressures, but become uniform at high pressures (Yoran et al., 1973). The descending limb of the curve is mainly due to diminished filament overlap and reduction in the number of cross bridges.

Force–Velocity Relationship

In contracting skeletal muscle, A. V. Hill found that the relationship between developed force and velocity of shortening was described by a displaced rectangular hyperbola,

$$(P + a) \times V = (P_o - P) \times b,$$

where P = load, and V = velocity of shortening (figure 7.5; Hill, 1970). When velocity is zero, force is maximal at P_o ($\equiv$ isometric contraction), while velocity is maximal (V_{max}) at near-zero load. Increasing load without change in inotropic state results in an increase in P_o but no change in V_{max}, while inotropic stimulation causes a rise in both parameters.

A. V. Hill's model includes a contractile element and a passive elastic component. When the muscle shortens, the contractile element stretches the series elastic component, which delays the rise in active tension. In skeletal muscle, passive tension is low at physiological sarcomere lengths, so that the model can be reduced to a single elastic element in series with the contractile element. Rapid stretch of the elastic element at

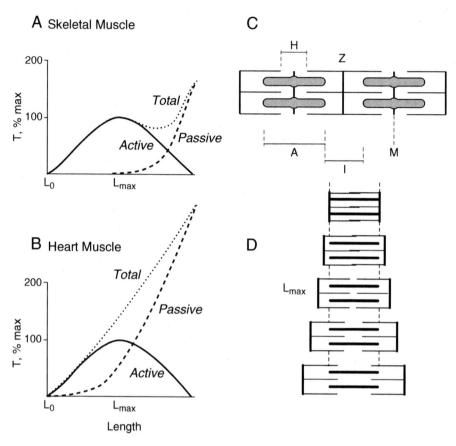

Figure 7.4. (A) Relationship in skeletal muscle between sarcomere length and active and passive tensions. (B) Same relationship in cardiac papillary muscle; active tension is total tension minus passive tension; L_{max}, length at maximum active tension ($\equiv100\%$). (C) Two adjoining sarcomeres, showing location of thick myosin and thin actin filaments, Z disks, A band, I band, and H zone. (D) Overlap between actin and myosin filaments at different initial lengths; the middle sarcomere corresponds to L_{max}. From Braunwald et al. (1967), with permission of Little Brown and Company, and Lippincott, Williams and Wilkins.

the start of contraction prevents the delayed rise in tension, which becomes maximal almost at once. This is termed the active state and is the same as the force developed during tetanus.

Some of the functional differences between cardiac and skeletal muscle are summarized below:

- Cardiac muscle has a long refractory period; while making it tetanus-proof, the active state is difficult to determine.
- The passive tension in cardiac muscle is high, so that load cannot be reduced sufficiently to determine V_{max}.

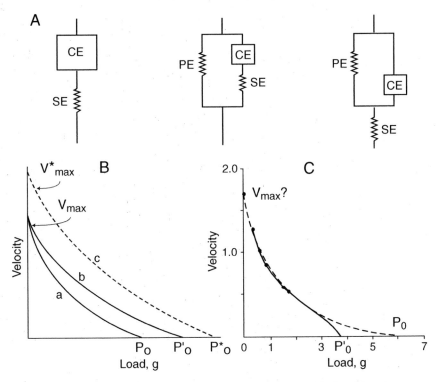

Figure 7.5. (A) Models of striated muscle, showing different distribution of tension on contractile elements (CE), series elastic element (SE), and parallel elastic elements (PE). (B) Force-velocity curves: (a) control, note V_{max} and P_0 intercepts; (b) raising initial muscle length increases isometric force to P'_0 but V_{max} unchanged; (c) inotropic stimulation shifts both V^*_{max} and P^*_0. (C) In papillary muscle, actual V_{max} is not at zero load and actual P'_0 deviates from rectangular hyperbola of Hill equation. (A) and (B) after Brady (1979); (C) after Brutsaert and Sonnenblick (1971).

- At high loads, the force–velocity relationship deviates from a rectangular hyperbola, so that deriving V_{max} by extrapolation is inaccurate.
- "Active state" in cardiac muscle develops much more slowly than in skeletal muscle (Brady, 1979).
- In cardiac muscle, every fiber is activated with every beat, and that force can only change through intrinsic and inotropic mechanisms. In skeletal muscle, force generation depends on its motor nerves and commonly increases through neural recruitment of more muscle fibers.
- Different genes regulate cardiac morphogenesis. In skeletal muscle, the developmental repertoire is controlled by the myoD homeodomain gene. In cardiac muscle, the homeodomain genes that affect formation of the heart tube and looping are related to the *Drosophila* gene *tinman* and include *Csx, Nkx 2.5,* and *Nkx 2.6.* Genes regulating cardiac morphogenesis after looping include portions of DNA that bind to the proteins eHAND and dHAND.

The high passive tension in cardiac muscle makes it difficult to determine V_{max}, and attempts to determine V_{max} and P_o by extrapolation have not been successful (Huxley, 1957; Braunwald et al., 1967; Brady, 1979; Braunwald and Ross, 1979; Brutsaert and Paulus, 1979; Parmley and Talbot, 1979).

Therefore, one may conclude that the Hill model applies to cardiac muscle only in a qualitative sense: Velocity is greater at low loads and developed force is maximal during isometric contraction (Van den Bos et al., 1973; Noble, 1977; Brady, 1979; Braunwald and Ross, 1979). From the practical viewpoint, the assessment of myocardial function in chronic hypertension is performed by determining myocardial mechanics and pump performance under controlled steady-state loading conditions in the normal myocardium and in the presence of LVH.

Inotropic Stimulation

Stimulation of cardiac β-ARs is associated with a stimulus-related increase in total force and the rate of LV pressure change (dP/dt) in the early part of the cardiac cycle and is followed by a more rapid rate of relaxation once contraction is over. Thus, both the increase and removal of cytosolic calcium is accentuated.

Stimulation of β-ARs activates G_s proteins, which in turn stimulate adenylyl cyclase and increase conversion of ATP to cyclic AMP (figure 7.6; Winegrad, 1982; Langer, 1992; Ishikawa and Homcy, 1997). Cyclic AMP activates protein kinase A, which

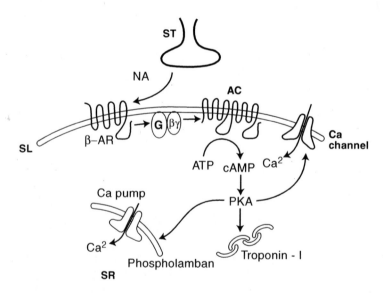

Figure 7.6. Noradrenaline (NA) stimulates β-AR, which is coupled to G-protein, increasing activity of adenylyl cyclase (AC), which increases cyclic AMP (cAMP) and phosphokinase A (PKA). The latter catalyzes several phosphorylation reactions, which increase calcium entry into cytosol from outside and from SR, with the latter regulated by phospholamban. ST, sympathetic terminal; SL, sarcolemma; SR, sarcoplasmic reticulum. From Ishikawa and Homcy (1997), with permission of *Circulation Research*, American Heart Association, and Lippincott, Williams and Wilkins.

catalyzes several phosphorylation reactions, some of which increase the rate and some the force of contraction. They include (1) phosphorylation of L-type Ca^{2+} channels, which enhances entry of Ca^{2+} into the cytosol; (2) phosphorylation of Tn-I, which alters responsiveness of contractile proteins (Winegrad, 1982); (3) phosphorylation of a 15 kDa sarcolemmal protein, which further increases Ca^{2+} entry through sarcolemmal pathways (Presti et al., 1985); and (4) phosphorylation of phospholamban, which regulates the SR calcium pump.

Phospholamban regulates inotropic state but not heart rate, as judged from results of targeted ablation of the phospholamban gene in mice (Luo et al., 1994). In these animals, basal dP/dt of the isolated heart was greater, the time to peak LV pressure was shorter, and relaxation was more rapid than normal. The effects are similar to those in normal hearts subjected to maximal β-AR stimulation. In phospholamban-deficient hearts, there is enhancement of activity and affinity for the calcium of their SR $Ca^{2+} -$ ATPase.

The cardiac β-ARs include β_1 and β_2 AR subtypes, in a ratio of approximately 3:1 (Koch et al., 1996). Inotropic effects can be evoked through each subtype, but stimulation of β_2-ARs brings additional mechanisms into play that increase Ca^{2+} (Xiao and Lakatta, 1993). In transgenic mice in which cardiac β_2-ARs are overexpressed, adenylyl cyclase and dP/dt$_{max}$ are already maximal under basal conditions. It suggests that stimulation of β_2-ARs acts on an earlier part of the pathway regulated by phospholamban (Koch et al., 1996).

Two autacoids, endothelin-1 (ET-1) and NO, which are produced by endocardial cells and myocytes, also modulate contractile performance. ET-1 increases peak tension and slows relaxation, similar to the effects of increasing preload (Brutsaert and Andries, 1992; Wang and Morgan, 1992; Brutsaert, 1993). Increasing preload also enhances synthesis of NO by the myocyte, which depresses ventricular contractility but increases the rate of relaxation through cGMP (Schulz et al., 1992; Ballignand et al., 1993). The rate of NO synthesis is greatest in myocytes of the inner LV wall layers, where circumferential stress is greatest (Pinsky et al., 1997).

Left Ventricular Geometry in EH

The diagnosis of LVH in hypertension has long been known to carry a poor prognosis (Sokolow and Perloff, 1961; Kannel, 1983; Levy et al., 1990; Levy 1991). In the early studies, performed 30–40 years ago, diagnosis of LVH was based on clinical, x-ray, and ECG criteria, and only 3–4% of the hypertensive population was diagnosed as having LVH. Since the introduction of echocardiography, the estimated prevalence of LVH has increased 10–15-fold, but prognosis is still poor (Devereux et al., 1983, 1987, 1994; Savage, 1987; Frohlich and Pfeffer, 1989; Levy et al., 1990). Cardiovascular mortality of hypertensives with LVH is about 70% above that of persons without LVH.

The Spectrum of LV Geometry

In normotensive individuals, LV geometry is influenced by age, sex, and several lifestyle factors. In adult males, LV mass index (LVMI) is about 15–20% greater than in females

(Savage, 1987; Devereux et al., 1994). LVMI and LV cavity dimensions increase with age, while transmitral E/A flow velocity ratio declines (Messerli et al., 1984; Laufer et al., 1989; Folkow and Svanborg, 1993; Lakatta, 1993).[2]

In exercise training, stroke and cavity volumes increase, while wall thickness (WT) is either thinner or unchanged (Jennings, Nelson, Dewar et al., 1986). Concentric LVH often develops in those who perform regular isometric exercise (e.g., professional weight lifters, wrestlers) (Spirito et al., 1994). In obesity, excess LVMI is linearly related to the excess body weight (Messerli, 1982). CO is raised and cavity dimensions are enlarged whether BP is normal or raised (Messerli, 1982; Mureddu et al., 1997).

Table 7.1 gives a spectrum of geometries calculated for a model spherical ventricle. Configurations A and B represent LV mass, cavity volume, and WT for sedentary normotensives and those engaged in exercise training; C, C_{in}, and C_{rm} include a range of concentric LVH and remodeling without an increase in LV mass, as noted in the vasculature (chapter 6); CE_1, CE_2, and CD are various types of eccentric hypertrophy. In chronic EH, the increases in WT/RI ratio restore average circumferential wall stress to normal. In configuration CD, the increase in WT is not sufficient to fully restore the stress.

Table 7.1. Changes in LV Geometry in Concentric LVH and Remodeling and in Eccentric LVH

Model	LV mass (g)	WT (cm)	RI (cm)	WT/RI ratio	BP (mmHg)	Circ. Stress (units)
A	152 (100%)	1.0	2.8794	0.3473	100	122.6
A^{acute}	152				150	184
B	176 (116%)	1.0	3.1405	0.3268	93	122.3
C	243 (160%)	1.415	2.8794	0.4914	150	122.5
C_{in}	181 (119%)	1.28	2.611	0.4902	150	122.9
C_{rm}	156.7 (103%)	1.22	2.4897	0.490	150	122.9
CE_1	290 (191%)	1.50	3.0598	0.490	150	122.9
CE_2	387.7 (255%)	1.615	3.3678	0.490	150	122.9
CD	339 (223)	1.50	3.3678	0.4454	150	137.7

Note: WT = wall thickness; RI = inner radius; LV = left ventricle; BP = blood pressure; Circ. Stress, circumferential wall stress; RI, inner cavity radius. Values in brackets under LV mass are percentages of A (normotensive control); B relates to changes in mild eccentric LVH in exercise training (Jennings et al., 1991). C, C_{in}, concentric LVH; C_{rm}, concentric LV remodeling; CE_1, CE_2, CD, eccentric LVH.

Source: Korner and Jennings (1998), with permission of the Journal of Hypertension and Lippincott, Williams and Wilkins.

Prevalence of LVH in EH

In hypertension, LV load is increased in everyone, yet not everyone has LVH. Part of the problem may be due to inaccuracies associated with the echocardiographic estimation of LVH. The heart chambers are first displayed in the two-dimensional mode and a region is then selected for scanning in M-mode format (Marshall et al., 1992). LV mass is calculated from measurements in one plane of the averaged value for WT and the internal dimensions. The shape of the LV is assumed to resemble a prolate ellipsoid of revolution and an algorithm is used to transform the measurements into LV mass (Marshall et al., 1992; Devereux and Roman, 1995; Devereux et al., 1997; Wikstrand, 1997). The "cube" formula of Devereux and Reichek (1977) is commonly used:

$$\text{LV mass (g)} = 1.04\,([\text{LVIDD} + \text{LVPWT} + \text{IVST}]^3 - \text{LVIDD}^3) - 13.6,$$

where LVIDD is the LV internal end-diastolic diameter in the midventricular region; LVPWT is the LV posterior wall thickness; IVST is the interventricular septal thickness; and 13.6 is an empirical correction factor to avoid overestimating LVMI.

LVH is diagnosed if LVMI (or an equivalent measure of LVH) $\geq$ the mean + 2 standard deviations (SDs) of a single measurement in normotensive controls. The estimated prevalence of LVH is greatest in the method with the smallest SD (Korner and Jennings, 1998). Cubing the measurements increases SD by a factor of about $(3 \times SD_{ave}^2)^{0.5}$, where SD_{ave} is the weighted average of the SD (percentage of their respective means) of the various terms in the formula. Another problem is the incongruity between assumed and actual LV geometry, which also enhances SD.[3] Last, the large spectrum of "normal" LV geometry due to lifestyle factors further inflates the normal SD.

With echocardiography, the SD of a single measurement of LVMI is high, which leads to underestimation of the prevalence of LVH, particularly when LVH is of mild and moderate degree (Culpepper et al., 1983; Devereux et al., 1994; Strauer et al., 1994; Devereux and Roman, 1995; Heesen et al., 1997). However, in severe hypertension, the prevalence is close to 100% (Devereux and Roman, 1995).

Some of the problems of estimation are illustrated in figure 7.7 (Laufer et al., 1989). The subjects had previously untreated mild and moderate EH. LVMIs were 9% and 26% greater, respectively, than in matched controls, but the overlap between the two groups was large; only 13% of those with mild EH and 25% of those with moderate EH fall were deemed to have LVH.

When the actual measurements in the single plane are used, the SDs are smaller and there is less overlap, for example, when using WT indexed for BSA (WT*) or WT/RI ratio. Their SDs are smaller and the estimated prevalence of structural abnormality ($\equiv$LVH) is 30% in mild hypertension and 55% in moderate hypertension (table 7.2).

Another approach has been to use multivariate discriminant function analysis, which employs the method of maximum likelihood to maximize pattern differences between groups that have been classified solely on the basis of BP measurements (Fisher, 1946; Norusis, 1986). Laufer et al. (1989) found the most useful discriminant functions were (1) those with two or more structural variables, for example, WT*, LVIDD, WT/RI; and (2) combinations of structural and functional variables (table 7.3). With this method, more people with mild and moderate EH are deemed to have LVH.

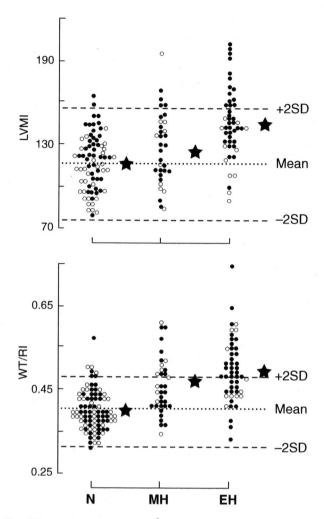

Figure 7.7. Top, LV mass index (LVMI, g/m² BSA) in 54 normotensive subjects (N), 24 with mild EH (MH), and 57 subjects with moderate EH. Bottom, WT/RI ratio in the same subjects, showing less overlap between hypertensives and controls. Males, closed circles; Females, open circles. From Laufer et al. (1989), with permission of *Hypertension*, American Heart Association, and Lippincott, Williams and Wilkins.

Echocardiographic estimates suggest that in EH, concentric and eccentric LVH occur with about the same frequency (Savage, 1987; Levy et al., 1990). In concentric hypertrophy and remodeling, LV mass is closer to normal than in eccentric hypertrophy (table 7.1). Hence, the chance of underestimating the prevalence of LVH is greater in concentric LVH. In turn, it suggests that its prevalence in EH may be greater than that of eccentric LVH.[4]

Nuclear magnetic resonance imaging (NMRI) is a more recent method for assessing LV mass, which is determined by numerical integration of serial LV slices without having to make assumptions about LV geometry. The SD ranges from 5% to 10% of

Table 7.2. Systolic and Diastolic BPs and Echocardiographically Determined Variables in Normotensives (N), Persons with Mild (MH), and Moderate EH (EH$_{mod}$)

Variable	Means ± SD			Prevalence[a]	
	N	MH	EH$_{mod}$	MH	EH$_{mod}$
SBP, mmHg	120 ± 11.3	144 ± 14.8	158 ± 24.9		
DBP, mmHg	77 ± 9.3	86 ± 9.2	99 ± 12.8		
LVMI, g/m^2	116	126*	143*	13%	25%
SD, %	± 18%	± 18%	± 18%	(5/38)	(14/57)
WT*, cm/1.8 m^2	1.0	1.09*	1.17*	29%	56%
SD, %	± 7.5%	± 9.7%	± 13.6%	(11/38)	(32)
WT/RI	0.40	0.47*	0.50*	37%	56%
SD, %	± 11%	± 15%	± 14%	(14/38)	(32/57)
LVIDD, cm/1.8 m^2	4.95	4.69	4.79	13%	4%
SD, %	± 7.6%	8.6%	8.0%	(5/38)	(2/57)
E/A*	1.87	1.45*	1.16*	12.5%	29%
SD, %	± 31%	40%	48%	(3/24)	(11/38)
FS, mm/s	0.36	0.39*	0.37	8.3%	8%
SD	± 18%	± 17.6%	± 20%	(4/36)	(4/50)

Note: Values are means ± standard deviations; SD expressed as %, percentage of mean.
[a]Prevalence is percentage of abnormal/total number in parentheses, e.g., 5 × 100/38 = 13%; value is "abnormal" if ≥ mean + 2 SD of normotensives. SBP, DBP, systolic and diastolic BP; LVMI, LV mass index; WT*, average wall thickness per 1.8 m^2 BSA; WT/RI, wall thickness/internal radius; LVIDD, LV internal end-diastolic diameter indexed to 1.8 m^2 BSA; E/A* ratio, transmitral blood flow velocity ratio early/atrial components indexed to 40 years of age; FS, fractional systolic shortening.
*$p < .01$ for difference from normotensive value.

Source: Laufer et al. (1989), with permission of *Hypertension*, American Heart Association, and Lippincott, Williams and Wilkins.

the mean of the normal group, which is well below the echocardiographic estimates (Missouris et al., 1996; Devereux et al., 1997). The main factor that has stopped the routine use of NMRI to date has been the higher cost. There is little doubt that for assessing LVMI accurately the method is superior to echocardiography. It needs to be used to reassess the LV changes in mild EH and for pharmacological investigations.

BP Accounts for Only Part of the Variance of LVMI

In the general population, BP and LVMI are linearly related with a substantial scatter about the regression line (Rowlands et al., 1982; Abi-Samra et al., 1983; Laufer et al., 1989). When clinic BP is used, only 9–16% of the LVMI variance is accounted for, which increases to 16–36% using ambulatory BP (Devereux et al., 1983). Some of the residual variance is accounted for by age, obesity, and exercise. Once these have been taken into consideration through stepwise multiple regression analysis, LVMI rises by only about 3–4% per 10 mmHg rise in systolic BP (Messerli et al., 1984).

Antihypertensive Therapy and Reversal of LVH

Regression of LVH due to antihypertensive therapy takes much longer than the few weeks it usually takes to normalize BP. When LVMI is increased by ~50% above the

Table 7.3. Results from Two Discriminant Function Analyses Using (1)
Two Variables (WT*, LVID*) and (2) Three Variables (WT*, FS, E/A¤)

	N	Mild EH	Moderate EH	p
Discriminant Function: WT, LVID**				
N	72%	20%	8%	<.001
n = 89				
Mild EH	29%	37%	34%	n.s.
n = 35				
Moderate EH	14%	16%	70%	<.001
n = 54				
Discriminant Function: WT, FS, E/A¤*				
N	82%	10%	8%	<.0001
n = 48				
Mild EH	26%	61%	13%	<.04
n = 23				
Moderate EH	22%	13%	65%	<.0001
n = 31				

Note: The number (*n*) of individuals correctly assigned to their particular group shown as percentage of *n* in each group.
n = number of subjects; WT*, average wall thickness indexed for BSA; LVID*, left ventricular internal diameter indexed for BSA; FS, fractional systolic shortening; E/A*, transmitral flow velocity ratio standardized by covariance to age 40 years. *p*, probability of significant between–group differences.

Source: Laufer et al. (1989), with permission of *Hypertension*, American Heart Association, and Lippincott, Williams and Wilkins.

normotensive mean, it may take months before any regression becomes detectable (Trimarco and Wikstrand, 1984; Korner et al., 1991; Dahlöf et al., 1992). This also occurs after aortic or mitral valve replacement (Dodge et al., 1974).

ACE inhibitors and AT_1 antagonists are said to be more effective in reducing LVMI compared to other antihypertensive drugs (Sen et al., 1977; Dahlöf and Hansson, 1992; Dahlöf et al., 1992; Devereux et al., 1994; Strauer et al., 1994). However, in more recent large trials the extent of the regression has been smaller than in the earlier studies (Jennings and Wong, 1997; Sheridan, 2000).

Intrinsic Mechanical Performance in LVH

In the in situ heart, contractile and pump properties are best assessed under steady-state controlled loading conditions (Sagawa, 1967; Van den Bos et al., 1973; Noresson et al., 1979; Broughton and Korner, 1980; Smolich et al., 1988a). Load is difficult to control adequately in intact animals and human subjects, which has encouraged investigators to search for "load-independent" indices of contractility. As with most holy grails, the search for such an index has proved illusory.

Isovolumetric Indices for Assessing Contractile Performance

About 80–90% of the ventricle's mechanical energy is developed during isovolumetric systole and the rest during ejection. Hence, the rate of change in LVP during isovolumetric contraction provides useful information about LV contractile properties. Three indices of contractility have been employed (figure 7.8) as follows:

- $(dP/dt)_{max}$ is the maximum rate of rise in LVP. It normally corresponds to activation of entire LV myocardium. If the aortic valve opens prematurely (e.g., at low BP), (dP/dt_{max}) no longer relates to tension development of the fully activated myocardium.
- $(dP/dt)_{DP40}$ is rate of rise in LVP at LVP of 40 mmHg above end-diastolic pressure. It occurs in early isovolumetric systole. It is never be affected by premature aortic valve opening (Mason et al., 1971). The index peaks long before maximum tension has developed.
- $(dP/dt/TP)_{max}$ is the maximum value of the ratio of [(dP/dt)/(instantaneous total LVP above atmospheric)]. It occurs early in isovolumetric systole and is lower when LAP is high (Broughton and Korner, 1980, 1983). It has been used to calculate contractile element velocity (Braunwald et al., 1967; Taylor et al., 1967), though the underlying assumptions have been disputed (Van den Bos et al., 1973). It is not an index of full myocardial activation.

Each index is affected load, but only $(dP/dt)_{max}$ is related to the full development of ventricular force; the indices $(dP/dt)_{DP40}$ and $(dP/dt/TP)_{max}$ occur earlier in isovolumetric systole and help in the interpretation of the significance of changes in $(dP/dt)_{max}$.

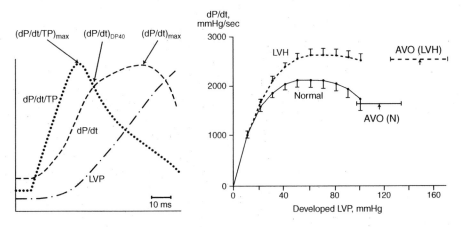

Figure 7.8. Left, left ventricular pressure (LVP, dot-dash line), rate of LVP rise (dP/dt, dashed line), and (dP/dt)/TP ratio (dotted line) during isovolumetric systole, where TP is total pressure above atmospheric. Arrows point to (from left): $(dP/dt/TP)_{max}$, (dP/dt_{DP40}), $(dP/dt)_{max}$. Right, relationship between developed LVP and dP/dt during isovolumetric systole (bars + 1 SEM of mean) from 9 normotensive (N) and 13 hypertensive LVH dogs (LVH). AVO, range of time of aortic valve opening in each group (arrow at mean). LAP constant at 15 mm-Hg, heart rate 150 bpm, autonomic blockade. From Broughton and Korner (1980, left), and (1983, right).

Intrinsic Properties

The experiments discussed below were performed in the in situ open chest dog heart preparation in which left atrial pressure (LAP), arterial BP, and heart rate were controlled independently during autonomic blockade, which eliminated BP-related reflexes (Broughton and Korner, 1980; Broughton, 1983). The preparation was used to compare the contractile properties of the LV of normal dogs with those with concentric LVH due to chronic renovascular hypertension (Broughton and Korner, 1983; Smolich et al., 1988b; Smolich, Weissberg, Friberg, Broughton et al., 1991).

In concentric LVH, basal $(dP/dt)_{max}$ is greater than in controls. Raising LAP while holding MAP and heart rate constant produced an increase in $(dP/dt)_{max}$ to a maximum at LAP ~20 mmHg (figure 7.9, top). At higher LAPs $(dP/dt)_{max}$ declined, which probably reflects inadequate coronary perfusion, since the descending limb was absent when MAP was allowed to rise.

The lower panel of figure 7.9 shows the effect of varying aortic diastolic BP (ADP) while LAP and heart rate remained constant: over the range of ADPs from 100 to 150 mmHg, $(dP/dt)_{max}$ remained unchanged in both normal and LVH dogs. In the LVH group, $(dP/dt)_{max}$ was 30–40% greater than in controls, which was approximately

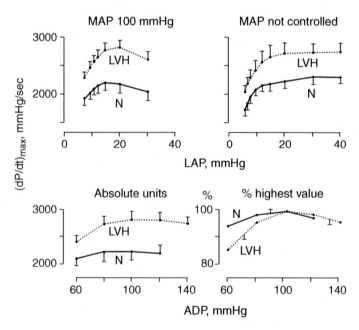

Figure 7.9. Upper panels: Effect of steady-state changes in left atrial pressure (LAP, mm-Hg) on $(dP/dt)_{max}$ in normal (N) and hypertensive LVH dogs; (left) mean arterial pressure (MAP) held at 100 mm-Hg; (right) MAP allowed to rise. Lower panels: (left) effect of step changes in aortic diastolic pressure (ADP, mmHg) on $(dP/dt)_{max}$ in N and LVH dogs; (right) results expressed as percentage of highest $(dP/dt)_{max}$; LAP, 15 mmHg. Heart rate 150 bpm and autonomic blockade in all groups. Adapted from Broughton and Korner (1983).

Table 7.4. Values of dP/dt_{max}, dP/dt_{DP40}, and $(dP/dt/TP)_{max}$ Measured at Aortic Diastolic BP (ADP) of 100 and 60 mmHg during Isovolumetric Systole in Normal and LVH Dogs

	Normal		LVH	
ADP, mmHg	100	60	100	60
dP/dt_{max}, mmHg/s	2200	2080	2800	2380*
	(100%)	(95%)	(100%)	(85%)*
dP/dt_{DP40}, mmHg/s	2020	2025	2500	2300*
	(100%)	(100%)	(100%)	(92)*
$(dP/dt/TP)_{max}$/s	46	46	47	44*
	(100%)	(100%)	(100%)	(94%)*

Notes: In both groups, LAP was held constant at 15 mmHg and heart paced at 150 bpm. Indices given in absolute units; percentages are value of each group at ADP 100 mmHg. *p < .05 for difference from value at 100 mmHg in the same group.

Source: Broughton and Korner (1983), with permission of *American Journal of Physiology* and American Physiological Society.

in proportion to the degree of LVH. It suggests close to normal contractile properties per gram of myocardium in LVH.

When ADP was reduced below 80–90 mmHg, it resulted in a decline in $(dP/dt)_{max}$ and in the early indices $(dP/dt)_{DP40}$ and $(dP/dt/TP)_{max}$ in LVH hearts (figure 7.9, bottom; table 7.4). This suggests myocardial depression. In contrast, in the normotensive controls there was a small reduction in $(dP/dt)_{max}$ while the early indices remained unchanged. Here there was no myocardial depression, but the reduction in $(dP/dt)_{max}$ suggests premature opening of the aortic valve.

Raising BP Does Not Increase Intrinsic Myocardial Contractility: There Is No Anrep Effect

The constancy of $(dP/dt)_{max}$ when ADP is raised from 100 to 150 mmHg (figure 7.9, bottom) is not in accord with the concept of homeometric regulation, also known as the Anrep effect (Sarnoff et al., 1960; Sarnoff and Mitchell, 1962). Acute elevation of BP was thought to increase intrinsic myocardial contractility in hypertension (Guyton and Coleman, 1967). However, most studies reporting such an increase have been in preparations with intact autonomic effectors and uncontrolled LV preload, in which the myocardium was often depressed prior to elevation of BP (Reeves et al., 1960; Wallace et al., 1963; Wildenthal et al., 1969; Monroe et al., 1972). The Anrep effect has not been observed under steady-state conditions in well-controlled preparations (Elzinga et al., 1977; Broughton and Korner, 1980, 1983; Smolich et al., 1988b).

Inotropic Stimulation

Stimulation of cardiac β-ARs with isoprenaline caused a four–fivefold increase in $(dP/dt)_{max}$ in the normal LV with heart rate held constant (figure 7.10).

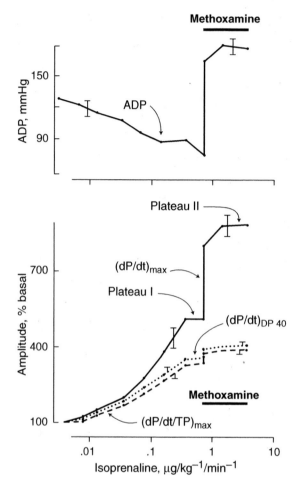

Figure 7.10. Effect of isoprenaline infusions (μg/kg/in) on (top) arterial diastolic pressure (ADP, mmHg); (bottom) $(dP/dt)_{max}$, $(dP/dt)_{DP40}$, and $(dP/dt/TP)_{max}$. After indices have stabilized, raising BP with methoxamine increases $(dP/dt)_{max}$ more than the other indices. Plateau I for $(dP/dt)_{max}$ is lower than plateau II because of early aortic valve opening at low BP. Data from Broughton and Korner (1980), with permission of *Cardiovascular Research* and Elsevier.

The accompanying fall in BP is due to the drug's peripheral vasodilator action on the skeletal muscle bed. After abolishing the hypotension by infusing the α_1-AR agonist methoxamine, $(dP/dt)_{max}$ increased further to 8–9 × basal. The drug has no cardiac inotropic effects and does not affect $(dP/dt)_{DP40}$, which excludes myocardial depression. Therefore the premature opening of the aortic valve at low arterial BP is what limits the initial $(dP/dt)_{max}$ response to isoprenaline.

With noradrenaline (NA) as the inotropic stimulus, the maximum increase in $(dP/dt)_{max}$ was 8–9 × basal in both normal and LVH hearts (figure 7.11). Absolute $(dP/dt)_{max}$ in LVH hearts was 30–40% greater than in controls, thus maintaining the difference observed at rest (Broughton and Korner, 1983). As long as myocardial blood supply is adequate, contractile function is normal in concentric hypertrophy.

Interestingly, in the LVH group dP/dt only exceeds the value in controls once iso-volumetric LVP has risen by 20–30 mmHg (figure 7.8, right). It suggests that in LVH

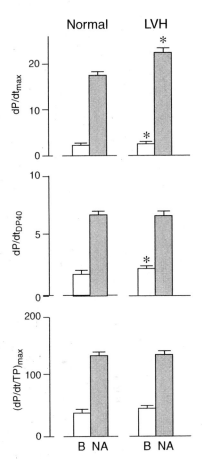

Figure 7.11. Effect of noradrenaline infusions (NA) in LVH and normal (N) dogs on $(dP/d)_{max}$, $(dP/dt)_{DP40}$ (mmHg/s $\times$ 1000^{-3}), and $(dP/dt/TP)_{max}$ (s^{-1}). B, basal; NA, maximum noradrenaline response (NA, 16 μg/kg/min). *$p <$ .05 for difference between the N and LVH groups. Adapted from Broughton (1983), Broughton and Korner (1983).

it takes longer to activate the myocardium and develop tension. This explains why during inotropic stimulation the increase in the early indices is smaller than in $(dP/dt)_{max}$.

LV Pump Performance Is Enhanced in Concentric LVH

Plots of end-systolic LVP versus end-systolic LV volume at different arterial BPs have shown that emptying of the LV is greater in LVH than in the normal heart (Smolich et al., 1988b). This accounts for the greater stroke volume in LVH at a given left atrial pressure (LAP) and constant heart rate in dogs and rats (Noresson et al., 1979; Broughton and Korner, 1986). This has been called the stroke volume amplifier.

Elzinga and Westerhof (1976) used the relationship between CO at constant heart rate and afterload in the isolated heart to quantify LV pump function. This has been used in autonomically blocked hypertensive dogs with LVH and in the isolated heart of SHR (figure 7.12; Noresson et al., 1979; Broughton and Korner, 1986). When LAP and heart rate are held constant, raising MAP results in a near-linear reduction in CO

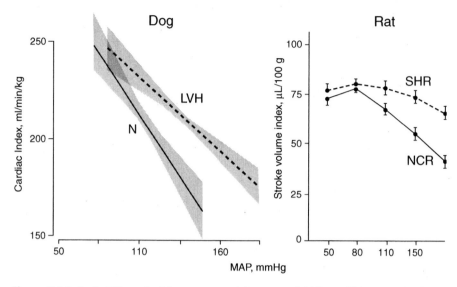

Figure 7.12. Left: Effect of raising mean arterial pressure (MAP, mmHg) on cardiac index (CI, mL/min/kg) in normal (N) and hypertensive LVH dogs (LAP 15 mmHg, heart rate 150 bpm, autonomic blockade; shading is + 1 SE). After Broughton and Korner (1985). Right: Rat isolated heart; effect of altering MAP on stroke volume index (μL/100 g body weight) in SHR and normal control rats (NCR). From Noresson et al. (1979).

(and stroke volume). The slope of the regression line is less steep in LVH, indicating that stroke volume is maintained better in this group than in that with normal LV.

Contractile and Pump Performance in EH

In persons with EH who have normal coronary arteries and concentric LVH, the LVMI is about 30% greater than in controls, with basal $(dP/dt)_{max}$ some 50% greater (figure 7.13; Strauer, 1979; Strauer et al., 1994). The greater difference in $(dP/dt)_{max}$ exceeds the rise found in automonically blocked dogs with LVH, in which the rise in $(dP/dt)_{max}$ was proportional to the degree of LVH. It suggests that in the patients with EH in whom there was an increase in cardiac SNA, intrinsic $(dP/dt)_{max}$ was probably close to normal.

In persons with EH, concentric LVH, and coronary disease, $(dP/dt)_{max}$ was still high, but there was some depression in ejection fraction (EF). Depression of EF becomes more pronounced with further LVH and dilation, which is considerably greater than the slight depression in $(dP/dt)_{max}$. EF is a valuable clinical test of pump performance, and its depression is usually associated with high LV end-diastolic pressure (Noble, 1977). Subjects with reduced EFs are close to heart failure; their markedly enhanced cardiac SNA boosts $(dP/dt)_{max}$ and masks the intrinsic depression of contractile function (Hasking et al., 1986).

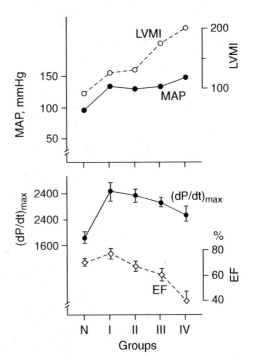

Figure 7.13. Data from normal human subjects (N) and three groups with EH: I, concentric LVH, no coronary disease; II, concentric LVH and obstruction of at least one major coronary artery; III, abnormal LV wall motion and coronary artery stenosis as in II; IV, more severe than III, with some LV failure. Scale on left refers to MAP (mmHg) and $(dP/dt)_{max}$, mmHg/sec (solid lines); scale on right refers to LV mass index, LVMI, g/m^2 BSA (determined by ventriculography) and ejection fraction, EF (percentage of normal, dashed lines). After Strauer (1979), with permission of *American Journal of Cardiology* and Elsevier.

A continuing increase in LV mass in subjects with hypertension and coronary disease is a grave prognostic sign (Frohlich and Pfeffer, 1989; Levy et al., 1990). What remains uncertain is the prognosis in the Group II subjects in figure 7.13.

Last, in eccentric LVH the pathways for myocardial excitation and repolarization are more dispersed than normal. This increases the probability of developing arrhythmias, particularly if cardiac SNA is high (Mayet et al., 1996; Topol, 1998).

Coronary and Myocyte Factors

Coronary inflow of blood into the LV myocardium occurs largely during diastole (Gregg, 1950; Marcus, 1983; Olsson and Bugni, 1986). In the RV, about half the coronary flow is in systole and half in diastole, as in other regional beds. Soon after birth, the number of LV myocardial capillaries becomes fixed (Hudlicka et al., 1992).

It has been suggested that during LV contraction the high tissue pressure during systole compresses the coronary arteries. Hoffman and Spaan (1990) found little evidence of this, but noted that the compression of intramural veins produced phasic changes in tissue blood volume. Possibly this could affect mitochondrial pO_2, which must be at least 2 mmHg for normal aerobic metabolism (Honig and Bourdeau-Martini, 1974).

About 40% of myocardial O_2 consumption (MV_{O2}) is used for generating tension during contraction, most of it during isovolumetric systole (Suga, 1990). The remainder is due to baseline metabolism, heat production, and the energy required for cellular transport processes. An increase in inotropic state elevates MV_{O2} (Feigl, 1983; Marcus, 1983).

Coronary Dilator Capacity

In hypertension, the structural R_1 vessel changes are similar to those in other beds (Strauer, 1979; Marcus, 1983; Friberg et al., 1985; Thybo et al., 1994). In LVH the dilatation of R_2 arterioles offsets the enhancement of constrictor tone, but at the cost of some reduction in the bed's capacity for further dilatation (figure 7.14; Strauer et al., 1994).[5] In uncomplicated EH the dilator reserve is reduced, and becomes further reduced by stenosis of the coronary arteries.

Once myocyte enlargement is too great or coronary blood flow too low for mitochondrial pO_2 to be maintained, ATP synthesis is depressed. This is associated with a decline in the LV's capacity to generate tension. Linzbach (1960) first proposed that at a critical level of myocyte hypertrophy of 70% or more, the large distance between capillaries would create diffusion difficulties. Linzbach's idea of a critical hypertrophy has held up well in both animals and humans. With the above degree of increase in LVMI there often is LV dilation, myocardial fibrosis, and clinical heart failure.

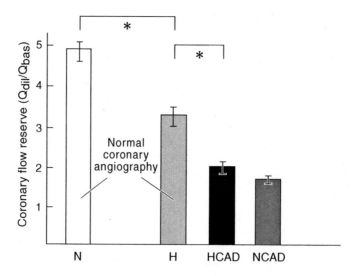

Figure 7.14. Coronary blood flow reserve is flow (Q) at maximum vasodilation divided by basal Q. Graph shows (1) normotensives with normal coronaries (N) and with coronary obstruction (NCAD); (2) hypertensives with normal coronaries (H) and with coronary obstruction (HCAD). *$p < .01$ for difference between groups. Redrawn from Strauer et al. (1994), with permission of Blackwell.

Transmural Coronary Blood Flow Distribution in LVH

Using the radioactive microsphere method in the in situ dog heart, Smolich, Weissberg, Friberg, Broughton et al. (1991) found that average myocardial blood flow was greater in hypertensive LVH than in normal dogs (figure 7.15). At ADP of 120 mmHg, the difference is most pronounced in the inner myocardial layers where circumferential stress is greatest (Grossman et al., 1975; Mirsky, 1979). It suggests that myocyte hypertrophy is greatest in the inner parts of the wall, as observed in other types of LVH (Hittinger et al., 1995; Iwase et al., 1996).[6]

When ADP was reduced from 140 to 100 mmHg, both LV workload and blood flow declined in each group (figure 7.15), while $(dP/dt)_{max}$ remained unchanged. This indicates that the myocardial O_2 supply was adequate at each workload. However, when ADP was lowered further to 80 and 60 mmHg, the reduction of blood flow was greater in the inner layers of the LVH compared to the normal heart (figure 7.15). Moreover, all the isovolumetric indices were depressed, which suggests an inadequate coronary O_2 supply (table 7.4). In the normal heart, ADP had to be reduced to about 30 mmHg before myocardial function became depressed (Broughton and Korner, 1983; Smolich et al., 1988a; Smolich, Weissberg, Friberg, Broughton et al., 1991).

The lower limit of the myogenic autoregulatory range increases in hypertension in proportion to the rise in resting BP (figure 6.9). In the coronary vasculature, this is best demonstrated in the RV, in which the R_1 vessel structural changes are similar to those supplying the LV, but the RV workload is virtually unaffected by the systemic BP (Tomanek et al., 1985; Wicker and Tarazi, 1985; Smolich, Weissberg, Friberg, and Korner, 1991). In the normal heart the myogenic response maintains RV blood flow unchanged between 120 and 60 mmHg, while in LVH RV blood flow begins to decline below 90–100 mmHg (Smolich, Weissberg, Friberg, and Korner, 1991).

Lowering BP in hypertensive humans and rats sometimes elicits myocardial depression and ECG abnormalities (Yagil et al., 1982; Friberg and Nordlander, 1986; Shimamatsu and Fouad-Tarazi, 1986; Pepi et al., 1988). This has raised concerns about precipitating myocardial ischemia by too great a therapeutic reduction in BP (Cruickshank et al., 1987; Cruickshank, 1988). However, clinical trials provide little support for this concern (Berglund et al., 1989; MacMahon, 1994). It may be that antihypertensive treatment quickly restores the BP limit of the myogenic response to normal.

Myocyte Hypertrophy and LV Structure and Function

In hypertension, adequacy of LV contractile activity and pump performance is more dependent on inotropic stimulation or the Frank-Starling mechanism than the normal heart (Feigl, 1983; Marcus, 1983). In the dilated LV, circumferential stress is greater, myocyte hypertrophy increases further, and repeated inadequacy of the coronary blood supply causes enhanced myocardial fibrosis (Pfeffer, Pfeffer, Fletcher et al., 1979; Engelmann et al., 1987; Capasso et al., 1990).

In SHR, the degree of LVH increases from birth until about 24 weeks of age (Hallbäck-Nordlander, 1980; Friberg and Nordlander, 1990; Korner et al., 1993). This is associated with an increase in LV force-generating capacity (figure 7.16; Pfeffer, Pfeffer, Fletcher et al., 1979; Pfeffer, Pfeffer, Fishbein et al., 1979; Pfeffer and Pfeffer, 1985).

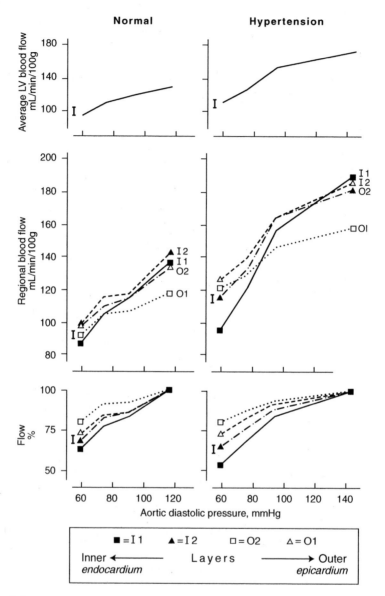

Figure 7.15. Effect of reducing aortic diastolic BP (mmHg) on LV blood flow (mL/min/100 g) in open-chest normal dogs (left) and hypertensive LVH dogs (right; constant LAP, heart rate, and autonomic blockade). Variables from above: (1) average LV myocardial blood flow; (2) blood flow in inner layers I1, I2, and outer layers O2, O1; (3) blood flow in the four layers expressed as percentage of initial value at highest BP. Redrawn from Smolich, Weissberg, Friberg, Broughton et al. (1991), with permission of *Hypertension*, American Heart Association, and Lippincott, Williams and Wilkins.

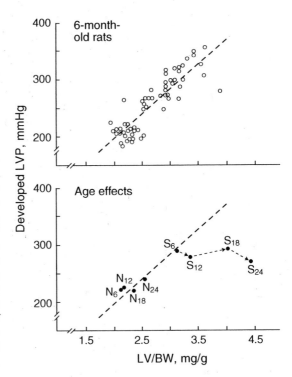

Figure 7.16. Top, relationship between peak LV pressure (LVP, mmHg) and LV weight/body weight ratio (LV/BW, mg/g) in 6-month-old rats, including WKY, SHR, and Dahl-S rats. Bottom, relation between peak LVP and LV/BW in normotensive WKY rats (N) and SHR (S) aged 6, 12, 18, and 24 months, as indicated in subscripts. Regression line (dashed line) from top graph has been superimposed and shows that in SHR over 6 months of age the increase in LV/BW no longer reflects the LVP-generating capacity found in younger rats in top graph. From Pfeffer and Pfeffer (1985), with permission of *Journal of Cardiovascular Pharmacology* and Lippincott, Williams and Wilkins.

LV dilation generally develops by the ages of 6–12 months, when LV force-generating capacity no longer keeps pace with continuing myocyte hypertrophy.

Focal myocardial necrosis and fibrosis develop once the critical myocyte volume of about 70% has been reached. The subepicardial wall layers are often affected first, despite the relatively low magnitude of circumferential stress in this region (Engelmann et al., 1987). The damage is a consequence of a coronary steal syndrome, where the hardest-working inner layer maintains its blood supply by drawing on that of the less active outer layer (figure 6.11). Apoptosis may play a role in the reduction of subepicardial myocytes (Hamet et al., 1995). However, in time focal myocyte necrosis and fibrosis develop in all layers (Rakusan et al., 1984; Engelmann et al., 1987; Capasso et al., 1990).

Cellular Mechanisms in Cardiac Hypertrophy

Physiological hypertrophy includes mainly age- and sex-related changes, while pathological hypertrophy is the result of pressure or volume overload.

Physiological Hypertrophy of Cardiac Myocytes

At birth, the cardiac myocytes are small and immature. In humans the capacity for myocyte proliferation is lost by 6–12 months, while in rats this occurs by 2–3 weeks

(Zak, 1974; Bugaisky et al., 1992; Hudlicka et al., 1992). From then on, growth is mediated solely through cell enlargement.[7]

In rats, a second nucleus develops in most myocytes over the first few months of life (Oparil et al., 1984). In humans, only 10–15% of myocytes are binucleate, while a high proportion are polyploidal. These changes are adaptations to the high levels of transcriptional activity required for synthesis of myocardial proteins at this time of life (Morgan et al., 1992).

From childhood to early adult life, LV and body growth rates are similar (Adams et al., 1989). In young adults, myocyte volume is about 10–20 times that at birth (Zak, 1974). Just under half the cell volume consists of myofibrils, while mitochondria occupy one third. The rest consists of SR, nucleus, and cytosol. The SR has longitudinal and transverse tubules that help bring about the almost synchronous activation of myofibrils after excitation of the sarcolemma. From then on, myocytes slowly increase in size throughout life.

Early in life, thyroid hormone, growth hormone (GH), adrenal steroids and sex hormones, insulin, and insulinlike growth factors (IGFs) all contribute to growth and differentiation and to the switching of isoforms of several myocardial proteins from fetal to adult types (Zak, 1974; Bugaisky et al., 1992; Hudlicka et al., 1992).

Thyroid hormone maintains myocyte integrity throughout life (Page and McCallister, 1973; Friberg et al., 1985). It plays a role in switching expression of contractile protein isoforms, for example, during exercise training (Rupp and Jacob, 1982; Rupp et al., 1984; Friberg et al., 1989).

GH mediates some of its effects through insulin, IGFs, and glucagon. It matches overall cardiac growth to that of the body. The link is apparent in genetically GH-deficient rats, in which lower body growth and heart growth are reduced in the same proportion, so that the heart weight/body weight ratio (HW/BW) ratio remains normal (Harrap et al., 1994). Conversely, in rats receiving GH injections, or in transgenic mice where GH is overexpressed in peripheral organs, body weight and heart weight increase in parallel without change in the HW/BW ratio (Harrap et al., 1988; Dilley and Schwartz, 1989). The extra growth is associated with elevation in CO and blood flow but no change in BP. This contrasts with human acromegaly, where hypertension is common (Cohen, 1974; Penney et al., 1985).

Changes in myocyte function associated with aging include a slow increase in cell length with the addition of sarcomeres at the end of each myocyte and gradual deterioration of contractile function (Fraticelli et al., 1989; Folkow and Svanborg, 1993; Lakatta, 1993). Similar pathological changes occur in heart failure (Gerdes et al., 1996). In old age, there is increased expression of fetal isoforms of many proteins, particularly in regions subjected to the greatest mechanical load (Eisenberg et al., 1985). Ventricular diastolic function alters due to impairment of the SR Ca^{2+} pump, which slows relaxation (Pfeffer, Pfeffer, Fishbein et al., 1979; Lundin et al., 1983; Friberg and Nordlander, 1990).

Pathological LV Hypertrophy

The subdivision into pressure and volume overload emphasizes the importance of hemodynamic signals, but other factors are also involved. The degree of LVH is usually greater in severe pressure overload than in volume overload (Olivetti et al., 1989).

Much information about pressure overload hypertrophy comes from loads of acute onset, such as 2K-1C hypertension or aortic banding. Synthesis of myocardial proteins and organelles starts within hours after the onset of overload (Page and McCallister, 1973; Morgan et al., 1992). The LV/BW ratio has increased within days, reaching a maximum in 2–3 weeks (Folkow et al., 1977; Folkow, 1978). In contrast, the rise in mechanical load and the LVH response in EH develop far more gradually.

Myocyte protein turnover is normally high, so that extra ribosomes are required in LVH for protein synthesis (Larson et al., 1993; Hannan et al., 1995; Luyken et al., 1996). The next priority is increased formation of new mitochondria, followed after 2–3 weeks by synthesis of myofibrillar proteins (Meerson et al., 1964; Page and McCallister, 1973; Meerson, 1974; Taylor et al., 1974; Ferrans and Rodriguez, 1987). Intercalated disk junctions also enlarge and new disks may develop in extensive hypertrophy (Yamamoto et al., 1996). There is increased expression of fetal isoforms of myosin light chain, skeletal muscle α-actin, and atrial and brain natriuretic peptides (ANP, b-NP; Chien et al., 1993; Murphy, 1996; Ohta et al., 1996).

The enlarged myocytes are of normal appearance (Taylor et al., 1974). Myofilaments, cytoskeletal structures, and extracellular collagen all increase in the same proportions as in the normal heart (Wikman-Coffelt et al., 1979; Ferrans and Rodriguez, 1987; Bugaisky et al., 1992; Hudlicka et al., 1992). Focal disorganization is a late development.

Intrinsic myocardial function is initially normal, with normal cross-bridge cycling rates, net Ca^{2+} fluxes, and ATP synthesis. When some of these intrinsic processes eventually become depressed, other mechanisms, notably sympathetic stimulation, may compensate for a substantial period (Gomez et al., 1997). In human cardiac failure, there is depression of the SR calcium-release channel, which is partly compensated through greater expression and activity of the Na^+-Ca^{2+} exchanger (Hasenfuss et al., 1994; Studer et al., 1994).

Regulatory Factors

In cardiac hypertrophy, there is enlargement of individual myocytes through parallel deposition of sarcomeres. The initial neurohumoral causes of EH produce LVH partly through the mechanical stimuli associated with pressure and volume overload, but there seems little doubt that the profile of neurohumoral stimuli itself affects the recruitment of growth factors that are mobilized in the tissues.

Mechanical Stimuli

Stretching cultured cardiac myocytes causes expression of myofibrillar proteins, ANP, and fetal MHC isoforms (Chien et al., 1993; Komuro and Yazaki, 1993). Stretch enhances the production of both local growth promoters (Ang II, ET-1, PDGFs) and growth inhibitors (NO, prostacyclins; Baker et al., 1992; Weber et al., 1994; Booz and Baker, 1996; Fareh et al., 1996; Sakai et al., 1996; Li and Brooks, 1997; Sadoshima and Izumo, 1997). Ang II promotes growth through stimulation of AT_1 receptors but also inhibits growth through stimulation of AT_2 receptors (Booz and Baker, 1996). As noted in chapter 6, even when average circumferential stress has been restored there remains a gradient across the wall, with the stress greatest along the inner layers where myocyte hypertrophy is most pronounced (Hittinger et al., 1995; Iwase et al., 1996; Mirsky, 1979).

Pressure overload mobilizes the local renin-angiotensin system, but there are alternative pathways. For example, in transgenic animals in which AT_1 receptors have been disrupted, the LVH develops in response to aortic banding even though these receptors are normally involved in the response (Harada et al., 1998).

LVH is greater in the presence of coronary disease (figure 7.13) since hypoxia lowers the threshold for the expression of the various factors involved. What is less clear is how eutrophic remodeling of the LV comes about. The most likely explanation is that during hypertrophy the net expansion of the myocyte mass is almost entirely in an inward direction, so that the WT/RI ratio can increase with a minimal increase in LV mass, as discussed in relation to figure 6.21.

Stimulation of ARs and Other G-Protein-Coupled Receptors

In cell culture studies, stimulation of α-ARs in the absence of mechanical stimuli produces myocyte hypertrophy (Simpson, 1983, 1985; Graham et al., 1996). Under in vivo conditions, the role of α-ARs on the heart is confounded by the peripheral vasoconstriction and elevation of BP which they induce.

ARs exist in two conformations, an inactive R form and an active R* form (Koch et al., 1996). When the agonist binds to R*, there is an increase in the proportion of receptors in the R* conformation. This also occurs when ARs are overexpressed, when effector activity may increase even in the absence of the agonist; for example, basal contractile activity increases when β_2-ARs are overexpressed (Koch et al., 1996).[8]

There are at least two α_1-AR subtypes, α_{1A} and α_{1B} (see Graham et al., 1996). In transgenic mice, overexpression of cardiac α_{1B}-ARs increases the proportion of receptors in the R* conformation, enhancing activity in the G_q protein-PLC pathway and giving rise to LVH without a rise in BP (Koch et al., 1996). LVH also occurs in spontaneous mutants in which cardiac α_{1B}-ARs are overexpressed. Similar LVH has been observed in transgenic mice with overexpression of myocardial AT_1 receptors (Hein et al., 1997). Both receptors couple to G_q proteins and activate the PLC pathway.

Multiple signaling pathways are the rule for the in vivo production of LVH. Uncoupling the connection between receptor and G_q protein in transgenic mice eliminates the cellular responses mediated through α_1-ARs, AT_1, and ET_A receptors and reduces the myocyte's diacetyl glycerol concentration (Akhter et al., 1998). However, basal LV/BW ratio is similar to that of the wild type (figure 7.17), which suggests that myocyte size is maintained through other pathways. However, the LVH response to aortic banding is markedly attenuated, indicating that the G_q-PLC pathway is essential for the full LVH response.

Experimental elevation of plasma Ang II causes LVH and myocyte hypertrophy, which also occurs when adding Ang II in culture, with attenuation of both responses by AT_1 antagonists (Baker et al., 1992; Lever and Harrap, 1992; Everett et al., 1994). Ang II binds to AT_1 and AT_2 receptors, which couple to other signaling pathways as well as to the G_q-PLC pathway (Sadoshima and Izumo, 1993b; Sadoshima et al., 1995). The angiotensinogen gene is upregulated in myocytes during mechanical stimulation, or when stimulated by glucocorticoids, thyroid hormone, and estrogens (Baker et al., 1992).

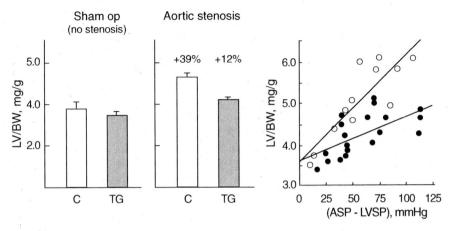

Figure 7.17. Mean LV/body weight ratios (LV/BW, mg/g) in control mice (C, open rectangles, open circles), and in transgenic mice (TG; gray rectangles, closed circles) with cardiac-specific disruption of receptor connection with Gq proteins. Left, after sham operation, LV/BW similar in C and TG mice, indicating that resting LV mass is maintained through other pathways. Middle, in aortic stenosis, LV/BW in C increased by 39%, but by only 12% in TG mice. Right, LV/BW is a function of systolic pressure gradient across aortic valve (ASP-LVSP, aortic systolic – LV systolic BP). Note steeper slope in C versus TG mice. From Akhter et al. (1998), with permission of American Association for the Advancement of Science.

The tissue conversion of Ang I to Ang II is carried out by ACE in some species, but by the enzyme chymase in others (Urata, Kinoshita et al., 1990; Urata et al., 1993; Liao and Husain, 1995; Wolny et al., 1997). Chymase is a serine protease that is located in cells of the myocardial interstitium including the mast cells, while ACE is present in normal amounts in endothelium.

Determinants of Expression of Master Genes for Hypertrophy

Figure 7.18 indicates schematically some of the factors that produce the coordinated synthesis of the myofibrillar and other muscle proteins in hypertrophy (Engelmann et al., 1989, 1993; Hudlicka et al., 1992; Schneider and Parker, 1992; Chien et al., 1993; Komuro and Yazaki, 1993; Sadoshima and Izumo., 1993a, 1993b; Brand and Schneider, 1996; Sadoshima and Izumo, 1997; Sadoshima et al., 1997; Sugden and Clerk, 1998; Olson and Molkentin, 1999; Sugden, 1999). Molkentin et al. (1998) suggested that a key step in the hypertrophy response is prolonged elevation of cytosolic Ca^{2+}, which, through a pathway including PKC, Ras, and a MAP kinase, activates the phosphatase calcineurin. In turn, calcineurin dephosphorylates the transcription factor $NFAT_3$ so that it can move into the nucleus, in which it causes expression of the genes for myocyte hypertrophy in conjunction with the transcription factor GATA4 and possibly others (Molkentin and Olson, 1997). In transgenic mice in which calcineurin is expressed throughout the heart, hypertrophy affects all the chambers and includes the full complement of myofilaments, regulatory proteins, cytoskeletal proteins, ANF, and so on (Molkentin et al., 1998; Molkentin, 2000). Calcineurin is inhibited by the

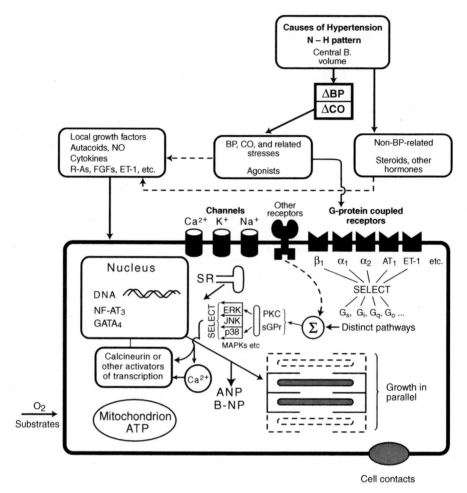

Figure 7.18. Functional neurohumoral (N-H) factors determine profile of local growth factors, autacoids, cytokines, and so on, which have hemodynamic and nonhemodynamic actions on myocytes. Myocyte enlargement requires activation of several signaling pathways including PKC (phosphokinase C) and small G proteins (e.g., Ras), which activate various MAP kinases such as ERK and JNK. This increases cytosolic Ca^{2+} and activates calcineurin and other factors, which allow transcription factors NF-AT$_3$ to enter the nucleus, causing hypertrophy in conjunction with GATA$_4$. Hypertrophy is through parallel addition of sarcomeres and an increase in other myocardial proteins, for example, atrial and brain natriuretic peptides (ANP, B-NP). SR, sarcoplasmic reticulum.

immunosuppressive drug cyclosporin A, which attenuates calcineurin-mediated hypertrophy.

For a short time it looked as though calcineurin might be the key to hypertrophy. However, it now appears that it is not essential in many types of hypertrophy. For instance, calcineurin has no effect on LVH in SHR or on LVH due to aortic banding

(Ding et al., 1999; Zhang et al., 1999). The calcineurin mechanism appears to be only one of several signaling pathways (figure 7.18; Olson and Molkentin, 1999; Sugden 1999).

Hypertension is one important side effect of cyclosporin A, which is administered for immunosuppressive action after cardiac transplantation. The elevation in BP almost always accompanies the immunosuppressive regimen, as observed in a study in which LV geometry was measured for 12 months after cardiac transplantation (Leenen et al., 1991). The hypertension was of mild to moderate degree despite antihypertensive treatment, but LVMI and WT decreased after the operation and there was no LVH at any time. The absence of LVH was thought to be due to the cardiac sympathetic denervation of the transplanted heart, but it could also be due to cyclosporin-induced inhibition of calcineurin.

Nonmyocyte Cells

While there are about twice as many nonmyocyte cells in the heart as there are myocytes, they only occupy 25–30% of the tissue volume (Weber and Brilla, 1991; Weber et al., 1994). The cells include fibroblasts, mast cells, macrophages, endocardial cells, and cells associated with the coronary vasculature. Fibroblasts secrete collagen into the extracellular matrix, which contains collagenases that degrade collagen as well as molecules that prevent degradation (Cleutjens, 1996).

There is linkage between type I and type III fibrillar collagen and the myocyte cytoskeleton, which contributes to the tissue's rigidity (Weber and Brilla, 1991; Cleutjens, 1996). The basement membranes of subendocardial myocytes have a backbone of type IV and type V collagen. Type VI collagen is largely extracellular and links the myocytes to extracellular tissue and adjoining cells, which helps to align sarcomeres within adjoining muscle bundles (Streeter, 1979; Ganote and Armstrong, 1993).

With a chronic increase in LV load, the collagen volume increases in parallel with myocyte enlargement (Keeley et al., 1991). When myocyte volume has increased by about 60–70%, the growth of fibrous tissue increases disproportionately and is most prominent near myocytes that have died (Weber and Brilla, 1991; Weber et al., 1994).

In culture, the same hormones and transmitters that elicit myocyte hypertrophy also induce proliferation of fibroblasts (e.g., Ang II, NA, mechanical stretch; Sadoshima et al., 1992, 1997; Sadoshima and Izumo, 1993a). Given that in the early stages of hypertrophy in vivo there is little early proliferation of fibroblasts, it suggests that at this time there may be factors inhibiting collagen secretion. Later, other signals come into play and promote proliferation of fibroblasts. These include protein serine/threonine kinases, known as stress-activated protein kinases; their activity increases after tissue damage (Force et al., 1996).

In experimental hypertension, high levels of aldosterone or other mineralocorticoids promote fibrosis, while spironolactone reduces this response (Weber et al., 1994). ACE inhibitors prevent collagen deposition, probably by increasing tissue bradykinin. They also partially reverse established fibrosis, as do calcium antagonists (Motz and Strauer, 1989; Eghbali et al., 1991; Keeley et al., 1991; Nicoletti et al., 1995; Ohta et al., 1996). Whether these drugs produce adequate inhibition of chymase in human LVH remains to be determined (Liao and Husain, 1995).

How the Heart Maintains Contractile Performance

There is a remarkable difference in physiological properties between cardiac and skeletal muscle, even though in both contraction is mediated through the interaction of actin and myosin. Skeletal muscle is activated more rapidly and its strength of contraction largely depends on the number of muscle fibers recruited by its motor innervation. Cardiac muscle has the same morphological appearance, but activation of the LV myocardium is slow, all muscle fibers are engaged at every beat, and its syncytial properties ensure synchronous coordinated contraction in response to rhythm generation by the cardiac pacemakers. Neural effector activity modulates this rhythm and does not initiate contraction as in skeletal muscle. The sympathetic nerves are the most important source of inotropic support through release of NA, while the chronotropic effects are mediated through the actions of both sympathetic and vagus nerves on the cardiac pacemakers.

In light of the above, it is clear that the contractile properties of cardiac and skeletal muscle are vastly different, notwithstanding all attempts to characterize them in the same way (Sonnenblick, 1962; Braunwald and Ross, 1979; Brutsaert and Paulus, 1979). Moreover, the hope of finding a load-independent index of contractility is a fantasy, since load is a major determinant of intrinsic myocardial contractility. Isovolumetric $(dP/dt)_{max}$ appears the best available index for characterizing ventricular contractile performance. In humans, the interpretation of the significance of a change has to draw on the results obtained in more controllable animal models.

In EH, cardiac contractile performance has to increase to match the progressive elevation of BP and TPR. This occurs through (1) sympathetic elevation of heart rate and inotropic support; (2) enhanced systolic emptying of the LV; (3) enhancement of filling pressure associated with elevation of central blood volume; and (4) development of LVH. In addition, vagal activity is reduced reflexly, as cardiopulmonary load increases (see chapter 9).

The first two are the main factors that enhance LV contractile performance in mild EH. In more severe EH, the development of LVH with normal contractile properties is the equivalent of additional inotropic support. LVH increases gradually over several years, with the slow progression suggesting only slight preponderance of growth-promoting signals over those inhibiting growth. About 40–50% of persons with mild EH have LVH, with the proportion rising to 100% in more severe grades of EH. In lean individuals the dominant pattern is concentric LVH or remodeling, though eventually eccentric changes develop as myocardial function deteriorates. In obese hypertensives, eccentric changes are already present in mild EH.

Cardiac performance depends on the coronary circulation's capacity to meet the LV's wide range of O_2 requirements, despite the structural and functional changes in its R_1 vessels and the impaired ascending vasodilation response (chapter 6). R_2 vessel dilation helps maintain coronary blood flow at rest and during moderate exercise. As myocardial hypoxia increases myocyte hypertrophy is enhanced, thus compounding the problem of O_2 supply. When myocyte size has increased by about 70%, coronary steal syndromes become a regular event. At first this may occur only transiently and rarely. As the frequency of steal syndrome increases, the result is considerable permanent focal damage, with depression of overall contractile performance. The heart comes to rely increasingly on the Frank-Starling mechanism for maintaining CO. This results in increasing LV dilation, more LVH, and cardiac failure.

In conclusion, the elevation of cardiac SNA in mild EH is part of the defense response. It helps the heart to maintain stroke output against the raised BP. Most persons with mild EH are likely to have some degree of LVH, but the effects on the myocardium are probably not uniform (Safar et al., 1979) and may be hard to detect. The subsequent progressive increase in LVH suggests that it is not the myocardium that limits cardiac performance, but the coronary vasculature. Gradual cardiac deterioration is a consequence of microcirculatory rarefaction after repeated exposures to steal syndromes in a metabolically active organ.

PART V

INTEGRATIVE ASPECTS OF NEURAL CIRCULATORY CONTROL

8

CNS Cardiovascular Pathways: Role of Fast and Slow Transmitters

The first part of this chapter gives a brief account of the cardiovascular pathways of the CNS, which were referred to briefly in chapter 2. However, the main aim is to provide an introductory framework for understanding the cardiovascular role of the fast and slow transmitter neurons.

As mentioned in chapter 2, the CNS endows the circulatory control system with adaptive properties, allowing it to alter its regulatory parameters under appropriate circumstances. For example, repeated aversive stimuli applied to the tail of the sea snail *Aplysia* strengthen the synapses by which it withdraws its gills in response to light touch. A serotonergic (5-HT) slow transmitter neuron plays a crucial role in this process of synaptic strengthening, which is called sensitization (Kandel, 2001). It is envisaged that a similar process strengthens synapses subserving the defense response to stress in persons genetically susceptible to EH, and it is important to know which neurons mediate these responses.

All the major cardiovascular effector responses in the CNS are mediated through neurons that release fast transmitters at their endings, such as glutamate. The responsiveness of the fast transmitter neurons is modulated by other neurons that release slow transmitters, such as monoamines. The slow transmitter neurons are interneurons that convey information between the various integrative sites and are thus closely involved in the tranformation of inputs to outputs. The modulatory action of some of the NA neurons is accentuated by the biotransformation of α-methyldopa within these neurons. α-Methyldopa is a well known centrally acting antihypertensive drug, and its action illustrates the importance of these modulatory mechanisms in the regulation of BP.

CNS Cardiovascular Pathways

Neurons are deemed to be "cardiovascular" if circulatory responses are evoked by localized stimulation or lesions, or if the neurons respond to changes in BP or to stimulation of arterial or cardiopulmonary baroreceptors.[1]

Autonomic Outputs and Bulbospinal Centers

The autonomic outputs include the parasympathetic cardiac vagal motoneurons, the sympathetic preganglionic motoneurons to the heart, to the various peripheral beds and to the adrenal medulla (figure 2.5). The vagal motoneurons are located in the nucleus ambiguus and the dorsal vagal motor nucleus of the medulla and innervate the heart and coronary vessels.

The sympathetic preganglionic motoneurons are located in the intermediolateral nucleus (IML) of the thoracolumbar segments of the spinal cord (Petras and Cummings, 1972). Their axons project to the sympathetic ganglia, from which the postganglionic nerves innervate the heart and the resistance vessels of various regional beds. The cells of the adrenal medulla are innervated directly by fibers from IML sympathetic motoneurons.

Integrative activity takes place at all levels of the neuraxis, including the spinal motoneurons and the premotor neurons of the rostral and caudal ventrolateral medulla (RVLM), the rostral ventromedial medulla, the caudal raphe nuclei, the hypothalamic paraventricular nucleus (PVN) and other hypothalamic nuclei, the midbrain periaqueductal gray region, and several others. Premotor neurons are defined on the basis of having at least some direct monosynaptic connections with the spinal motoneurons, but all premotor neurons also make polysynaptic connections with the latter (Dampney, 1994a). Higher centers such as the thalamus, cortex, and limbic regions play important roles in cardiovascular regulation. Their role has not been given as much weight as that of the hindbrain region involved in baroreflexes.

The RVLM neurons are an important source of normal resting sympathetic tone (Dampney, 1994a, 1994b). They receive afferent projections from many sources including projections from the arterial and cardiopulmonary baroreceptors, respiratory receptors, and many others. Their afferents synapse in the nucleus tractus solitarii (NTS), and their projections reach RVLM via the caudal ventrolateral medulla (Chalmers and Pilowsky, 1991; Chalmers, 1998; Blessing, 1997). However, resting sympathetic tone also comes from sources above the pons, and from hypothalamic nuclei, various hindbrain and midbrain centers, and many regions from forebrain and cerebellum, which synapse in RLVM neurons (Richter and Spyer, 1990; Dampney, 1994a; Pilowsky, 1995).[2]

Forebrain, Diencephalon, Midbrain, and Cerebellum

The responses to virtually all circulatory disturbances depend on the integrative activity in several neuron groups in different parts of the brain. This has been demonstrated by labeling neurons with Fos, the protein product of the c-*fos* gene, which is expressed soon after excitation of a particular neuron (Dampney and Horiuchi, 2003).

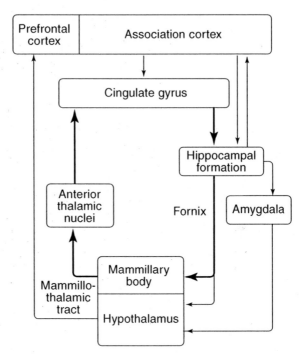

Figure 8.1. Main brain regions in neural circuit for emotion. The thick lines are the circuit originally proposed by Papez (1937), while more recent additions are shown as fine lines. The hippocampal formation is the hippocampus, entorhinal cortex, and subiculum. From Kupferman (1991), with permission of McGraw-Hill, New York.

The cortex exerts both excitatory and inhibitory influences on subcortical centers. For example, the primary motor cortex is the source of widespread autonomic excitation at the start of exercise (Clarke et al., 1968). Inhibitory influences play a role in matching and modulating the neural outputs in response to sensory stimuli. Their importance is dramatically illustrated in the "thalamic" preparation in which the neocortex and rhinencephalon have been removed. In thalamic animals, a mildly painful stimulus, a sudden touch or noise, often evokes a so-called sham rage response:[3] The animal arches its back, hisses and snarls and moves, while its pupils dilate and BP and heart rate increase (Cannon and Britton, 1925; Bard, 1928; Bard and Mountcastle, 1948; Korner et al., 1969). Sham rage illustrates that forebrain structures normally restrain excessive subcortical responses to mild stimuli. The major sources of inhibition are the orbitoinsular cortex, the anterior temporal cortex, and the cingulate gyrus (Kennard, 1945; Wall and Davis, 1951; Wall and Pribram, 1951; Löfving, 1961; Hoff et al., 1963; Folkow and Neil, 1971; Smith and DeVito, 1984; Folkow, 1987; Cechetto and Saper, 1990). Stimulation of these regions inhibits sympathetic activity and often somatic movement. These inhibitory systems have become particularly powerful in primates in conjunction with their massive forebrain development (see chapters 11, 14). Their role may be very important in affective regulation.

James Papez (1937) was the first to propose a neural circuit for expressing emotions. It includes regions of the neocortex, limbic system, and hypothalamus (figure 8.1). The limbic system includes the phylogenetically primitive cortex around the upper part of the brainstem, that is, the cingulate gyrus, subcallosal gyrus, the hippocampal formation, amygdala, septum, nucleus accumbens (which is part of

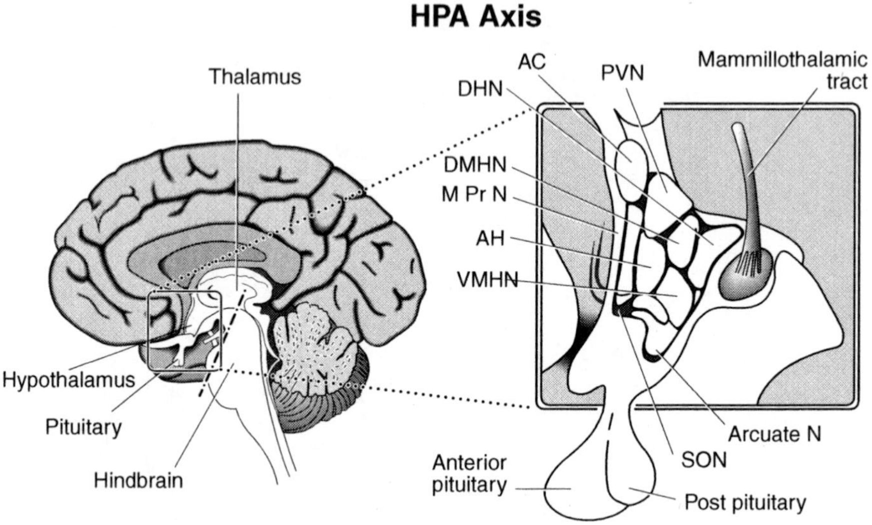

HPA Axis

Figure 8.2. Left, sketch of hypothalamus and pituitary gland. Right, enlarged medial view of main hypothalamic nuclei and lobes of pituitary gland. AC, anterior commissure; PVN, paraventricular nucleus; M Pr N, medial preoptic nucleus; VMHN, ventromedial hypothalamic nucleus; AH, anterior hypothalamic nucleus; SON, supraoptic nucleus; DHN, DMHN, dorsal and dorsomedial hypothalamic nucleus. Adapted from Kupferman (1991) and Niewenhuys et al. (1981).

the corpus striatum), and the orbitofrontal cortex (MacLean, 1970; Kupferman, 1991; Rosenzweig et al., 1996).

In mammals, the systemic effects of the defense response are evoked from the dorsomedial hypothalamic nucleus and PVN (figure 8.2). Other PVN subnuclei release peptides that affect pituitary hormone secretion (Kupferman, 1991; Reichlin, 1992; de Wardener, 2001). They include corticotropin-releasing hormone (CRH), which increases secretion by the anterior pituitary of adrenocorticotrophic hormone (ACTH); the latter, in turn, increases secretion of adrenal glucocorticoids. Local actions of CRH raise BP and heart rate (Fisher and Brown, 1983) and influence neuroendocrine activity in several parts of the brain (Swanson et al., 1983).

Other hypothalamic centers regulate body temperature, fluid volume, electrolyte composition, and metabolic activity, each of which affects cardiovascular function. The suprachiasmatic nuclei of the anterior hypothalamus contain the neurons that generate circadian rhythms which adjust many body functions, including BP, to the sleep-waking cycle (Moore-Ede, 1986; Moore, 1999).

Some specialized neuron groups known as circumventricular organs are located in regions where the blood-brain barrier is somewhat deficient, allowing certain molecules to gain access to the CNS. The circumventricular organs include the area postrema at the lower end of the fourth ventricle, the subfornical organ, and the organum vasculosum of the lamina terminalis in the anteroventral regions of the third ventricle (AV3V; figure 8.3; Brody et al., 1983; Ferrario et al., 1987; Johnson and Loewy, 1990).

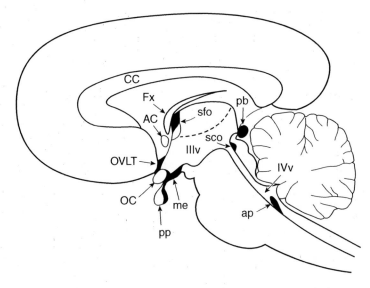

Figure 8.3. Sagittal view of brain showing circumventricular organs (black areas) that surround the 3rd and 4th ventricles. They lack a blood-brain barrier and have a rich blood supply. AC, anterior commissure; ap, area postrema; CC, corpus callosum; Fx, fornix; me, mesencephalon; OC, optic chiasma; OVLT, organum vasculosum of lamina terminalis; pb, pineal body; pp, posterior pituitary; sco, subcommissural organ; sfo, subfornical organ. From Landas et al. (1985), with permission of *Neuroscience Letters* and Elsevier.

Afferent Mechanisms

Afferent inputs that elicit cardiovascular responses include (1) segmental spinal afferents; (2) NTS afferents in the 9th and 10th cranial nerves; and (3) somatosensory, visual, auditory, and behavior-related inputs providing information about the environment (figure 2.15). The segmental inputs come from receptors in skin, bones, joints, skeletal muscle, viscera, and blood vessels (Koizumi and Brooks, 1972; Simon, 1974; Malliani, 1982; Rowell, 1983, 1993; Stella and Zanchetti, 1991; Sato et al., 1997). They include nociceptors, thermoreceptors, cardiac and aortic sympathetic afferents, skeletal muscle chemoreceptors, and renal chemoreceptors and mechanoreceptors. Their fibers synapse in the dorsal horn of each segment. They influence the sympathetic motoneurons through a short segmental pathway and through a long polysynaptic loop that reaches the spinal motoneurons via synapses in the NTS and other supraspinal centers.

The 9th and 10th cranial nerves carry afferent fibers from the arterial, cardiac, and pulmonary baroreceptors, the arterial chemoreceptors, lung inflation receptors, and various visceral inputs (Paintal, 1971, 1973; Kirchheim, 1976; Spyer, 1981, 1990; Daly, 1986). Each synapses in a distinctive part of the NTS, from which they project to centers in the hindbrain, diencephalon, and forebrain.

Somatosensory, visual, auditory, olfactory, and various other afferents provide information about the environment. They are processed by thalamus, cortex, and limbic system, which play a crucial role in the recognition of stressful stimuli (Rosenzweig et al., 1996; Gazzaniga, 1997).

The cerebellum has long been thought to play a role in cardiovascular regulation, but exactly what it does has been obscured by the many studies performed under anesthesia. It plays a role in ANS regulation in exercise, which is closely linked to the regulation of skeletal muscle movements (chapter 10). Its role in exercise provides a model for its wider role as an information comparator in disturbances where the relative size of two or more afferent inputs determines the effector response.

Determinants of Resting Sympathetic Tone

From the effects of localized electrical stimulation or lesions on resting BP, it was thought at one time that the medullary pressor region (also known as the lateral tegmental field) was the source of resting sympathetic tone (Wang and Ranson, 1939; Alexander, 1946). However, with electrical stimulation or lesions one cannot distinguish whether the maneuvers affect the neuronal cell bodies or merely nerve fibers passing through the region (Dampney, 1994b).

This became possible with the use of localized microinjections of chemical substances (e.g., transmitters, neurotoxins), which act only on cell bodies (Feldberg and Guertzenstein, 1976; Goodchild et al., 1982). These suggested that much of resting spinal sympathetic tone in anesthetized animals came largely from the subretrofacial nucleus in the RVLM region (Dampney, 1981, 1994a; Dampney et al., 1985; Granata et al., 1985; Pilowsky et al., 1985; Dean and Coote, 1986; McAllen, 1986; McAllen and Dampney, 1989). Acute destruction of these neurons causes a large fall in BP, as after acute spinal transection. As with the latter, there is usually some recovery after a few days (Cochrane and Nathan, 1989).

It has been suggested (1) that these neurons are a region of high spontaneous pacemaker activity (Haselton and Guyenet, 1989; Guyenet, 1990; Guyenet and Koshiya, 1995), (2) that they may be metabolically active (Dampney and Moon, 1980; Sun, Jeske, and Reis, 1992), and (3) that they receive much input from other regions (Gebber, 1990, 2001).

In anesthetized animals, BP does not usually alter after infracollicular decerebration (Korner et al., 1969, 1972; Yamori and Okamoto, 1969), which is why it was thought that these regions are not a source of tonic vasomotor tone. However, absence of such changes could be simply due to the loss of both excitatory and inhibitory tonic suprapontine influences following decerebration.

This is illustrated by studies showing that ablation of PVN causes a fall in BP in normal and hypertensive rats (Ciriello et al., 1984; Herzig et al., 1991; Takeda et al., 1991). More recently, large and prolonged falls in BP and lumbar SNA have been elicited by localized microinjection of the GABAergic agonist muscimol into the PVN of SHR and WKY (figure 8.4; Allen, 2002). The fall in SNA was greater in SHR than in WKY, which has implications for the pathogenesis of SHR hypertension (chapter 16).

Medullary Compression a Cause of EH?

Janetta (1980, and Janetta et al., 1985) found that patients undergoing surgery for trigeminal neuralgia often had pulsatile vascular loops that made contact with the RVLM region. Surgical decompression in hypertensive patients with these contacts

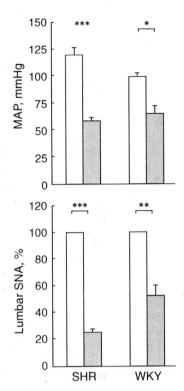

Figure 8.4. Mean arterial pressure (MAP, mmHg) and lumbar sympathetic nerve activity (SNA, percentage of preinjection control) before and 5–8 minutes after bilateral microinjection of GABA agonist muscimol (1–1.5 mmoles/side) in PVN of SHR and WKY rats. Results are means ± SEMs; *, **, ***, for $p = .05, .01, .001$ for pre- and postinjection differences. From Allen (2002), with permission of *Hypertension*, American Heart Association, and Lippincott, Williams and Wilkins.

elicited long-term falls in BP. Janetta's findings have been confirmed by several investigators (Naraghi et al., 1994, 1997; Morimoto et al., 1999; Gajjar et al., 2000). It raises the question whether medullary compression of this region causes EH or whether compression might be a consequence of EH. In a well-designed case control study, Hohenbleicher et al. (2001) confirmed the greater prevalence of neurovascular contacts in hypertensives compared to normotensives (39% vs. 25%, $p < .05$). However, in hypertensives with vascular contacts, the BP was identical to that of the hypertensives in whom vascular contacts were absent.

The effect of decompression in the neurosurgical patients certainly suggests that BP was higher in those with vascular contacts. With sufficient compression, one would expect BP to rise in normotensives not genetically predisposed to EH. But the suggestion that this might be a specific cause of EH is made tenuous by finding closely similar BPs in the two subgroups of hypertensive patients in Hohenbleicher's study. It suggests that the neurosurgical patients had a mixed background of high BP genes and that some rise in BP is a nonspecific consequence of vascular compression.

Synaptic Transmission

Neurons communicate through release of transmitters, which are packaged into membrane-bound organelles and transported to the axon terminals (Jahn and

Sudhof, 1994; Bloom, 1996; Bennett, 2001). Specialized proteins regulate transmitter storage in the vesicles and its release into the synaptic cleft. Upon release, transmitters bind to and stimulate specific receptors on the postsynaptic membrane of the adjoining neuron.

Fast Synaptic Transmission

Fast transmitters operate directly gated ion channels and mediate their full action within about 1 ms after release, allowing rapid coordination of effector responses. Glutamate is the most common fast excitatory transmitter. It binds to a specific receptor on a cation channel on the postsynaptic membrane, which is what determines the rapidity of its reponse (Kandel and Schwartz, 1991). Glutamate receptors include the kainate and kainate-quisqualate A receptors, which have similar properties and permit the passage of Na^+ and K^+ but not of Ca^{2+} (figure 8.5). Both are stimulated to the same extent by the glutamate agonist AMPA (α-amino-3-hydroxy-5-methyl-4-isoxazole proprionic acid) and are often termed AMPA receptors. Another receptor is the NMDA receptor, which is selectively activated by the agonist N-methyl-d-aspartate and allows passage of Na^+, K^+, and Ca^{2+} ions. At the normal membrane potential of about -65 mV, the channel is plugged by extracellular Mg^{2+}, which keeps it closed when glutamate binds to the receptor. For the channel to function the plug has to be extruded, which requires depolarization of the membrane by 20–30 mV. This usually occurs through release of an excitatory transmitter from another neuron. The NMDA receptor can be regarded as a "logic" gate, which operates only when the two events occur coincidentally (Kandel and Schwartz, 1991; Glynn, 1999). Glutamate also acts

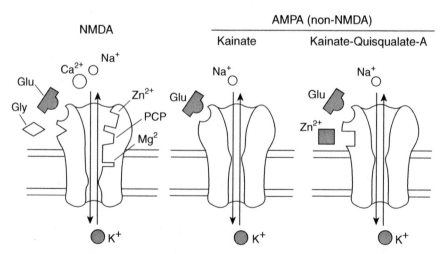

Figure 8.5. Three types of glutamate receptors that regulate directly gated ionic channels. The NMDA receptor is on a channel permeable to Ca^{2+}, Na^+, and K^+, with binding sites for glutamate (Glu), Mg^{2+}, Zn^{2+}, and glycine (gly) and phencyclidine (PCP). The other receptors are on the kainate and kainate-quisqualate channels, both of which are only permeable to Na^+ and K^+. After Kandel and Schwartz (1991), with permission of McGraw-Hill, New York.

on a fourth "metabotropic" receptor, through which it modulates responsiveness of adjoining neurons like a slow transmitter (chapter 10).

The fast inhibitory transmitters GABA and glycine act on receptors that are located on an anionic channel when gated Cl^- ions flow into the neuron and hyperpolarize the membrane. Inhibitory synapses are most abundant on the neuron's cell body where they are favorably placed to override the effects of excitatory dendritic inputs.

Slow Synaptic Transmission

The slow transmitters include the biogenic amines (e.g., NA) and small peptides, such as Ang II, arginine vasopressin (AVP), and atrial natriuretic peptide (ANP). The latency of slow transmitters is about 100 ms and their duration of action is rather prolonged (Kandel and Schwartz, 1991; Schwartz and Kandel, 1991; Glynn, 1999; Greengard, 2001).

After binding to its receptor, the transmitter starts a cascade of biochemical reactions that may increase the production of second messengers (e.g., cAMP, cGMP, diacylglycerol, Ca^{2+} ions), or activate various protein kinases which affect the properties of receptors, voltage-gated ion channels, ionic pumps, and various transcription factors (figure 8.6; Greengard, 2001). The net effect may be to alter the amount of transmitter released by an action potential. In addition, phosphorylation of the receptors often alters the neuron's responsiveness to other neurotransmitters.

Greengard (2001) discovered that phosphorylation of a single site on a regulatory protein in neostriatal neurons profoundly affects DA signaling. Stimulation of the D1 receptors increases production of cAMP and activates phosphokinase A (PKA); the result is phosphorylation of threonine-34 (Thr-34) on the regulatory protein DARPP-32 (dopamine cAMP-regulated phosphoprotein, molecular weight 32 kD). This changes DARPP-32 from an inactive molecule into an inhibitor of protein phosphatase 1 (PP1), thereby enhancing phosphorylation of neurotransmitter receptors, ion channels, and transcription factors. Stimulation of the D2 receptors has the opposite effect and prevents an increase in cAMP while increasing cytosolic Ca^{2+}. The latter activates other phosphatases (e.g., PP2), which dephosphorylate the DARPP-32 molecule at Thr-34, reversing the D1-mediated effects.

In his Nobel lecture, Greengard (2001) discussed the modulation of fast transmission by slow transmitter neurons as follows:

> The differences . . . seem amazing between the lack of complexity of fast synaptic transmission in which there is a single ligand-operated ion channel and the enormously complicated pathways underlying slow synaptic transmission. However when one thinks of fast synaptic transmission as being the hardware of the brain and slow synaptic transmission as being the software that controls fast transmission, the molecular basis by which nerve cells communicate with each other makes more sense (p. 1029).

Cardiovascular Effector Responses Are Mediated by Fast Transmitters

All the major cardiovascular effector responses in the CNS are due to release of fast transmitters (Chalmers and Pilowsky, 1991; Dampney, 1994a). Of the descending

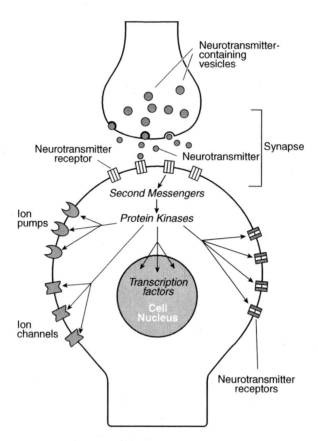

Figure 8.6. Some of the signaling pathways associated with slow synaptic transmission, as discussed in text. From Greengard (2001), with permission of American Association for the Advancement of Science.

bulbospinal fibers to the spinal sympathetic motoneurons, about 65% are excitatory and release glutamate, and 35% are inhibitory and release GABA (Llewellyn-Smith et al., 1992).

Neurally produced nitric oxide (NO) can also modulate activity of fast transmitter neurons in a number of regions, such as the RVLM and cerebellum (Gally et al., 1990; Garthwaite, 1991; Hope et al., 1991). For example, in RVLM neurons NO enhances the inhibitory action of GABA (Kishi et al., 2002).

Strengthening of Synaptic Transmission (Sensitization) in *Aplysia, Drosophila,* and Humans

Reference has been made in earlier chapters that the hypothalamic defense response, which accounts for the early elevation of BP, is evoked more readily in persons with EH than in normotensives. The process by which this comes about is a consequence of repeated presentation of stressful stimuli in susceptible individuals. The process is analogous to learning and is the result of alterations in transmission and structural changes in specific synapses. Chapter 2 referred briefly to synaptic strengthening in the sea snail *Aplysia*, where repeated aversive conditioning lowers the response threshold of the gill withdrawal reflex (Kandel, 2001). Analogous mechanisms subserve mammalian learning and memory and play a role in the development of EH.

Cellular Mechanisms of Sensitization in *Aplysia*

After the skin is gently touched, the siphon and gill are reflexly withrawn into the mantle cavity for greater protection. Sensitization occurs after repeatedly applying painful electric shocks to the tail, which reduces the threshold to touch, so that larger and more prolonged reflex responses are evoked (figures 2.23, 2.24; Kandel, 2001).

The neural circuit subserving the response consists of 24 sensory neurons from the siphon connected to 6 gill motoneurons. The activity of a serotonergic (5-HT) interneuron is crucial in altering the responsiveness of synapses between sensory and motoneurons. Its activity increases production of cAMP and phosphokinase A (PKA), causing an increase in Ca^{2+} at the presynaptic terminal (figure 8.7). The reflex response is enhanced by a greater release of glutamate at the synapse at each nerve impulse.

The effects of tail shock can be simulated by microinjecting 5-HT into a sensory neuron maintained in cell culture. Several puffs of 5-HT increase activity of PKA and of mitogen-activated protein kinase, which cause expression of the CREB-1 gene and other genes responsible for synthesis of synaptic proteins (figure 8.7). The new synaptic connections are responsible for long-term enhancement of the reflex response. The new connections develop solely at synapses with 5-HT nerves.

Analogous Changes in Mammalian Neurons

Similar neuronal changes in mammals were first discovered in the pathways subserving memory. In mammals, a network of neurons in the hippocampus and temporal lobe plays a crucial role for memories of places and objects. Following repeated presentation of a stimulus, long-term potentiation (LTP) of the excitatory postsynaptic potential (EPSP) develops in this circuit (figure 8.8), which is an electrophysiological marker of the synaptic changes just considered in *Aplysia* (Kandel and Schwartz, 1991; Kandel, 2001). Glutamate stimulation of NMDA receptors gives rise to LTPs and accompanies memory storage in hippocampal CA1 neurons. Conversely, NMDA antagonists abolish LTPs and memory storage (Glynn, 1999; Kandel, 2001).[4] In transgenic mice in which PKA activity has been reduced there are fewer and shorter LTPs, which are associated with a deficit in long-term spatial memory.

The converse of eliciting an LTP is the induction of long-term depression (LTD) of synaptic transmission, which is another mechanism that plays a role in memory (Rosenzweig et al., 1996). It signifies a long-lasting decrease in the EPSPs and is evoked by low-frequency afferent stimulation of NMDA receptors and is also associated with raised cytosolic Ca^{2+}. However, the amount of Ca^{2+} that enters the neuron is less than with LTPs. LTPs require high-frequency stimulation, which gives rise to a large surge of Ca^{2+} in the postsynaptic neuron, increased activation of protein kinases, and phosphorylation of synaptic proteins. LTDs are associated with

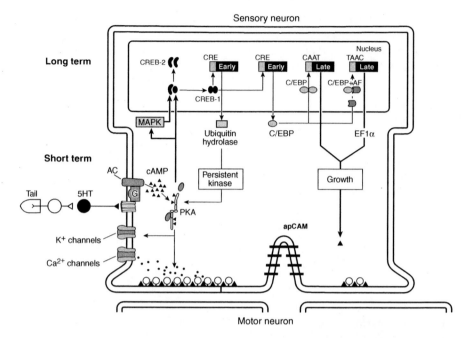

Figure 8.7. Sketch of sensory neurons of *Aplysia*: One tail shock causes transient 5-HT release, which activates adenylyl cyclase (AC) and increases cAMP. The result is recruitment of protein kinase A (PKA). The latter's regulatory subunits (rods) separate from the catalytic subunits (ovals), causing phosphorylation of channels and exocytosis machinery in presynaptic membrane, which enhances glutamate release. The upper part of the diagram shows long-term effects of repeated tail stimuli: After further rises in cAMP mitogen activated protein kinase (MAPK) is formed and acts on the nucleus to activate transcription factor CREB-1 and to remove repressive action on CREB-1 by CREB-2. CREB-1 causes expression of several "early" genes, including a ubiquitin hydrolase, which regulates proteolysis of the regulatory subunit of PKA, which results in persistent phosphorylation of the latter's substrate proteins. Other genes produce growth of new synaptic connections. From Kandel (2001), with permission of American Association for the Advancement of Science.

activation of protein phosphatases, which dephosphorylate synaptic proteins. Thus, the state of phosphorylation of synaptic proteins determines whether the stimulus elicits an LTP or an LTD.

Aversive Conditioning in *Drosophila*

Benzer and colleagues used an avoidance paradigm to determine the role of genetic factors in the fruit fly *Drosophila*'s capacity to learn from past experience (Benzer, 1973; Quinn et al., 1974; Dudai et al., 1976). Some 40 flies were placed into a cylinder connected to two tubes, each of which contained a distinctive odor to which the flies were similarly attracted. In one tube the fly received an electric shock soon after entry, while no shock was administered on entering the other tube (Quinn et al., 1974).

About 90% of wild-type flies quickly learn to avoid the tube in which they receive the shock. However, some flies never learn despite their excellent sense of smell.

Figure 8.8. Top, three hippocampal pathways from which long-term potentiation (LTP) of the excitatory postsynaptic potential (EPSP) can be induced are (1) the perforant pathway from the subiculum, which has excitatory connections with granule cells in dentate gyrus; (2) the mossy fiber pathway connects the latter neurons to the pyramidal cells in area CA3; and (3) the Schaffer collateral pathway connects the pyramidal cells of the CA3 region with those of the CA1 region. Bottom, early and late changes in LTP in Schaffer collateral pathway. A single stimulus train for 1 second at 100 Hz elicits an LTP that lasts ~2 hours; four trains at 10-minute intervals evokes LTP of more than 24 hours duration. From Kandel (2001), with permission of American Association for the Advancement of Science.

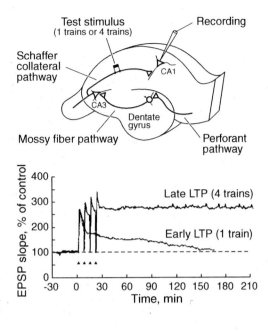

These mutants have lost the function of one or more genes that regulate the transmitter and synaptic changes in figure 8.7 (Dudai et al., 1976; Tully, 1987; Dudai, 1988). For example, one mutant with poor learning skills could not express the dopa decarboxylase gene, which is required for the synthesis of 5-HT and DA.

Role of Monoaminergic Neurons

Monoaminergic neurons include the catecholaminergic and serotonergic neurons, which are part of the reticular formation of the brainstem. Up to the 1940s, reticular neurons were regarded as playing a rather nonspecific role in the coordination of arousal, alertness, and attention in other neural systems (Moruzzi and Magoun, 1949; Scheibel et al., 1955; Scheibel and Scheibel, 1967). From the 1960s onward, as the distinctive anatomical and biochemical features of the various monoaminergic neuron groups were identified, it gradually emerged that they also have distinctive functional roles (Falck and Hillarp, 1959; Dahlström and Fuxe, 1964, 1965; Ungerstedt, 1971; Aston-Jones and Bloom, 1981; Aghajanian and Vandermaelen, 1986; Björklund and Lindvall, 1986; Cooper et al., 1991; Jacobs and Azmitia, 1992; Pilowsky et al., 1995). In the cardiovascular system, their functions appear to be quite specific, as discussed later in this chapter.

Anatomical Aspects

The monoaminergic neurons include the NA and adrenaline-containing neurons, the DA neurons, and the 5-HT neurons. The cell bodies of the DA neurons are in the midbrain and diencephalon, while those of the NA, adrenergic, and 5-HT neurons are located in discrete cell groups in the medulla and pons.

NA and Adrenaline Neurons

The NA neurons are classified into discrete A1 to A7 neuron groups (figure 8.9; Dahlström and Fuxe, 1964, 1965; Ungerstedt, 1971). There are some 10,000 NA neurons in the rat, of which ~50% are in the locus ceruleus (LC, A6) and the dorsal part of the subceruleus (A7), 30–35% are in the lateral tegmental group (A1, A5, and the ventral part of A7), and the rest are in the dorsomedial group.

Ascending NA fibers from the LC and part of A7 go to the cerebral cortex, hippocampus, thalamus, amygdala, septum, stria terminalis, and the hypothalamus and midbrain via the dorsal NA bundle. Fibers from A1, A2, A5, and part of A7 go mainly to the hypothalamus via the ventral NA bundle (Björklund and Lindvall, 1986). The two NA bundles are readily identifiable at the border of the pons and midbrain and carry the entire NA innervation to suprapontine parts of the brain. Sectioning both bundles does not affect the DA neurons.

Most descending NA fibers of cardiovascular significance come from the A5 and A6+A7 neurons (Neil and Loewy, 1982; Korner, Badoer and Head, 1987; Coote, 1988; Loewy, 1990). In addition, NA neurons from LC innervate the cerebellum and several hindbrain cell groups, including other monoaminergic neurons (Aghajanian and Vandermaelen, 1986; Foote et al., 1983; Jacobs and Azmitia, 1992).

The adrenaline neurons are mostly in C1 neurons in RVLM, in which they are cotransmitters in about 60% of glutaminergic neurons. C2 neurons are in the dorsal medulla close to NTS and A2 neurons and send axons to the hypothalamus and pontine and medullary centers (Cooper et al., 1991; Goldstein, 1992).

DA Neurons

DA neurons are the most numerous of the CA neurons and are found in the midbrain and diencephalon (figure 8.9. They lack dopamine-β-hydroxylase (DβH), which converts DA to NA (figure 5.12). DA neurons are localized in the A9 neurons in the substantia nigra and in the A8 and A10 cells in the ventral tegmental area of the midbrain. The A11 to A15 neurons are in the hypothalamus and pituitary region and regulate functions of the hypothalamopituitary axis; the A16 and A17 groups are present in the retina and olfactory bulb (Cooper et al., 1991).

The midbrain DA neurons have long axons that project to the neostriatum (caudate nucleus, putamen), the limbic cortex (including cingulate and entorhinal areas), the septum, nucleus accumbens, amygdaloid complex, piriform cortex, and prefrontal cortex (Björklund and Lindvall, 1986; Cooper et al., 1991; Goldstein, 1992).

Serotonergic Neurons

Serotonergic neurons are part of the midline raphe and adjacent nuclei of the brainstem (figure 8.9). The B1, B2, and B3 groups are the most caudal and send descending fibers to the spinal cord. The B4, B5, and B6 groups project to hindbrain and

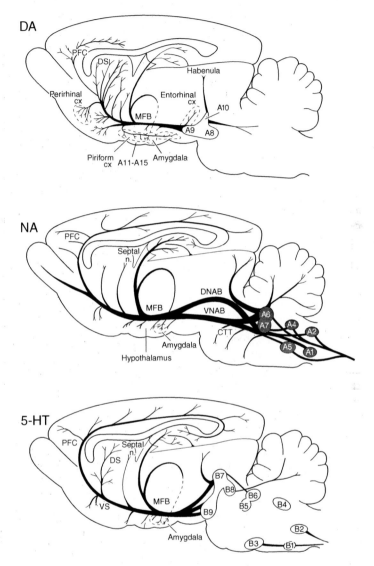

Figure 8.9. Sketch of main central monoaminergic groups. Top, dopaminergic (DA) neuron groups and distribution of their axons to diencephalon and forebrain. Note midbrain location of A8–A10 cell bodies, and hypothalamic location of A11–A15 neurons. MFB, medial forebrain bundle; DS, dorsal striatum. Middle, A1–A7 are main NA cell groups with axon projections to diencephalon, forebrain, cerebellum, hindbrain regions, and spinal cord. A6 is locus ceruleus; DNAB and VNAB, dorsal and ventral ascending NA bundles. Bottom, B1–B9 are serotonergic (5-HT) neuron groups, with projections to similar regions innervated by NA neurons; B4–B9 are 5-HT cell groups in median raphe nucleus. From Robbins and Everitt (1995), with permission of MIT Press.

cerebellum, while B7, B8, and B9 send ascending fibers to the hypothalamus, preoptic region, cortex, hippocampus, septum, olfactory tubercle, and amygdala and to the caudate nucleus and putamen (Grant and Stumpf, 1975; Jacobs and Azmitia, 1992; Pilowsky et al., 1995).

General Functional Aspects

Monoaminergic neurons are present in all vertebrate species (Björklund and Lindvall, 1986). This suggests a fundamental importance in adaptive and evolutionary terms. They participate in many types of regulation, such as arousal and sleep, learning, memory and conditioning, sensory and motor functions, eating and drinking behavior, and so on (Foote et al., 1983; Jacobs and Azmitia, 1992; Robbins and Everitt, 1995). Serious diseases such as Parkinson's disease and schizophrenia may result from DA neuron malfunction, while defective signaling of CA or 5-HT neurons has been implicated in depressive illness and other mood disorders.

The activity of NA neurons in LC and dorsal raphe 5-HT neurons is closely tied to the sleep-waking cycle (Jacobs, 1987). In addition, LC neurons respond briskly to novel and noxious somatosensory stimuli, althought this may wane when stimuli are repeatedly presented.

After local application of NA to the cerebral cortex, the rate of firing of cortical neurons is reduced, making it easier to recognize new stimuli against a less noisy background (Foote et al., 1983). The behavioral response is often influenced by past experience. For example, when NA is applied to the dentate gyrus of the hippocampus, an auditory signal elicits an increase in firing of the dentate neurons if the animal has learned to associate the signal with imminent presentation of food; otherwise, firing tends to decrease (Segal and Bloom, 1976).

There is evidence that selective lesions of the dorsal NA bundle have significant effects on learning. For example, after such lesions in rats, functions such as eating, drinking, and somatic movement remain normal even though the animals are no longer able to learn new rules about discriminating between signals that provide cues about the tasks to be performed. Interestingly, they generally retain the rules learned before the lesion (Robbins and Everitt, 1995).

DA neurons, like NA neurons, are also activated by novel stimuli. The DA system optimizes the function of the prefrontal lobe during arousal and regulates the sensory input from thalamus to cortex. It comes into play when the animal has learned to expect a reward (chapter 10; Schultz, 1992; Schultz et al., 1997; Carlsson et al., 1997; Carlsson, 2001; Fiorillo et al., 2003).

Methods for Determining Cardiovascular Role

The discharge of single NA neurons in groups A5, A6, and A7 alters in response to changes in MAP, blood volume, arterial hypoxia, and pain (Elam et al., 1981, 1984, 1985, 1986; Andrade and Aghajanian, 1982). This suggests that the neurons receive projections from afferents from the cardiovascular, respiratory, and somatosensory systems. However, it has proved difficult to relate the findings to alterations in effector responses.

Another method involves destruction of central CA terminals (i.e., NA and DA terminals) by i.c.v. administration of the selective neurotoxin 6-hydroxydopamine (6-OHDA). The chronic effects of this on resting MAP and heart rate were minimal, thus providing no clue about how the modulatory circulatory actions of these neurons affect cardiovascular regulation by the CNS.

However, during the first few hours after administration of the neurotoxin to awake animals there are marked changes in BP and heart rate (Korner, Oliver, Reynoldson et al., 1978; Head and Korner, 1980; Korner and Angus, 1981; Korner and Head, 1981; Head and de Jong, 1986; Korner, Badoer, and Head, 1987). These are due to neurotoxin-induced NA and DA release from the central terminals.[5] This has helped to determine which fast transmitter pathway is the target of the modulatory actions.

Similar large changes in BP and heart rate occur after i.c.v. injection of specific serotonergic neurotoxins (e.g., 5,6- and 5,7-dihydroxytryptamine, 5,6- and 5,7-DHT), which are due to release of 5-HT (Baumgarten and Björklund, 1976; Head and Korner, 1982; Wolf and Bobik, 1988). After giving either 6-OHDA or 5,6-DHT, the phase of transmitter release is followed by gradual destruction of the relevant neuron terminals. The absence of long-term changes when this process is complete may be due to the compensatory changes in the activity of other pathways.

Effects of DA and NA Neuron Activity on BP, Heart Rate, and the Defense Response

In conscious rabbits, an i.c.v. injection of 6-OHDA elicits a rise in BP and a fall in heart rate due to central CA release, with the peak response occurring about 2.5 hours after injection (figure 8.10, left). In contrast, in pontine (infracollicularly decerebrate) rabbits, neurotoxin-induced CA release causes falls in BP and heart rate of relatively short duration (figure 8.10, middle).[6] Similar changes are evoked in sinoaortically denervated (SAD) animals with intact brain, in which an early BP fall is followed by a late rise as in normal rabbits (figure 8.10, right; Korner, Head, and Badoer, 1984). Thus the late rise in BP in intact animals is mediated through a suprapontine pathway, while the absence of an early fall in BP is due to buffering by baroreflexes.

In intact animals and in pontine rabbits, the bradycardia is largely due to increased vagal excitation. In contrast, the heart rate changes in SAD rabbits are almost entirely due to changes in cardiac SNA (Korner et al., 1987).

Administration of the neurotoxin causes chronic depletion of brain NA and DA, but resting BP and heart rate are close to preinjection levels after 1 to 2 weeks (Chalmers and Reid, 1972; Korner, Reynoldson, Head et al., 1979; Korner and Head, 1981; Head et al., 1983). The absence of a significant change in BP is due to the fact that although 6-OHDA destroys most cardiovascularly relevant terminals, some neurons' modulatory influences are pressor while others are depressor. For example, localized bilateral transection of the spinal NA pathway elicits a long-term elevation of MAP by ~ 10 mmHg, indicating that this pathway normally inhibits constrictor tone (Elghozi et al., 1989).

The large cardiovascular changes due to CA release are prevented by prior i.c.v. injection of 6-OHDA given several days earlier. Moreover, there is no further depletion

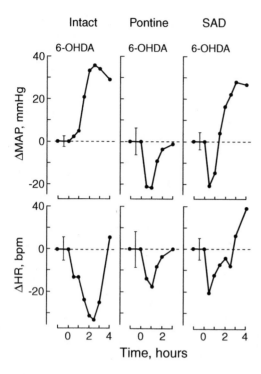

Figure 8.10. Effects of catecholamine release on mean arterial pressure (ΔMAP, mmHg) and heart rate (ΔHR, beats/min) in awake rabbits, injected at time 0 with 6-OHDA (600 μg/kg, i.c.v.) through intracisternal catheter. Left, intact animals; middle, pontine rabbits; right, rabbits with previous sinoaortic denervation (SAD). Bar on left ± 1 SEM for a single time interval. From Korner, Head, and Badoer (1984), with permission of *Journal of Cardiovascular Pharmacology* and Lippincott, Williams and Wilkins.

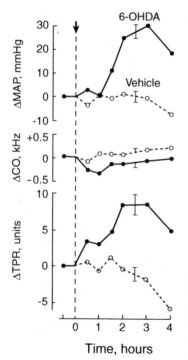

Figure 8.11. Changes in mean arterial pressure (ΔMAP, mmHg), cardiac output (ΔCO, kHz Doppler shift), and total peripheral resistance (ΔTPR, units) in awake rabbits over 4 hours after i.c.v. injection of 6-OHDA (600 μg/kg) or ascorbic acid vehicle. Based on data from Korner, Oliver et al. (1978).

of transmitter after the second dose of neurotoxin (Korner and Head, 1981; Head and Korner, 1982).

Significance of CA-Induced Pressor Effect

The late rise in BP after i.c.v. 6-OHDA is due to an increase in TPR (figure 8.11; Korner, Oliver et al., 1978). At the peak response, the renal and gastrointestinal Vas Rs are raised and blood flows are reduced, while skeletal muscle Vas R is little altered but blood flow is raised (figure 8.12).

The peripheral pattern induced by transmitter release resembles the defense response. The absence of clear muscle vasodilation may be due to a more marked elevation of plasma adrenaline than that evoked by stress (figure 5.4). Nevertheless, the pattern suggests that the CA neurons modulate target neurons in the hypothalamus (chapter 11).

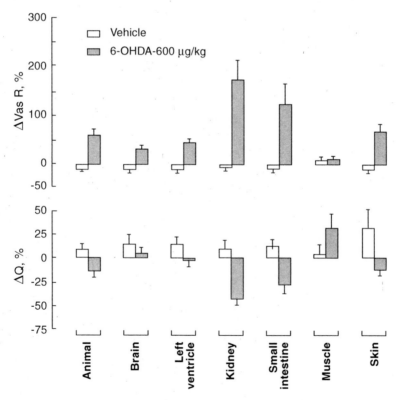

Figure 8.12. Changes in blood flow (ΔQ) and vascular resistance (ΔVas R) of awake rabbits at 2.5 hours after i.c.v. injections of 6-OHDA (600 μg/kg) (shaded) or ascorbic acid vehicle (clear). CO (whole animal) and blood flows in brain, left ventricle, kidney, small intestine, skeletal muscle, and skin determined by radioactive microsphere method. From Korner, Oliver et al. (1978), with permission of *European Journal of Pharmacology* and Elsevier.

Role of DA and NA Neurons

Whether the pressor and heart rate responses are due to DA or NA release can be determined by sectioning the dorsal and ventral ascending NA bundles. This removes the entire NA innervation to suprapontine target neurons, while leaving the DA innervation intact (Van den Buuse, Versteeg, and De Jong, 1984; Van den Buuse, 1991, 1993). Three to four weeks were allowed after the lesion for the fibers to degenerate: The rabbits were then injected with 600 μg/kg 6-OHDA i.c.v. to observe whether the effects of transmitter release had altered from the normal response determined in sham-operated animals (Van den Buuse et al., 1991). Two groups of rabbits were studied: one with intact arterial baroreceptors (nondenervated rabbits) and another in which SAD had been performed 1–2 weeks before injecting the neurotoxin (figure 8.13, left two panels).

The MAP responses of the nondenervated rabbits after the bundle lesions were unchanged, but the bradycardia was completely abolished (figure 8.13, left panel). Similarly, in SAD rabbits the MAP changes were unaffected but the sympathetically mediated tachycardia was enhanced (figure 8.13, second panel).

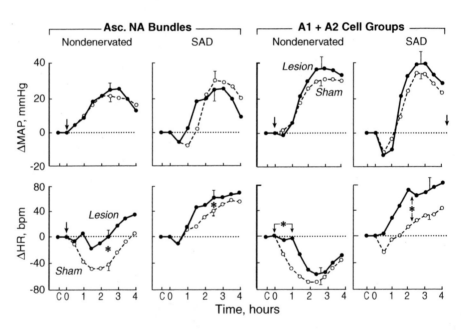

Figure 8.13. Left two panels, effects of CA release induced by i.c.v. 6-OHDA (600 μg/kg) at arrow, on ΔMAP and ΔHR 4 weeks after section of dorsal and ventral ascending NA bundles or sham operation following acute central CA release in awake nondenervated and SAD rabbits. Right two panels, effects of 6-OHDA-induced CA release on ΔMAP and ΔHR following bilateral electrolytic lesions of A1 + A2 NA cell groups or sham operation performed 3–4 weeks earlier. *$p < .05$ for Δ between lesioned and sham groups during early and late response components. From, left, Van den Buuse et al. (1991), and, right, Korner, Badoer, and Head (1987).

It follows that (1) the pressor effect and regional Vas R changes are largely due to DA modulation of the defense pathway; (2) the bradycardia in nondenervated rabbits is due to NA modulation of the cardiac vagus through a suprapontine loop; (3) SAD has little effect on the rise in MAP but enhances the sympathetically mediated tachycardia.

Role of Individual NA Neuron Groups

To test the role of individual NA neuron groups on the transmitter release response, bilateral electrolytic lesions (or sham operations) of the A1, A2, A1+A2, A5, and A6+A7 NA neuron groups were performed (Badoer et al., 1987; Korner, Badoer and Head, 1987); 3–4 weeks were allowed for the fibers to degenerate, at the end of which an injection of 600 μg/kg 6-OHDA i.c.v. was administered to determine whether any of the lesions had induced changes from the normal transmitter release response. As before, the effects of the lesions or sham operation were examined in animals with intact baroreceptors (nondenervated rabbits) and in SAD rabbits.

BP Responses

In sham-operated rabbits, an early fall in BP was observed only in SAD animals (figure 8.14). The fall emanated from the A5 and the A6+A7 neuron groups, since the BP fall was abolished after lesions of these regions.

A5 and A6+A7 lesions also had significant but small effects on the late peak pressor response (figure 8.14). After A5 lesions there was a small attenuation of the peak but only nondenervated animals were affected. After A6+A7 lesions, a similar attenuation occurred only in SAD rabbits (figures 8.14, 8.15).

Thus, each of the above group of neurons has a small tonic effect on BP mediated through bulbospinal pathways, which has been modelled in figure 8.16. It is assumed that the A5 and A6+A7 groups each have two neuron populations, one affecting the vasodilator pathway from RVLM to the spinal sympathetic motoneurons and the other affecting the constrictor pathway.[7] After ablating A5 neurons, the neurotoxin-induce NA release affects the A6+A7 neurons by resetting the entire time-ΔMAP curve by a few mmHg below normal (figure 8.15, left panel). The A6+A7 NA neurons are assumed to receive input from low-threshold arterial and cardiac baroreceptors, so that when the BP rises during transmitter release bulbospinal constrictor tone is inhibited slightly. This gives the impression of attenuation of the late pressor maximum, even though the trough peak amplitude is not affected. SAD abolishes the feedback, which accounts for the minimal change in peak BP in SAD rabbits.

After A6+A7 lesions, NA release affects the A5 neurons, which are assumed to receive input from high-threshold arterial and cardiopulmonary baroreceptors. Hence modulation of BP occurs only in the latter part of the observation period, with slight inhibition of both constrictor and dilator pathways. The result is little change from the normal BP response. In SAD rabbits, there still is feedback from cardiopulmonary baroreceptors, which are assumed to inhibit only the constrictor pathway, resulting in slight attenuation of the BP peak.

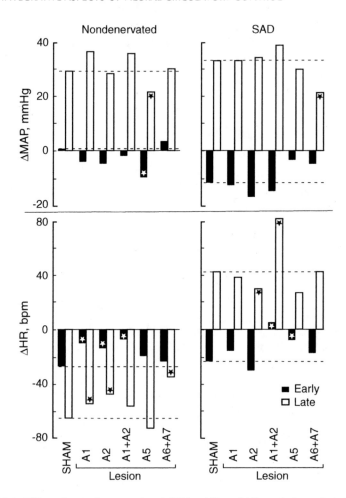

Figure 8.14. Effects in nondenervated and SAD rabbits of bilateral electrolytic lesions of various NA neuron groups or sham operations performed 3–4 weeks earlier, on ΔMAP and ΔHR induced by 6-OHDA-mediated CA release. The neuron groups lesioned were A1, A2, A1+A2, A5, and A6+A7 NA neurons. Early responses (black bar) are measurements 0.5 hours after 6-OHDA; late responses (clear bar) are averages between 3 and 3.5 hours after 6-OHDA. Horizontal dashed lines are average early and late responses after sham operation. *$p < .05$ for Δ between lesioned and sham response. From Korner, Badoer, and Head (1987), with permission of *Brain Research* and Elsevier.

Heart Rate Responses

In nondenervated rabbits, the vagal bradycardia that normally occurs during the first hour of transmitter release is evoked by a minimal rise in BP (figures 8.10, 8.13, left). This suggests marked vagal facilitation in response to the baroreceptor input (Korner, 1979a). A1+A2 lesions abolish this component of the heart response, which is also

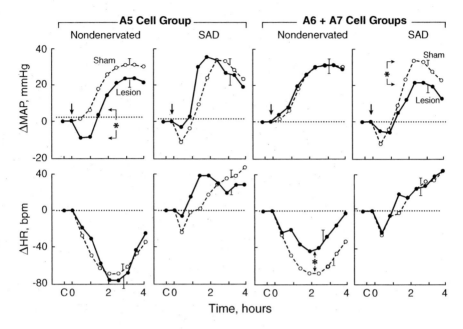

Figure 8.15. Time course of ΔMAP and ΔHR in awake nondenervated and SAD rabbits in response to i.c.v. 6-OHDA-induced CA transmitter release, injected at arrow. Bilateral ablation of A5 neurons or of A6 + A7 neurons or sham operation performed 3–4 weeks earlier; *$p < .05$ for difference between lesioned and sham groups. From Korner, Badoer, and Head (1987), with permission of *Brain Research* and Elsevier.

abolished by lesions of the dorsal and ventral ascending bundles (Fig.8.13, third panel cf with first panel). The facilitation of vagal activity thus occurs through a loop from NTS A1 and A2 neurons to the hypothalamus and back from the hypothalamus to the medullary vagal motoneurons.

The late component of vagal bradycardia is abolished by the bundle lesions but is little affected by ablation of A1+A2. Other NA inputs affect this component, with input from A5 neurons probably playing a major role (figure 8.15).

Effects of 5-HT Neurons on BP and Heart Rate

After i.c.v. injection of 5,6-DHT, the transmitter release response consists of a rise in heart rate and a bimodal rise in BP (figure 8.17; Korner and Head, 1981; Head and Korner, 1982). The early and late BP components are mediated respectively through bulbospinal and suprapontine pathways. The creatinine sulfate vehicle also has a pressor effect, so that the "true" early BP component is about half the actual response. The rise in heart rate is due to reduction in resting vagal activity.

Interaction between CA and 5-HT Pathways

Prior destruction of 5-HT neurons has virtually no effect on the BP and heart rate changes induced by 6-OHDA-induced CA release (figure 8.18). However, prior

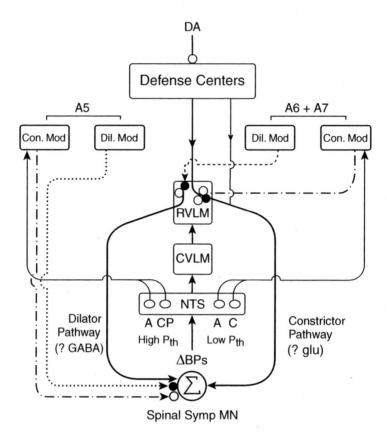

Figure 8.16. Model of how lesions of A5 and A6+A7 NA neurons alter BP following 6-OHDA-induced CA release: The initial fall in BP is through NA modulation of dilator pathway activity, while late rise is due to modulation by DA neurons of bulbospinal constrictor activity originating in hypothalamus (black circle, cell bodies of both sets of neurons in RVLM). A5 and A6+A7 neurons each have two population: one modulating the dilator pathway (Dil. Mod) and the other modulating the constrictor pathway (Con. Mod; open circles, sites of modulation). Dil. Mod neurons do not receive input from baroreceptors, while A6+A7 Con. Mod neurons receive projections from low-threshold arterial and cardiac baroreceptors (A, CP, Low P_{th}) and modulate fast transmission in the bulbospinal constrictor pathway. A5 Con. Mod neurons receive input from high-threshold arterial and cardiopulmonary baroreceptors (A, CP, High P_{th}) and modulate both constrictor and dilator pathways at high BP.

destruction of CA neurons abolishes the 5-HT-induced late pressor component, while the rise in heart rate is reduced by half. Thus, the ascending monoaminergic pathway subserving the peak pressor response has a 5-HT neuron in series with a DA neuron (figure 8.19).

In contrast, the descending 5-HT and NA fibers have opposing independent effects on BP. The heart rate changes suggest a series-parallel arrangement, whereby some 5-HT neurons inhibit NA neurons to reduce vagal tone, while other 5-HT and NA pathways, respectively, reduce and increase vagal tone independently.

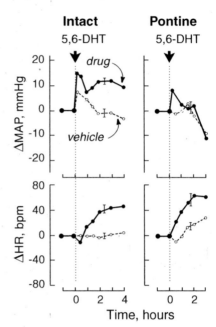

Figure 8.17. Left, average MAP (mmHg) and HR (bpm, beats/min) responses in awake rabbits injected with i.c.v. 5,6-DHT (633 μg/kg) or creatinine sulfate vehicle at arrow. Right, responses in pontine preparation. From Head and Korner (1982).

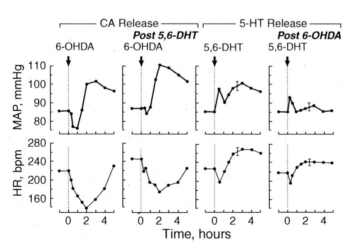

Figure 8.18. Left panels: Average ΔMAP (mmHg) and ΔHR (bpm, beats/min) in awake rabbits in response to 6-OHDA (600 μg/kg i.c.v. at arrows). In first panel, responses of previously untreated rabbits. Those in second panel had received 5,6-DHT (633 μg/kg i.c.v.) 7 days earlier. Right panels: First panel shows effect of i.c.v. 5,6-DHT in previously untreated rabbits. Those in second panel had received i.c.v. 6-OHDA injected 7 days earlier, and the small early rise in MAP is due to creatinine sulfate vehicle. From Korner and Head (1981), with permission of *Journal of the Autonomic Nervous System* and Elsevier.

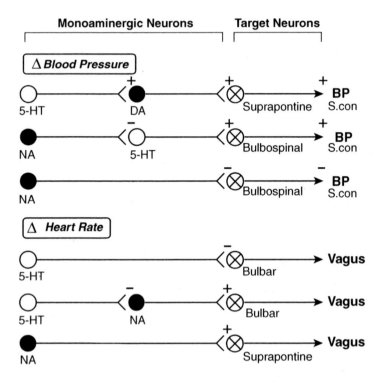

Figure 8.19. Schema shows series parallel arrangement by which modulatory DA, NA, and 5-HT neurons affect target neurons that release fast transmitters in suprapontine and bulbospinal centers, which alter BP and heart rate. S.con., sympathetic constrictor nerves. The afferents to monoaminergic neurons come from cardiovascular and other afferent sources.

Modulation of Cardiac Baroreflex Properties

During NA transmitter release, the vagal bradycardia component of the reflex is facilitated during rises in BP, as evident from the steeper slope and higher bradycardia plateau of the reflex function curve (figure 8.20, left; Korner, Reynoldson et al., 1979; Korner and Head, 1981).[8] The long-term effects of destruction of the NA terminals are directionally opposite to the acute effects, with attenuation of the vagal response.

Similarly, 5-HT release inhibits vagal efferent activity (figure 8.20, right; Korner and Head, 1981; Head and Korner, 1982). After loss of 5-HT terminals, the chronic changes in reflex properties are directionally opposite to the acute effects, with facilitation of the vagal response.

Therefore, the properties of the reflex 1 to 2 weeks after destruction of the NA terminals are like the acute effects of 5-HT release, while after destruction of 5-HT terminals the properties are like the acute effects of NA release. This suggests that the NA and 5-HT neurons modulate vagal motoneuron responsiveness on a moment-to-moment basis through the parallel arrangement shown in figure 8.19. This is of practical significance in EH, where the attenuation of vagal responsiveness occurs in response to chronic elevation of the cardiopulmonary load.

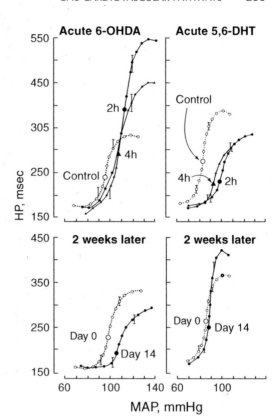

Figure 8.20. Top, cardiac baroreflex curves relating MAP to heart period (HP): measurements before (control) and 2 and 4 hours after 6-OHDA- or 5,6-DHT-induced transmitter release. NA release facilitates BP-related cardiac vagal activity as assessed from changes in slope and upper plateau, while 5-HT release inhibits these responses. Bottom, chronic effects 2 weeks after destruction of NA and 5-HT terminals: After destruction of CA terminals, vagal changes resemble those of acute 5-HT release, while response after destruction of 5-HT terminals similar to effects of acute NA release. From Korner and Head (1981), with permission of *Journal of the Autonomic Nervous System* and Elsevier.

Catecholaminergic Modulation in Hypertension

In SHR hypertension the high BP has a neural basis, with DA neurons playing an important role in its pathogenesis. Corresponding information about DA neurons in EH is not available, but central NA neuron activity is enhanced.

Role of DA Neurons in SHR Hypertension

Increased hypothalamic responsiveness in SHR raises peripheral sympathoadrenal activity in early life, causing a rapid rise in BP (chapter 16). Haeusler and colleagues were the first to observe that the rise in BP was greatly attenuated by 6-OHDA-induced destruction of central CA neurons in young SHR (Haeusler et al., 1972; Haeusler, 1976). They thought that the attenuation was due to the destruction of NA fibers. However, Van den Buuse and colleagues subsequently provided strong evidence that it was the loss of DA neurons that suppressed the hypertension (figure 8.21; Van den Buuse, De Kloet et al., 1984; Van den Buuse, Versteeg et al., 1984; Van den Buuse et al., 1986).

They showed that localized destruction of the ascending NA bundles had no effect on the hypertension and neither did central administration of the neurotoxin DSP-4

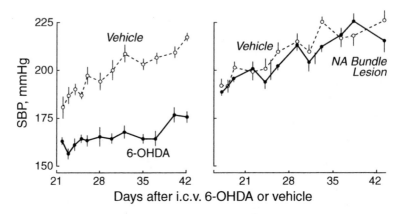

Figure 8.21. Left, changes in systolic BP (SBP, mmHg) during development of hypertension in 5–6-week-old SHR (open circles, dashed lines) are attenuated by i.c.v. 6-OHDA injection. Right, localized destruction of dorsal and ventral ascending NA bundles has no effect on hypertension, suggesting that the latter is due to modulation by DA neurons. Based on Van den Buuse, De Kloet et al. (1984) and Van den Buuse (1985).

(N-chlorethyl-N-2 bromobenzylamine HCl), which causes more specific destruction of NA terminals and has no effect on DA terminals. In contrast, significant attenuation of the hypertension was produced by electrolytic lesions of DA neurons in the substantia nigra (Van den Buuse et al., 1986).

Further support for the idea that DA neurons plays a role in SHR hypertension came from experiments on the effects of i.c.v. 6-OHDA in the presence of reuptake blockers with different affinities for the NA and DA uptake pumps. The greater a blocker's affinity for a particular pump, the less neurotoxin enters the terminals and the smaller the number of terminals destroyed. Desipramine has a greater affinity for the NA reuptake pump, which allows 6-OHDA to enter DA terminals freely, so that there is long-term attenuation of the hypertension. In contrast, the affinity of the blocker GBR-1299 for the DA pump is pronounced, so that little 6-OHDA enters DA terminals and the hypertension develops normally.

Thus, the modulation by DA neurons produces development of SHR hypertension. This accords with the findings in rabbits that DA neurons are important in eliciting an acute cardiovascular defense response.

Role of NA Neurons in EH

In humans, one jugular vein drains blood from the hindbrain, hypothalamus, and several subcortical structures, while the other drains blood from the cerebral cortex. The NA spillover of the former comes from the central NA neurons, rather than from the sympathetic terminals to blood vessels (Ferrier et al., 1993; Lambert et al., 1994, 1995; Esler, 1995).

In a population of volunteers that included persons with EH and normal subjects, there was a positive relationship between central NA neuron activity and renal and

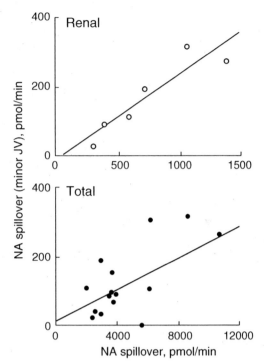

Figure 8.22. Relationship between NA spillover into jugular vein (JV) that reflects central NA neuron activity, and total (average) and renal NA spillover rates. From Ferrier et al. (1993), with permission of *Journal of Hypertension* and Lippincott, Williams and Wilkins.

average peripheral SNA (figure 8.22). It raises the question whether the central NA neurons evoked the elevation of peripheral SNA or whether the high peripheral SNA was responsible for the central changes.

Assuming that the findings in rabbits apply also to humans, it is likely that the NA neurons in humans receive baroreceptor afferents in accordance with the model in figure 8.16. With an elevated cardiopulmonary load in EH, the relationships in figure 8.22 suggest that the raised central NA activity is a consequence of the raised cardiopulmonary load rather than the cause of the raised SNA.

Central Actions of α-Methyldopa

α-Methyldopa (α-MD) is a centrally acting antihypertensive drug that has been in use since the 1960s (Oates et al., 1960). It undergoes biotransformation to α-methyl NA in central NA neurons and this molecule displaces transmitter NA in the axon terminals. α-Methyl NA and residual NA in the NA neurons stimulates hindbrain α_2-ARs, which lowers BP (van Zwieten, 1999).

At a near-maximal i.c.v. dose of α-MD, the fall in MAP is due to reduction of TPR and CO, with each accounting for about half the response (Badoer et al., 1983). About 75% of the fall in heart rate is due to increased vagal activity, while 25% is due to inhibition of cardiac SNA (Kobinger, 1984; Korner, Head, Bobik et al., 1985). The heart rate changes are mediated through the suprapontine loop from the A1 and A2 neuron groups to the hypothalamus and back to the medulla and spinal cord. They are

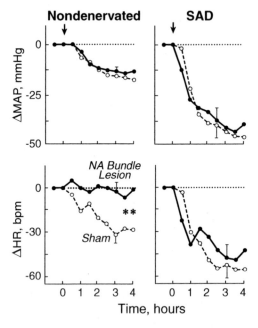

Figure 8.23. Effect of previous dorsal plus ventral ascending NA bundle lesions (Lesion) or sham operation (Sham) on MAP (mmHg) and HR (beats/min) responses to i.c.v. α-MD (0.4 mg/kg) in awake rabbits. Left panels, nondenervated rabbits with intact arterial baroreceptors; right, animals with sinoaortic denervation (SAD). From Van den Buuse et al. (1991), with permission of *Brain Research* and Elsevier.

abolished after chronic sectioning of the dorsal and ventral NA bundles (figure 8.23, left; Van den Buuse et al., 1991). The bundle lesion has no effect on the fall in MAP, which is in accord with the drug's largely bulbospinal site of action (Van Zwieten, 1999; Head and Burke, 2000). In SAD rabbits, the falls in MAP and heart rate are about twice as great as in animals with intact arterial baroreceptors, indicating that the drug's action in the intact organism is limited by the baroreflexes (figure 8.23, right).

The hypotensive action of α-MD is abolished after 6-OHDA-induced destruction of central CA terminals, which attenuates the bradycardia (figure 8.24, middle panel; Day et al., 1973; Finch and Haeusler, 1973; Head et al., 1983). Furthermore, the effects of α-MD are reduced to about half by prior destruction of 5-HT terminals (figure 8.24, right panel).

α-MD is rapidly taken up by 5-HT neurons and it was thought that it inhibited 5-HT synthesis, reducing transmitter stores (Stone and Porter, 1967). However, this has not been observed in brain synaptosomes rich in 5-HT (Wolf and Bobik, 1989).

A more likely mechanism is suggested by figure 8.19, illustrating how 5-HT and NA neurons affect BP. About 50% of NA neurons, which modulate sympathetic constrictor tone at bulbospinal level, inhibit bulbospinal target neurons directly, while the other 50% do this by first inhibiting a 5-HT neuron. This explains why destruction of NA terminals completely eliminates the antihypertensive action of α-MD, while destruction of 5-HT terminals eliminates only half the response (Korner, Head, Bobik et al., 1984).

Last, the rate of conversion of i.c.v. α-MD to α-methyl NA was studied in the different NA neuron groups (Bobik et al., 1988). It was most rapid in A1, A2, and A5 neuron groups and was somewhat less marked in A6 neurons.[9]

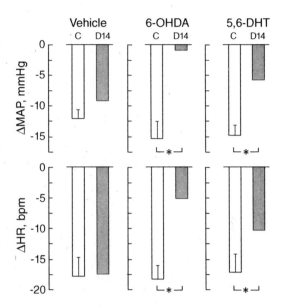

Figure 8.24. Average changes in MAP (mmHg) and HR (beats/min) 3–4 hours after i.c.v. α-methyl dopa (0.4 mg/kg). Control responses (C) on day 0, clear bars; shaded bars, responses on day 14 after i.c.v. vehicle (left panel), 6-OHDA (600 µg/kg; middle panel), and 5,6-DHT (633 µg/kg; right panel). *$p < .01$ for Δ between day 0 and 14 responses. From Head et al. (1983), with permission of *Journal of Cardiovascular Pharmacology* and Lippincott, Williams and Wilkins.

The above supports the hypothesis that α-MD lowers BP by increasing activity of A5 and A6+A7 neurons and enhances activity in the bulbospinal dilator pathway in figure 8.16. The BP fall is moderated by baroreflex-induced elevation of activity in the constrictor pathway. α-MD-induced bradycardia is mediated through increased A1 and A2 neuron activity, which facilitates development of bradycardia through the suprapontine loop despite the large fall in BP.

Integration and Communication within the Central Controller

Integration of information of cardiovascular relevance occurs at all levels of the neuraxis from cortex to spinal cord. Because of the excessive emphasis on baroreflexes by many cardiovascular neuroscientists, it is sometimes forgotten that circulatory regulation of autonomic function is closely linked to most regulatory functions performed by brain. For example, autonomic regulation in exercise is closely linked to the control of skeletal muscle movement (chapter 10). In EH, the elevation of sympathoadrenal activity depends on the nature and intensity of the stress, many behavioral factors, lifestyles, and diets (chapters 11–14). Even when regulation in response to pressure perturbations is entirely through baroreflexes, the autonomic responses are always determined by the sum of the inputs from the arterial, cardiac, and pulmonary baroreceptors, and not just by those of one group of baroreceptors (chapter 9).

A given disturbance usually activates several sensory inputs, which in turn affect activity of a whole network of cardiovascular neurons. It is the network that performs the integrations which determine the autonomic output pattern. With some disturbances the integration is not only based on the immediate input profile but often takes into account previous analagous events stored in memory. This makes for fairly complex relationships between inputs and neurohumoral outputs. Some of the complexities arise from the modulatory effects of slow transmitter neurons, which play a key role in the transformation of inputs to outputs. To use Greengard's analogy, the network's target neuron hardware functions appropriately only when programmed by the software of the slow transmitter neurons. The latter neurons provide the control system with its adaptive characteristics and determine both the short-term and long-term alterations of many of its parameters. Hence the focus in this chapter on some of their cardiovascular actions.

Cardiovascular Role of Neurons Releasing Fast and Slow Transmitters

Over the last 15 years, it has become clear that all major autonomic effector patterns generated in the hypothalamus and hindbrain excite the sympathetic motoneurons of the spinal cord and the vagal motoneurons through premotor neurons that release fast transmitters (Chalmers and Pilowsky, 1991; DiMicco et al., 1992; Dampney, 1994a; Dampney et al., 2002; Pilowsky and Goodchild, 2002). Their rapidity of action ensures synchronization of the different effector components of the overall autonomic pattern.

Discussion of the cardiovascular effects of the slow transmitter neurons in this chapter has been limited to the DA, NA, and 5-HT neurons mainly because the responses elicited by specific neurotoxin-induced transmitter release have provided better clues about the fast transmitter target neurons on which they act than previous methods.

An acute increase in activity of DA neurons modulates hypothalamic target neurons through which the defense pattern of sympathoadrenal activity is evoked. The DA neurons receive information from the prefrontal cortex about the nature and intensity of the stress. This is conveyed to the target neurons located in at least two major cell groups in the hypothalamus and in midbrain neurons of the periaqueductal gray region (chapter 11). Ascending fibers from 5-HT neurons also provide additional input to DA neurons, through which the defense response can also be evoked (figure 8.19). Some of the afferent information to the 5-HT neurons may come from the cerebellum, in the latter's role as a regulator of the autonomic response to exercise. The DA neurons are also involved in a pathway from the renal chemoreceptors to the hypothalamus that elevates BP (chapter 15). Changes in ascending NA neuron fiber activity has also been observed in renal hypertension (chapter 15), but from the current analysis of CA release NA neurons probably carry information from baroreceptors, which may moderate the magnitude of the defense response.

The main NA neurons affecting BP are located in the A5 and A6+A7 cell groups, and their net effect is to lower BP through the bulbospinal depressor pathway. This is opposed by the pressor action of descending 5-HT axons.

Cardiac slowing results from increased modulatory activity of ascending fibers from the NA neurons in the A1 and A2 groups. Their actions enhance vagal excitation and inhibit cardiac SNA. The pathway extends from A1 and A2 to PVN in the hypothalamus (A. Allen, personal communication), from which fast transmitter neurons descend to the vagal and cardiac sympathetic motoneurons in the hindbrain and spinal cord. Cardiac slowing mediated through the same mechanism can be elicited by strong stimulation of the arterial chemoreceptors (Korner, Shaw, West et al., 1973) and by α-MD and clonidine (Badoer et al., 1983; Korner, Head and Badoer, 1984; Korner, Head, Bobik et al., 1984). NA neurons from A5 also increase vagal excitation through a direct hindbrain pathway, which cause less facilitation than increased activity in the long loop via the hypothalamus.

The A1 and A2 neurons facilitate the effects of BP changes on the vagus, while 5-HT neurons inhibit cardiac vagal activity. The modulation may occur from moment to moment in response to alterations in afferent profile in normal animals. More important, the inhibitory modulatory action through 5-HT neurons is responsible for the vagal deficit during chronic elevation in cardiopulmonary load in hypertension (chapter 9). Almost identical inhibition of vagal activity is produced by i.c.v. CRH (Fisher, 1989), which may contribute to the rapid inhibition of vagal tone during heavy exercise.

The model in figure 8.16 also explains the antihypertensive action of α-MD. It is assumed that the fall in BP occurs through the main modulatory action of α-methyl NA plus NA in the A5, A6, and A7 neurons, causing the fall in BP through increased activity in the bulbospinal dilator pathway. The fall in BP is moderated through the baroreflex by increased constrictor activity brought about through the other NA neuron populations in the above regions. α-MD also causes cardiac depression through A1 and A2 NA neurons, which masks the counterregulatory rise in heart rate that would normally occur through baroreflexes in response to peripheral vasodilation. Clinically, α-MD is a very effective antihypertensive drug. One major side effect is somnolence, which is why it went out of fashion. Its action on the CNS is quite nonspecific, like that of so many other antihypertensive drugs.

Synaptic Strengthening (Sensitization)

A striking characteristic of persons with EH is the low stress threshold for eliciting the defense response. A similar low threshold also contributes to SHR hypertension. The best available model of this type of synaptic strengthening is that produced by repeated aversive stimuli on the gill withdrawal reflex in *Aplysia*, which Kandel used as a paradigm for learning. The critical step in the sensitization process is the increased activity of a 5-HT neuron, as a result of which biochemical changes in the nerve terminal increase the amount of fast transmitter released and later increase the synaptic input to the motoneuron through the growth of new synaptic contacts (figure 8.7). Once sensitization has developed, the gill remains withdrawn for prolonged periods in the virtual absence of stimuli.

As noted in chapter 5, in mild EH the elevation of the BP is due to a sustained defense response. In rabbits and rats, this pattern is evoked through modulatory activity by DA neurons. Assuming that these neurons also mediate the response in humans, their repeated stimulation will sensitize the defense pathway, as discussed in chapter 11. The finding by Esler's group that central NA neuron activity is raised in persons with EH is likely to be due to elevation in cardiopulmonary load, causing rises in A6+A7 neuron groups in accordance with the model in figure 8.16.

Concluding Comments

Clearly, more analysis is needed to define the major fast transmitter pathways that link the autonomic premotor neuron groups to each other as well as to the vagal and sympathetic motoneuron outputs. In addition, more is required to characterize the nature of the inputs that determine the activity of slow transmitter neurons. Some of these neurons that terminate on a given target neuron may alter transmitter release at the synapse, while others may change the responsiveness of receptors and channels subserving other functions. It allows a given target neuron to respond in diverse ways to quite a number of inputs.

Last, it seems pertinent to ask how a relatively small number of monoaminergic or peptidergic neurons of a given type are not only important in circulatory regulation, but also perform many regulatory functions pertaining to other systems. Although the role of the monoaminergic neurons in circulatory control and in SHR hypertension has long been known, it has been the somewhat fortuitous findings associated with transmitter release that have shown the importance of these neurons in the generation of specific autonomic patterns. In chapter 9, it will become evident that their effect on baroreflex properties occurs in response to specific cardiovascular inputs, while chapter 11 discusses their role as an information channel from the thalamocortical system to the ANS, which is the neural mechanism that initiates EH in response to an adverse environment. The various monoaminergic neurons are also important modulators of the level of arousal of the thalamocortical system and of many of its other activities. Probably only a small fraction of each group of monoaminergic neurons, say 10–20%, may be committed to the cardiovascular system, while the rest subserves other regulatory functions.

9

Whole-Organism Baroreflexes

In the classic analysis of baroreceptor reflexes, the idea was to examine circulatory and neural responses emanating from an isolated receptor zone in anesthetized animals, for example, from the carotid sinus baroreceptors (Heymans and Neil, 1958; Angell-James and Daly, 1970; Linden, 1973; Paintal, 1973; Mancia et al., 1976; Abboud and Thames, 1983; Daly, 1986). Much of the current understanding of regulation of the ANS is based on experiments of this type. However, accumulating data about the responses of individual reflexes and trying to resynthesize the behavior of the intact organism has proved virtually impossible.

A different approach is outlined in this chapter. After a brief review of receptor properties, "whole-organism" baroreflexes are characterized and their properties compared in healthy normotensives and persons with chronic hypertension. A neuronal network in the CNS receives simultaneous information from the arterial, cardiac, and pulmonary baroreceptors. Since the circulation is a closed-loop hydraulic system, any disturbance affecting BP engages all of the baroreceptors to varying degrees. Combinations of baroreceptor afferents project to slow transmitter interneurons, which alter the responsiveness of the fast transmitter pathways to the vagal and sympathetic motoneurons (chapter 8). In chronic hypertension, whole-organism cardiac and constrictor baroreflexes have different properties than subjects with normal BP, and one objective has been to examine some of the mechanisms responsible for the changes in their properties.

The effectiveness with which baroreflexes maintain BP varies, as illustrated in different types of tissue hypoxia. This is due to changes in relative magnitude of the inputs from the arterial, cardiac, and pulmonary baroreceptors. Some of these factors contribute to the modest increase in BP variability in hypertension, though other factors such as the R_1 vessel structural changes also play a role. The last topic examines and questions the basis of the still widely held belief that baroreflex dysfunction is a cause of EH (Eckberg and Sleight, 1992).

Cardiovascular Baroreceptors

Afferent nerves from the arterial, cardiac, and pulmonary baroreceptors reach the CNS through the 9th and 10th cranial nerves (Spyer, 1981, 1990). Additional information about BP comes through segmental spinal inputs through the sympathetic afferent nerves (Malliani, 1982). All baroreceptors are mechanoreceptors and adapt to long-term changes in BP. This is responsible for their relatively normal function in chronic hypertension.

Properties of Arterial, Cardiac, and Pulmonary Baroreceptors

Arterial Baroreceptors

The carotid sinus and aortic arch baroreceptors provide information about mean arterial pressure (MAP), pulse pressure, and arterial dP/dt. Some of the arterial baroreceptors in each receptor zone give rise to myelinated A-fibers, while others give rise to the more slowly conducting unmyelinated C-fibers. Both A- and C-fiber baroreceptors discharge in response to deformation forces in the vascular wall (Kirchheim, 1976; Brown, 1980; Andresen and Yang, 1989; Koushanpour, 1991; Chapleau et al., 1995).

The pressure threshold (P_{th}) of A-fiber baroreceptors is low and, once exceeded, causes a rapid rise in discharge to a saturation plateau (figure 9.1). In C-fiber barore-ceptors, P_{th} is higher and their discharge rises more gradually (Kirchheim, 1976; Coleridge and Coleridge, 1980; Seagard et al., 1990).

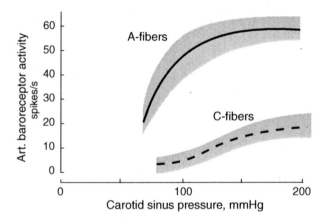

Figure 9.1. Relationship between BP and discharge in isolated arterial baroreceptor A- and C-fibers. Line shows average responses and shading is at ±1 SEM. Based on data in Kirchheim (1976) and Seagard et al. (1990).

Cardiac and Pulmonary Baroreceptors

Most atrial baroreceptors are located close to the venoatrial junctions. One group discharges with a prominent burst of activity related to the atrial a wave. In others, often termed volume receptors, the discharge increases in parallel with the v wave (Gauer and Henry, 1963; Paintal, 1971, 1973; Linden, 1973; Thorén et al., 1976, 1979). Ventricular baroreceptors are largely C-fibers of fairly high P_{th} (Thorén et al., 1979, 1986; Coleridge and Coleridge, 1980). Their BP responsiveness is increased by several chemical agents, such as veratrum alkaloids, bradykinin, and prostaglandins. Most pulmonary artery baroreceptors also have C-fiber afferents; P_{th} is high and their discharge is sparse and irregular (Coleridge et al., 1964a, 1964b; Paintal, 1971).

Last, baroreceptors associated with the sympathetic afferent nerves are located in the heart, coronary arteries, and large thoracic vessels and mostly give rise to C-fibers (Malliani, 1982). Reflex effects occur only in response to large changes in transmural BP or exposure to chemical agents (Coleridge and Coleridge, 1979).

Rapid Resetting of Arterial Baroreceptors

Arterial baroreceptors are relatively slowly adapting mechanoreceptors: The sharp increase in firing rate that follows a step increase in BP takes 1–1.5 minutes to subside (Sleight et al., 1977, Koushanpour, 1991). The rate of adaptation depends on the hysteresis properties of the arterial wall and on changes in the receptor's ionic conductances.

When resting BP has risen or fallen to a new steady level, the P_{th} of A-fiber arterial baroreceptors rapidly resets in the same direction (Coleridge et al., 1981; Dorward et al., 1982). After 15–30 minutes, P_{th} has shifted by 0.2–0.5 mmHg per mmHg resting BP (Schultz et al., 1985; Andresen and Yang, 1989; Chapleau et al., 1989; Seagard et al., 1992). However, BP sensitivity (gain) of the receptor remains unchanged (figure 9.2, middle; Coleridge et al., 1981; Dorward et al., 1982). There is also a change in the relationship between BP and receptor firing pattern (figure 9.2, top), raising the question of the duration of the brain's memory for a previous BP level (Dorward and Korner, 1987). Given the partial nature of rapid resetting of A-fiber baroreceptors, some memory is probably retained at the receptor level for longer than the approximately 60 seconds it takes to develop a stable discharge (Burke et al., 1986). C-fiber baroreceptors reset more gradually, allowing the brain to recognize a change in their discharge from a previous level for at least several hours. The mechanisms contributing to resetting include hysteresis of the wall (Coleridge et al., 1984) and the effects of wall tension and stretch that alter the receptor's generator potential and ionic conductances (Brown, 1980; Heesch et al., 1984; Munch and Brown, 1985; Sachs, 1987; Andresen and Yang, 1989; Chapleau et al., 1995).

Rapid baroreceptor resetting maximizes the information content received by the brain about arterial BP and extends the BP range over which baroreflexes operate at high gain (Dorward et al., 1982; Dorward and Korner, 1987). Rapid resetting generally results in a greater shift in reflex P_{th} than the P_{th} at the arterial baroreceptor level (Dorward et al., 1982, 1985; Burke et al., 1986). This applies even when the reflex is evoked from an isolated carotid sinus after eliminating the other baroreceptors (Drummond and

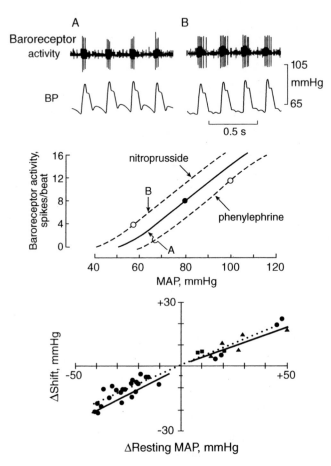

Figure 9.2. Top, arterial pressure pulse and A-fiber baroreceptor unit discharge at points A and B of the control and nitroprusside curves in anesthetized rabbits. Fifteen minutes after resetting, the discharge pattern has altered for the same MAP and pressure pulse. Middle, relationship between MAP (mmHg) and A-fiber aortic baroreceptor unit discharge (spikes/beat) under control conditions (solid line) and after sustained changes in resting MAP produced by IV infusions of nitroprusside or phenylephrine (dashed lines); circles are mean resting MAPs. Bottom, relationship between change in resting MAP during nitroprusside and phenylephrine infusions (abscissa) and shift in receptor function curves (ordinate). From Dorward et al. (1982) and Dorward and Korner (1987).

Seagard, 1996). It suggests that incoming discharge contains more information than that pertaining to the alterations in MAP.

Baroreceptor Resetting in Chronic Hypertension

In chronic hypertension, the BP sensitivity of the arterial baroreceptors is reduced (figure 9.3), which is partly due to the low distensibility of the arterial wall (Angell-James, 1973; Brown et al., 1976; Sapru and Wang, 1976). The increase in P_{th} of the

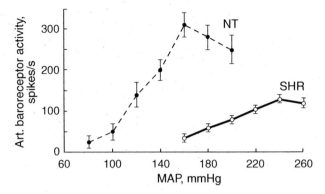

Figure 9.3. Relationship between MAP (mmHg) and aortic baroreceptor discharge (spikes/s) in SHR and normotensive rats during stepwise increments in BP held for about 30 seconds; values, means ± SEMs). Note higher P_{th} and lower slope in SHR hypertension. From Sapru and Wang (1976), with permission of the *American Journal of Physiology* and American Physiological Society.

arterial baroreceptors is close to the rise in resting BP; that is, resetting (adaptation) is complete (McCubbin et al., 1956; Kezdi, 1962; Angell-James, 1973; Angell-James and Lumley, 1974; Sleight et al., 1977; Brown, 1980; Krieger et al., 1982). This takes about 2 days for A-fiber P_{th} in acute experimental hypertension (Krieger et al., 1982; Krieger, 1989). The change is more gradual in arterial C-fiber baroreceptors (Thorén et al., 1983). In chronic hypertension, the information received by the brain about changes in MAP is probably similar to that received when BP is normal, but there may be differences in discharge related to the alterations in pulse pressure (figures 4.3 and 5.6).

There has been controversy whether P_{th} of cardiac and pulmonary baroreceptors is also reset in chronic hypertension (Thorén et al., 1979; Coleridge and Coleridge, 1980; Ricksten et al., 1981). In all chronic hypertension, cardiopulmonary load (central BPs and blood volumes) is raised and, as discussed later in this chapter, there is no doubt that the raised load is responsible for long-term changes in reflex properties. This is not really a matter of whether the receptors have or have not become adapted, for eventually all receptors adapt. The signaling of raised load affects the phasic pulsatile information received by the brain. In addition, there are also changes in the relative magnitude of inputs from the arterial baroreceptors on the one hand and the cardiac and pulmonary baroreceptors on the other, which contribute to the differences in reflex properties.

In conclusion, because rapid resetting is only partial the CNS recognizes for some time a change in input from the arterial baroreceptors as a change from a previous reference level. The main advantage of the partial resetting is to maximize the gain of the reflex response. In chronic hypertension, the receptors have become completely adapted. This is responsible for the effectiveness of minimizing BP variability in hypertension, which is only slightly impaired. Elevation in central load is signaled by changes in pulsatile characteristics of the receptor discharge and by changes in the relative magnitude of the inputs from the arterial and cardiopulmonary receptors.

Cardiac Baroreflexes in Hypertension

In hypertension, vagal responsiveness to rises in BP is subnormal, and this is an indicator of future cardiovascular risk and mortality (Eckberg and Sleight, 1992; Osterziel et al., 1995; La Rovere et al., 1998; Kardos et al., 2001; Ziegler et al., 2001; Head, 2002; Lantelme et al., 2002). Although this makes the underlying mechanisms a matter of obvious interest, they have been the subject of little experimental analysis.

Methods for Studying Cardiac Baroreflexes

Study methods include the rapid ramp method and a number of steady-state methods.

Ramp Methods

Injecting an IV bolus of a constrictor drug causes a ramp rise in BP, which evokes reflex cardiac slowing (Smyth et al., 1969; Pickering et al., 1972; Mancia et al., 1976; Mancia and Mark, 1983; Eckberg and Sleight, 1992). The systolic BP (SBP) of a given beat is linearly related to the heart period (HP, pulse interval) of the succeeding beat (figure 9.4). The slope of the regression line is a measure of baroreflex sensitivity (BRS) or gain. The lengthening of HP is mostly due to increases in vagal efferent activity, because the vagus has a faster response time than the sympathetic nerves (Glick and Braunwald, 1965; Scher and Young, 1970). BRS is significantly reduced in chronic hypertension (figure 9.4), signifying vagal impairment (Sleight, 1974, 1991). BRS is also reduced in older people independently of hypertension (Gribbin et al., 1971; Eckberg and Sleight, 1992).

If vasodilator drugs are injected, the resulting fall in BP is also linearly related to the evoked falls in HP (tachycardia; Pickering et al., 1972). The slope generally differs from that elicited by constrictor drugs.

Various "spontaneous" ramp methods have been developed in which BP and HP (or heart rate) are recorded for several minutes and BRS determined automatically from the spontaneous fluctuations, using computer techniques (Parati et al., 1990; Eckberg and Sleight, 1992; Parlow et al., 1995; Ziegler et al., 2001; Laude et al., 2004). In one method, the computer selects spontaneous sequences of three or more rises in SBP and the corresponding HP changes and calculates average BRS from the regression line derived from all such sequences. Another method uses cross-spectral analysis to determine the frequency range over which BP and HP are most highly correlated: Only these data are used to calculate average BRS. There is reasonable agreement between estimates of BRS by spontaneous and conventional ramp methods. These methods are finding increasing clinical use because of the prognostic significance of the result (Laude et al., 2004).

Steady-State Methods

With steady-state methods, the BP-induced alterations in HP (or heart rate) are due to changes in both vagal and sympathetic effector activity (Korner, West et al., 1972; Korner et al., 1974; West and Korner, 1974). MAP is altered by brief IV infusions of

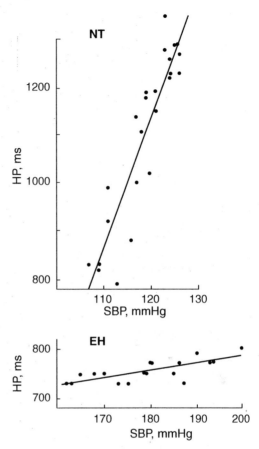

Figure 9.4. Blood pressure ramp after bolus injection of pressor drug, showing linear relationship between systolic BP (SBP, mmHg) and heart period (HP, ms) in normotensive subject (NT, top) and in subject with EH (bottom). From Bristow et al. (1969), with permission of *Circulation*, American Heart Association, and Lippincott, Williams and Wilkins.

different concentrations of vasoactive drugs, alternating between vasoconstrictor and vasodilator drugs with a rest pause between injections.[1] Another way is to examine the responses to slow ramp rises or falls in BP (1–2 mmHg/s; Dorward et al., 1985). A given ΔMAP induces directionally similar changes in cardiac and pulmonary BPs, so that ΔMAP serves as an index of a more elaborate BP profile (Korner et al., 1972; Korner, West et al., 1974). In animals, the reflex can be evoked by altering BP by inflating previously implanted perivascular aortic and inferior vena cava balloons.

The relationship between MAP and HP (or heart rate) is described by a four-parameter sigmoid logistic function (figure 9.5). The parameters are: (1) the lower plateau (P_1); (2) the effector response range between plateaus (P_2); (3) the average gain (G_{av}), which is the slope of the steep part of the curve and equals $P_2 \times P_3/4.56$, where P_3 is the coefficient of curvature, also known as the range-independent gain; (4) the median BP (BP_{50}; P_4) (Korner, 1989; Head, 1995). For markedly asymmetric curves, a five-parameter logistic function provides a better fit (Ricketts and Head, 1999).

A small step rise in MAP from resting alters HP (or heart rate) through a reciprocal rise in vagal activity and reduction in cardiac SNA. As ΔMAP rises, the vagal changes become more pronounced, with the response at the plateau entirely vagal.

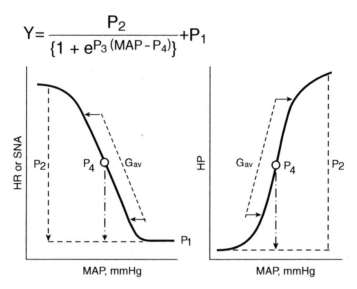

$$Y = \frac{P_2}{\{1 + e^{P_3 (MAP - P_4)}\}} + P_1$$

Figure 9.5. Logistic function curves relating mean arterial pressure (MAP, mmHg) to heart period (HP, ms, right) and to heart rate (HR, beats/min) or sympathetic nerve activity (SNA, units, left). Curve parameters are: P_1 = lower plateau; P_2 = HR or HP range; P_3 (not shown) = curvature coefficient, that is, normalized (range-independent) gain; P_4 = BP_{50}, that is, MAP at midpoint between upper and lower plateaus; G_{av} = average gain over ±1 standard deviation from BP_{50}.

The converse occurs with falls in MAP, where the tachycardia plateau is almost entirely due to sympathetic excitation.

Either HP or heart rate can be used as the dependent variable. The HP scale accentuates differences in bradycardia plateaus between hypertensives and normotensives, which is useful in studies on the vagal deficit in hypertension. The heart rate scale gives equal weight to both effector components, permitting assessment of their relative magnitude.

Cardiac Baroreflex Properties in Hypertension

In EH, the vagal bradycardia plateau becomes increasingly attenuated as resting BP rises, while the tachycardia plateau is unaffected (figure 9.6; Korner, West et al., 1974). G_{av} is markedly depressed in those with severe EH but is either normal or raised when hypertension is mild. In older subjects, the vagal bradycardia plateau, G_{av}, and the HP range are all more depressed than in the corresponding groups of younger normotensives and persons with EH (table 9.1). Vagal impairment occurs in most types of chronic hypertension in humans and animals, suggesting that it is a nonspecific consequence of the high BP (Korner, 1989; Eckberg and Sleight, 1992).

In SHR, the time course of development of the vagal deficit can be determined more accurately than in human cross-sectional studies (figure 9.7; Head and Adams, 1988, 1992). At 6 weeks of age, hypertension is still mild and the bradycardia and tachycardia

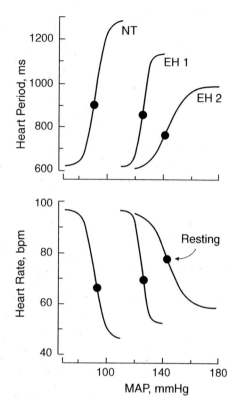

Figure 9.6. Top, baroreflex curve relating mean arterial pressure (MAP, mmHg) to heart period (HP, ms) in 18–30-year-old healthy normal subjects (NT) and age-matched subjects with mild and more severe EH (EH 1, EH 2). Bottom, same data plotted as the MAP-heart rate (beats/min) relationship. Circles along curve are resting values. From Korner and Head (1992), with permission of Birkhäuser (Springer-Verlag).

Table 9.1. Mean Resting Values and Parameters of MAP-HP Curve in Young and Older Normotensive Subjects (NT) and Persons with Mild and Moderate/Severe EH (EH_1, EH_2)

Variable	<30 Years Old			>30 Years Old		
	NT	EH_1	EH_2	NT	EH_1	EH_2
Age, yrs	23.6	26.4	25.2	43.9	39.1	47
MAP, mmHg	92	125*	142*	99	126*	151*
PP, mmHg	53	68*	70*	57	70*	90*
Bradycardia plateau, ms	1280	1110*	960*	1030	910*	800*
BP_{50}, mmHg	92	125*	143*	101	124*	154*
HP Range, ms	670	520*	397*	371	322	173*
G_{av}, ms/mmHg	41	49 ns	13*	21	13*	11*
n	14	5	4	9	11	4

Note: MAP, mean arterial pressure; PP, pulse pressure; HP, heart period (milliseconds, ms); BP_{50}, median blood pressure; HP range, HP range between plateaus; G_{av}, average gain. *$p < .05$ for difference from NT.

Source: Korner, West et al. (1974) with permission of *Clinical and Experimental Pharmacology and Physiology* and Blackwell.

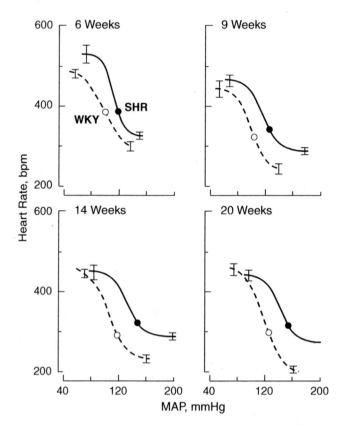

Figure 9.7. Average relationship between MAP (mmHg) and heart rate (beats/min) in SHR (solid) and WKY rats (dashed lines) at ages 6, 9, 14, and 20 weeks. From Head and Adams (1992), with permission of *Clinical and Experimental Pharmacology and Physiology* and Blackwell.

plateaus are similar to those in WKY, while G_{av} is significantly greater. There is increasing attenuation of the bradycardia plateau and depression of G_{av} from the age of 9 weeks onward, as BP continues to increase.

Determinants of Cardiac Baroreflex Properties

During alterations in cardiopulmonary load, the information from arterial, cardiac, and pulmonary baroreceptors is transmitted from NTS to the vagal and sympathetic motoneurons through NA and 5-HT interneurons (chapter 8). In addition, peripheral vagal ganglionic transmission is affected by changes in plasma Ang II (see below). Sinoaortic denervation (SAD) reduces the heart rate range by 90–95% (table 9.2), suggesting that the cardiopulmonary baroreceptors modulate the effects mediated through the arterial baroreceptors (Korner et al., 1972; Korner, Shaw, West et al., 1973; Blombery and Korner, 1979).[2]

Unfortunately, the role of the cardiac and pulmonary baroreceptors cannot be assessed by classic denervation methods, because the afferent and efferent fibers travel

Table 9.2. Resting Values and Parameters of MAP-Heart Rate (HR) Function Curves in Awake Sham-Operated Rabbits, and in Rabbits Subjected to Bilateral Removal of Aortic Nerves, Carotid Sinus Nerves, and Sinoaortic Denervation, Operated 6–8 days Previously

Variable	Sham-op	AN Den	CS Den	SAD
Tachy plateau, bpm	353	324	338	295
Brady plateau, bpm	170	206	245	281
HR range, bpm	183	118	93	14
G_{av}, bpm/mmHg	12.2	3.5	4.7	~0
MAP ± sem, mmHg	85 ± 1.4	97* ± 2.1	108* ± 2.8	110* ± 4.5
Resting HR, bpm	223	250	287	283
n	6	5	7	5

Note: n = number of rabbits; Tachy, tachycardia; Brady, bradycardia; AN Den, aortic nerve denervation; CS Den, carotid sinus nerve denervation; SAD, sinoaortic denervation; HR, heart rate; MAP, mean arterial pressure; sem, standard error of mean. *$p < .05$ for difference from sham-operated rabbits.

Source: Adapted from Blombery and Korner (1979).

in the same vagus nerve. Hence their role has to be determined indirectly. One way is to raise BP beyond the plateaus, which evokes additional bradycardia (figure 9.8). The nonlinearity of the function curve suggests that as the intravascular BPs are raised, additional pressure-sensitive receptors come into play. These have turned out to be high-threshold cardiac and pulmonary baroreceptors, the BP responsiveness of which is enhanced by atrial natriuretic peptide (ANP) (Ludbrook, 1984; Korner and Head, 1992; Woods et al., 1994).

Another approach has been to compare the reflex properties when the reflex is evoked by the perivascular balloon and vasoactive drug methods. For a given change in MAP, the change in cardiopulmonary load is greater with the balloon cuff method than with the drug method. During aortic cuff inflation, the upstream arterial segment becomes less compliant, so that the changes in arterial pulse pressure and cardiac and pulmonary BPs are greater than those elicited by constrictor drugs which act on downstream resistance vessels. Similarly, a given fall in ΔMAP is accompanied by greater falls in cardiopulmonary BP, CO, and arterial pulse pressure with IVC balloon cuff inflation than with vasodilator drugs (Korner et al., 1972; Korner, West, and Shaw, 1973; Korner, West et al., 1974).

This approach was first used in two genetically distinct rabbit strains, selected on the basis of difference in BRS during steady-state rises in BP (Weinstock and Rosin, 1984; Weinstock et al., 1984, 1986).

With all autonomic effectors intact, the heart rate range between the plateaus was smaller with the cuff method than with the drug method, which was largely due to differences in the vagal responses of both groups of rabbits (figures 9.9, 9.10; Weinstock et al., 1988). Cuff-induced rises in MAP elicited less vagal excitation than the same ΔMAP evoked with the drug method, suggesting that the vagal deficit (i.e., attenuation of the vagal plateau) was due to the greater cardiopulmonary load. Moreover, the tachycardia plateau was slightly smaller with the cuff method than with the drug method. However, when only the sympathetic nerves were working, the cuff method evoked more tachycardia than the drug method. It follows that in the intact animal,

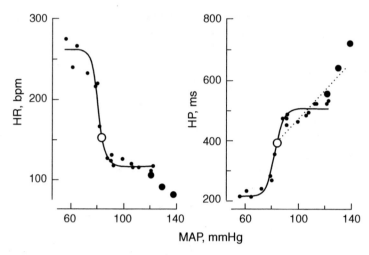

Figure 9.8. MAP-HR (left) and MAP-HP (right) relationships in one rabbit; small circles are data points and are responses to brief IV infusions of phenylephrine and sodium nitroprusside with BP alternately raised and lowered around resting values. Open circles, average resting values. Raising MAP beyond bradycardia plateau evoked more bradycardia (large black circles). The nonlinearity in the curves suggests additional afferent input. From Weinstock et al. (1988), with permission of *American Journal of Physiology* and American Physiological Society.

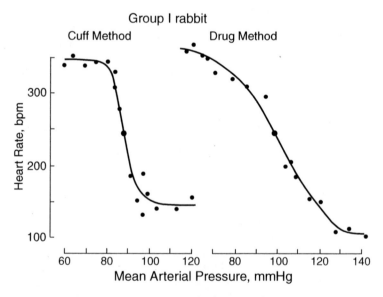

Figure 9.9. Relationships between mean arterial pressure (mmHg) and heart rate (beats/min) in one Group I rabbit, showing differences in properties when reflex evoked by cuff method (left) and by drug method (right). From Weinstock et al. (1988), with permission of *American Journal of Physiology* and American Physiological Society.

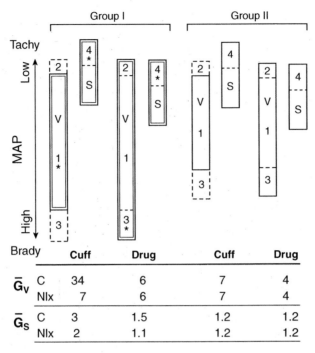

		Cuff	Drug	Cuff	Drug
$\bar{G}_V$	C	34	6	7	4
	Nlx	7	6	7	4
$\bar{G}_S$	C	3	1.5	1.2	1.2
	Nlx	2	1.1	1.2	1.2

Figure 9.10. Subdivisions of vagal (V) and sympathetic (S) heart rate ranges in Group I and II rabbits, for reflex evoked by cuff and drug methods in the same animal. Table gives vagal and sympathetic components of gain (G_v, G_s) under control conditions (C) and during naloxone (Nlx). Segment 1 is largest component of V; segments 2, 3, and 4 defined from response differences between the two methods. Solid lines, actual heart rate ranges with each method; dashed lines, segments not responsive to cuff-induced changes in BP. Asterisk denotes responsiveness of some segments to naloxone (Group I only). Further discussion in text. After Weinstock et al. (1988).

the greater rise in SNA evoked by lowering BP with the cuff method is offset by some residual vagal tone (figure 9.10). In contrast, lowering BP with vasoactive drugs results in a tachycardia plateau that is entirely due to sympathetic excitation, while vagal tone has fallen to zero.

The greatest method-related difference between Group I and II rabbits was in their G_{av} responses (figure 9.10). In Group I, cuff-induced G_{av} was 6 times the value with the drug method, while in Group II the increase in G_{av} was only 1.8 times as great as with the drug method.

Partitioning the Vagal and Sympathetic Heart Rate Ranges

The largest part of the vagal range in each group of rabbits is segment 1 (figure 9.10); segments 2 and 3 are the differences in vagal responses elicited by the cuff and drug method at low and high MAPs, respectively. Vagal neurons in segment 3 do not respond to cuff-induced rises in BP, but they do respond to drug-induced BP rises.

Only Group I rabbits responded to naloxone, which (1) reduced vagal G_{av} with the cuff method, and (2) eliminated segment 3 with the drug method (figure 9.10). Naloxone also eliminated segment 4 of the sympathetic motoneuron pool with both methods.

Although Group II rabbits did not respond to naloxone, the method-related effects on the vagal and sympathetic components of the heart rate range were closely similar (figure 9.10). It suggests that their neuron pools are organized in a similar fashion, apart from not having an opiate interneuron.

Modeling the Input-Output Relationship

It is assumed that the action of cardiopulmonary baroreceptors on this reflex depends on the integrity of the arterial baroreceptors (table 9.2; Korner et al., 1972; Korner, Shaw, West et al., 1973; Blombery and Korner, 1979; Faris et al., 1980). A corollary is that method-related response differences are due to interactions between the various groups of baroreceptors (Weinstock et al., 1988). A further assumption is that afferent information is transmitted from the NTS to the vagal and sympathetic motoneurons through: (1) a noradrenergic (NA) interneuron which enhances vagal effector activity, and (2) a serotonergic (5-HT) interneuron which inhibits the vagus (see figure 8.20). The last assumption is that in Group I rabbits a naloxone-sensitive synapse in the NTS region reinforces the action of the NA neuron.

Model D in figure 9.11 explains the changes in reflex properties due to small rises in cardiopulmonary load induced by vasoactive drugs. The afferent inputs to the vagal motoneurons include (1) low-threshold arterial baroreceptors that project to segment 1; and (2) low-threshold arterial and cardiac baroreceptors that project to segment 3 via the NA interneuron. Modest elevation in BP engages the low-threshold arterial and cardiac baroreceptors, which enhance G_{av} through segment 1 and increase activity in segment 3. Lowering BP reduces vagal activity to zero and raises sympathetic activity.

The general Model G (figure 9.12) explains the changes in response to a larger range of cardiopulmonary loads. The afferent input comes from low-, medium-, and high-threshold arterial, cardiac, and pulmonary baroreceptors. As before, segment 1 receives a direct projection from arterial baroreceptors and indirect projections from low- and medium-threshold arterial and cardiac baroreceptors through the opiate neuron linked to the NA interneuron.[3] The 5-HT interneuron receives projections from medium- and high-threshold arterial, cardiac, and pulmonary baroreceptors.

A cuff-induced moderate rise in cardiopulmonary load stimulates the 5-HT neuron mildly, inhibiting segment 3 and accounting for the attenuated bradycardia plateau at high BPs. At the same time, the input from arterial and cardiac baroreceptors of low and medium threshold stimulates the NA interneuron, exciting segment 1 and raising G_{av}. A further rise in cardiopulmonary load stimulates the 5-HT neuron more strongly, inhibiting the NA neuron completely. This leaves the arterial baroreceptors as the sole input to segment 1, while high-threshold baroreceptors inhibit segments 3 and 2.

Relating Group I to Group II Findings and to Other Rabbit Strains and Species

The greater vagal heart rate range in Group I suggests that its vagal motoneurons are either more numerous or more active than those in Group II. The drug and cuff methods

Figure 9.11. Model D, showing effects of modest changes in BP on vagal and sympathetic motoneuron pools (VMN, SMN). ΔBP alters afferent activity of low-threshold (lt) arterial and cardiac baroreceptors, which affect NTS neurons: arterial baroreceptor projections go (1) directly to VMN and SMN; (2) arterial and cardiac baroreceptor projections go to VMN via a noradrenergic (NA) neuron. A mild increase in load activates segment 3 through the NA neuron, raising G_{av}, which is prevented by naloxone in Group I rabbits; *, naloxone-sensitive segment. Similar changes in segment 3 occur in other rabbits but are unaffected by naloxone. Plasma Ang II concentration affects vagal ganglionic transmission (see figure 9.13).

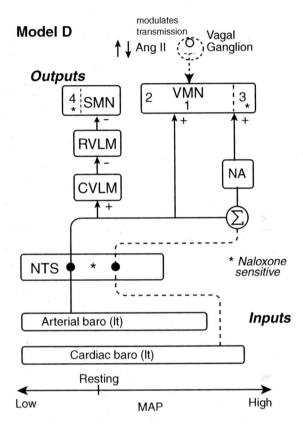

have similar effects on vagal and sympathetic segments in each strain, suggesting similar relationships between input and output. Nevertheless, the effects of naloxone on G_{av} and other segments of the motoneuron pool of Group I rabbits strengthens the case that some of the method-related differences are due to interactions between the various afferent inputs. The opiate synapse is responsible for the high BP sensitivity of G_{av} in Group I. It is absent in Group II, where the still significant but smaller enhancement of G_{av} may be due to NA interneuron activity in the absence of the opiate neuron.

Group I and Group II rabbits were bred originally from the New Zealand White strain. Similar method-related differences to those observed in Group II were seen in other New Zealand White rabbits and in a multicolored English strain (Faris et al., 1980; Kingwell et al., 1991). In mild EH and in early SHR hypertension, G_{av} is often raised while the vagal bradycardia plateau is either normal or only slightly depressed (Figures 9.6, 9.7). When hypertension becomes severe, the bradycardia plateau and G_{av} are both depressed, and G_{av} approaches the low gain of the arterial baroreceptors in chronic hypertension (figure 9.3; Angell-James, 1973; Angell-James and Lumley, 1974; Sapru and Wang, 1976; Brown, 1980; Ichikawa et al., 1995). It appears that the predictions of Model G apply to other mammalian species.

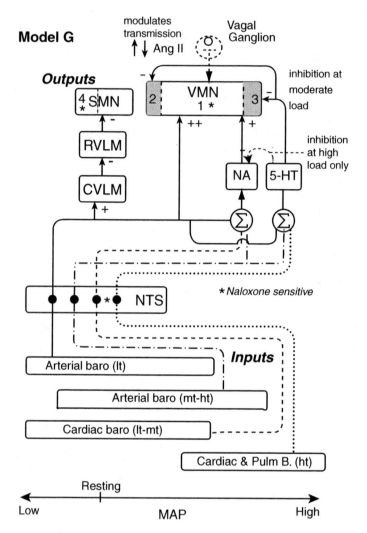

Figure 9.12. Model G describes effect of greater range of loads on vagal and sympathetic motoneuron pools (VMN, SMN). The afferents include low-, medium-, and high-threshold arterial and cardiac baroreceptors (lt, mt, ht) and mt and ht pulmonary baroreceptors. VMNs and SMNs receive direct projections from arterial baroreceptors, while vagus receives the combinations of arterial, cardiac, and pulmonary baroreceptors as shown. The NA neuron receives input from lt arterial and cardiac baroreceptors, while the 5-HT neuron receives input from mt and ht baroreceptors. At mild to moderate cardiopulmonary loads, G_{av} increases through the NA neuron, while the 5-HT neuron inhibits segment 3. At greater load, the 5-HT neuron inhibits the NA neuron, leaving the arterial baroreceptors as the sole input to VMN. Changes in plasma Ang II alter vagal ganglionic transmission. CVLM, RVLM, caudal and rostral ventrolateral medulla; *, naloxone-sensitive (Group I only).

Effect of Ang II on Vagal Deficit

Changes in plasma Ang II concentration have long been known to affect baroreflex properties, but there has been controversy whether this occurs through CNS or peripheral mechanisms.

Peripheral and Central Effects of Ang II on the Vagal Component of the Reflex

Scroop and Lowe (1968, 1969) infused Ang II into the vertebral artery and found that it depressed vagal function. Later, Potter (1982) found that Ang II depressed the vagus through a peripheral action. Angus (unpublished data) examined the latter action in the isolated guinea pig atrium preparation: Low concentrations of Ang II (10^{-11} and 10^{-10} M) depressed the bradycardia evoked by electrical stimulation of the peripheral vagus nerve, but had no effect on the bradycardia response evoked by field stimulation of vagal nerve terminals (figure 9.13). The above concentrations are equivalent to plasma Ang II levels of 20 to 200 pg/mL. The findings suggest that a small increase in Ang II depresses vagal ganglionic transmission but has no effect on presynaptic receptors on the vagal nerve endings.

In awake rabbits, IV infusions of Ang II at rates of 50 and 100 ng/kg/min depressed G_{av} by ~40%, but caused little change in the bradycardia plateau (figure 9.14, left; Korner, 1988). When Ang II was given by the i.c.v. route, BP rose and caused resetting of the function curve,[4] with little change in other parameters (figure 9.14, right); peripheral PRA and PRC declined in a dose-related manner, which may be

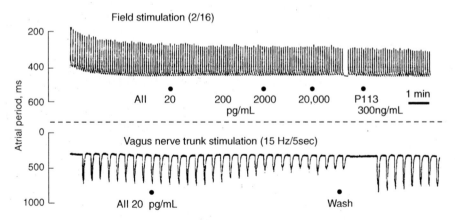

Figure 9.13. Lower trace, in isolated guinea pig atrium, electrical stimulation of right vagus for 5 seconds every 30 seconds (5–15 Hz; duration 0.5–1 ms; supramaximal voltage) increases atrial period (slows rate), with low concentrations of Ang II (AII) attenuating response. Upper trace, electrical field pulses delivered in atrial refractory period depolarize sympathetic and vagal varicosities (Angus and Harvey, 1981); propranolol (10^{-7}) prevents sympathetic responses; bradycardia occurs within the atrial interval in which field pulse is delivered but is unaffected by Ang II or saralasin (P113). Thus, Ang II inhibits vagal ganglionic transmission but has no effect on prejunctional receptors at vagal terminals. Courtesy of Professor James Angus.

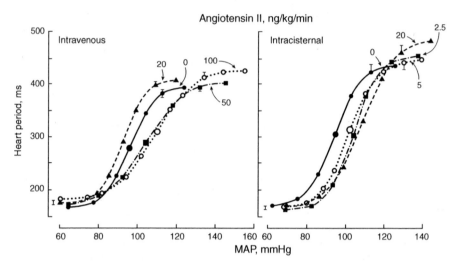

Figure 9.14. Left, average cuff-induced MAP-HP curves from 5 awake rabbits during IV Ang II infusion at rates of 0, 20, 50, and 100 ng/kg/min. G_{av} reduced at higher doses, but bradycardia plateau unaffected. Right, MAP-HP curves from 6 rabbits infused with i.c.v. Ang II at rates of 0, 2.5, 5.0, and 20 ng/kg/min. Resting MAP rose at all doses, plasma renin concentration (PRC) declined slightly, but G_{av} and vagal plateau unaffected. From Korner and Oliver, unpublished data.

either a reflex response or a direct effect of the raised BP on the renal barostat (Davis and Freeman, 1976; Dampney et al., 1979). It may account for the minimal changes in reflex parameters (see below).

Thus, small rises in plasma Ang II depress vagal ganglionic transmission and reduce G_{av}. Centrally administered Ang II has no direct effect on vagal function but raises BP through its effect on central constrictor pathways (Bickerton and Buckley, 1961; Ferrario et al., 1987; Brody et al., 1991; Phillips, 2000).

Reducing and Inducing the Vagal Deficit

The vagal deficit is altered by antihypertensive treatment, administration of vasoactive drugs, renal hypertension, and changes in dietary salt. In some of the above there are changes in both cardiopulmonary load and plasma Ang II.

Antihypertensive Treatment

In theory, if high cardiopulmonary load was the cause of the vagal deficit, its reduction should improve vagal function. However, the effects of antihypertensive treatment have been highly variable, with improvement often evident only when treatment succeeded in causing regression of LVH (Grassi et al., 1988; Head and Adams, 1992).

In Goldblatt 2K-1C hypertension, the vagal deficit is rapidly induced, in parallel with rises in BP and plasma Ang II (Jones and Floras, 1982). Surgical cure of experimental wrap hypertension restored vagal function as well as BP (Fletcher et al., 1976; Fletcher, 1984). Removal of the renal artery clip after several weeks of high BP rapidly lowers BP, but its effects on vagal function have varied: In one study, restoration of function was rapid (Jones and Floras, 1982), while in another this took 2–3 weeks (Edmunds et al., 1990), with no obvious reason for the difference.

In most experiments, antihypertensive treatment has been discontinued for 1–2 weeks before examining the reflex properties, by which time cardiopulmonary load is likely to have risen again. In order to avoid this, it is necessary to determine the reflex properties within 12 or 24 hours following the last treatment.

This was done in hypertensive cellophane-wrapped rabbits in which treatment with a β-blocker + diuretic began 6 weeks after wrapping.[5] Treatment lowered MAP and blood volume in wrapped rabbits and restored vagal function, but 2 weeks after stopping therapy the vagal deficit was reestablished (figure 9.15, left; table 9.3; Korner, 1982, 1989; Blake, 1983). In other rabbits, treatment was instituted 8 weeks after wrapping, and vagal function was completely restored after 2 weeks of therapy (figure 9.15, right).

Thus, as predicted by Model G, lowering cardiopulmonary load promptly restores vagal function. In hypertensive rabbits, the short period of treatment lowered MAP and blood volume but had no effect on LVH.

Effect of Vasodilator and Vasoconstrictor Drugs

A short period (say 30 minutes) of IV infusion of a vasodilator drug reduces cardiopulmonary load but raises PRA, while the reverse changes are evoked by vasoconstrictors.

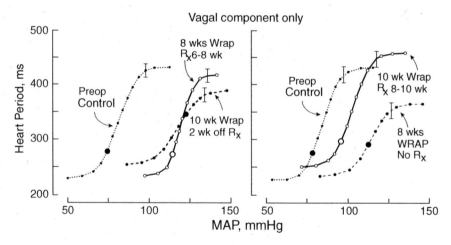

Figure 9.15. MAP-HP curves of vagal component of cardiac baroreflex in renal cellophane-wrapped rabbits before and after treatment with timolol (4 mg/kg/day) and frusemide 2 mg/kg/day), given up to day of test. Left, results from six rabbits showing (1) preoperative control; (2) treatment from 6–8 weeks after wrapping restored vagal function; (3) treatment discontinued between 8 and 10 weeks, when vagal deficit returned. Right, results in six different rabbits showing (1) control; (2) 8 weeks after wrapping without treatment; (3) treatment from 8 to 10 weeks restored vagal function. Large circles in each sigmoid curve are resting values. Data from Korner (1989), with permission of *Clinical and Experimental Pharmacology and Physiology* and Blackwell.

Table 9.3. Average Mean Arterial Pressure and Blood Volume (mL) at Baseline and the End of 6, 8, and 10 Weeks after Operation in 6 Wrapped and 6 Sham-Operated Rabbits

Variable	Baseline	6 Weeks	8 Weeks (T&F)	10 Weeks
MAP				
W	70	123	115*	127
S	78	77	75	79
CO				
W	598	661	633	650
S	694	651	555	738
B.Vol				
W	110	118	98*	—
S	138	129	106*	—

Note: MAP, mean arterial pressure, mmHg; B.Vol, blood volume, mL; T & F, timolol 4 mg/kg, twice/day i.m.; frusemide, 2 mg/kg/day i.m. *$p < .01$ for difference between weeks (6 and 10) vs. week 8 for MAP, and between weeks 6 vs. 8 for blood volume. The animals received timolol and frusemide between 6 and 8 weeks.

Source: Blake (1983).

In order to distinguish the effects of load from those of Ang II, the reflex was examined before and during administration of an Ang II antagonist or an ACE inhibitor.

Sodium nitroprusside infusion produced dose-related falls in MAP and TPR and rises in PRA and PRC (table 9.4; figure 9.16, top; Korner et al., 1981).[6] At the highest dose, the bradycardia plateau and G_{av} were depressed; the falls in MAP and TPR were greater in the presence of captopril, but the attenuation of the vagal plateau was about half that observed with nitroprusside alone. It follows that reduction in load in the intact animal produces a small reduction in HP range, while the elevation of Ang II causes a decrease in G_{av} and further reduction in HP range.

Table 9.4. Hemodynamic, Heart Rate, and Plasma Renin Concentrations (PRC) in 5 Conscious Rabbits during IV Infusions of Sodium Nitroprusside Given in the Absence of Captopril on One Day and during IV Infusions of Captopril on Another

	No Captopril			Captopril[a]		
NP, μg/kg/min	0	2.5	5	0	2.5	5
MAP, mmHg	91	82*	76*	88	69**	60*,**
CO, kHz	2.8	3.1	3.1	2.8	2.8	2.6
TPR, units	31.8	27.5*	26.2*	31.2	25.2*	22.6*,**
HR, bpm	242	263*	273*	248	283*	302*,**
PRC, ng/ml/hour	4.9	6.0*	7.2*	—	—	—

Note: The experiments in columns 2–4 and columns 5–7 were performed 7–10 days apart in the same animals; NP, nitroprusside infused for 30 min, before cardiac baroreflex measurements. *$p < .05$ for significant Δ from control. **$p < .05$ for greater change than without captopril. [a]Captopril, infused by 10 μg/kg/min IV, starting 20 min before NP and continuing through experiment.

Source: Unpublished data of Korner, Oliver, and Casley (1981).

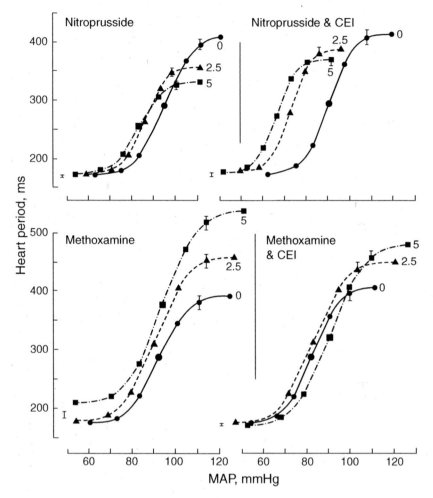

Figure 9.16. Average MAP-HP cardiac baroreflex curves (cuff method) from seven awake rabbits studied on four occasions at 5–8 day intervals. Top left, during IV infusions of sodium nitroprusside at 0 (solid line), 2.5 (dashed line), and 5.0 (dot-dash line) μg/kg/min. Top right, same IV nitroprusside infusions in the presence of converting enzyme inhibitor captopril (CEI; 10 μg/kg/min). Lower left, IV methoxamine was given at 0, 2.5, and 5 μg/g/min and (lower right) methoxamine plus captopril. Nitroprusside and methoxamine started 30 minutes before reflex studies; captopril started 20 minutes before the start of vasoactive drugs. From Korner and Oliver, unpublished data.

Methoxamine infusion increased TPR and lowered PRA and PRC (table 9.5). Both the bradycardia plateau and G_{av} were raised, and these changes were less pronounced in the presence of captopril (figure 9.16, bottom). Thus, the modest rise in load caused a small increase in HP range and vagal plateau in the intact animal, which were enhanced by the associated reduction in plasma Ang II.

Table 9.5. Hemodynamic, Heart Rate, and PRC Changes in 5 Awake Rabbits during IV Infusions of Methoxamine Given without Captopril on One Day and during Infusions of Captopril on Another

	No Captopril			Captopril[a]		
Methoxamine µg/kg/min	0	2.5	5	0	2.5	5
MAP, mmHg	90	89	90	80	79	86
CO, kHz	2.7	2.6	2.0*	2.7	2.6	2.3
TPR, units	35.8	37	48.2*	30.2	31	37.8*
HR, bpm	224	212	173*	259	246	224*
PRC, ng/ml/hour	5.9	2.4*	1.7*	—	—	—

Note: Abbreviations and protocol as in table 9.4. *$p < .05$ from corresponding control.
[a]Captopril, infused by 10 µg/kg/min IV, starting 20 min before methoxamine and continued through experiment.

Source: Unpublished data of Korner, Oliver, and Casley (1981).

In conclusion, small changes in cardiopulmonary load and plasma Ang II affect the reflex properties independently. The load-related changes affect mainly vagal segment 3 (figure 9.10).

Effects of Dietary Salt Intake in Normal and Hypertensive Rabbits

Six weeks after renal cellophane wrapping or sham operation, the wrapped rabbits had severe hypertension, which was accompanied by LVH and a 20% reduction in glomerular filtration rate (Korner, Oliver, and Casley, 1980; Korner et al., 1981). Subsequently, each animal was maintained on low, normal, and high salt (i.e., on 0.5, 5, and 50 mmol sodium/day), receiving each diet for a period of 2 weeks.[7] There were rises in PRA and PRC on low salt, and corresponding decreases on high salt, with the changes more pronounced in the hypertensive rabbits (table 9.6). At the end of each 2-week period, reflex properties and hemodynamics were examined before and during administration of saralasin, a nonselective Ang II receptor antagonist.[8]

On the high-salt diet, the MAP of hypertensive rabbits was 40 mmHg above that of controls, while CO, stroke volume, and blood volume were all significantly greater and PRA and PRC were more depressed (table 9.6). The bradycardia plateau and G_{av} were both depressed compared to controls (figure 9.17). Since the reflex properties were little affected by saralasin, the difference between the groups was mainly due to the greater cardiopulmonary load in the wrapped rabbits.

Switching hypertensive rabbits from high to low salt caused a 10 mmHg fall in resting MAP, that is, by 25% of the original excess BP. Blood volume declined by ~5%, bringing CO and stroke volume into the normal range. G_{av} increased at the lower cardiopulmonary load despite the rise in Ang II. Last, vagal function was completely restored by saralasin, bringing G_{av} and the bradycardia plateau close to normal.

In normotensive controls, the switch from high to low salt had little effect on hemodynamics but raised Ang II. This was largely responsible for the attenuated bradycardia plateau in intact rabbits (figure 9.17). Thus the high cardiopulmonary

Table 9.6. Effects on Hemodynamics, Plasma Renin Activity, and G_{av} in Sham-Operated and Renal Cellophane Wrapped Rabbits at the End of 2-Week Periods on Low, Normal, and High Salt Diets, before and during Administration of Saralasin

| | Sham Operation | | | | | | Renal Wrap | | | | | |
| | No Drug | | | Saralasin | | | No Drug | | | Saralasin | | |
	L	N	H	L	N	H	L	N	H	L	N	H
MAP[a]	86	90	90	77	80	86	122*	132	137	110	125	123
CO	592	636	574	609	604	580	604	705	737**	665	704	718
SV	2.3	2.4	2.1	—	—	—	2.4	2.4	2.7**	—	—	—
TPR	14.5	14.1	15.6	12.6	13.2	14.8	20.2	18.7	18.5	16.5	17.8	17.1
G_{av}	7.8	9.4	8.3	10.7	10.5	9.20	6.9	5.28**	4.57**	9.11	6.84**	5.69**
PRA	2.91	2.21	1.90	—	—	—	4.45	2.37	1.58	—	—	—
log PRA	0.45*	0.34	0.24*	—	—	—	0.55*	0.31	0.11*	—	—	—

Note: L, low salt diet, 0.5 mmol Na/day; N, normal salt, 5 mmol Na/day; H, high salt, 50 mmol Na/day; MAP, mean arterial pressure, mmHg; CO, cardiac output, mL/min (thermodilution); SV, stroke volume, mL; TPR, total peripheral resistance, units; G_{av}, average gain, ms/mmHg; PRA plasma renin activity, ng Ang I/mL/hour. *$p < .05$ for Δ from normal salt; **$p < .05$ for from sham group.

[a]All MAPs in wrapped rabbits greater than in corresponding controls.

Source: Korner, Oliver, and Casley (1980), Korner (1988), and unpublished data.

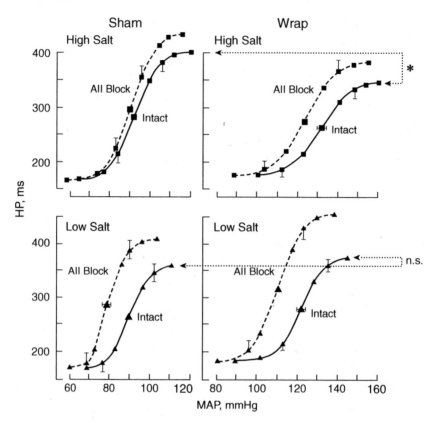

Figure 9.17. Average MAP-HP cardiac baroreflex curves obtained with the cuff method in renal cellophane wrapped or sham-operated rabbits after a 2-week period on high salt and low salt. Curves were obtained before (solid lines, intact) and during IV infusion of saralasin, at 6 μg/kg/min (dashed lines, AII block). From Korner et al. (1981), with permission of *Acta Physiologica Scandinavica* and Blackwell.

load in chronic hypertension causes substantial vagal depression, which is modulated further by diet-induced changes in plasma Ang II.

Sympathetic Constrictor Baroreflexes

The renal sympathetic baroreflex is a prototype of constrictor reflexes. Over the physiological BP range, its gain depends on interactions between arterial and cardiac baroreceptors, while specific cardiac and pulmonary baroreceptors account for the nonlinearities observed at high and low BPs. In EH and SHR hypertension, the gain of sympathetic constrictor reflexes is greater than in normotensives due to their higher resting SNA.

Renal Sympathetic Baroreflex

The function curves were derived in awake rabbits with a previously implanted renal nerve electrode, perivascular aortic and vena cava balloons, and a pericardial catheter for instilling procaine into the pericardial cavity. The procaine is a local anesthetic that blocks transmission in the cardiac nerves (Dorward et al., 1985; Burke and Dorward, 1988).

The function curve has a central sigmoidal component, with nonlinearities in renal SNA (RSNA) responses to, respectively, large falls and rises in intravascular BPs (figure 9.18, curve *aco*). Reducing BP below resting causes a steep rise in RSNA to an upper plateau, which is followed by a sharp decline in RSNA at an MAP at or below ~50 mmHg, which is called the hypotensive reversal response. The reversal response is prevented by administration of naloxone through its action on an opiate synapse in the CNS (Schadt and Gadis, 1985; Evans et al., 1989; Korner, unpublished data). Conversely, when raising BP above resting RSNA declines first to a lower plateau, rising again above MAPs of 110 mmHg, which is called the hypertensive reversal response.

After intrapericardial instillation of procaine to remove cardiac baroreceptor influences, the response to lowering BP is a steeper rise in RSNA while the hypotensive reversal response is abolished (figure 9.18, curve *ao*). However, during rises in BP the RSNA response is the same as in normal rabbits.

Sinoaortic denervation eliminates the steep part of the sigmoid curve, so that lowering the BP below resting causes a more gradual rise in RSNA (curve *co*).[9] However, when MAP is increased above ~90 mmHg, the action of cardiac receptors inhibits

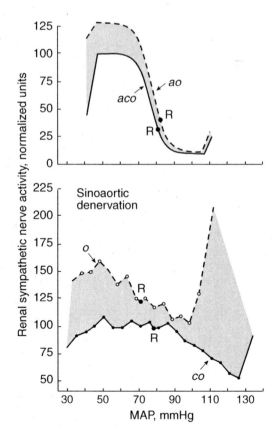

Figure 9.18. Top, relationship between MAP (mmHg) and renal sympathetic nerve activity (RSNA, units) in awake rabbits. Curve *aco*, arterial, cardiac, and other baroreceptor afferents working; *ao*, arterial and other baroreceptors working after procaine block of cardiac nerves. Bottom, MAP-RSNA curves about 24 hours after sinoaortic denervation; curve *co*, cardiac and other receptors working; *o*, other receptors working after blocking cardiac nerves with procaine. From Dorward et al. (1985), with permission of *Circulation Research*, American Heart Association, and Lippincott, Williams and Wilkins.

RSNA, and this is abolished by procaine (curve o). Remarkably, after procaine the hypertensive reversal response is markedly enhanced. The afferent mechanisms are uncertain but are probably tissue chemoreceptors in the kidney and skeletal muscle, which are stimulated by lower body ischemia during aortic balloon inflation (see chapters 10 and 15).

In summary, progressive unloading of the arterial baroreceptors normally causes an increase in RSNA to a maximum at the plateau. The net action of the cardiac baroreceptors is to limit the increase in RSNA through an opiate slow transmitter neuron; the latter's inhibitory action becomes maximal at the hypotensive reversal response. However, the action of cardiac receptors is not uniform (Paintal, 1971, 1973; Linden, 1973): Some inhibit RSNA when unloaded, while unloading others accentuates the arterial baroreceptor-mediated rise in RSNA (see Nonhypotensive Hemorrhage). At very high arterial BPs and cardiopulmonary loads, the high-threshold cardiac and pulmonary baroreceptors inhibit RSNA; normally this is masked by low-threshold baroreceptors and by other afferents that mediate the hypertensive reversal response.

Acute Hypertension Depresses the Baroreflex

Raising resting MAP by 30–45 mmHg depressed the entire renal baroreflex (Dorward et al., 1990). Half the inhibition was due to cardiac baroreceptor influences, but naloxone had no effect on the response, suggesting that the receptors were different from those mediating the hypotensive reversal response. They are probably high-threshold LV baroreceptors, pulmonary baroreceptors, and sympathetic afferents (Churchill and Cope, 1929; Mancia et al., 1975, 1976; Thorén et al., 1976; Malliani, 1982; Undesser et al., 1985; Kunze, 1986).

A large acute rise in BP raises central blood volume and LV wall stress, which appears to be an important factor in the reflex response. The latter is close to normal in chronic hypertension with LVH, when wall stress is also normal.

Constrictor Reflexes in EH and SHR Hypertension

Grassi, Cattaneo et al. (1998) studied the muscle sympathetic baroreflex in persons with mild and moderate EH and in age-matched normotensives. The changes in muscle SNA (ΔMSNA) were expressed as percentages of each group's resting value, giving a gain (slope) in EH similar to that observed in persons with normal BP (figure 9.19, bottom). However, resting MSNA is raised in EH (chapter 5) and when allowance is made for this, there is significant elevation of the gain of the baroreflex (figure 9.19, top).

This also applies to the difference in renal baroreflex function curves between SHR and WKY. Huang and Leenen (1994) found that the ΔMAP-ΔRSNA function curves were virtually superimposable when ΔRSNAs were expressed as percentages of each group's resting values. However, resting RSNA is greater in SHR (chapter 16) and when this is allowed for the RSNA range and G_{av} is significantly greater than in WKY.

Baroreflex Changes Evoked by Stimulating the Defense Area

Electrical stimulation of the hypothalamic defense region in dogs markedly enhanced renal and mesenteric Vas responses evoked by altering BP in the isolated carotid sinus

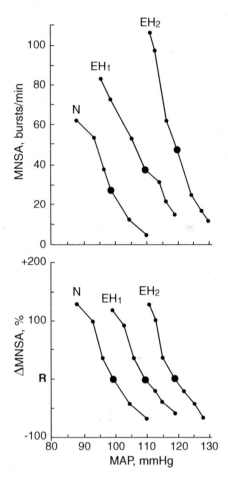

Figure 9.19. Top, relationship between MAP (mmHg) and muscle SNA (MSNA, bursts/min) in normotensives, persons with mild and moderate to severe EH (EH$_1$, EH$_2$); resting MSNA in hypertension (solid circles). Resting MSNA and slope (G$_{av}$) both raised in EH. Bottom, same results with MSNA expressed as percentage of each group's resting value, when slopes are similar in all groups. Adapted from Grassi, Cattaneo et al. (1998).

preparation (Kumada et al., 1975). Similar changes have been induced in RSNA function curves in rats (Wilson et al., 1971).

Mild air jet stress is a natural stimulus that elicits the hypothalamic defense response. A stimulus intensity that increases RSNA by ~100% in SHR has virtually no effect in WKY rats (figure 9.20, left; Thorén and Lundin, 1983). When resting RSNA is depressed by raising BP, air jet stimulation still evokes substantial elevation in RSNA in SHR (figure 9.20, middle). The different response threshold in SHR and WKY is genetically determined (figure 3.10; DiBona et al., 1996). The resulting F$_2$ population provides a model of genetically determined response variation to an environmental stimulus.

Disturbances That Engage the ANS Mainly Through Baroreflexes

Certain disturbances evoke autonomic changes almost entirely through baroreflexes, but the effectiveness of the regulation is not as stereotyped as this might suggest.

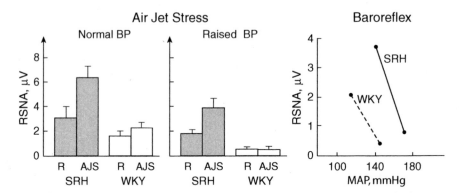

Figure 9.20. Left, renal sympathetic nerve activity (RSNA, μV) in SHR and WKY rats, at rest (R) and during air jet stress (AJS). RSNA increased by ~100% in SHR but altered little in WKY. Middle, raising BP by infusing phenylephrine lowered resting SNA in both strains, but AJS still caused elevation in SHR. Right panel, note steeper slope of MAP-RSNA relationship in SHR than in WKY. After Thorén and Lundin (1983), with permission of Springer-Verlag, Berlin.

How tightly BP is regulated depends on whether loading and unloading of the different groups of baroreceptors is concordant (directionally similar) or discordant, when, for example, the disturbance may cause unloading of the arterial baroreceptors and loading of the cardiac and pulmonary baroreceptors.

Nonhypotensive Hemorrhage

In experiments in awake instrumented rabbits, blood was removed through an indwelling catheter at about 3% of the blood volume per minute until the BP fell abruptly, marking the transition from the nonhypotensive to the hypotensive phase of hemorrhage (figure 9.21, left; Korner et al., 1990; Oliver et al., 1990; Courneya and Korner, 1991). The fall in BP is due to active sympathetic inhibition arising from left ventricular receptors that contribute to the hypotensive reversal response (Öberg and White, 1970; Öberg and Thorén, 1972). Like the latter, the transition can be delayed by naloxone (Thorén, 1979; Ludbrook and Rutter, 1988; Schadt and Ludbrook, 1991).

After 20% of the blood volume had been removed, MAP was only 3.7% below baseline before hemorrhage. This contrasts with a 55.3% fall in BP under the open-loop conditions of neurohumoral blockade (NHB), which eliminates the actions of the ANS and AVP and Ang II (Korner et al., 1990).[10] The gain of the BP control system is 15 (55.3/3.7), indicating 96% compensation for the open-loop effect of the disturbance.

The difference in total peripheral conductance (TPC) between intact and NHB rabbits provides a measure of net vasoconstriction (figure 9.21, right). The vasoconstriction included the renal, mesenteric, and hindquarter beds.[11] The neurohumoral changes were almost entirely through the ANS, while plasma levels of AVP and Ang II barely altered until after the transition to the hypotensive phase (Korner et al., 1990; Oliver et al., 1990; Courneya et al., 1991). Heart rate increased by 34% with about 60% of the response due to an increase in cardiac SNA, providing some inotropic support.

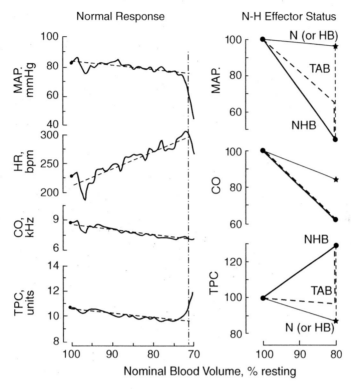

Figure 9.21. Left, record from awake rabbit bled at 4 mL/min, showing linear relationships between nominal blood volume (% BV remaining) and MAP (mmHg), heart rate (HR, bpm), cardiac output (CO, kHz Doppler shift), and total peripheral conductance (TPC, units). During initial nonhypotensive phase, decline in MAP is small and is followed by sudden drop in MAP and HR and a rise in TPC during transition to hypotensive phase. Right, average normalized responses (% of prehemorrhage value) during removal of 20% blood volume in eight rabbits in which effector function was normal (N); hormonal block (HB) of actions Ang II and AVP; total autonomic block (TAB); neurohumoral block (NHB). Rise in TPC during NHB indicates local vasodilation. From Korner et al. (1990), with permission of *American Journal of Physiology* and American Physiological Society.

The constrictor drive due to unloading of arterial and cardiac baroreceptors was in the ratio of 2.5:1 arterial:cardiac influence (Courneya and Korner, 1991). During this phase of hemorrhage, the upper plateau of the RSNA function curve is depressed by about 10%, and this increases after intrapericardial procaine (figure 9.22; Burke and Dorward, 1988). Clearly, in the intact animal unloading this group of cardiac barore-ceptors potentiates the rise in RSNA mediated through unloading of the arterial baroreceptors.[12]

The transition to the hypotensive phase marks a major change in the state of the BP control system: ANS control is switched off and is replaced by hormonal regulation through AVP and Ang II. Although the hormones are powerful vasoconstrictors, they are less effective in the short-term maintenance of MAP than the ANS (Korner et al., 1990).

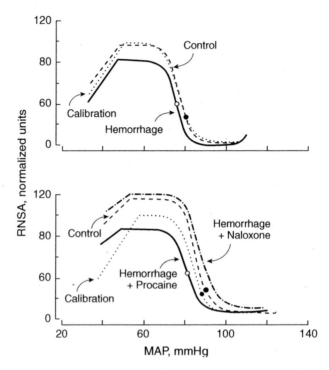

Figure 9.22. Average MAP-RSNA curves in awake rabbits showing response after removing 18% of the blood volume. Dotted line, initial reference calibration; dashed line, control; solid line, during hemorrhage; dot-dash line, hemorrhage plus naloxone. Note mild depression of upper plateau in top panel, which is greater after procaine block of cardiac nerves in bottom panel, suggesting that in intact rabbits unloading this group of cardiac receptors reinforces effects of arterial baroreceptor unloading on RSNA. Depression during hemorrhage abolished by naloxone. Data from Burke and Dorward (1988).

In contrast to the ANS, the hormones only provide minimal cardiac support, which is why BP remains low during the hypotensive phase.[13]

Primary Tissue Hypoxia Due to Inhalation of Carbon Monoxide

Inhalation of 0.2% carbon monoxide in 21% O_2 reduces arterial O_2 capacity by approximately 50%, causing a fall in tissue pO_2 without change in arterial pO_2 (Korner, 1965b; Chalmers et al., 1967a; Korner, 1970). The tissue hypoxia dilates the resistance vessels, causing a substantial fall in MAP and raising local blood flow, CO, and cardiac filling pressures.

The fall in MAP suggests a less effective regulation than in nonhypotensive hemorrhage (figure 9.23). The BP control system has a gain of about 2 and corrects for only half the fall in MAP observed under open-loop conditions. The fall in BP suggests

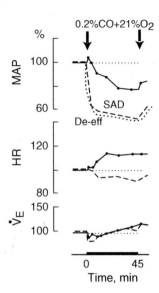

Figure 9.23. Effect of inhalation of 0.2% carbon monoxide in 21% O_2 (between arrows) in awake rabbits on mean arterial pressure (MAP), heart rate (HR), and respiratory minute volume (V_E), expressed as % of resting. All afferents intact, solid line; after sinoaortic denervation (SAD), dashes; after total autonomic block (de-eff), dotted lines. Average arterial pO_2 was normal, while mixed venous pO_2 was low. Adapted from Korner (1965b) and Chalmers et al. (1967a).

unloading of the arterial baroreceptors, while the high central filling pressures will raise cardiopulmonary baroreceptor discharge. The directionally dissimilar signals from the two groups of baroreceptors are responsible for the lower gain of the control system.

Valsalva Maneuver in EH

The Valsalva maneuver has long been used as a qualitative test of autonomic function (Cohn et al., 1963; Braunwald, 1965; Sharpey-Schafer, 1965; Korner, West et al., 1973; Eckberg and Sleight, 1992). Hamilton et al.'s (1936) classic paper describes four phases. Phases 1 and 3 are at the beginning and end of voluntary forced expiration when there are small transient changes in BP and heart rate; during phase 2 expiratory pressure remains steady, while MAP and heart rate rise to plateaus; phase 4 follows the end of forced expiration when there is the well-known BP overshoot and bradycardia (figure 9.24).

Korner, Tonkin, and Uther (1976, 1979) compared the phase 2 responses in persons with EH and normotensives. The rise in expiratory pressure (EP) increases intrathoracic and intraabdominal pressures, shifting blood volume from thorax and abdomen into the limb veins. This results in decline in CO and arterial pulse pressure and unloading of the arterial and cardiopulmonary baroreceptors, which evoke autonomic responses similar to those in nonhypotensive hemorrhage. The effects of graded EPs on hemodynamics and heart rate were examined under the following conditions: (1) with intact effectors, (2) during cardiac effector blockade with atropine and propranolol, and (3) during total autonomic blockade (TAB; Korner, Tonkin, and Uther, 1979).

Responses in Normotensive Subjects

Normotensive responses included EP-related falls in CO, and rises in MAP, right atrial, and peripheral vein pressures (RAP; figure 9.25). In addition, there were EP-related

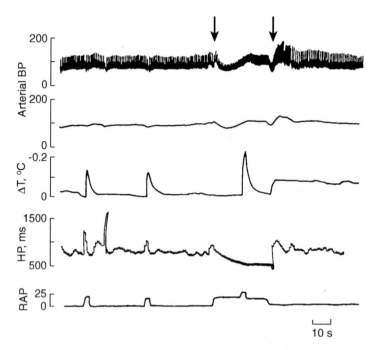

Figure 9.24. Record from normotensive subject showing changes during Valsalva maneuver, in which expiratory pressure of 30 mmHg was maintained for 30 seconds (between arrows). From top: (1) pulsatile arterial BP; (2) mean arterial BP, mmHg; (3) changes in pulmonary artery temperatures (°C) during three thermodilution curves: two before and one during phase 2; an increase in area ≡ fall in CO; (4) heart period (HP, ms); and (5) RAP, right atrial pressure, mmHg; transients are tap-turning artifacts. From Korner, Tonkin, and Uther (1976), with permission of *Journal of Applied Physiology* and American Physiological Society.

rises in TPR and heart rate (figure 9.26). Atropine and propranolol abolished the rises in heart rate, while the fall in MAP during TAB was pronounced and the rise in TPR was abolished (figure 9.27). Because the maneuver is so brief, tissue hypoxia is small, accounting for the absence of peripheral vasodilation during TAB.[14] Hence, the EP-related rise in TPR is a measure of sympathetic constrictor activity.

The rise in MAP during the Valsalva maneuver contrasts with the small fall in MAP during nonhypotensive hemorrhage, although there is concordant unloading of arterial and cardiopulmonary baroreceptors in both disturbances. The rise in BP is due to the central command associated with the voluntary forced expiratory effort during the Valsalva maneuver, which enhances the baroreflex-mediated autonomic changes (chapter 10).

Changes in EH

With intact effectors, the EP-related fall in CO is the same as in normotensives, but the rise in MAP is small or absent (figure 9.25). This may be partly due to arterial baroreceptor impairment in EH, though the excellent maintenance of BP during the

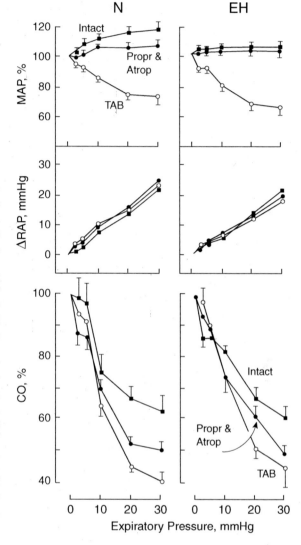

Figure 9.25. Hemodynamic responses near the end of phase 2 of the Valsalva maneuver in normotensives (N; MAP range 79–90 mmHg) and persons with EH (MAP range 115–165 mmHg), (1) with ANS intact (squares); (2) in presence of propranolol + atropine (Propr & Atrop, black circles); and (3) during total autonomic blockade (TAB, open circles). Results in each case show relationship between expiratory pressure (mmHg) and (from top) ΔMAP (% of resting), Δ right atrial preessure (ΔRAP, mmHg), ΔCO (% of resting). From Korner, Tonkin, and Uther (1979), with permission of *Clinical and Experimental Pharmacology and Physiology* and Blackwell.

maneuver casts doubt on this explanation, since the nonarterial baroreceptors appear to be making up for the impairment.

As indicated in figure 9.26, the relationship of EP to ΔTPR is similar in normotensives with intact effectors and during cardiac autonomic blockade. However, this is not the case in persons with EH, in whom the rise in TPR during elevation in EP is significantly greater in the presence of cardiac blockade than with intact effectors (figure 9.26, top). In EH, the rise in TPR is smaller with effectors intact because they secrete enough adrenaline to cause vasodilation. This masks the neural rise in TPR, which only becomes manifest in the presence of atropine and propranolol, with the propranolol doing the unmasking (see below, Valsalva-like Reflex in Awake Rabbits).

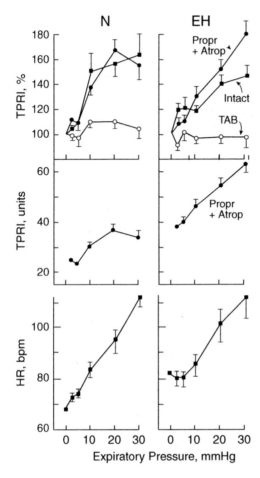

Figure 9.26. Relationships in same groups as in figure 9.25, between expiratory pressure (mmHg) near end of phase 2 of the Valsalva maneuver and (top) total peripheral resistance index (TPRI, % of resting); (middle) TPRI in resistance units while on propranolol + atropine (Propr + Atrop); (bottom) heart rate (HR, bpm). Abbreviations as in figure 9.25. From Korner, Tonkin, and Uther (1979), with permission of *Clinical and Experimental Pharmacology and Physiology* and Blackwell.

The secretion of adrenaline is a component of the defense response in persons with EH. Its secretion suggests that the Valsalva maneuver is perceived by them as more stressful than by normal subjects.

During cardiac blockade, the elevation of TPR units in persons with EH was 24 units compared with 14 units in normotensives, which is a 70% difference. The greater effect is in accord with the raised resting SNA in EH and the action of the structural vascular amplifier.

Valsalva-like Reflex in Awake Rabbits

A reflex was induced by simultaneously applying a Valsalva pressure (VP) to a tracheotomy-respiratory valve assembly and to a small cuff wrapped around thorax and abdomen (Blombery and Korner, 1982). The circulatory response closely resembles that in humans, except that MAP does not rise in rabbits, in which breathing continues during the maneuver.

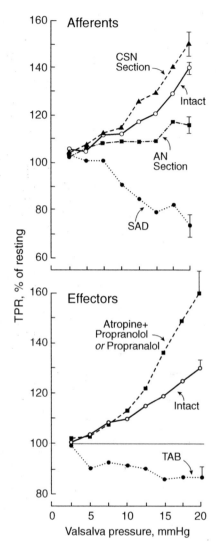

Figure 9.27. Relationships between Valsalva pressure (mmHg) and total peripheral resistance (TPR, % of baseline), top, 7–10 days after (1) sham operation; (2) bilateral carotid sinus nerve (CSN) section; (3) bilateral aortic nerve (AN) section; and (4) sinoaortic denervation (SAD). Bottom, responses in different groups of rabbits in which (1) all effectors were working, intact; (2) on atropine + propranolol; (3) on propranolol alone; and (4) during total autonomic blockade (TAB). Based on Blombery (1978) and Blombery and Korner (1982).

Rabbits also secrete adrenaline during the maneuver and their TPR response is enhanced in the presence of atropine + propranolol, and by propranolol alone (figure 9.27, bottom; Korner, Blombery et al., 1976; Blombery, 1978; Blombery and Korner, 1982). To the rabbits, the increase in VP is unexpected and appears to be mildly stressful, in contrast to the voluntary response in normal humans. SAD abolishes systemic vasoconstriction during the maneuver, highlighting the role of baroreflexes in circulatory regulation (figure 9.27, top).

In summary, the autonomic response to the Valsalva maneuver depends on unloading of the arterial and cardiopulmonary baroreceptors plus a central command mechanism related to the voluntary forced expiratory effort. In EH, the α-AR neural constrictor response is enhanced, but is masked by stress-related adrenaline secretion. It suggests that in EH the defense response is superimposed on the Valsalva reflex.

Determinants of BP Variability in EH

BP variability is usually assessed from analysis of continuous 24 hour BP recording (O'Brien, 1994). In one method, the mean values and standard deviations (SDs) are determined for every half hour, with the average SD taken as index of diurnal BP variability (Mancia et al., 1983). The latter increases with severity of EH and with age. In subjects with moderate and severe hypertension, the variability is about 30% and 70% greater than in age-matched normotensives (Mancia et al., 1983; Floras et al., 1988; Mancia, 1990; Eckberg and Sleight, 1992).

In normal individuals, the circadian changes and the daytime differences between work and home environments are the largest sources of BP variability. Both are raised in persons with EH (figure 4.7; Pickering et al., 1992; Pickering, 1995). BP variability is inversely related to cardiac BRS, and the impaired cardiac baroreflex has been considered to be the main reason for the raised variability (Mancia et al., 1983; Floras et al., 1988). However, the vagal depression that underlies the low BRS is a function of high cardiopulmonary load, that is, of the severity of hypertension. In contrast, the gain of sympathetic constrictor reflexes is usually enhanced.

The chief determinants of the raised variability in EH are the enhanced responsiveness of the defense pathways and the amplification of Vas R due to the R_1 vessel structural changes. These account for most of the increase in the diurnal range of BP changes in EH (figure 4.7). The vagal deficit makes a small additional contribution to the enhanced BP variability; at very high loads, constrictor reflexes are also depressed and the overall baroreflex contribution to variability increases.

Does Baroreflex Dysfunction Cause Hypertension?

The possibility has often been raised that baroreflex dysfunction is a major cause of EH (e.g., Eckberg and Sleight, 1992). To determine whether this belief has substance, one might seek answers to the following questions: (1) Does SAD or denervation of cardiopulmonary baroreceptors disinhibit SNA sufficiently to raise BP? (2) Do long-term alterations in input of one group of baroreceptors affect resting BP? (3) Is SHR hypertension due to faulty signaling in the central baroreflex pathways? (4) What is the mechanism of the fulminating lethal hypertension that has been reported following electrolytic lesions of the baroreflex pathways?

Effect of Baroreceptor Denervation

Eberhard Koch (1931) was the first to propose that impaired arterial baroreceptor function disinhibited the vasomotor center, thereby increasing SNA and BP. He had observed that BP in rabbits was raised several days after SAD (Koch and Mies, 1929). This was confirmed by some investigators (Kremer et al., 1933; Korner, 1965a; Chalmers et al., 1967b; Korner, 1970; Korner, Shaw, West et al., 1973; Chalmers and Reid, 1972; Ito and Scher, 1981; Bishop et al., 1987; Persson et al., 1988), but not by others (Koch and Mattonet, 1934; Cowley et al., 1973; Cornish and Gilmore, 1985; Geer et al., 1986).

Cowley et al. (1973) were the first to record BP continuously over 24 hour periods in awake dogs: They found that SAD did not alter average MAP, but that BP variability had increased considerably. They concluded that baroreflexes had no long-term effect on resting BP and that the earlier findings that SAD caused a rise in BP had been due to inadequate sampling of BP.

However, there is a significant body of experience suggesting that daytime MAP is significantly raised by ~20 mmHg for at least 6–8 days after SAD; in addition, definite but smaller rises in MAP occur after selective denervation of the carotid and aortic baroreceptors (e.g., table 9.2; Korner, 1965a, 1970; Chalmers et al., 1967b; Korner, Shaw, West et al., 1973; Blombery and Korner, 1982; Snell et al., 1986). It seems therefore that there is at least transient daytime disinhibition for several days which later becomes suppressed. Similarly, chronic labile hypertension has occurred in humans after neck surgery or radiotherapy involving both carotid sinuses (for references, see Heusser et al., 2005). The corollary is that nocturnal MAP is reduced, which would make the above findings consistent with those of Cowley et al. (1973).

The most comprehensive analysis of the effects of denervation of various combinations of baroreceptors has been performed in trained awake dogs, using 1 hour recording sessions that were repeated several times per week for many weeks (table 9.7; Persson et al., 1988).

SAD did not cause a permanent rise in BP, in agreement with Cowley et al. (1973), but MAP was often raised for several days. BP was also unchanged after denervation of cardiopulmonary baroreceptors, but each procedure increased BP variability. Only after combined sinoaortic plus cardiopulmonary baroreceptor denervation was there a long-term rise in MAP by about 20 mmHg. This was accompanied by substantial increases in BP variability and elevation in heart rate and PRA. The variability was partly due to very large slow arterial BP oscillations (figure 9.28).

Thus, in order to raise resting BP, virtually the entire input from all the baroreceptors has to be dismantled to cause sufficient disinhibition of SNA. The procedure is associated with much greater BP variability than is found in EH. The suppression of

Table 9.7. Means ($\pm$SEM) of Mean Arterial Pressure (MAP, mmHg), Standard Deviation of MAP(SD_{MAP}), Heart Rate (HR, bpm), and Plasma Renin Activity (PRA, ng Ang I/m/hour) in Trained Foxhounds

	MAP	SD_{MAP}	HR	PRA
Sham (10)	100 $\pm$ 1.5	8.2 $\pm$ 0.6	84 $\pm$ 3.5	0.9 $\pm$ 0.2
CPD (5)	99 $\pm$ 2.9	11.2 $\pm$ 0.8	94 $\pm$ 7.7	1.1 $\pm$ 0.7
ABD (6)	100 $\pm$ 3.1	9.4 $\pm$ 0.8	76 $\pm$ 5.9	1.0 $\pm$ 0.2
SAD (5)	101 $\pm$ 3.1	12.7 $\pm$ 1.4	96 $\pm$ 7.6	0.8 $\pm$ 0.3
CPSAD (7)	120 $\pm$ 4.6	26.1 $\pm$ 1.7	118 $\pm$ 3.7	3.6 $\pm$ 0.9

Note: CPD, cardiopulmonary denervation; ABD, aortic baroreceptor denervation; SAD, sinoaortic denervation; CPSAD, cardiopulmonary denervation + SAD; numbers in parentheses in column 1 are number of dogs. Data collected over at least 3 weeks with several recording sessions per week, each of 60 minutes duration.

Source: Persson et al. (1988), with permission of *European Journal of Physiology* (Pflüger's Archiv) and Springer-Verlag.

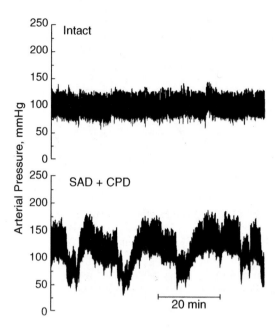

Figure 9.28. Arterial pressure recordings in awake dog (Intact) and after combined sinoaortic and cardiopulmonary denervation (SAD + CPD) in same animal, in which there were large BP oscillations of average cycle length of 17 minutes determined by spectral analysis. After Persson et al. (1990), with permission of *American Journal of Physiology* and American Physiological Society.

transient disinhibition of SNA after SAD alone is a gradual process that depends on the input from cardiac and pulmonary baroreceptors to the CNS.

Chronic Changes in Arterial Baroreceptor Input

The arterial baroreceptors adapt to a long-term change in resting BP, which allows them to maintain BP about almost any resting level. This is in accord with the absence of long-term systemic BP rise following SAD, which is equivalent to complete unloading of the arterial baroreceptors.

A quasi-isolated carotid sinus preparation has been developed in conscious dogs, the unloading of which produced a rise in BP over several days (Thrasher, 2002). This was done by reducing BP of one innervated carotid sinus using a perivascular balloon in the common carotid, while the other carotid sinus and aortic arch baroreceptors had been previously denervated. The low sinus pressure was maintained despite elevation of systemic BP, and carotid sinus pulse pressure was also reduced.

After reducing carotid sinus pressure, the systemic MAP rose by 23 mmHg. This was maintained for 7 days and was accompanied by elevation of heart rate and PRA. Removing the clamp restored systemic MAP to the initial baseline level. However, in a later study when observations were continued for several weeks, systemic BP returned to within a few mmHg of the baseline value (Thrasher, 2005a, 2005b).

Thus the early disinhibition of SNA is similar to the many arterial baroreceptor denervation studies discussed earlier. As high BP was not maintained permanently, it seems plausible that the same nonarterial baroreceptors and CNS mechanisms that restore BP after SAD were responsible for the later suppression of SNA.

Another approach was used by Lohmeier et al. (2004). They applied phasic bilateral near-maximal electrical stimuli to both carotid sinuses for a period of 7 days, which caused MAP to fall by some 30 mmHg, which was associated with falls in heart rate and plasma NA.

The phasic signals emanating from the arterial baroreceptors remained constant for 7 days, which suggests that the central pathways did not adapt. It would be interesting to determine whether there was any buffering through baroreflexes, similar to that occurring during central administration of α-MD (figure 8.23).

Is SHR Hypertension Caused by Faulty Baroreflex Signaling?

An abnormality in RVLM signaling in the baroreflex pathway has been proposed as a cause of SHR hypertension (Chalmers, 1998). The activity in RVLM neurons was assessed by counting the number of neurons that expressed Fos, the protein product of the "immediate early" gene c-fos (chapter 8; Dragunow and Faull, 1989; Morgan and Curran, 1991; Dampney and Horiuchi, 2003).

At rest, Fos expression in RVLM neurons was about twice as great in SHR as in WKY (Chalmers et al., 1994). Lowering BP for about 1 hour with nitroprusside elicited a six-sevenfold increase in Fos expression in WKY but had no effect on Fos expression in SHR (Minson et al., 1994, 1995). This was thought to indicate that the capacity to inhibit RVLM neurons was reduced in SHR, thus explaining their high BP.

Later experiments by the same investigators found that that baroreflex function is normal (Minson et al., 1996). Fos-labeling of spinal sympathetic motoneurons was greater in SHR than in WKY, both at rest and during nitroprusside-induced reduction in BP (figure 9.29). This agrees with results of direct assessment of renal baroreflex properties in SHR, which show no functional impairment (Thorén and Lundin, 1983; Huang and Leenen, 1992).

However, this still leaves unexplained why Fos expression does not increase in RLVM neurons during a fall in BP. It may be that during increased hypothalamic activity the incoming information about baroreceptor unloading elicits a different pattern of gene expression.

Anodal Lesions and Hypertension

Fulminating hypertension has been reported after production of large anodal lesions in the NTS (Reis et al., 1975). These produced far greater rises in BP than did combined peripheral arterial plus cardiopulmonary baroreceptor denervation. Very large rises in BP have also been reported after anodal lesions of A1 NA neurons (Blessing et al., 1981) and after anodal lesions of the rostral hypothalamus (Gauthier et al., 1981). All of the lesions caused a near 100% mortality.

The above lesions were made through stainless steel electrodes, and the ferric ions deposited in the tissue around the lesion excited nearby pressor neurons (Whishaw and Robinson, 1974; Head et al., 1987). Hypertension did not occur after cathodal lesions or when gold or platinum electrodes were used to make anodal lesions (Head et al., 1987). These bizarre rises in BP are experimental artifacts that have nothing to do with baroreflexes.

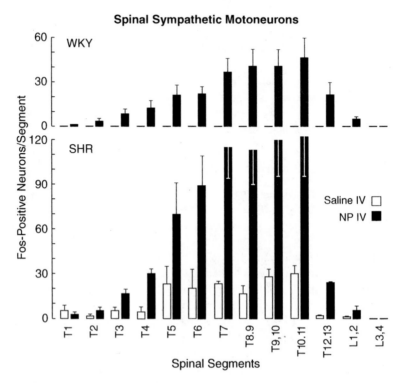

Figure 9.29. Graphs showing number of Fos-positive immunoreactive neurons per spinal segment after saline infusion (open bars) and after nitroprusside (NP) infusion in thoracic and lumbar spinal segments of WKY and SHR (black bars). Note greater number of Fos-positive neurons in SHR during both saline and NP infusions. From Minson et al. (1996), with permission of *Hypertension*, American Heart Association, and Lippincott, Williams and Wilkins.

Baroreflexes, Adaptive Circulatory Control, and EH

Baroreflexes are the chief moment-to-moment arterial BP regulators but also exert some tonic effects. Their main function is to reduce BP variability about the prevailing resting BP. They contribute to "system identification" and participate in major parameter adjustments when there are changes in the state of the adaptive control system. The baroreflex pathways have extensive interconnections with many groups of central neurons, including the regions responsible for long-term BP rises in EH, which, in turn, influence the BP responsiveness of the baroreflex pathways.

Their role in reducing BP variability depends mainly on the capacity of the arterial baroreceptors to adapt to a new level of resting BP within several days, which enables them to correct perturbations at relatively high gain. The process begins within 1–2 minutes after the onset of the pressure change, when it is called rapid resetting. However, rapid resetting affects mainly A-fiber baroreceptors, so that changes in C-fiber discharge through incoming BP-related signals can be recognized for some time as a change from a previous reference level. Once all the baroreceptors have become fully adapted, the neural component of the system reduces moment-to-moment BP variability almost as well as normally.

The arterial baroreceptors are the preeminent group of pressure-sensitive receptors, but they are best regarded as being the first among (almost) equals. The nonarterial baroreceptors affect the gain of the regulatory feedback system, which depends on the direction and magnitude of their activity in relation to that of the arterial baroreceptors. Nonarterial and arterial baroreceptors converge on common slow transmitter interneurons, which allows the former to compensate, at least partially, for the low BP sensitivity of the carotid sinus and aortic baroreceptors in severe chronic hypertension. Clearly the properties of specific slow transmitter neurons are important determinants of how well a loss of arterial baroreceptor gain is compensated in the operation of the overall baroreflex system. Some slow transmitter neurons must also be involved in suppressing the transient disinhibition of SNA that follows SAD. These safety mechanisms make the baroreflex network preeminent for reducing BP variability but at the same time make it an unlikely primary source for long-term elevation of BP.

In EH, there is some increase in BP variability related to the severity of hypertension. In moderate EH, the vagal impairment of the cardiac baroreflex makes a small contribution to the greater BP variability, with the main increase due to hypothalamic hyperresponsiveness and the structural amplification of Vas R. When cardiopulmonary load becomes very high (e.g., in obesity) sympathetic constrictor baroreflexes are also depressed. At that stage, baroreflexes make a larger contribution to BP variability than in mild and moderate EH.

Reference has been made (1) to classic analysis of individual baroreflexes; (2) to whole-organism baroreflexes, in which there are central interactions between the different groups of baroreceptors; and (3) to more elaborate circulatory disturbances where baroreceptors also affect the evoked autonomic responses.

Classic reflex analysis from an isolated baroreceptor zone at best represents a fragment of how baroreflexes function in the whole organism. However, these preparations are valuable for characterizing baroreceptor properties and have been used extensively for this purpose (Brown, 1980; Andresen and Yang, 1989; Koushanpour, 1991). They probably could be used more extensively for mapping the CNS projections from particular baroreceptors to major neuron groups involved in cardiovascular integration.

In whole-organism baroreflexes, the emphasis is on interactions between the various groups of baroreceptors. In the MAP range of about ±10 mmHg about resting, the main interaction is between low-threshold arterial and cardiac baroreceptors, while at very low and high arterial BPs the high-threshold cardiac and pulmonary baroreceptors assume greater importance (figure 9.30).

The cardiac vagal deficit is an example of tonically mediated compound baroreflex influences in chronic hypertension. The elevated cardiopulmonary load engages medium- and high-threshold arterial, cardiac, and pulmonary baroreceptors, which adapt relatively little to high loads at each heartbeat, in contrast to A-fiber baroreceptors. The deficit is accentuated by elevation in plasma Ang II, which depresses vagal ganglionic transmission, while reduction in Ang II, for example in low-renin hypertension, moderates the effect of raised cardiopulmonary load. The results of computerized methods for deriving BRS from spontaneous variation are a valuable clinical indicator of future cardiovascular risk.

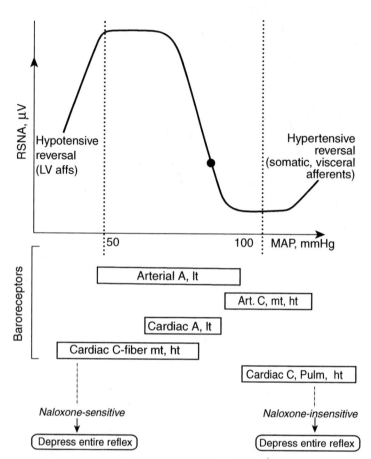

Figure 9.30.   Schema relating components of MAP-RSNA function curve to operating range of main baroreceptor groups, each classified as having low, medium, and high thresholds (lt, mt, and ht). Arterial (Art) and cardiac baroreceptors include A- and C-fiber receptors. Interactions in center are between lt arterial, and lt and mt cardiac baroreceptors. At low MAP (and ≡ cardiac BPs), net cardiac receptor inhibitory influence gives rise to naloxone-sensitive hypotensive reversal response. At high MAP, the depression evident in curve *co* in figure 9.19 is due to drive from ht cardiac and pulmonary (Pulm) baroreceptors. Hypertensive reversal response mediated through tissue chemoreceptors and possibly other somatic and visceral afferents.

In EH and SHR hypertension, the elevation of G_{av} and of the response range of sympathetic constrictor baroreflexes is a specific parameter change in neural types of high BP. The changes are a consequence of the effect of hypothalamic hyperresponsiveness on resting SNA. At very high cardiopulmonary loads, constrictor baroreflexes are also tonically inhibited (figure 9.30), for example, in gross obesity, well above the loads that elicit the vagal deficit (chapter 13).

The third approach considered here has been the assessment of the contribution made by specific baroreceptors to autonomic responses elicited by circulatory disturbances.

The perturbations discussed in this chapter have been chosen because of the large contribution made by the baroreflexes to the autonomic responses. Nonhypotensive hemorrhage is an example in which baroreflexes maintain BP most effectively through simultaneous unloading of low-threshold arterial and cardiac baroreceptors. Similar unloading of the two sets of baroreceptors accounts for the high gain of the regulatory system during the Valsalva maneuver or when assuming the upright posture, in both of which BP is maintained close to baseline during the disturbance. In contrast, during carbon monoxide hypoxia BP is not as well maintained and the low gain of the system is due to discordant effects on low-threshold arterial baroreceptors that are unloaded, while there is increased loading of the low-threshold cardiopulmonary baroreceptors.

In the Valsalva maneuver, the profile of baroreceptor changes is similar to that in nonhypotensive hemorrhage. In EH, the neural effect on TPR at high EP is 70% greater than in normotensives, which is due partly to greater resting SNA and partly to the action of the structural R_1 vessel amplifier. Both effects are partially masked by adrenaline secretion, which is a marker of the defense response.

Baroreflexes play some role in all perturbations that affect BP, though their contribution is not always as great as the disturbance selected in this chapter. In normal persons, the rise in BP during phase 2 of the Valsalva maneuver is a manifestation of the effects of voluntary central command to maintain the expiratory pressure, which enhances the baroreflex constrictor effects.

In conclusion, baroreflexes are the main regulators of BP. What is remarkable in EH is not that BP variability is greater than normal, but that the change is relatively modest. This is only possible because of the close central interactions of the inputs from the arterial, cardiac, and pulmonary baroreceptors. This helps to maintain regulatory function in EH and other types of chronic hypertension close to normal depite the marked changes in arterial wall properties in which some of the baroreceptors are embedded.

10

Exercise Training and Its Long-Term Effects on Blood Pressure: Linkage to Somatic Movement

Muscular exercise begins as a voluntary act, emanating from the cerebral cortex. The cerebellum compares the planned somatic movement with its actual execution by the musculature, adjusting discrepancies as they arise and storing them in memory for future reference.

The exercising muscles depend on cardiorespiratory performance for an adequate supply of O_2 and glucose. Hence one would expect the mechanisms regulating somatic movement during exercise to be closely linked with those involved in cardiovascular control.

The immediate consequence of muscle contraction is vasodilation in the active muscle. The associated autonomic response is evoked by cortical command signals related to those that initiate movement, with modulation by feedback from the active muscles and the baroreflexes (Astrand and Rodahl, 1986; Rowell, 1993). The pattern of the autonomic changes is a variant of the defense response, but the effect of regular exercise training is to reduce the resting BP between sessions. This makes exercise training a worthwhile nonpharmacological treatment of EH (World Health Organization, 1989; Arakawa, 1993; Jennings and Kingwell, 1994; Fagard and Amery, 1995). The BP-lowering effect of exercise also occurs in healthy normotensive subjects, so that it has a potential role in the prevention of EH.

Circulatory and Respiratory Changes during Exercise

The type of activity required to lower BP is submaximal aerobic exercise (figures 4.12, 4.13). Aerobic exercise includes walking, running, swimming, and bicycling, while anaerobic exercise includes weight lifting, wrestling, and isometric exercise. The type of aerobic exercise required to significantly lower BP is associated with some accumulation of anaerobic metabolites in muscle, but their concentration is below that accumulating in anaerobic exercise.

Haemodynamic and Respiratory Changes

For a given type of exercise, the rise in respiratory minute volume and in SBP, pulse pressure, and CO are all linearly related to the rate of work.

Blood Pressure

At the start of exercise at a moderate work rate the BP increases within seconds, reaching a plateau after 3–4 minutes (figure 10.1). The rise in SBP ranges from 20 to 70 mmHg, depending on the rate of work, with heart rate increasing in parallel; DBP generally decreases slightly or remains unchanged (Korner, 1947, 1952a). At the end of moderate submaximal exercise, SBP reaches the baseline resting value in 3–5 minutes, but then falls further by 10–20 mmHg; this is accompanied by falls in MSNA and plasma NA (Bennett et al., 1984; Cleroux et al., 1992; Coats et al., 1989; Floras et al., 1989). The low values of all these variables are maintained for ∼1 hour, after which there is gradual recovery over 2–3 hours.

Blood Flow and Respiratory Changes in Steady-State Exercise

In moderate to heavy exercise, CO increases up to three-sixfold. Most of the increase goes to the active skeletal muscle bed, and coronary blood flow also increases (figure 10.2; Wade and Bishop, 1962; Rowell, 1974, 1993; Astrand and Rodahl, 1986). There are parallel rises in total O_2 consumption and respiratory minute volume

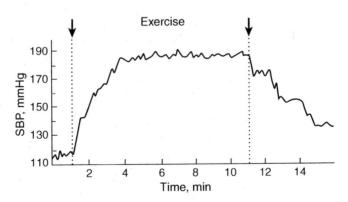

Figure 10.1. Average time–systolic BP (SBP, mmHg) relationship during steady exercise (between arrows) and subsequent recovery in 21 subjects (age range 19–26 years). The rate of work was 2.35 watt/kg body weight. From Korner (1952a).

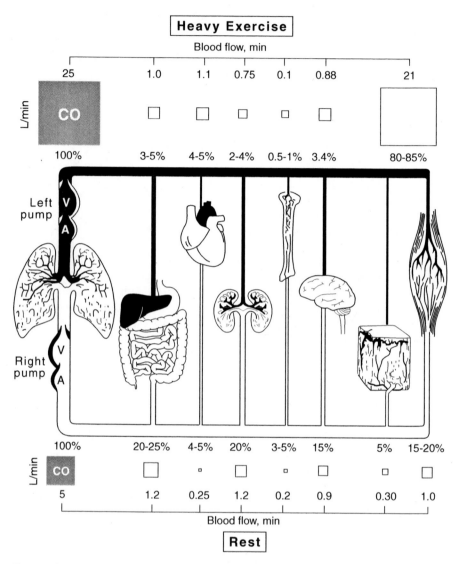

Figure 10.2. Diagram illustrating cardiac output (CO) and its distribution to gastrointestinal, coronary, renal, bone, brain, skin, and muscle beds beds at rest (bottom) and during near-maximal exercise. Blood flows expressed in L/min and also as percentage CO. Blood flow to fat not shown. From Astrand and Rodahl (1986), with permission of McGraw-Hill Book Company, New York.

(Haldane and Priestley, 1935; Astrand and Christensen, 1963; Dejours, 1963; Nielsen and Asmussen, 1963).

   These changes are accompanied by marked vasoconstriction in the renal, gastrointestinal, and nonactive muscle beds (Wade and Bishop, 1962; Rowell, 1993). Skin also constricts except in hot weather or if body temperature rises too much (Rowell, 1974).

The gastrointestinal vasoconstriction helps shift blood volume from the abdomen to the cardiopulmonary compartment, which, together with the muscle pump action of contracting muscles, maintains high central filling pressures and a high CO.

Assuming MAP values at rest and during exercise of, respectively, 100 and 150 mmHg, the TPR during exercise is only about 30% of resting TPR. This indicates the importance of vasodilation in the active muscles in the elevation of CO and SBP.

Autonomic Changes and Functional Sympatholysis

At high rates of work the cardiac vagal effector tone rapidly falls to zero, while cardiac SNA increases (Cunningham et al., 1972; Jennings et al., 1981; Rowell, 1993). Constrictor SNA rises in the renal, gastrointestinal, skin, and nonactive skeletal muscle beds.

Local vasodilation in active muscle and myocardium is due to the effects of local hypoxia, adenosine and ATP, endothelial NO (and EDHF), and nitrothiol compounds (chapter 6). In humans and dogs, plasma adrenaline concentration does not rise during exercise, but it does in rabbits (Blair et al., 1961; Donald and Shepherd, 1963; Whelan, 1967; Péronnet et al., 1981; Ludbrook and Graham, 1984).

Although constrictor tone increases markedly in the nonactive skeletal muscle bed, there is no corresponding rise in contracting muscle, which is known as functional sympatholysis. This was thought at one time to be due to the dilator actions of tissue hypoxia and muscle metabolites on the VSM cells, masking neural vasoconstriction (Remensnyder et al., 1962; Burcher and Garlick, 1973). However, more recent evidence suggests that in contracting muscle the expression of neural NOS (nNOS) increases, causing an increase in formation of NO, which prevents vasoconstriction (Thomas and Victor, 1997; Thomas et al., 1998; Stamler and Meissner, 2001).

This is illustrated in figure 10.3 (top), where contraction of skeletal muscle prevents the vasoconstriction that is evoked in resting muscle by local application of NA or by stimulation of sympathetic nerves. In contrast, little nNOS is expressed in skeletal muscle of *mdx* mice,[1] in which vasoconstriction can be evoked by NA. Vasoconstriction can also be evoked in mice in which the nNOS gene has been disrupted (figure 10.3, bottom and middle panels). Thomas et al. (1998) have suggested that the insensitivity to vasoconstrictor stimuli is due to reduction in the influx of Ca^{2+} into VSM cells. How NO is formed in contracting muscle is still uncertain. One possibility is that it is formed in response to ACh released from the somatic motor nerve terminals.

Changes in ANP and PRA

During bicycle exercise at 60% of maximum work capacity (W_{max},) the rise in plasma ANP is greater in persons with EH than in normotensives, while the rise in PRA is smaller (figure 10.4; Sudhir et al., 1988). The difference in responses appears to be due to the greater rise in the central cardiopulmonary pressures of hypertensives, in whom the cardiopulmonary load is already high at rest. The additional rise in load during exercise is probably responsible for the 25% lower value of W_{max} in persons with EH compared to that of normotensives. The lower threshold for developing dyspnea may limit the amount of exercise that persons with EH tolerate.

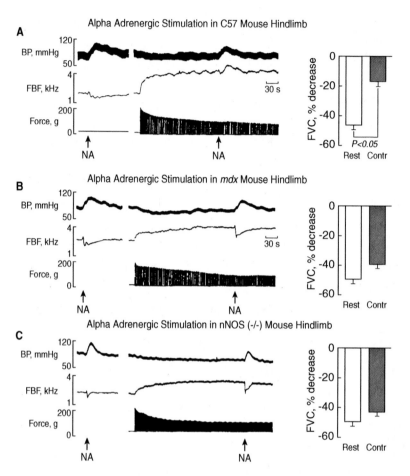

Figure 10.3. Left panel, recordings in mice of arterial BP (mmHg), femoral blood flow (FBF, kHz Doppler shift), and force of electrically induced contraction in gastrocnemius muscle (g). (A) In C57 mouse, intraarterial noradrenaline (NA) at arrow causes vasoconstriction at rest, but not during contraction. (B) NA does not induce vasoconstriction during muscle contraction in *mdx* mouse in which NO is low. (C) There is no vasoconstriction in nNOS knockout mouse for the same reason. Right panel, NA-mediated decreases in femoral vascular conductance (FVC, %) at rest (clear bars), and during contraction (shaded bars) in the various mouse strains. From Stamler and Meissner (2001) and Thomas et al. (1998).

Mechanisms of Circulatory Control during Exercise

The prime determinants of autonomic changes during exercise are central command and muscle chemoreceptor activity, while baroreflex parameters also alter.

Central Command

Exercise is a voluntary act and therefore the autonomic and respiratory changes are unlikely to be initiated by peripheral sensory stimuli. This was recognized by

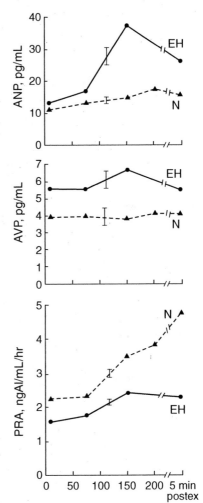

Figure 10.4. Average time course of changes during and after exercise in plasma concentrations of atrial natriuretic peptide (ANP, pg/mL), arginine vasopressin (AVP, pg/mL), and in plasma renin activity (PRA, ngAngI/mL/hour) in persons with essential hypertension (EH; $n = 13$, solid lines) and normal subjects (N; $n = 8$, dashed lines). The exercise was raised gradually up to W_{max}. From Sudhir et al. (1988), with permission of *Journal of Human Hypertension* and Nature Publishing Group.

Johansson (1895) and later by Krogh and Lindhard (1913, 1917), who hypothesized that the CNS must be the source of the almost immediate rises in heart rate and respiration at the start of exercise. To many investigators, "central command" was an unfamiliar concept, differing from the more traditional reflex responses evoked by changes in activity of specific afferents (Houk, 1988; Rowell, 1993).

An experiment by Gandevia et al. (1993) provides a convincing demonstration of the cortical origins of central command. The subjects were human volunteers, who were artificially ventilated after having had their skeletal muscles paralyzed with a curare-like drug. They were asked to reproduce the effort required to perform graded isometric arm exercises that they had performed earlier in the laboratory. Remarkably, this evoked graded rises in BP and heart rate in the absence of any muscle movement or contraction (figure 10.5). Presumably, activation of central command occurred by recalling the previous experiences from memory. In exercise, the changes probably arise from

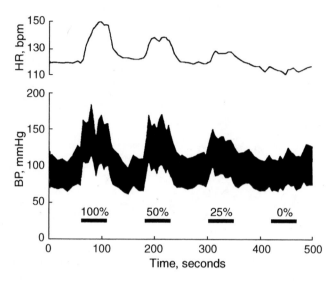

Figure 10.5. Changes in heart rate (bpm) and BP (mmHg) during attempted voluntary movements in a paralyzed, mechanically ventilated human volunteer. The bars indicate attempts to
perform 100%, 50%, 25%, and 0% of maximum isometric forearm contraction, as previously
performed in the laboratory. From Gandevia et al. (1993), with permission of the *Journal of
Physiology* (London) and Blackwell.

the motor and prefrontal cortical regions (Clarke et al., 1968; Hohimer et al., 1979;
Smith, Astley, DeVito et al., 1980).

Gandevia's work on central command was inspired by earlier experiments by his
mentor Ian McCloskey, in which the subjects were asked to maintain the tension in
the triceps muscle constant during isometric arm exercise (Goodwin et al., 1972).
Triceps tension could be altered without the subject being aware of it, by applying an
ultrasonic vibratory stimulus to the biceps tendon, which stimulates muscle spindle
afferents, so that tension is reduced reflexly in the triceps. To maintain the desired
triceps tension, the subject has to increase central command, which causes greater
rises in heart rate, BP, and respiration than when the tension is maintained without
the vibratory stimulus.

A Discontinuity after Sprint Exercise

During a short sprint, the rise in BP is largely dependent on central command and
when exercise stops there is a sudden fall in BP (figure 10.6; Korner, 1952a). This BP
trough was first described by Sir Thomas Lewis and coworkers in British soldiers
during World War I, who were being investigated for battle fatigue (Cotton et al.,
1915–1917). They concluded that the trough was probably a normal phenomenon.[2]

From the regulatory viewpoint, the sudden BP drop is due to a discontinuity in
regulation during the sprint between the end of central command and the start of excitatory drive from muscle chemoreceptors. During this interval there is pooling of blood
in the previously active limbs, while constriction increases slowly in the nonactive

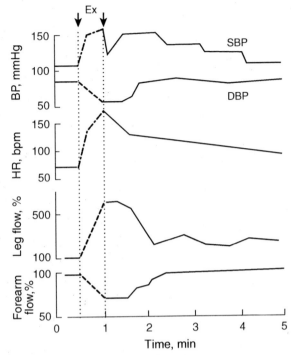

Figure 10.6. Average time course of changes during (between arrows) and after exercise in systolic and diastolic BP (SBP, DBP, mmHg), heart rate (HR, beats/min), leg and forearm blood flows (% of resting), measured by impedance plethysmography in 21 medical students (15 men, 6 women). The exercise was 30-second bicycle sprint at an average rate of work of 6.8 watt/kg body weight. From Korner (1952a).

muscles (figure 10.6). The subsequent rise in postexercise SBP is due to systemic vasoconstriction mediated through the interaction of muscle chemoreceptors and baroreflexes. In steady-state exercise, there is no corresponding regulatory discontinuity and virtually no BP trough at the end of exercise (figure 10.1).

Muscle Chemoreflex

The muscle chemoreflex is elicited by anaerobic metabolites in the active muscles and helps to raise BP during and after exercise. It was discovered by Alam and Smirk (1937a, 1937b; 1938), who found that after occluding the limb circulation with a BP cuff, the rises in BP and heart rate during exercise were greater than normal. Moreover, the BP remained raised after exercise for as long as the limbs remained occluded. Merely occluding the limbs without exercise had little effect on BP. Later, the afferent nerves mediating the reflex were found to be small myelinated and unmyelinated fibers from skeletal muscle (Coote et al., 1971; McCloskey and Mitchell, 1972).

Exercising an ischemic limb is painful, which is why Alam and Smirk used very low rates of work in their experiments. But even then it is difficult to differentiate an exercise-related rise in BP from the effects of pain. However, if the limbs are occluded only after exercise, pain is slight and the changes are largely due to exercise (Korner, 1952b; Rowell et al., 1976).[3]

After heavy or moderate sprint exercise, bilateral occlusion of both limbs causes persistent elevation of BP (figure 10.7). Muscle SNA is also raised (Mark et al., 1985; Rowell, 1993).

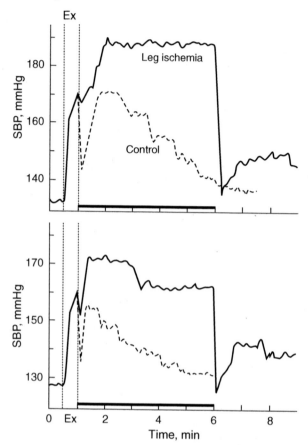

Figure 10.7. Top, effects of two 30-second sprints on postexercise SBP (mmHg) in the same subject: (1) with free lower limb circulation (dashed lines); and (2) during postexercise obstruction of lower limb circulation (bar at bottom), which maintained raised SBP until occlusion was removed. Exercise performed between dotted lines at 6.82 watt/kg. Bottom, similar experiments in another subject performed at 3.84 watt/kg. From Korner (1952b).

In contrast to the sustained elevation of BP during limb occlusion after exercise, respiration and heart rate recover rapidly (figure 10.8, control; Freund et al., 1979). It suggests that respiratory regulation during exercise is linked almost entirely to central command. This also applies to the vagal component of the heart rate response, which recovers rapidly, while cardiac SNA remains raised just like BP (O'Leary, 1991).

Further clarification of the role of the muscle chemoreflex comes from a study on the effects of lumbar peridural anesthesia (Freund et al., 1979). The anesthetic blocks conduction not only of sensory but also of motor nerves, and the resulting motor weakness makes it more difficult to maintain the same level of exercise than normally. Accordingly, during exercise a greater effort is required to maintain exercise, which enhances the rises in BP, heart rate, and respiration (figure 10.8, middle). However, once exercise is over the BP recovers rapidly despite limb occlusion, because of the sensory block from muscle afferents. As the anesthetic begins to wear off, conduction of the motor nerves recovers more rapidly than that of the sensory nerves: Now no extra effort is required to maintain the desired rate of work during exercise, and the BP

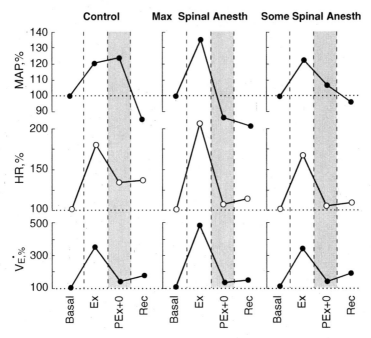

Figure 10.8. Results in one subject studied under control conditions (left, Control); during maximum peridural spinal anesthesia (middle, Max Spinal Anesth); some time later when motor deficit no longer present but sensory conduction was still blocked (right, Some Spinal Anesth). On each occasion, MAP (mmHg), heart rate (HR), and minute ventilation (V_E) were measured before exercise (basal), during exercise (Ex), postexercise with limbs occluded (PEx+O), and at recovery (Rec). Data from Freund et al. (1979).

and other responses are the same as under control conditions. But after exercise, BP still recovers rapidly despite limb occlusion, since the sensory nerves are still blocked (figure 10.8, right).

In conclusion, at the time of maximal peridural anesthesia, the greater effort of central command enhances the cardiorespiratory responses during exercise, which occurs in parallel with recruitment of additional skeletal motor units to maintain the desired rate of work (see Hobbs and Gandevia, 1985).[4] The study also demonstrates the importance of muscle chemoreceptor activity in circulatory regulation after exercise.

Heart Rate and Renal SNA Changes and Resetting of Baroreflex Properties

The rise in heart rate during exercise is due to elevation in cardiac SNA and reduction in vagal activity (Jennings et al., 1981). The influence on the vagus is illustrated by the progressive decline in BRS with gradually rising rates of work (figure 10.9; Cunningham et al., 1972).

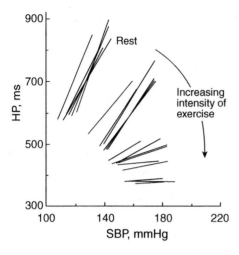

Figure 10.9. Successive BP-heart period (HP, ms) ramps in one subject, obtained under resting conditions and during exercise at gradually increasing work rates, when slope of ramp (≡ BRS, baroreflex sensitivity) approaches zero as vagal tone is abolished. Adapted from Cunningham et al. (1970, 1972).

Interpreting Changes in Reflex Properties

Changes in the baroreflex function curve parameters elicited by a disturbance permit inferences whether or not particular groups of autonomic motoneurons receive connections from cardiovascular baroreceptors (Korner, Shaw, West et al., 1973; Korner, 1979a). For example, when only the plateaus alter without changes in BP-related parameters, the effect is mediated through motoneurons not receiving baroreceptor projections (figure 10.10, top). When only the BP-related parameters alter

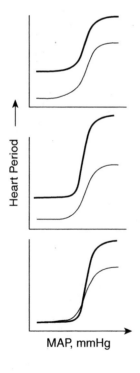

Figure 10.10. Changes in baroreflex parameters during circulatory disturbance permit inferences whether or not motoneurons receive input from the baroreceptors, as illustrated in MAP–heart period function curves. Top, disturbance produces similar shifts in plateaus, but no change in BP-related parameters, suggesting that it acts on motoneurons independent of baroreflex pathways. Bottom, the changes are entirely BP related, suggesting that the disturbance acts entirely on the baroreflex pathways. Middle, the disturbance produces uneven changes in plateaus and changes in BP-related parameters, suggesting that some motoneurons receive input from the baroreceptors while others do not. From Korner, Shaw, West et al. (1973), with permission of *Circulation Research*, American Heart Association and Lippincott, Williams and Wilkins.

(e.g., G_{av} and the response range) the change occurs through motoneurons that receive baroreceptor projections (figure 10.10, bottom). When the shifts in the two plateaus are unequal and there are also changes in BP-related parameters, both types of motoneurons are involved (figure 10.10, middle).

Effect of Exercise on Cardiac and Renal Baroreflex Properties

In trained rats, exercising on a treadmill the changes in properties of the MAP-heart rate baroreflex during exercise include elevation in both plateaus of the curve and substantial depression of the heart rate range (figure 10.11, bottom; Miki et al., 2003). The investigators did not examine the effects on the vagal and sympathetic components, but work in humans suggests that during exercise vagal activity is suppressed, leaving mainly sympathetic function intact. Hence, the appropriate comparison for assessing the effect of exercise on G_{av} is with the resting sympathetic component of G_{av}.[5]

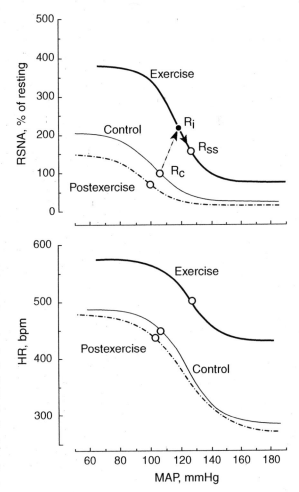

Figure 10.11. Top, renal sympathetic baroreflex curves relating MAP (mmHg) to renal SNA (RSNA, % of resting) in trained rats; control (fine continuous line), during treadmill exercise (bold line), and 30 minutes postexercise (dot-dash line). Open circles, starting values for each period. Exercise alters both plateaus, G_{av} and RSNA range; arrow points from resting control (R_c) to hypothetical initial value during exercise (R_i), which is greater than during steady state (R_{ss}). Reflex depressed after exercise. Bottom, cardiac baroreflex relating MAP and to rate (HR, bpm) under control conditions, during and after exercise. The large reduction in HR range during exercise suggests that vagal tone abolished and reflex mediated mainly through cardiac sympathetic, as discussed in text. Adapted from Miki et al. (2003), with permission of *Journal of Physiology* (London) and Blackwell.

On this assumption, G_{av} during exercise is about double resting sympathetic G_{av}, which is in accord with renal baroreflex changes.

The changes in renal sympathetic baroreflex properties are shown in figure 10.11 (top). During exercise, the renal sympathetic nerve activity (RSNA) range and G_{av} were about twice the corresponding resting values. These parameter changes are similar to those associated with the defense response (Kumada et al., 1975; Iriki et al., 1977a; Thorén and Lundin, 1983). The shifts in the plateaus were unequal, with the shift in the lower plateau providing the best estimate of BP-independent changes during exercise. Thus, the rise in RSNA during exercise is partly mediated through sympathetic motoneurons that receive projections from the baroreceptors, and partly through motoneurons that do not. The corollary is that only some of the rise in RSNA during exercise can be inhibited through the baroreflex, which is similar to what Lundin and Thorén (1983) observed in SHR when examining the effect of air jet stress on BP (figure 9.20).

One hour after exercise the cardiac baroreflex properties had recovered, including the vagal component (figure 10.11). However, the renal baroreflex was markedly depressed.

Arterial and Cardiac Baroreceptors and the BP Response

In animals with intact afferents, BP rises during exercise, but in animals with sinoaortic denervation (SAD), the BP falls (Walgenbach and Donald, 1983; Ludbrook and Graham, 1984). This suggests that baroreflexes contribute to the normal rise in BP. What has puzzled investigators is why central command and muscle chemoreceptors are not able to raise the BP during exercise even without the arterial baroreceptors.

Ludbrook and Graham (1984) performed a factorial experiment in rabbits to examine how the arterial and cardiac baroreceptors influenced BP during treadmill exercise (figure 10.12).[6] With all afferents intact (group *aco*), MAP, CO, and heart rate all rose during exercise, while TPRI declined, as in humans. After cardiac receptor denervation with procaine (group *ao*), the rises in CO and heart rate and the fall in TPRI were attenuated and ΔBP differed only slightly from normal. After arterial baroreceptor denervation (groups *co*, *o*), MAP and TPRI fell and the rises in CO and heart rate were attenuated, with the changes greatest when SAD was combined with cardiac receptor denervation (group *o*).

Ludbrook and Graham explained the intact animal's responses by suggesting that baroreflex function was completely suppressed at the start of exercise but recovered later on. However, we now know that only vagal function is suppressed, but not the sympathetic baroreflexes (figure 10.11). Nor was there full appreciation of the large contribution of the role of elevation of CO to the rise in BP.

Hence, an alternative explanation seems necessary. Assuming that changes in baroreflex parameters soon after the start of exercise are similar to those in figure 10.11, RSNA will increase initially from a resting value of 100 units to a hypothetical value of 210 units (R_i), which equals the average of the shifts in lower and upper plateaus. As BP rises to its steady-state value, the moderating effect of the renal baroreflex reduces RSNA from 210 to 170 units (R_{ss}). This is characteristic of a feed-forward system with negative feedback (chapter 2).[7] At no time is there inhibition of sympathetic baroreflexes.

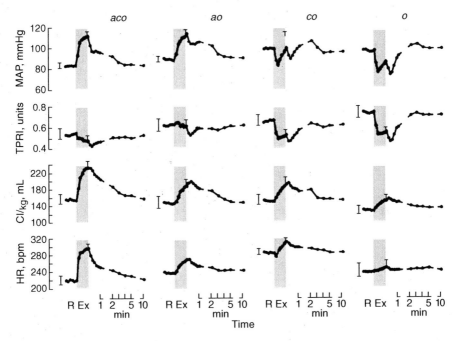

Figure 10.12. Effects of arterial and cardiac baroreceptors on (from top) MAP (mmHg), total peripheral resistance index (TPRI, mmHg/mL/kg), cardiac index (CI, mL/min/kg), heart rate (HR, bpm) in trained rabbits at rest (R), during 60-second treadmill exercise (Ex), and after exercise. Italic letters over panels indicate which afferents are functioning: *a*, arterial baroreceptors; *c*, cardiac baroreceptors; *o*, other nonbaroreceptor inputs. Bars are 2 × SEMs at rest and SEM at the end of exercise. From Ludbrook and Graham (1984), with permission of *American Journal of Physiology* and American Physiological Society.

Why Baroreflex Function Is Necessary for the Rise in BP

The rise in BP is first due to vasodilation in the active muscles, which accounts for much of the increase in CO. This is complemented by the rise in constrictor and cardiac SNA, which limits the fall in TPRI, enhancing cardiac filling pressures and providing inotropic and chronotropic support to the heart through elevation of cardiac SNA.

About one third of the steady-state rise in constrictor SNA during exercise is mediated through sympathetic motoneurons without baroreceptor input, while the remainder depends on motoneurons that receive baroreceptor input. The latter component is lost after SAD, and the baroreflex-independent component is too small to make the required hemodynamic adjustments. Moreover, after SAD there is reduced cardiac, vasoconstrictor, and venomotor support, resulting in a smaller rise in CO than in intact animals. In turn, the attenuated CO response determines a greater than normal fall in tissue pO_2 in the active skeletal muscle bed. Together, these factors account for the greater fall in MAP and TPRI.

In conclusion, central command and muscle chemoreceptor afferents are the primary sources of elevation of SNA during exercise. However, much of the rise in BP depends on their interaction with baroreflexes.

Long-Term Effects of Regular Exercise Training

The antihypertensive effect of regular exercise depends on the rate of work at each session and the frequency of sessions. In some studies, no antihypertensive action between training sessions has been observed, which has been mostly due to training at either too high or too low rates of work (figure 4.13; Jennings and Kingwell, 1994).

Circulatory, Autonomic, and Other Changes

The antihypertensive effect of exercise was first observed in Dahl-S rats and then in SHR (Rapp, 1982; Tipton et al., 1983, 1984). Later Jennings, Nelson, Nestel et al. (1986) showed that exercise training produced a long-term fall in BP between sessions in sedentary normotensive subjects. Soon afterward this was also found to occur in persons with EH (figure 4.17; Nelson et al., 1986).

The study of Jennings, Nelson, Nestel et al. (1986) examined the changes in each subject at four levels of habitual activity, each lasting 4 weeks: (1) normal sedentary activity; (2) subnormal activity, which included a very quiet period in hospital; (3) normal activity plus 30 minutes' bicycle exercise 3 times per week at 60–70% of W_{max}; and (4) normal activity plus exercise 7 times per week at the above rate of work. The order of the activity levels was varied according to a Latin-square experimental design to eliminate bias. Measurements were made at the end of each 4-week period, at least 48 hours after the last bout of exercise. Body weight and salt intake were maintained constant throughout.

At subsedentary levels of activity, the resting hemodynamic variables remained the same as during the sedentary phase, but there were significant changes after 4 weeks of regular exercise performed 3 times per week and 7 times per week: Resting MAP, TPRI, and heart rate all fell below the corresponding sedentary values, while CI increased (figure 10.13). Maximum O_2 consumption increased, which suggests an enlarged area of the previously active skeletal muscle bed.[8]

Long-Term Effects on SNA

After training 3 times per week, resting SNA between bouts of exercise was below the sedentary level, with the greatest falls in renal (42%) and muscle (40%) outflows; total (average) NA spillover fell by 24% and cardiac NA spillover did not change (Meredith et al., 1991; Grassi et al., 1994).[9] However, there was a small depression of the sympathetic component of the MAP-heart rate baroreflex curve (Kingwell et al., 1992); reports of changes in vagal components have been variable and inconclusive (Bedford and Tipton, 1987; Smith et al., 1988; Somers et al., 1991; Grassi et al., 1994). Plasma NA declined but plasma adrenaline did not alter (Jennings, Nelson, Nestel et al., 1986).

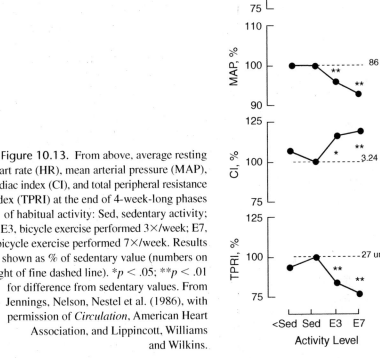

Figure 10.13. From above, average resting heart rate (HR), mean arterial pressure (MAP), cardiac index (CI), and total peripheral resistance index (TPRI) at the end of 4-week-long phases of habitual activity: Sed, sedentary activity; E3, bicycle exercise performed 3×/week; E7, bicycle exercise performed 7×/week. Results shown as % of sedentary value (numbers on right of fine dashed line). *$p < .05$; **$p < .01$ for difference from sedentary values. From Jennings, Nelson, Nestel et al. (1986), with permission of *Circulation*, American Heart Association, and Lippincott, Williams and Wilkins.

These findings are consistent with observations in rabbits on the effects of 8 weeks of exercise training. This resulted in marked depression of renal and cardiac baroreflexes, with reduction in G_{av} and renal SNA and heart rate ranges (figure 10.14; DiCarlo and Bishop, 1988). The depression of the heart rate range was greater than in humans, but the renal changes were of the same order of magnitude.

Time Course of Changes during Training and Detraining

The good news is that the effect of exercise training on BP becomes apparent rapidly. By the third session of exercise training (at 60% of W_{max} 3 times per week), resting BP had fallen below the sedentary value, reaching a nadir by the end of the second week (figure 10.15; Meredith et al., 1990). The time course of the changes in TPRI, CO, and O_2 consumption was similar, but there was a lag before plasma NA and heart rate started to fall. On resuming a sedentary lifestyle (detraining phase), the recovery of BP and the other variables preceded recovery of plasma NA. It took 4 weeks from the end of training for all variables to return to the initial levels.

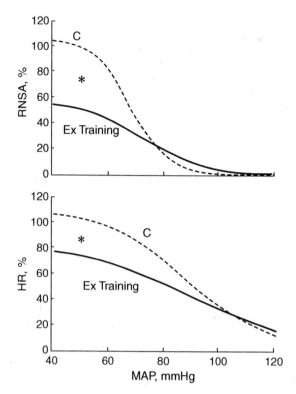

Figure 10.14. Renal and cardiac baroreflex curves relating MAP to renal sympathetic nerve activity (RSNA) and heart rate (HR) in two groups of rabbits (1) at the end of 8 weeks of treadmill exercise training (Ex training); (2) sedentary controls (C). In each group, MAP was expressed in mmHg, while RSNA and HR were expressed as a percentage of each group's upper plateau (=100%) before the start of 8 weeks of training. *$p < .05$ for difference between control and trained rabbits. Resting values in control and trained groups were, respectively, MAP: 74, 74 mmHg; HR: 257, 213* bpm; plasma volume: 45, 54*; body weight: 2.4, 2.8*. From DiCarlo and Bishop (1988), with permission of *American Journal of Physiology* and American Physiological Society.

The findings suggest that the peripheral changes that result in widening of the active muscle bed initiate the fall in BP. The decline in plasma NA starts later and reflects depression of sympathetic baroreflexes.

Exercise in Management of Mild Hypertension

Submaximal exercise as the sole treatment of EH has been mainly used to lower BP in patients with mild established EH. Jennings, Nelson, Dewar et al. (1986) performed a small study in 13 previously untreated subjects with EH whose baseline SBP/DBP averaged 157/102 mmHg over a 6-week observation period. After another month of sedentary activity, this had declined to 144/97 mmHg. In response to a bicycle ergometer exercise regimen at 60–70% of W_{max} performed 3 times per week, BP fell to 133/86 mmHg after 4 weeks and was 128/86 mmHg after 12 months of exercise. Two patients eventually required antihypertensive drug therapy, one after 15 months and one after 21 months.

Figure 10.16 shows BP data from another patient with mild EH. This indicates that exercise is indeed the cause of the fall in BP. She was initially treated with antihypertensive drugs, which were stopped after 5 months. Her BP rose rapidly over the next 4 weeks, but fell when exercise was performed at 65% of W_{max} 3 times per week, falling further on a daily regimen. BP rose when exercise was stopped and was subsequently maintained in the normal range by the 3 times per week regimen.

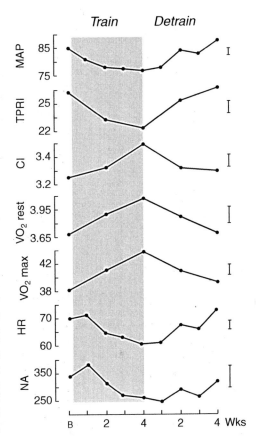

Figure 10.15. Average changes in circulatory, metabolic, and autonomic variables in 10 normotensive subjects during 4 weeks of training (standard bicycle exercise) and 4 weeks of detraining. Variables (from above): mean arterial pressure (MAP, mmHg); total peripheral resistance index (TPRI, units/m^2); cardiac index (CI, L/min/m^2); resting O$_2$ consumption (VO$_2$ rest, mL/min/kg); maximum O$_2$ consumption, O$_2$ consumption at W$_{max}$ (VO$_2$ max, mL/min/kg); heart rate (HR, bpm); NA (plasma noradrenaline concentration, pg/mL). Bars are least significant difference. From Meredith et al. (1990), with permission of *Journal of Hypertension* and Lippincott, Williams and Wilkins.

Unfortunately, the experiment ended when the subject broke her leg. It took several months after that before pharmacotherapy had to be recommenced.

Responses to Various Types of Aerobic Exercise

All the above studies have described the effects of bicycle exercise, in which quantification of the work rate is so easily performed. Long-term lowering of resting BP between training sessions also occurs in response to training when performing treadmill exercise and walking and swimming.

At low rates of work, the reduction in BP is only about 2–3 mmHg. For optimum BP reduction: (1) the rate of work should be 50–70% of the person's W$_{max}$; the use of W$_{max}$ normalizes variation in work capacity between individuals and groups; (2) a session should be of 30–40 minutes' duration and repeated not more than 3–4 times per week; and (3) exercise training should, if appropriate, be combined with weight reduction (see chapter 4; Arakawa, 1993; Kingwell and Jennings, 1993; Jennings and Kingwell, 1994; Reid et al., 1994; Georgiades et al., 2000).

When exercise is the sole nonpharmacological intervention, the reduction in MAP has ranged from 5–11 mmHg (average 7.5 mmHg; table 10.1). However, the falls

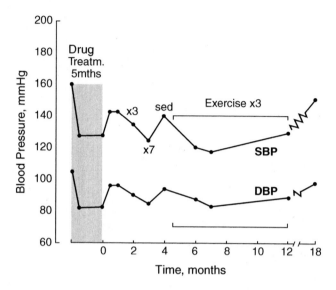

Figure 10.16. Supine resting systolic and diastolic BP (SBP, DBP mmHg) in one patient treated first with antihypertensive drugs (shading). Medication was stopped and after 1 month's sedentary activity, exercise was carried out at 65% of W_{max} at 3 or 7×/week as described in text. From Korner, Jennings, Esler, Anderson et al. (1987), with permission of Elsevier.

in MAP are nearly twice as great (figure 4.23) when exercise is performed together with a program of body weight reduction in overweight persons (Reid et al., 1994; Georgiades et al., 2000).

A Study in Which There Was No Antihypertensive Effect

Assessment of the effects of exercise was based on the responses of two groups: A treatment group performed regular bicycle ergometer exercise at 80–85% of W_{max},

Table 10.1. Examples of Long-Term Reduction in Mean Arterial Pressure (MAP) Due to Exercise Training (50–70% of W_{max} for 30–40 minutes, 3–4×/week)

Intervention (duration, months)	MAP, mmHg			
	n	Start	End	Reference
Bicycle exercise (12)	13	112	101	Jennings et al., 1986a
Bicycle exercise (12)	8	112	107	Jennings et al., 1991
Treadmill exercise (6)	16	104	97	Somers et al., 1991
Bicycle exercise (3)	7	101	95	Reid et al., 1994
Bicycle ex + weight ↓ (3)	9	102	89	Reid et al., 1994
Weight ↓ only (3)	7	95	89	Reid et al., 1994
Treadmill exercise (6)	44	109	103	Georgiades et al., 2000
Treadmill ex + weight ↓ (6)	36	110	94	Georgiades et al., 2000

Note: Two studies compared the effects of exercise alone with those of exercise plus weight reduction.

while a parallel control group performed "light (bicycle ergometer) exercise against zero resistance . . . , to allow for the familiarisation effects on blood pressure" (Cox et al., 1993; Cox, 1994; Beilin, 1994). The high rate of work in the treatment group was one contributing factor to the small magnitude of the long-term reduction in BP. BP also declined in the zero-load group, so that there was little difference between their responses. Hence the authors concluded that regular exercise had little or no long-term effect.

The authors were puzzled by the BP response in the zero-load group and commented that "very light exercise against zero resistance might involve some cardiovascular changes, leading to a fall in BP independently of a training effect" (Beilin, 1994, p. S76). Probably the zero-load exercise makes significant demands on central command, which alter with training. The exercise group performed near-maximal rather than submaximal exercise, where little fall in BP would normally be expected. At that intensity, the exercise becomes stressful and tends to raise BP (see below).

It follows that when using exercise for the nonpharmacological treatment of EH, only work intensities below 70% of W_{max} are effective. In addition, only sedentary subjects are the appropriate reference group. Last, there are advantages in using more than a single intensity of exercise before making recommendations about nonpharmacological interventions.

Exercise Training and Stress

One of the two studies considered below discusses the effects of exercise training during the stressful Antarctic winter. The second study was performed in obese persons with EH and relates to the effect of exercise training on the hemodynamic responses.

Exercise Training in Antarctica

The effects of exercise training during the summer and winter months in Antarctica were briefly discussed in chapter 4 (Jennings et al., 1989; Jennings, Deakin et al., 1991).[10] In the summer, virtually every day involves some vigorous outdoor activity, which accounts for the low daytime BPs of expedition members. Therefore it is not surprising that adding the standard exercise regimen has no further effect on their resting BPs (figure 4.16; table 10.2). However, during the winter the inclement weather makes outdoor activities virtually impossible, so that everyone is housebound and sedentary. Most expedition members find this frustrating and stressful: They become irritated by their colleagues; alcohol consumption is often excessive; they feel trapped and lose their sense of autonomy. Their normal sedentary daytime MAP is about 12 mmHg greater than in summer. Performing the standard bicycle training under these circumstances restores resting BPs to the summer value.

Probably the rise in daytime BP in the absence of exercise was due not only to the sedentary lifestyle but also to the increased chronic psychosocial stress and high alcohol consumption (chapter 11). Anecdotally, the subjects' perception of stress appeared to be reduced by exercise, but no formal analysis was undertaken about whether they were less irritable and quarrelsome and whether their sense of well-being had increased.

Table 10.2. Ambulatory Daytime BPs in 13 Members of the Australian National Antarctic Expedition during Winter and Summer, When Each Subject Was Studied during Three 4-Week Periods

	Winter			Summer		
BP, mmHg	NW	3× Ex/Week	7× Ex/Week	NW	3× Ex/Week	7× Ex/Week
SBP	161	140*	143*	140	138	138
DBP	94	90*	88*	87	84	85
MAP	116	107*	106*	104	102	103

Note: Systolic, diastolic, mean BP (SBP, DBP, MAP, mmHg); NW, normal work for time of year.
*$p < .05$ for Δ in resting BP from NW.
(1) performing normal work without exercise training (NW); (2) performing NW and standard bicycle exercise 3×/week at about 60% of W_{max}; (3) as in (2), except that exercise was performed 7× Ex/week.

Source: Jennings, Deakin et al. (1989, 1991).

Exercise Training and Acute Stress Tests

The study was performed in previously untreated obese persons with mild EH or high normal BPs (Georgiades et al., 2000). They were randomly assigned to one of three groups: (1) exercise training alone, (2) exercise training plus weight reduction, and (3) sedentary controls. After 6 months on each regimen, resting hemodynamics and the responses to four short stress tests were compared in the various groups. The stress tests included: (1) a public speech on a controversial topic; (2) an anger interview in which subjects spoke about a recent interpersonal episode that had made them angry; (3) a mirror image tracing test in which a star, viewed in a mirror, had to be drawn as many times as possible in the time available; (4) a cold pressor test, in which the right leg was immersed into a bucket of ice water for a certain time. The tests are all mental challenges, while pain is a feature of the cold pressor test.

The circulatory findings are summarized in table 10.3. After 6 months of training, resting BP, heart rate, and TPR were reduced, while CO was greater than in corresponding sedentary controls. The changes in those subjected to exercise plus weight reduction were greater than in those performing only exercise.

The four stress tests evoked virtually the same rises BP in the exercising and control members of all three groups (table 10.3). However, this does not mean that exercise did not elicit autonomic changes. Because there often were reciprocal changes in CO and TPR, it suggests that in this particular context BP changes are not ideal for differentiating the groups.

In the control group, TPR fell in three out of the four stress tests (speech, anger, and cold pressor), which suggests that adrenaline secretion masked SNA-mediated vasoconstriction in the muscle bed (figure 5.17).[11] The fall was attenuated in all the exercising groups, which could mean either attenuation or enhancement of the relationship. In the mirror trace test, the TPR increased indicating peripheral constriction, and this was attenuated in the exercising groups, supporting the idea that exercise attenuates the responses to all the stress tests. Giving propranolol might have helped differentiate between the controls and exercising subjects (cf. figures 9.26, 9.27); better still, direct

Table 10.3. Average Resting Circulatory Variables and Changes during a Public Speech (PS), Anger Interview (AI), Mirror Trace Test (MT), and Cold Pressor Test (CP)

Variable	Group	Rest	PS	AI	MT	CP
	C	143	+31	+31	+31	+25
SBP, mmHg	E	129*	+36	+28	+27	+28
	E + Wt ↓	127*	+34	+28	+32	+30
	C	88	+14	+11	+17	+13
DBP, mmHg	E	83*	+16	+14	+16	+16
	E + Wt ↓	79*	+16	+14	+17	+18
	C	4.73	+2.47	+1.83	−0.5	+0.86
CO, L/min	E	5.47	+2.22	+2.17	+0.3	+1.21
	E+Wt ↓	5.72	+2.22	+1.61	+0.3	+1.04
	C	2007	−405	−356	+405	−117
TPR, units	E	1684*	−203	−195	+295	+4
	E + Wt ↓	1477*	−166*	−121*	+202*	+33*

Note: SBP, systolic BP; DBP, diastolic BP; CO, cardiac output; TPR, total peripheral resistance. + or − indicates change from resting.
*$p < .05$ for Δ from control group.
All subjects were initially overweight with high normal BP or mild EH and had been allocated for 6 months to one of the following groups: (1) sedentary controls (C); (2) regular treadmill exercise (Ex); (3) regular exercise plus weight reduction (Ex + Wt ↓).

Source: Georgiades et al. (2000).

measurements of plasma NA and adrenaline might have helped in interpreting the effects of the stress tests.

Conclusion

The Antarctic study is a serendipitous natural experiment in which moderate stress is superimposed on an enforced sedentary lifestyle. Under these conditions, exercise training completely abolishes the net rise in resting BP. It appears that exercise also antagonizes the perception of stress, although more objective measurements are required before this can become a definitive conclusion. The study of Georgiades et al. (2000) also suggests that exercise attenuated the autonomic effects of stress, but this requires confirmation by more direct methods. However, the study clearly showed that not only did exercise training reduce resting BP between bouts of exercise, but also that the levels reached during acute stress tests are below those observed in the absence of exercise training.

Strenuous Exercise Training Is a Simple Stress Model

When exercise is performed at rates of work above 75% of W_{max}, anaerobic metabolites accumulate to a greater degree in the active muscles than at lower work rates. This causes the subject some discomfort and requires greater effort to maintain the rate of work at the desired level. Both the factors contribute to the nonlinearity of the BP-work relationship (figure 4.13; Jennings, Deakin et al., 1991; Kingwell and Jennings, 1993; Jennings and Kingwell, 1994; Tipton et al., 1984). The perception of the stressful nature of the exercise under these circumstances contrasts with the "feel-good" emotions associated with submaximal work rates.

The above nonlinearities had been observed earlier in SHR (Tipton et al., 1984). Treadmill exercise was performed 5 days per week from the age of 4 weeks onward and BPs were measured at 12 and 24 weeks of age (table 10.4). In rats exercising at 40–60% of W_{max}, SBP was 12 mmHg lower than in nonexercising SHR by 24 weeks of age. However, SBP was 13 mmHg higher than in controls when exercise was performed at work rates $\geq 75\%$ of W_{max}.

Training and Cardiovascular Structural Changes

In all these experiments, exercise training was performed at work rates that produce optimal lowering of BP.

Skeletal Muscle

In the active muscles, the capillary density increases, together with the number of capillaries per muscle fiber. Maximum blood flow rises in parallel with maximum O_2 consumption (Andersen and Henriksson, 1977; Brodal et al., 1977; Clausen, 1977; Hermansen and Wachtlová, 1971). These changes are mostly due to the opening up of existing capillaries and resistance vessels (Hudlicka, 1991; Hudlicka et al., 1992).

Table 10.4. Systolic Blood Pressure (SBP, mmHg) in 12- and 24-Week-Old Male (m) and Female (f) SHR

	SBP, mmHg	
Grade of Exercise and Status	12 Weeks	24 Weeks
Moderate exercise		
UTr, m	166	184
Tr, m	153*	174*
UTr, f	159	187
Tr, f	144*	173*
Severe exercise		
UTr, m	164	208
Tr, m	166	221**
UTr, f	152	192
Tr, f	155	205**

Note: Tr, trained; UTr, untrained; m, male; f, female; *$p < .05$ for Δ(Tr–UTr); **$p < .05$ for Δ(Tr–UTr).

Groups included rats performing treadmill exercise at 40–60% of W_{max} and more severe exercise (>75% W_{max}) 3–4 ×/week from age of 4 weeks onward and corresponding groups of untrained rats.

Source: Tipton et al. (1983).

In addition, forearm dilator responsiveness to intraarterial ACh is enhanced (Kingwell and Jennings, 1993, 1998; Kingwell et al., 1996).

Heart and Arteries

Twelve months of standard bicycle training at 60% of W_{max} for 30–40 minutes 3 times per week produced modest LV structural changes in persons with mild EH (Jennings, Nelson, Dewar et al., 1986). Wall thickness and the ratio of wall thickness to internal radius decreased, while the internal radius increased. These changes are due to mild chronic central volume overload.

Training increases arterial distensibility (Cameron and Dart, 1994; Kingwell et al., 1997). This is most quantifiable in animal studies in which the arterial elastic properties have been assessed in vitro (Folkow and Löfving, 1956; Safar et al., 1983; Folkow and Karlström, 1984; Benetos and Safar, 1993; Mulvany and Aalkjaer, 1990; London and Levy, 1993). In WKY rats given free access to an exercise wheel, prodigious amounts of daily exercise training were performed between the ages of 4 and 20 weeks, which increased aortic distensibility by 15% and increased internal radius by 5% (Kingwell et al., 1998). These are very substantial changes. In contrast, aortic distensibility did not change in SHR, which were not inclined to perform nearly as much work. Probably at work rates that produce optimal lowering of BP, there is a small increase in aortic distensibility.

Circulatory Regulation during and after Exercise: A Role for the Cerebellum?

Central command and afferents in active muscle are the prime regulators of skeletal muscle movement during exercise, and their effects are coordinated by the cerebellum. The same inputs are also responsible for the autonomic changes, so that the cerebellum is probably also involved in these adjustments. A role for the cerebellum in circulatory control has long been suspected (Moruzzi, 1940; Lisander, 1970; Lisander and Martner, 1971; Bradley, Ghelarducci et al., 1987; Bradley, Pascoe et al., 1987; Bradley, Paton et al., 1987; Miura and Takayama, 1988; Paton and Spyer, 1992). This was based on large circulatory effects evoked by stimulation or lesions of cerebellar structures and the ability to modulate the hypothalamic defense response by cerebellar stimulation. Almost all this work was performed in anesthetized or decerebrate preparations, so that the physiological circumstances under which the cerebellum might be involved have been shrouded in mystery.

During exercise, the autonomic changes are linked closely to skeletal muscle performance. The cerebellum balances the information from the various afferent mechanisms, which has immediate consequences for the somatic motor system and the ANS, both during and after exercise.

Cardiovascular Regulation during Exercise

At the start of moderate aerobic exercise, active skeletal muscle contraction gives rise to vasodilation. At the same time, signals from the CNS give rise to elevation of SNA to the heart, renal, gastrointestinal, skin, and nonactive muscle beds (figure 10.17). Cardiac vagal tone is abolished,[12] while the raised cardiac SNA provides the heart with inotropic and chronotropic support. The autonomic pattern is a variant of the defense response to mental stress, in which the rises in SNA are similar, but skeletal muscle vasodilation and cardiac vagal inhibition are smaller.

Part of the BP rise during exercise is nonautonomic due to the high CO that is mainly caused by the vasodilation in the active muscle, which is accentuated by the NO-mediated functional sympatholysis. Blocking SNA in only the active muscles is a remarkable regulatory feat, of which control engineers would be proud.

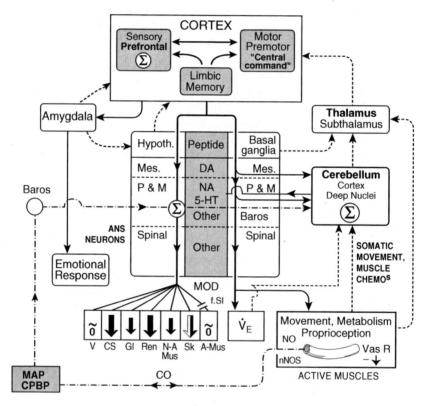

Figure 10.17. Schema of circulatory control during exercise. Somatic movement, autonomic activity, and respiration are all regulated in response to central command, with feedback from active skeletal muscle, with cerebellum playing a coordinating role. Slow transmitter neurons that modulate target neurons are shown in shaded column in center. Hypertension generates a circulatory pattern that is a variant of the defense response: inhibition of vagal motoneurons (V) and increases in SNA in cardiac (CS), gastrointestinal (GI), renal (Ren), and nonactive muscle (N-A Mus) outflows; size of the black arrows related to magnitude of ΔSNA-mediated constriction. Skin either constricts or dilates, depending on thermoregulatory demands. Local metabolic dilation in active muscle (−) is reinforced by NO. The increases in MAP and cardiopulmonary BP (CPBP) during exercise moderate the rises in SNA through reset baroreflexes. Hypoth., hypothalamus; Mes., mesencephalon; P & M, pons and medulla; nNOS, neural nitric oxide synthase; Vas R, vascular resistance. Further discussion in text.

Central command is high during exercise, with its sympathoexcitatory effects determining the responses in conjunction with the increasing discharge of the muscle chemoreceptors. The latter warn the brain to slow down if somatic motor activity becomes excessive. The cerebellum compares the magnitude of central command and the afferent activity from active muscle, and adjusts somatic motor activity on the basis of this comparison. A similar cerebellar operation probably contributes to the rise in SNA and resetting of the baroreflex properties through specific NA and 5-HT slow transmitter neurons.

Interactions between Central Command, Muscle Chemoreceptors, and Baroreflexes

Central command can raise BP by calling on past experiences from memory (figure 10.5). However, normally it acts in conjunction with peripheral signals from the active muscles, as illustrated during peridural anesthesia (figure 10.9).

The hypothalamic defense area increases SNA during exercise through two pathways: A less powerful pathway is independent of baroreceptor influences, while the more powerful pathway alters baroreflex properties, thereby contributing substantially to the elevation of BP. Both sets of changes probably depend on cerebellar assessment of the relative magnitude of central command and muscle chemoreceptor activity (figure 10.17).

Determinants of Circulatory Changes between Training Sessions

After the first bicycle exercise session at 50–70% of W_{max}, a short period of vasodilation in the previously active muscles is accompanied by slight depression of constrictor baroreflexes. Together these factors account for the slightly lower BP that is present for 1–2 hours from the end of exercise. Central command ceases immediately at the end of exercise, and muscle chemoreceptor discharge stops within 3–5 minutes. Hence, what maintains the mild depression of constrictor baroreflexes probably relates to CNS changes affecting synaptic transmission toward the end of the preceding exercise.

In successive bouts of exercise at the identical rate of work, the size of the active muscle bed increases, mainly in response to progressively greater skeletal muscle hypertrophy. The neural signals also change progressively. Central command draws increasingly on past experience, so that the initial autonomic adjustments in figure 10.11 occur rapidly. However, with practice less cortical effort is required to maintain the rate of work and central command tends to diminish from the high initial value as exercise continues. In contrast, muscle chemoreceptor discharge gradually increases as usual, because the rate of accumulation of anaerobic metabolites alters little from session to session. It is the changes in the ratio of central command to muscle chemoreceptor activity that increase baroreflex depression and cause reduction in TPR and BP between training sessions. This type of operation is exactly in line with normal function of the cerebellum, as discussed below.

However, when training is performed at near-maximal rates of work, BP rises between exercise sessions. Because of the discomfort and stress, a greater effort is required of central command to maintain exercise. From the subject's viewpoint, it is quite a stressful experience.

A Role for the Cerebellum in Circulatory Control?

The cerebellar cortex and deep nuclei contain nearly 50% of all neurons in the CNS. Its cortical cytoarchitecture is uniform, which suggests that its operations may be relatively stereotyped. Its role in maintaining postural balance is well known. It also coordinates planning and execution of somatic movements, the learning of motor skills, and Pavlovian conditioning of muscle reflexes (Eccles et al., 1967; Ito, 1984; Thompson, 1990; Ghez, 1991).

The cerebellar cortex has five types of neurons (stellate, basket, Purkinje, Golgi, and granule cells) arranged in three layers—an outer molecular layer, the Purkinje cell layer, and an inner granule cell layer (figure 10.18). The molecular layer includes the parallel fibers that are the axons of the granule cells, and the stellate and basket cells. The Purkinje cells are large GABAergic neurons; their dendrites extend into the molecular layer, while their axons are the sole output of the cerebellar cortex, which modulates the activity of neurons in the deep nuclei.

The mossy fibers and the climbing fibers originate from neurons in various brainstem nuclei and are the major afferents to the cerebellum. Each stimulates the deep nuclei before acting on the Purkinje cells (figure 10.19). Other interconnections between many cerebellar regions and the brainstem are through 5-HT and NA neurons from, respectively, the raphe and locus ceruleus cell groups.

The mossy fibers synapse with the granule cells and innervate the Purkinje cells through the parallel fibers (figure 10.18). They discharge at high spontaneous rates and raise Purkinje neuron firing to 50–100 spikes per second in response to sensory stimuli and voluntary movement.

All the climbing fibers come from inferior olivary neurons that receive input from the motor cortex (figure 10.18). Their synapses with Purkinje neurons are very powerful: A single action potential of the climbing fiber elicits so-called complex spikes in Purkinje cells, consisting of a large EPSP followed by a burst of smaller action potentials. However, the spontaneous rate of discharge of climbing fibers is slow, so that they have little direct effect on Purkinje cell discharge. Their main role is to modulate the latter's responsiveness to the input from the mossy fibers.

The cerebellum has three distinct functional regions: (1) the vestibulocerebellum in the flocculonodular lobe, which regulates eye movement, posture, and balance; (2) the spinocerebellum, which includes the midline and intermediate parts of each hemisphere—it receives input from the limb muscles and its output helps in the execution of limb movement by modulating the activity of the fastigial nucleus and the nucleus interpositus; and (3) the cerebrocerebellum is the largest part of the cerebellum and is located in the lateral part of each hemisphere; its input comes from nuclei in the pons which relay information from the cerebral cortex and the basal ganglia, and its output projects back to the motor and premotor cortex via the dentate nucleus and thalamus (figure 10.18).

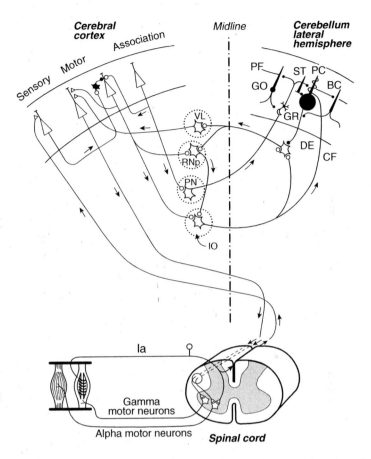

Figure 10.18. Schematic diagram of neural circuit for regulation and learning of skeletal muscle movement, in which lateral cerebellar hemisphere plays a major role. Many parallel fibers provide input to each Purkinje cell, but only a single climbing fiber makes contact with a given Purkinje cell. CF, climbing fiber; BC, basket cell; GO, Golgi cell; GR, granule cell; MF, mossy fiber; PC, Purkinje cell; PF, parallel fiber; ST, stellate cell; DE, dentate nucleus; IO, inferior olivary nucleus; PN, pontine nuclei; RNp, parvocellular part of red nucleus; VL, ventrolateral thalamic nucleus. From Kawato (1995), with permission of MIT Press.

Information originating from the sensory cortex and hippocampal formation is processed by the basal ganglia and cerebrocerebellum, which give rise to the commands for movement by neurons in the premotor and motor areas of the cortex (figure 10.17). The spinocerebellum receives details of the commands and corrects them in the light of peripheral feedback. Eventually the adjusted motor programs are stored in cortical and subcortical regions for future use.

The hypothesis is that the same cortical motor commands that evoke skeletal muscle movement also elicit the autonomic changes (figure 10.17). They reach the hypothalamus (1) from the prefrontal cortex via midbrain DA neurons, and (2) from the cerebellum via NA and 5-HT neurons (figure 10.17). The prefrontal cortex evaluates the

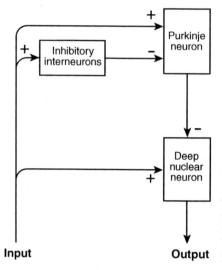

Input **Output**

Figure 10.19. Schema showing that major inputs to cerebellum first excite neurons in deep cerebellar nuclei and then either inhibit or enhance Purkinje neuron discharge. This further modifies discharge of deep nuclei. From Ghez (1991), with permission of McGraw-Hill, New York.

motor commands in the light of other sensory and behavioral information, while the cerebellum relates them to skeletal muscle afferent activity. Not all of the latter relevant to somatic movement is important for the autonomic adjustments, which depend mainly on muscle chemoreceptor activity.

On the basis of theoretical modeling, Marr (1969) and Albus (1971) proposed independently that the strength of the parallel fiber synapses is modified by the activity of the climbing fibers and that this is important in the learning of motor skills. Such modulation also plays a role in associative (Pavlovian) conditioning of skeletal muscle reflexes (chapter 11; Ito, 1984, 1989; Thompson, 1990; Bartha and Thompson, 1995; Kawato, 1995).

Long-term depression (LTD) of synaptic transmission between parallel fibers and Purkinje cells occurs when the rates of discharge of those mossy and climbing fibers that are associated with a particular movement increase simultaneously (Ito, 1984; 1989). Exercise induces LTD of Purkinje cells when central command and muscle afferent activity increase simultaneously, which affects both somatic and autonomic activity: The LTD disinhibits the underlying deep nuclei, as a result of which somatic motoneuron activity and SNA both increase. A considerable amount of progress has been made on identifying the cellular mechanisms that give rise to LTD in Purkinje neurons (Ito et al., 1982; Crepel and Audinat, 1991; Linden and Connor, 1991; Crepel et al., 1995).[13]

Long-term potentiation (LTP) of Purkinje cell synapses develops when the discharge of mossy fibers is increasing while that of climbing fibers is either falling or remains unchanged (Kawato, 1995). LTP increases Purkinje neuron discharge, which produces more inhibition of the deep nuclei and reduces the discharge of their projections to the cortex.

LTP will increase during successive training sessions as central command declines in the course of each session, while muscle chemoreceptor activity increases.

The resulting greater inhibition of the deep nuclei could reduce discharge of 5-HT neurons in series with DA neurons (figure 8.19) lowering discharge from the hypothalamic defense area neurons that affect activity of cardiac and constrictor baroreflexes. Depression of these reflexes then becomes manifest between sessions. Alternatively, BP could be lowered through NA neurons acting on bulbospinal pathways similar to the effects of α-MD, which is independent of the defense area.

LTP at Purkinje cell synapses could also explain the reduction of RSNA that occurs after its initial rise during several minutes of electrical stimulation of sciatic nerve afferents. On stopping stimulation, RSNA becomes depressed for some 20–60 minutes (Shyu et al., 1984; Hoffmann and Thorén, 1986; Kenney et al., 1991).

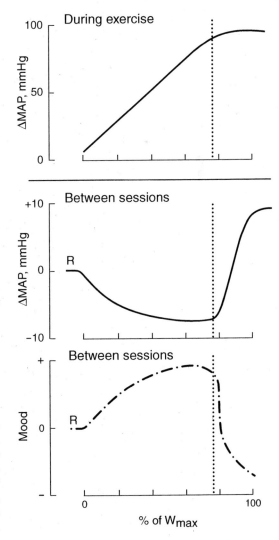

Figure 10.20. Top, during each bout of steady-state exercise of standard length and intensity, the change in systolic BP (SBP) depends on the rate of work (% of person's W_{max}). Middle and bottom panels, when training is performed regularly at less than 75% W_{max} (vertical dotted line), MAP between bouts of exercise falls below the sedentary value, and feelings about training are generally positive. If training is greater than 75% W_{max}, MAP often rises above sedentary value, which is often associated with negative, stressful emotions.

Neural activity from the amygdala could also contribute to the postexercise autonomic changes. For example, the prefrontal cortex will interpret the feel-good emotions associated with submaximal exercise differently than the stress associated with near-maximal exercise, which has the opposite effects on defense pathway responsiveness.

In summary, the close linkage between skeletal muscle and autonomic responses during exercise makes a prima facie case that the cerebellum coordinates both functions. The long-term postexercise changes due to training depend on what happens during exercise in each session. A major difference between the altered responsiveness to both submaximal and near-maximal exercise is the greater reversibility than the changes associated with mental stress. This may be more apparent than real. The autonomic effects of mental stress are also reversible in normal persons, but much less so in persons with EH, who develop structural synaptic changes as in *Aplysia* and mammalian memory neurons. These involve DA neuron synapses linking cortex and hypothalamus. It suggests that LTP and LTD changes involving synapses with cerebellar Purkinje cells may be solely functional without development of new synaptic contacts.

Regular Exercise Training: Potential for Preventing EH

Exercise is a self-imposed challenge. Performing 30 minutes of submaximal exercise at 50–70% of W_{max} is within most people's capacity and, indeed, often becomes addictive. The rise in BP is linearly related to the rate of work, when normalized in terms of the person's W_{max} (figure 10.20, top). The major inputs to the control system are central command and afferents from active skeletal muscles, both of which alter baroreflex properties. The cerebellum is a comparator of the major inputs and optimizes somatic motor and autonomic responses.

Regular training reduces resting BP and SNA, and often generates positive emotions (figure 10.20, middle and bottom). In contrast, resting BP tends to rise when training involves near-maximal exercise, which may cause pain and muscle injury. A working hypothesis is that the brain evaluates submaximal and near-maximal exercise differently, with distinctive slow transmitter neurons depressing or increasing resting SNA.

Lack of exercise training may be a factor in the pathogenesis of EH. EH first becomes manifest in young adulthood or early middle age, when the level of habitual physical activity often diminishes suddenly. Hence, continuing regular exercise training in that age group merits promotion as a public health measure for the prevention of EH. Reversing EH becomes much more difficult once hypertension has become established, in view of the cardiac, vascular, and neural structural changes.

PART VI

THE BRAIN AS THE SOURCE OF LIFESTYLE-RELATED HYPERTENSION

11

Psychosocial Stress and Hypertension

Life is stressful and stress is experienced quite frequently by almost everyone. However, there is considerable variation in the perception of stress: A given stimulus that is mildly stressful to some is regarded as very stressful by others. Only a relatively small proportion of persons who feel chronically stressed go on to develop EH, which suggests greater sensitivity of their neural pathways mediating the cardiovascular responses to stress, since there is little to suggest that the lives of those with EH are more stressful than those of persons with normal BPs.

From the data discussed in chapters 4 and 5, it seems likely that stress plays a major role in the pathogenesis of EH. Its role as a potential cause is always mentioned in textbooks and in compendia on hypertension, but the proposal has generally been received with muted enthusiasm (Swales, 1994c; Laragh and Brenner, 1995; Kaplan, 2002). One reason may be that the perception of stress involves the cortex, memory, and many of the higher functions of the CNS. This area has tended to be neglected by cardiovascular physiologists, although it has been of great interest to behavioral neuroscientists.

Accordingly, this chapter examines the relationship between stress and autonomic, hormonal, behavioral, and somatic motor responses from available knowledge in the various fields. This includes the pathways through which stress is perceived and the extent of enhancement of the autonomic responses in EH. Discussion of the long-term effects of psychosocial and mental stressors in animals and humans illustrates the role of day-to-day environmental and lifestyle factors and the importance of genetic mechanisms.

Stress arises when the brain is uncertain whether an environmental challenge is within the subject's capacity to meet it (Frankenhaeuser, 1987; McEwen, 1994).

Stress-generating situations (i.e., stressors) include natural disasters, adversarial confrontation, physical danger, accidents, socioeconomic hardship, job loss, life events such as divorce or death of a loved one, and a large range of other mental challenges. The perception of stress depends on how an individual views the environment.

Each person probably has a maximum capacity for meeting stress-related challenges with an adequate functional performance. The problem has been to find a scale for expressing this capacity that allows for the large individual variation. As noted in chapter 10, exercise training provides a model for this, since normalizing work rate in terms of an individual's maximum work capacity (W_{max}) gives relatively uniform physiological and emotional responses in those engaged in exercise training.

Regular exercise also illustrates that long-term effects on BP and SNA follow repeated exposure to excessive stressors. Elevation of SNA is the main initiator of the hypertension, contrasting with very intense stresses in which glucocorticoid hormones are raised while BP and SNA are normal or low (McEwen, 1994; Folkow, 1987).

CNS Pathways Mediating Responses to Psychosocial Stress

The detection of stressful stimuli at conscious and subconscious levels involves the thalamus and cortical and subcortical neuron populations. The end result is a change in activity of specific sets of slow transmitter neurons that determine the autonomic and emotional responses through the hypothalamus and amygdala.

Sensory Processing: Role of Thalamus, Cortex, and Subcortical Mechanisms

The brain must recognize a mental challenge such as a hostile act or imminent danger. Sometimes a particular person or environment reminds one of an unpleasant past experience. This depends on integrating the information presented through many sensory modalities. In addition, the assessment of the challenge includes taking account of the likely risks and rewards of a particular course of action. All these factors contribute to the perception of stress.

Figure 11.1 shows the main CNS pathways involved. Incoming sensory information flows through the thalamus and the sensory and prefrontal cortex and is compared with analogous information in the memory stores of the hippocampus and the various cortical, limbic, and cerebellar regions. If the stimulus is deemed to be stressful, it results in increased activity of DA, 5-HT, or other slow transmitter neurons that modulate target neuron responsiveness in the hypothalamus and amygdala; the latter extracts information necessary for expressing the emotional response (Smith and DeVito, 1984; Gray, 1994; LeDoux, 1994). The sensory input to the cortex is also influenced by the DA neurons. Under quiescent conditions, the action of the corpus striatum on the thalamus limits its sensory input to the cortex. DA neuron activity counteracts these effects, and the resulting rise in sensory input increases the level of arousal (Carlsson et al., 1997; Carlsson, 2001).

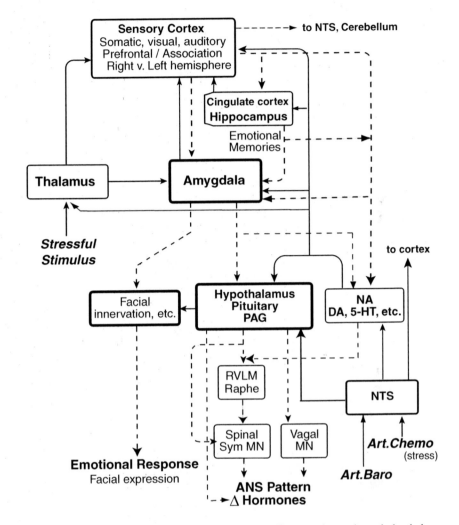

Figure 11.1. Stress is recognized through a complex afferent pathway through the thalamus, sensory cortex, and prefrontal cortex. These have reciprocal connections with cingulate cortex, hippocampal formation, and amygdala but also nucleus tractus solitarius (NTS) and cerebellum. Descending pathways effect responsiveness of target neurons in the hypothalamus, periaqueductal gray (PAG), and amygdala through various slow transmitter neurons (e.g., DA, 5-HT). The defense pattern is generated in the hypothalamus and midbrain, which affects activity of vagal and sympathetic motoneurons partly through hindbrain neurons subserving baroreflexes. Strong stimulation of the arterial chemoreceptors can give rise to a variant defense response (chapter 14). Ascending pathways, solid lines; descending pathways, dashed lines. Art.Baro, arterial baroreceptors; Art.Chemo, arterial chemoreceptors; RVLM, rostral ventrolateral medulla; Spinal Sym MN, spinal sympathetic motoneurons; NA, DA, 5-HT, noradrenergic, dopaminergic, and serotonergic neuron groups.

The brain's response to a stressor depends on integration of the associated visual, auditory, and somatosensory information by the corresponding primary and higher order cortical association areas (Darian-Smith, 1982; Mountcastle, 1984; Darian-Smith et al., 1996; Rosenzweig et al., 1996). The thalamocortical system can integrate this type of complex inputs very rapidly and accurately and distinguish them from related inputs (Edelman, 1989; Edelman and Tononi, 2000). Moreover, Edelman's theory of neuronal group selection allows for variation between individuals of how such complex stimuli are perceived. This arises through differences in neural connections in different components of the network, which is why the theory is also known as neural Darwinism. It helps explain why an adverse stimulus may appear to be more adverse to some than to others.

The cortical information flows to the prefrontal cortex as a coded and simplified version of the original inputs (Goldman-Rakic, 1987). That the simplification is considerable is suggested by the similarity of neuroendocrine responses evoked by very disparate stressors.

Prefrontal cortical neurons communicate with the neuron populations subserving learning and memory. The neuronal networks formed in this way are in accord with Hebb's original ideas about perception and can be visualized by positron emission tomography (Drevets and Raichle, 1994; Roland et al., 1997). For example, the network for memorizing a face from photographs includes the primary and secondary visual cortex of each hemisphere, the right hippocampus and medial temporal cortex, and the left prefrontal cortex. Recalling the face from memory works through most of the original network plus a number of additional regions (Grady et al., 1995). The networks provide the means of taking numerous interactions into account during the integration process.

Adaptive social behavior depends on the integrity of the prefrontal cortex: Small localized lesions in this region give rise to serious behavioral disorders that usually do not affect vision, hearing, language, and basic reasoning capacity (table 11.1; Damasio, 1994). Subjects with such lesions have diminished inhibitory control over social behavior; they are distracted easily and may have difficulty formulating new ideas. Their attitudes toward people and environmental stimuli are often flat and negative.

In contrast, when the prefrontal cortex is optimally stimulated, we see enhancement of performance and social functioning, sometimes referred to as the executive syndrome (Rosenzweig et al., 1996). During the depressive phase in bipolar disorders this region is underactivated, while during the manic phase it becomes overactivated (Damasio, 1997; Drevets et al., 1997). In animals, raising midbrain DA neuron activity simulates the executive syndrome (Le Moal and Simon, 1991). Something analogous was first studied by Olds and Milner (1954) in their classic operant conditioning experiments on self-stimulation in rats: Pressing a lever mildly stimulates the ascending tracts to the hypothalamus, limbic, and prefrontal regions, including those from DA neurons (figure 11.2). The animals appear to find these stimuli highly rewarding and become addicted to them.

Something rather similar occurs in heavy smokers who become addicted to this type of reward. The effect of smoking on their BP was studied in a group of young adults who habitually smoked more than 20 cigarettes per day (Groppelli et al., 1992). On one occasion, following nighttime abstinence from smoking, they were

Table 11.1. Some Characteristics of Regional Prefrontal Syndrome
Following Localized Lesions

Dorsolateral Lesion (Dysexecutive Type)	Orbitofrontal Lesion (Disinhibited Type)	Mediofrontal Lesion (Apathetic Type)
Diminished judgment, planning, insight, and temporal organization Cognitive impersistence Motor programming deficits (may include aphasia and apraxia) Diminished self-care	Stimulus-driven behavior Diminished social insight Distractibility/Emotional lability	Diminished spontaneity Diminished verbal output (including mutism) Diminished motor behavior (including akinesis) Urinary incontinence Lower extremity weakness and sensory loss Increased response latency

Source: Rosenzweig et al. (1996), with permission of Sinauer Associates.

asked to smoke their first four cigarettes of the day after getting up in the morning. The first cigarette elicited the greatest rises in SBP, DBP, and heart rate, but the other cigarettes also elicited significant rises (figure 11.3). Their smaller magnitude was due to long-lasting elevation of BP and sympathoadrenal activity after each cigarette (Cryer et al., 1976). After each cigarette there was relatively little BP recovery, resulting in a cumulative rise in MAP of ~15 mmHg during that hour. On another occasion,

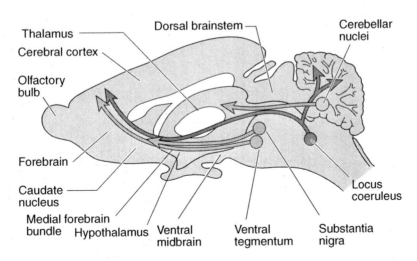

Figure 11.2. Pathways involved in self-stimulation experiments in rats of Olds and Milner (1954). Large circles show placements of the stimulating electrodes in different experiments; these were activated by the rat by pressing a lever. The arrows on the ascending tracts point to the targets of the reward circuits, including ascending tracts from DA and other monoaminergic neurons. From Rosenzweig et al. (1996), with permission of Sinauer Associates.

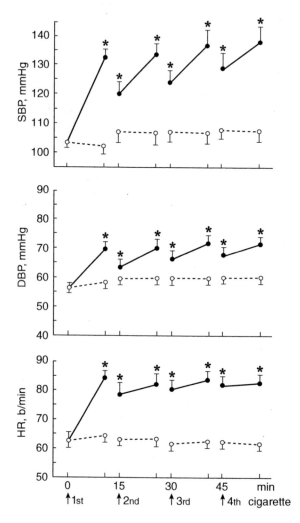

Figure 11.3. Effect of smoking four cigarettes at 15-minute intervals on systolic and diastolic BP (SBP, DBP, mmHg) and heart rate (HR, beats/min); closed circles and solid lines show changes at start and end of smoking; open circles, changes in another experiment at corresponding times during the nonsmoking hour. The progressive elevation of BP reflects the persistence of autonomic effects after each cigarette. From Groppelli et al. (1992), with permission of *Journal of Hypertension* and Lippincott, Williams and Wilkins.

the subjects' ambulatory BPs were measured over an 8-hour period while smoking ad libitum; on a smoking day MAP was 5–10 mmHg higher than on a nonsmoking day (table 11.2).

Memory

Memory serves as a reference for interpreting a stressor's significance. The ease with which a particular memory is recalled depends on how vividly it was first presented and the frequency of subsequent stimulation. Encoded memories are stored initially in the hippocampal formation and in the neocortical sensory areas associated with each modality. In time the importance of the hippocampal formation diminishes, except for topographical memory, for which the hippocampus remains the chief repository (Glynn, 1999). Memory recall is through the establishment of neuronal networks between specific regions of the two hemispheres; for example, the network

Table 11.2. Results from 10 Heavy Smokers, Showing Differences
in Ambulatory BPs and Heart Rate Between an 8-Hour "Smoking" Day
and Another 8-Hour "Nonsmoking" Day

Variable	Δ (S − NS) ± SEM	p
SBP, mmHg	5.2 ± 1.7	*
DBP, mmHg	6.4 ± 1.1	*
MAP, mmHg	5.9 ± 1.3	*
HR/min	8.0 ± 3.0	*

Note: SBP, systolic BP; DBP, diastolic BP; MAP, mean arterial BP; HR, heart rate/min; Δ (S − NS), difference between smoking and nonsmoking day, within subjects.
*p for Δ < .01.

Source: Groppelli et al. (1992).

for recalling a precise route to a destination includes the right hippocampus and left prefrontal cortex (Maguire et al., 1998).

The Hypothalamus and the Defense Response

Hess was the first to describe a coordinated pattern of increased sympathoadrenal activity, muscle movement, and vocalization evoked by electrical stimulation of the hypothalamus of conscious cats (Hess and Brugger, 1943; Hess, 1957). The animals acted as if warding off an aggressor, hence the term *Abwehrreaktion* or defense response.

As discussed in earlier chapters, the pattern elicited by acute stressors (e.g., mental stress, aerobic exercise) includes rises in BP, heart rate, and CO, vasoconstriction of the renal, gastrointestinal, and skin beds, and vasodilation in the skeletal muscle bed that are largely mediated through the ANS. The same pattern is present in the resting circulation of persons with EH.

Since Hess's work, many investigators have stimulated the hypothalamus electrically to localize the sources of the autonomic pattern and to trace the descending projections (Eliasson et al., 1951; Abrahams et al., 1960, 1964; Feigl et al., 1964; Zanchetti et al., 1976; Hilton, 1982; Hilton and Marshall, 1982; Jordan, 1990). However, for localizing the sources of the pattern, electrical stimulation provides ambiguous answers because both cell bodies and fibers of passage are stimulated. When chemical stimuli came into use, it was found that with glutamate exploration of the hypothalamus there were very few sites from which the defense response could be elicited, except with large amounts of amino acid, which is not ideal (Lipski et al., 1988). In contrast, microinjections of glutamate into the periaqueductal gray (PAG) region of the midbrain readily evoked the defense response. This raised the possibility that the PAG could be the site of the command neurons for this autonomic pattern (Carrive et al., 1987; Bandler and Carrive, 1988).

However, this now appears unlikely. DiMicco and colleagues evoked the defense response from discrete regions of the dorsomedial hypothalamic nucleus (DMHN) by injecting the GABA antagonist bicuculline (figure 11.4; Schmidt and DiMicco, 1984; Sample and DiMicco, 1987; DiMicco et al., 1992). Their findings suggest that

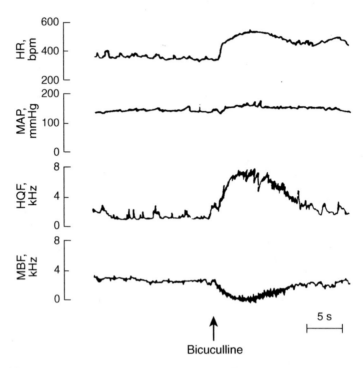

Figure 11.4. Effects of bilateral microinjection of the GABA antagonist bicuculline methiodide (20 pmol/250 nL) into the dorsomedial hypothalamic nucleus of a conscious rat. Variables (from top): heart rate (HR, beats/min), MAP (mmHg), hindquarter and mesenteric blood flows (HQBF, MBF, kHz Doppler shift). Note marked elevation of heart rate and limb blood flow (↓ HQ Vas R) and reduction in mesenteric blood flow (↑ mesenteric Vas R). From DiMicco et al. (1992), with permission of Birkhäuser and Springer-Verlag.

the DHMN neurons are normally inhibited by forebrain mechanisms, with removal of the inhibition and unmasking their activity. Once the exact site was known, the response could be elicited by microinjecting small amounts of glutamate (DiMicco et al., 1992). The paraventricular nucleus (PVN) is another region from which elevation of constrictor SNA can be evoked, though not usually increased secretion of adrenaline (Dampney, 1994a; Dampney et al., 2002; Dampney, personal communication; Horiuchi et al., 2005).

Variants of the Defense Response

Variant forms of the defense response are evoked by mental stress, aerobic exercise, strong stimulation of the arterial chemoreceptors, and nasopharyngeal stimulation associated with apnea. EH is a chronic variant of the stress-related defense pattern.

In all of the above responses, there is SNA-mediated vasoconstriction in renal, mesenteric, and skeletal muscle beds. The vasoconstriction in the muscle bed is masked by adrenaline-mediated vasodilation during acute mental stress and strong arterial chemoreceptor stimulation, and in EH, when there is a phasic increase in the level of stress (Fukuda and Kobayashi, 1961; Chalmers et al., 1966; Uther et al., 1970; Schramm et al., 1971; Hjemdahl et al., 1984; Freyschuss et al., 1988). In exercise, the muscle vasoconstriction is blocked by the effects of an increase in NO in the active musculature (chapter 10) and adrenaline secretion is generally absent.

There is also a range of heart rate responses. With mental stress, exercise, and in EH the heart rate increases, but there are differences in the degree of cardiac sympathetic and vagal involvement. In contrast, in the presence of strong chemoreceptor stimulation or apnea, there is bradycardia through vagal excitation and reduction in cardiac SNA (chapter 14).

Hypothalamic Mapping

The question arises whether these variant responses are mediated through somewhat different hypothalamic neuron populations. To try to answer this and to investigate the role of baroreflexes on these responses, the hypothalamus was mapped in two groups of anesthetized rabbits, one with intact arterial baroreceptors, while sinoaortic denervation (SAD) had been performed earlier in the other (Korner et al., 1983). In half the animals of each group mapping was performed with electrical stimulation, while glutamate was used (100–200 nL of 0.5 M per injection) in the other half.

As expected, of the sites from which electrical stimulation evoked mesenteric constriction or hindlimb dilation, fewer than 30% responded to glutamate (figure 11.5; table 11.3).[1] The glutamate-sensitive sites were mostly in the medial part of the hypothalamus, while the lateral hypothalamus was the most common source of the pattern during electrical stimulation. With arterial baroreceptors, intact glutamate-sensitive sites were present throughout the length of the medial hypothalamus, while after SAD responsive sites were present mainly in the anterior half. The findings suggest that in the intact animal the various stressors engage somewhat different neuron populations, probably extending beyond DMHN and PVN. In addition, the autonomic responses are modulated by baroreflexes, as observed during exercise.

Long-Term Hypothalamic Stimulation Causes Hypertension

In a pioneering study, Folkow and Rubinstein (1966) stimulated the hypothalamus of 9–12-week-old Sprague-Dawley rats for a period of several weeks. Weak stimuli were applied intermittently during the night when the rats are normally active. This raised BP, increased the level of alertness, and enhanced exploratory behavior.

MAP increased gradually during 9 weeks of stimulation, rising by ~15 mmHg above the baseline of unstimulated controls (figure 11.6). At the end of that time, stimulation was stopped and BP rapidly declined. Stimulation was resumed 1 week later, and now the BP rise was more rapid than on the first occasion. The gradual nature of the first rise in BP suggests that inhibitory mechanisms moderated the initial rise in BP. Their smaller magnitude on the second occasion could have been due to sensitization of the defense pathway or to amplification associated with cardiovascular hypertrophy, which is more likely.

Mesenteric constriction/Hindlimb dilation

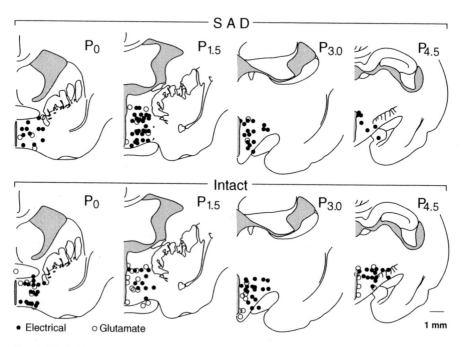

Figure 11.5. Hypothalamic stimulation sites from which the peripheral vascular component of defense response could be evoked (i.e., $\uparrow$ mesenteric Vas R, $\downarrow$ hindquarter Vas R by $\geq 10\%$ of resting). Mapping performed in four transverse planes at P_0, $P_{1.5}$, $P_{3.0}$, and $P_{4.5}$, where suffix is distance from bregma in millimeters in the anterior-posterior plane (Girgis and Shih-Chang, 1981). Separate groups were used for: (1) electrical stimulation through fine steel needles (50–100 μA, rectangular pulses of 0.25–0.5 ms, 60/s; black circles); (2) local injections of glutamate (0.5 M, 100–200 nL; clear circles). In half the rabbits arterial baroreceptors were intact and in half sinoaortic denervation (SAD) had been performed 1–2 weeks earlier. All experiments under alfathesin anesthesia. Number of rabbits 23, with 5–6 per subgroup. From Korner et al. (1983); diagram courtesy of B. K. Evans, J. Oliver, J. Aberdeen, J. Cassel, and P. Korner.

Acute Stresses in Animals and Humans

Animals

An ingenious preparation was devised by Zanchetti and colleagues, in which a conscious instrumented test cat was confronted by an aggressor cat with an electrode implanted in its midbrain (Adams et al., 1968, 1969; Mancia et al., 1972; Zanchetti et al., 1976). On stimulation, the aggressor cat struck out involuntarily at the test cat but could not hit it because a partition separated the two animals. The test cat responded to the simulated attacks in one of three ways: (1) with the classic defense pattern following a loud meow and limb movements; (2) with uniform moderate vasoconstriction

Table 11.3. Patterns of Changes in Mesenteric and Hindquarter Conductance (MC, HC) Showing Number of Responses Evoked during Electrical and Glutamate Stimulation in Intact and Sinoaortically Denervated Anesthetized Rabbits

Electrical Stimulation							Glutamate Stimulation						
MC ↑	↑	0	↓	↓	↓	0	↑	↑	0	↓	↓	↓	0
HC ↑	0	↑	↑	↓	0	0	↑	0	↑	↑	↓	0	0

A. Intact Art. Baroreceptors

P_{00}	6	0	14	24	1	2	33	1	3	4	6	0	2	69
P_{15}	6	0	18	31	0	0	30	1	1	6	13	2	3	64
P_{30}	3	0	15	28	0	4	32	2	0	10	7	0	2	76
P_{45}	5	1	18	25	2	6	32	0	3	7	7	1	6	86
Σ	20	1	65	108	3	12	127	4	7	27	33	3	13	295

B. Sinoaortic Denervation

P_{00}	31	3	20	17	2	5	20	16	3	7	4	1	3	80
P_{15}	26	2	31	28	2	5	20	17	2	14	6	1	3	99
P_{30}	14	1	5	8	6	4	9	3	2	1	2	3	0	47
P_{45}	25	0	21	21	17	7	18	8	3	11	0	5	8	88
Σ	96	6	77	74	25	18	61	44	10	33	12	10	14	314

Note: MC, HC, mesenteric, hindquarter conductance; ↑ increased conductance, i.e., vasodilatation; 0, no change; ↓, decreased conductance, i.e., vasoconstriction; P, A-P position relative to bregma; 00, bregma; 15, 30, 45 ≡ 1.5, 3.0, 4.5 mm. There were 5–6 rabbits in each of the 4 groups.

Source: Unpublished data of B. K. Evans, J. Oliver, J. Aberdeen, J. Cassel, and P. Korner.

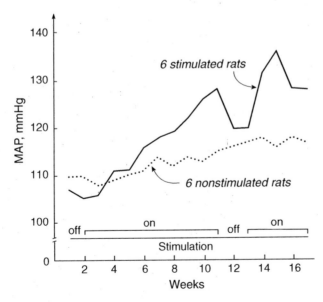

Figure 11.6. Effects of electrical stimulation through implanted electrodes on BP in six Sprague-Dawley and a similar number of unstimulated controls. Note gradual initial BP rise, followed by return to control on stopping stimulation (off) and more rapid rise on resuming stimulation. From Folkow and Rubinstein (1966), with permission of *Acta Physiologica Scandinavica* and Blackwell.

and a rise in heart rate; and (3) by becoming immobile, which was associated with mild vasoconstriction and bradycardia.

Thus, one response consisted of somatic movement and an autonomic response similar to that during exercise. In the absence of movement, vasoconstriction was more uniform and included the muscle bed.

Another stressor consisted of blowing air at an animal's face for a few minutes, which elicited the full defense response (DiBona, 1991). Repeating the stress four times at 15-minute intervals caused only slight attenuation of the rise in BP.

Acute Responses in Humans

Mental stress tests, such as mental arithmetic or word conflict tests, readily evoke the defense response in normotensive (and hypertensive) subjects, particularly when the test is performed at some speed (Falkner, 1987; Mancia and Parati, 1987; Herd, 1991). In one early study the subjects had to perform mental arithmetic under trying circumstances, which raised BP and CO and caused renal vasoconstriction and forearm muscle vasodilation (figure 11.7, left; Brod et al., 1959).

A less contrived situation was the natural stress experienced by American college students preparing for a forthcoming examination (Frankenhaeuser, 1978). Ten days before the examination their urinary excretion of NA and adrenaline started to rise gradually, peaking dramatically on the day of the test (figure 11.8). A similar stress study was done with applicants to a training course for aspiring army parachutists (Ursin et al., 1978). On the first day, their plasma catecholamines and glucocorticoids were, respectively, about 50% and 100% above baseline. However, the rises were much smaller by the second day and were absent by the fifth jump. The subjects rapidly became habituated to jumping after the initial anxieties and fears turned out to be groundless.

Is the Defence Pathway Sensitized in EH?

In EH, as the pathways subserving the defense response become sensitized, the sympathetic responses to a given stressor become greater than in normotensives. In addition, the responses outlast the stimulus, in accordance with the LTP model in *Aplysia*.

Figure 11.7 is a comparison of the circulatory responses to mental arithmetic in normotensives and persons with EH (Brod et al., 1959). When the responses were expressed as percentage changes of each group's resting value, there were no obvious differences between the groups. However, when the results are expressed as actual Vas R changes, the rise in renal Vas R was 1.69 times greater in those with EH than in normotensives (table 11.4). Assuming a structural amplification factor of 1.35, the results suggest additional neural enhancement of Vas R. In the muscle bed, the fall in actual Vas R was similar in the two groups. However, when allowance is made for structural amplification, the reduction in Vas R was smaller in EH than in normotensives (24 vs. 35 units). From the dose-response curves in figure 5.6, this could signify increases in SNA or in plasma adrenaline in EH, or in both. In the absence of measuring the sympathoadrenal changes, this makes the result indeterminate. However, the strongest evidence favoring sensitization of the CNS pathways

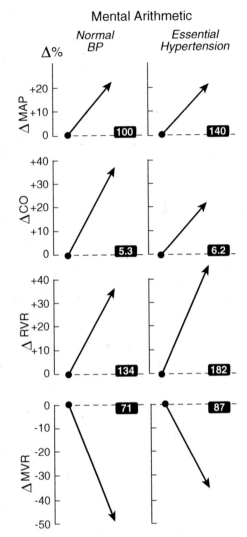

Figure 11.7. Changes in mean arterial pressure (ΔMAP), cardiac output (ΔCO), and renal and forearm muscle vascular resistances (ΔRVR, ΔMVR) during mental arithmetic for 15 minutes in 10 subjects with EH and 8 healthy normotensives. Responses given as percentage of resting in each group; numbers on baseline are actual resting values. Adapted from Brod et al. (1959).

in EH is that after stopping mental arithmetic, renal Vas R and heart rate remained raised for longer in EH (33 minutes) than in normotensives (10 minutes; cf. figure 2.10; Brod, 1963).

This is in accord with data from earlier chapters. For example, a word conflict test caused renal vasoconstriction in persons with EH but elicited little change in normotensives (figure 3.13). In another example, adrenaline secretion was superimposed on the Valsalva-induced TPR response in persons with EH but not in normotensives (figure 9.26).

Nevertheless, the sensitization of the defense pathway in EH appears to be considerably smaller than in *Aplysia* or in mammalian memory neurons. If true, this would

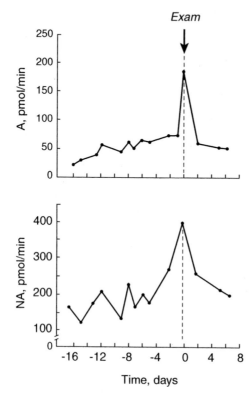

Figure 11.8. Urinary excretion of adrenaline (A, pmol/min) and noradrenaline (NA, pmol/min) before, during, and after a college examination. From Rosenzweig et al. (1996), based on Frankenhaeuser (1978), with permission of Sinauer Associates.

suggest somewhat different cellular mechanisms from those in figure 8.7. An alternative explanation is that the true synaptic changes are greater than suggested by the data in table 11.4, but that they are masked by inhibitory mechanisms. These could include baroreflexes and the great inhibitory system from the cortex surrounding the insula, which limits the magnitude of hypothalamic autonomic responses (chapter 8).

The latter explanation appears to be correct. In arterial hypoxia, strong stimulation of the arterial chemoreceptors excites hypothalamic defense neurons that elevate constrictor SNA, but the excitation is largely suppressed by forebrain inhibitory signals linked to lung inflation until respiration becomes compromised (chapter 14; Korner et al., 1968). Using this model, Somers et al. (1988) found that in response to moderate arterial hypoxia the increase in muscle sympathetic nerve activity (MSNA) in those with EH was two to three times that of normotensives (figure 11.9), while the rises in respiration, MAP, and heart rate were similar in both groups.[2] However, by superimposing voluntary apnea on hypoxia, the rise in MSNA in persons with EH became 13 times that of normotensives. The apnea disinhibits the hypothalamic neurons that are normally suppressed by respiration, thereby unmasking the hyperresponsiveness associated with EH.

In conclusion, there is evidence of considerable sensitization of the defense pathway in EH. However, the resulting hyperresponsiveness is normally partially inhibited by the great forebrain inhibitory system emanating from the insula and surrounding regions.

Table 11.4. Changes in Vascular Resistance (Vas R) Units in Renal and Muscle Beds during Mental Arithmetic Stress Test from Brod's Data in Figure 11.7

	NORMOTENSIVE	EH
Resting MAP, mmHg	100	140
Resting renal Vas R, units	134	182
Test renal Vas R, units	182	263
Δ (Test-rest) adjust by 1/1.35	48	81
		60
Sympathetic component in EH		(60 − 48) = 12
Resting muscle Vas R, units	71	87
Test muscle Vas R, units	36	55
Δ (Test-rest), units adjust by 1/1.35	−35	−32
		−24
Sympathetic component in EH		(−24 + 35) = 12

Note: The greater rise in renal Vas R in persons with EH than in normotensives is due to (1) a greater rise in SNA, and (2) a 1.35-fold enhancement by the structural vascular amplifier.

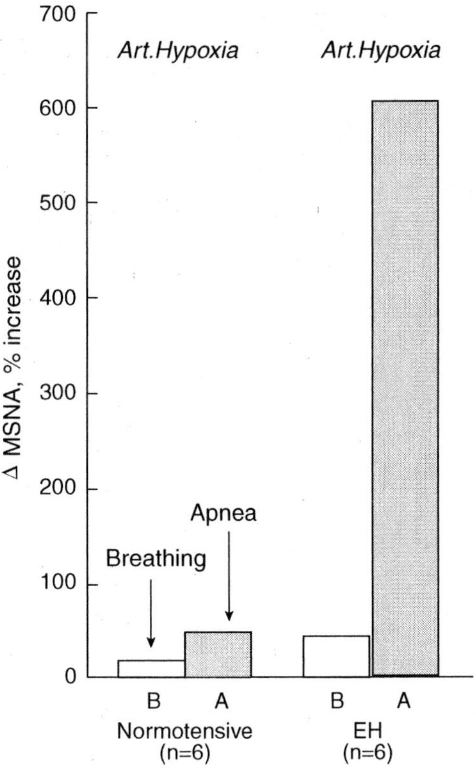

Figure 11.9. Increases in muscle SNA (ΔMSNA, % of resting) in 6 normotensives and 6 persons with mild EH during isocapnic arterial hypoxia while hyperventilating (open bars) and when voluntary apnea was superimposed (shaded bars). From Somers et al. (1988), with permission of *Hypertension*, American Heart Association, and Lippincott, Williams and Wilkins.

This may be the reason for the slow development of EH when compared to the rate of development of mammalian memory associated with learning.

Amygdala and the Expression of Emotions

Emotions and feelings evoked by stress can be regarded as distinctive CNS outputs, similar to those mediated through the ANS. In his famous book *The Expression of the Emotions in Man and Animals*, Charles Darwin (1872) suggested that animals could express emotions just like humans, which ran counter to what was widely believed at the time. Darwin thought that the associated facial expressions communicated information of survival value to other animals. According to Ekman (1998), similar emotional and facial responses are found from a young age in all human societies and cultures.

Plutchik (1994) has classified emotions into contrasting pairs, including joy and sadness, acceptance and disgust, anger and fear, and excitation and relaxation. Rage, grief, amazement, vigilance, apprehension, and ecstasy are regarded as mixtures of the above (Rosenzweig et al., 1996). The type of emotion may be obvious from the subject's demeanor, but often emotions are private and subjective (Mandler, 1987; Damasio, 1994; Rosenzweig et al., 1996; Glynn, 1999). In addition to the emotions that are evoked in response to a stimulus or situation, there is always a level of background feeling even in the absence of categorical emotions.

The perception of emotions still challenges behavioral neuroscientists. Some 100 years ago, William James and Carl Lange thought that they were inseparable from the accompanying autonomic activity and skeletal muscle movements. The James-Lange theory of emotions was criticized by Cannon (1915), who thought that the brain could generate emotions independently of these motor accompaniments. He argued that quadriplegic subjects experience emotions in the absence of normal effector responses. However, their facial expressions are often associated with emotions, which is in accord with the James-Lange theory. Later, Schachter suggested that the brain interprets feelings and emotions in the context of environmental and internal events (Schachter and Singer, 1962; Schachter, 1971).

Damasio (1994, 1997) has emphasized that psychosocial interactions and many decisions are distorted in the absence of normally expressed emotions. From a discussion of the role of the amygdala considered below, emotions are probably best regarded as a separate neural output, which is generated through its own cortical and subcortical neuronal network. As mentioned in chapter 3, patients with Down syndrome are virtually EH-proof because they tend to underestimate stress intensity, while persons with EH tend to interpret stress in the opposite way, which plays a role in the enhanced autonomic changes.

Role of the Amygdala

The amygdala plays a crucial role for the expression of emotional responses (LeDoux, 1994; Glynn, 1999). It has several nuclei that receive input from the thalamus, sensory and prefrontal cortex, and from the hippocampus (figure 11.10; Turner et al., 1980; Smith and DeVito, 1984).

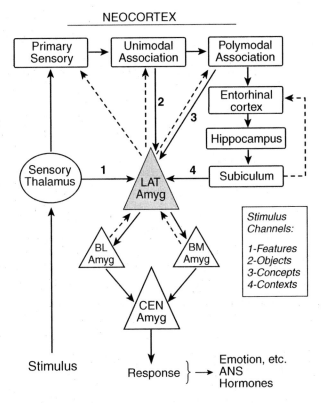

Figure 11.10. Amygdala pathways for fear conditioning. The lateral nucleus (LAT Amyg) receives input from thalamus (1), neocortex (2), including higher order association areas (3), and hippocampal formation (4). In the amygdala, the lateral nucleus is connected to the central nucleus (CEN Amyg) via basolateral and basomedial nuclei (BL Amyg, BM Amyg). When CS is a simple cue, fear conditioning is through either pathways 1 or 2; when conditioning depends on discrimination between related stimuli, the cortical pathway is essential. Pathway 3 is from the medial prefrontal cortex; pathway 4 provides information about particular places. The output from central nucleus contributes to the emotional responses. From LeDoux (1994), with permission of MIT Press.

The amygdala's role was elegantly demonstrated in a "split-brain" experiment in which the right and left hemispheres are separated by sectioning the corpus callosum and optic chiasma (Sperry, 1968). After the operation, visual information to each amygdala comes from the eye on the same side. Downer (1961) used the split-brain preparation in a monkey with only one functioning amygdala. This monkey became wild and aggressive when the experimenter approached the cage, but if the eye projecting to the functioning amygdala was covered, the animal was tame and ate raisins from the experimenter's hand, but reverted to its wild behavior when the cover was removed.

LeDoux (1994) studied the neural mechanisms associated with the conditioned fear response in rats. The animals had been trained to associate an auditory signal with a mild electric shock applied soon afterward through the wire floor of the cage. At the first trial the shock made the rat jump. Once the rat learned the association between sound and shock, it responded to the sound with immobility (freezing) and a rise in BP. The sound is the conditioned stimulus (CS), while the shock is the unconditioned stimulus (UCS). The UCS always elicits a response, even in a naive rat. In contrast, normally no response is evoked by the CS until the animal has learned to associate it with the UCS. This is known as associative learning or classical Pavlovian conditioning.

Any sensory signal can be paired in this way. As LeDoux (1994) stated, "The stimuli that normally activate the hard-wired responses are those that have acquired meaning through evolutionary rather than through individual learning. . . . Conditioning opens up this channel . . . to new environmental events" (p. 1050).

The pathway activated by the sound goes from the auditory and prefrontal cortex to the lateral amygdaloid nucleus. The amygdala receives topographical input from the hippocampus about the rat's location in the cage when it receives the shock. The lateral nucleus projects to the central amygdaloid nucleus, which provides input to the hypothalamus for stress-induced renal vasoconstriction (Koepke et al., 1987). The sound-induced freezing behavior and rise in BP are, surprisingly, not affected by ablation of the auditory cortex. This is because the amygdala also receives a direct auditory input from the medial geniculate body in the thalamus, in addition to that received through the auditory cortex (figure 11.10).

This does not mean that the auditory cortex is redundant. Its role in the conditioned response was investigated by Jarrell et al. (1987), who trained intact rabbits to respond to two auditory tones of widely different pitch. One tone was always followed by the shock and elicited immobility and bradycardia, while the other tone never provoked a shock, so that there was no accompanying response. After ablation of the auditory cortex, both tones evoked bradycardia. Thus, the brain responded indiscriminately to sound when only the thalamic input was operational. The cortical discrimination in the intact animal ensures that appropriate behavioral and circulatory responses occur only in response to the sound stimulus specifically associated with the shock.

Emotions and Personality Factors in the Context of the Defense Response

The emotion evoked by stress is assumed to be mediated through an independent pathway, although it is influenced by accompanying neuroendocrine and motor changes. For example, increased secretion of androgens enhances aggressive behavior.

Do emotions and attitudes in persons with EH differ from those expressed by normotensive subjects? A large number of studies performed over the last 30–40 years have shown that, compared to normotensives, persons with EH tend to be more assertive, have higher levels of anxiety and defensiveness, show more repressed anger and feelings of depression, and have a greater capacity for self-deception (Brodman et al., 1949; Edwards, 1959; Cattell and Schreier, 1967; Hambling, 1951; Kalis et al., 1961; Torgersen and Kringlen, 1971; Shapiro, 1972; Pilowsky et al., 1973;

Markovitz et al., 1991; Pickering, 1994; Everson et al., 2000; Rutledge and Linden, 2000; Räikkönen et al., 2001; Ohira et al., 2002). In hypertensive women, there is a strong association between depressive symptoms and BP: Changes from low to high depressive symptoms over a 10-year period were associated with an SBP difference of about 10 mmHg and a DBP difference of about 3 mmHg (Räikkönen et al., 2001).

Conditioned Stimuli Can Elicit Defense Response

Smith and colleagues trained young baboons to recognize the association between various tasks to be performed and particular visual and auditory cues, which had no cardiovascular effects prior to training (Smith et al., 1979; Smith, Astley, DeVito et al., 1980; Smith, Astley, Hohimer et al., 1980; Smith and DeVito, 1984). The learning process was accelerated by giving the animal a small food reward (e.g., a drop of fruit juice) when the task was performed correctly.

Once trained, the animal performed leg exercise on a stationary bicycle as long as a particular light was on, or pressed a lever in response to another light. The monkey had also learned to associate a particular sound (CS) with a painful electric shock (UCS), which was delivered 60 seconds after the tone. On a typical day, the appropriate light set the monkey exercising, but when the sound CS came on the animal stopped and ignored the light, responding instead with the defense pattern well ahead of the UCS (figure 11.11).

After lesioning the hypothalamic area from which the defense pattern had been evoked and following recovery from the operation, it was no longer possible to evoke the defense response with either the CS or UCS (figure 11.11; Smith, Astley, DeVito et al., 1980; Smith and DeVito, 1984). However, the normal cardiovascular response to exercise was largely retained, which suggests that the variant defense responses are generated through somewhat different hypothalamic neuron populations.

The cerebellum also plays a role in the Pavlovian conditioning of somatic motor reflexes, such as the rabbit eyeblink reflex. The animal learns to recognize the association between an auditory CS and a puff of air on the cornea (UCS), until the CS alone eventually evokes the reflex (Thompson, 1990; Bartha and Thompson, 1995; Rosenzweig et al., 1996). The elements of the cerebellar circuitry involved have been well defined, with the sound input acting through the mossy fibers and projecting to the same Purkinje neurons as the UCS, which excites the corresponding climbing fibers. Blowing air on the face also evokes the defense response (DiBona, 1989; Burke, Malpas, and Head, 1998). Hence, it is probable that the cerebellum plays a role in the learning process that associates the sound CS with the UCS, which occurs in conjunction with memory neurons in the hippocampus and sensory cortex, all of which play important roles in Pavlovian conditioning (Thompson, 1990; Rosenzweig et al., 1996).

Pavlovian conditioning also plays a role in extending the number of neutral stimuli that help recall a stressful situation. They also give rise to the corresponding autonomic responses and play a role in the development of EH.

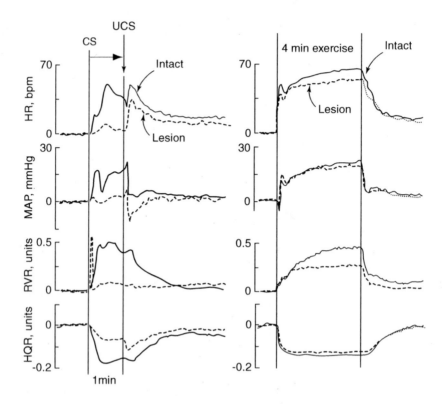

Figure 11.11. Left, effects of conditioned sound stimulus (CS) and unconditioned stimulus (UCS, painful electric shock given 1 minute later) in awake baboons. Solid lines, average changes from control; variables: heart rate (HR, bpm), mean arterial pressure (MAP, mmHg), renal and hindquarter vascular resistance (RVR, HQR, units). CS evokes responses long before UCS. Dashed lines show effects after electrolytic lesions of hypothalamic defense area, which largely abolished responses. Right, responses to leg exercise when monkey was prompted by a visual cue. Note similarity to defense pattern, but response only slightly affected by lesion. Adapted from Smith, Astley, DeVito et al. (1980) and Smith and DeVito (1984).

Role of Slow Transmitter Neurons

The outcome of the sensory analysis by the thalamus and cortex and memory circuits, integrated over time, is conveyed to the hypothalamus and amygdala by excitatory or inhibitory slow transmitter interneurons (figure 11.12). The excitatory interneurons probably include DA neurons and 5-HT neurons, with the latter evoking the defense response both indirectly (figure 8.19) and through direct effects on 5-HT receptors located on DMHN and PVN neurons (Horiuchi et al., 2005).

DA neurons enhance cortical arousal by regulating the sensory input from thalamus to cortex (figure 11.13; Carlsson et al., 1997; Carlsson, 2001). However, their main action in EH and in SHR hypertension is probably through DA receptors on hypothalamic and PAG neurons through the connections between prefrontal cortex,

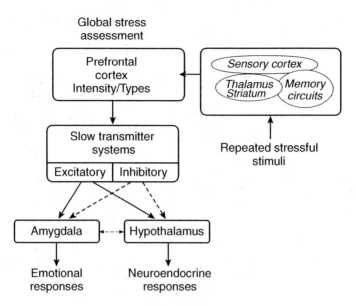

Figure 11.12. Stressful stimuli are processed by thalamus, sensory cortex, and memory circuits, and prefrontal cortex perceives this as stress intensity integrated over a period of days or weeks. Either excitatory or inhibitory slow transmitter neurons may be activated, with different effects on target neurons.

midbrain DA neurons, and hypothalamus (figure 11.12; Le Moal and Simon, 1991). In addition, DA neuron activity is enhanced in expectation of a reward. Normally, in monkeys DA neurons discharge at a slow steady rate that increases briefly if the animal receives an unexpected drop of fruit juice (Schultz, 1992). Subsequently, once the animal has learned the association between a number of visual cues and the chances of receiving a reward, they develop characteristic firing patterns (Fiorillo et al., 2003). When a cue tells the animal that a reward will always be forthcoming, this elicits a short burst of DA neuron activity. On the other hand, the neurons stay silent

Figure 11.13. Schema suggesting that dopaminergic neurons regulate sensory input from thalamus to cortex by disinhibiting the normal inhibitory action of the striatum on the thalamus, increasing the level of arousal, which is mediated through glutamate. From Carlsson (1988, 2001), with permission of Native Publishing Group and American Association for the Advancement of Science.

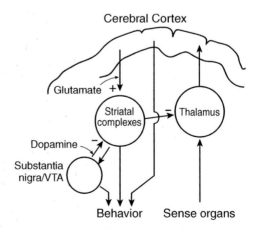

when another cue indicates that there will be no reward. Disparate cues that leave uncertain whether or not there will be a reward evoke a short burst of neuron activity followed by a steady rise in discharge at a rate related to the likelihood of receiving a reward. In recent years, it has become clear that the most powerful learning occurs in relation to uncertain reward schedules. In relation to the defense response, uncertainty reduces the threshold for eliciting the effector responses to a given stressor.

Stress-Related Stimulus-Response Relationships

The responses to stress depend on its nature and intensity. This raises two questions: (1) Why do diverse stressors evoke similar neuroendocrine responses? and (2) How does the brain gauge intensity of stress?

The brain can discriminate between different types of stress. However, since many stressors give rise to similar autonomic, hormonal, and emotional responses, it is likely that the incoming information is simplified. As a first approximation, the perceived stress intensity appears to be closely related to the subject's neurohumoral responses.

Thus, stress is subjective, where a stimulus that is mildly stressful to subject A may be very stressful to subject B. As Mandler (1987, p. 219) states, "when riding on a roller-coaster, whether the ride seems joyful or dreadful depends on the company, past experience and whether we feel secure or in imminent danger." Even when a person feels that the challenge can be met, there usually remains uncertainty about whether the proposed plan of action will be effective. However, when the stress intensity appears excessive, the subject will expect almost certain defeat.

A scale based on subjective assessment of stress intensity is similar to the use of normalizing the work rate during exercise in terms of the subject's W_{max} (chapter 10). The subjective nature of stress was recognized by George Orwell in the novel *1984*, where the interrogator of the totalitarian regime subjects each political dissident to the individual's own personalized nightmare, that is, the most stressful experience for that particular subject.

Figure 11.14 relates five categories of subjective perception of stress intensity to changes in SNA, plasma adrenaline, glucocorticoids, and BP responses. In terms of the differences in psychological makeup between normotensives and hypertensives, an intensity regarded by the former as mild (intensity 1) may be regarded by those with EH as moderate (intensity 2 or 3), with corresponding differences in their effector responses.

The stress-intensity SNA, BP, and mood relationships are nonlinear with marked reduction from their maxima as stress becomes very high (intensity 5). The threshold for rises in plasma adrenaline is somewhat greater than for SNA. It accords with other findings that SNA and adrenaline secretion are regulated independently (Uther et al., 1970; Dodt et al., 1997). Plasma glucocorticoids increase gradually in response to mild to moderate stress intensities, but even these relatively small changes are important because they reduce NO synthesis. However, when stress intensity becomes very high glucocorticoid secretion increases dramatically. This mobilizes metabolic resources for immediate use while at the same time depressing the immune system (McEwen, 1994, 1998). They may also play a role in depressing SNA (Dodt et al., 2000).

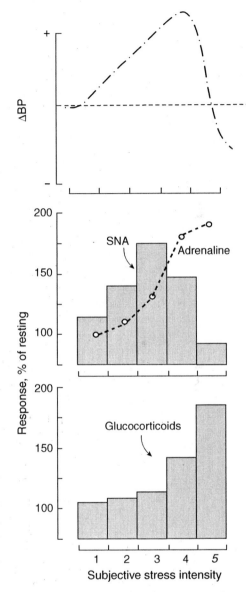

Figure 11.14. Relationship between subjective stress intensity and (1) changes in BP from baseline (+, −); (2) sympathetic neural activity (SNA) and plasma adrenaline; and (3) plasma glucocorticoid concentration, all as percentage of baseline. Stress intensity: 1, mild; 2, moderate; 3, moderately severe; 4, severe; 5, very severe.

Panic attacks are an example of severe stress, fortunately mostly of brief duration, which leave the subject weak and exhausted: Plasma adrenaline is markedly raised while SNA is often normal, suggesting regulation through different mechanisms (Wilkinson et al., 1998).

It follows that only stress intensities associated with elevation of SNA are of relevance in the initiation of EH. This accords with Walter Cannon's views about the role of the sympathetic nervous system in emergencies. The subject's positive mood changes at moderately severe intensities of stress, when despite a lot of effort to meet the challenge, the outcome becomes increasingly uncertain. When stress intensity is very severe, the organism may suffer pathological injury. Such very high stress intensities were used by Hans Selye in his experimental work on stress. They define the limits of an organism's adaptive capacity, but have little relevance to the pathogenesis of EH.

Cardiovascular Effects of Chronic Stress in Animals

In some of the early studies on psychosocial interactions in rodent populations, the stress resulted from territorial and sexual rivalries between males. In other studies using aversive conditioning paradigms, the stress arose from the animal's capacity to meet challenges over which it had little control.

Life in the Rodent Wild West

James Henry's pioneering work on BP in mouse populations straddled the boundaries of psychology and physiology (Henry et al., 1967, 1971, 1972; Henry and Cassel, 1969). A laboratory village consisted of about 30–40 male and female mice of a particular strain, which were housed in boxes that were accessed through a limited number of narrow passages. Social interactions were obligatory to access the food and water supply.

The mice took up residence when they were 4 months old, having lived in isolation in small cages from the time of weaning. As a result, their social skills were minimal, making them ill prepared for communal life. There was much fighting in some of the strains, which gave rise to hypertension, while in other strains there was little aggressive behavior and little change in BP.

In the aggressive CBA strain, fighting was considerable, with frequent evidence of fresh tail bites in most animals. The average rise in SBP was ~30 mmHg above the level of control rats living in isolation cages and was due to increased sympathoadrenal activity; the BP changes in males were about double those in females (figure 11.15, top; Henry et al., 1971). On returning to isolation cages after 6 months of communal life, there was some decline in SBP over 2–3 months, but at the end of that time it was still above that of controls.

The fighting and hypertension are a consequence of the sexually driven aggressive behavior of the males. Both were greatly reduced in another group of young males, which had been castrated while still in isolation. However, fighting broke out again and BP rose when these mice received daily injections of methyl testosterone (Henry and Cassel, 1969).

Other mice of the same strain were placed in the population cages from the time of weaning and acquired better social skills. As a result, the fighting was less intense, and the rise in SBP in males was about half that observed in socially naive mice (figure 11.15, bottom). The female mice remained normotensive and gave birth to a greater number of surviving pups.

Some mouse strains are intrinsically docile, and their interaction with other mice was accompanied by little aggressive behavior. When placed into population cages, their BPs remained close to those of controls.

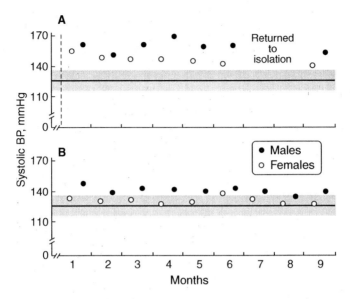

Figure 11.15. Top, average systolic BPs of 17 male and 17 female CBA mice, which had lived in isolation until 4 months of age, then spent 6 months in population cage before again being isolated (black circles, males; open circles, females). Solid line and shading (mean SBP ± 1 SD): data from control mice living in isolation cages from weaning over entire period. Dashed vertical line: start of communal life. Bottom, when the males and females lived together from weaning, their social skills improved, resulting in about half the rise in BP. Adapted from Henry et al. (1972).

Studies in Rats

Harrap et al. (1984) tried to confirm the above observations in rats, using a similar experimental design. After 3 months of social isolation following weaning, 30–40 male and female rats lived for 8 weeks in similar population cages. Controls included (1) socially isolated rats; and 2) 4–5 rats of the same sex housed in a standard cage, in which BPs and plasma NA were lower than in (1). The three strains examined included WKY, Sprague-Dawley, and borderline hypertensive rats (BHR; F_1 hybrids from female WKY × male SHR crosses, see chapter 3).

None of the above strains developed hypertension. Fighting and injuries were common and were most marked in BHR, which developed cardiac hypertrophy and elevation of plasma NA, while plasma corticosterone was significantly depressed.

Social Instability in Smaller Populations

Henry was surprised by the absence of hypertension and in his subsequent work on rats adapted a design devised by the French behavioral physiologist Mormède (Mormède et al., 1990; Mormède, 1997).[3] The animals were housed in smaller population cages holding only 8–10 rats of both sexes. The stress arose from frequently changing group membership (Henry et al., 1993). This was done in so-called unstable populations, in which one male rat was moved to another cage every few days and replaced by another male. In stable populations, there were no changes of rats throughout the study period. As an additional control, pairs of males and females of the same strain were housed in a single small cage.

BPs were measured in the males of three strains: (1) the WKHA rat, which is hyperactive but friendly (Hendley and Ohlsson, 1991); (2) the Sprague-Dawley rat, which is moderately peaceful; and (3) the Long-Evans rat, which is very aggressive. It is tempting to make the human analogies where (1) is extroverted and social, (2) is quiet and somewhat introverted, and (3) is aggressive and possessive.

In WKHA rats, the SBP remained the same as in the stable and unstable populations and in paired controls (figure 11.16). In Sprague-Dawley rats, the SBP increased by 10 mmHg in the unstable group but remained the same in the stable colonies as in paired controls. The largest BP rise of 20 mmHg was observed in the unstable Long-Evans rats, in which the fierce fighting between some of the animals resulted

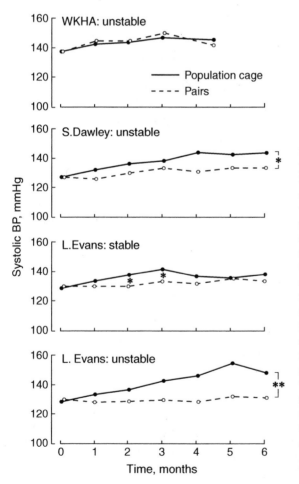

Figure 11.16. Mean SBPs of male rats living in small population cages holding 8–10 rats of both sexes (black circles, solid lines); controls were male-female pairs living in small cages. In the stable colonies, membership did not change over 6 months. In unstable colonies, a male was often exchanged with a male from another cage. WKHA rats are hyperactive but do not fight; Sprague-Dawley rats compete and scratch but do not bite; Long-Evans rats are aggressive and bite readily. $*p < .01$, $**p < .001$, for significant difference from controls. After Henry et al. (1993), with permission of *Hypertension*, American Heart Association, and Lippincott, Williams and Wilkins.

in several deaths. In the stable Long-Evans populations, there was only a small rise in BP during the first few months, which had subsided toward the end of the study (figure 11.16).

Significance of Studies on Territorial and Sexual Conflict

The responses to the territorial and sexual rivalries between males are manifestations of some of the most basic instincts related to species survival. The different strains varied in their aggressive behavior, probably due to genetic factors. However, the average BP responses of a given strain often mask the variation in responses within the population, which requires looking at the outcomes of the fights between individual animals.

Individual Variation within a Given Strain

Each fight has a winner and a loser. In some strains, the group dynamics remain stable once the identity of the dominant and subordinate animals has been established. In others in which the males are evenly matched in strength and aggression, it may be more difficult to categorize the population.

During sporadic fights, the BP rise in the winner tends to be less than in the loser, as in figure 11.17 (Henry et al, 1995; Fokkema, 1985; Fokkema and Koolhaas, 1985).[4] Remarkably, in a second contrived laboratory confrontation arranged several weeks later, the identical BP responses were elicited in each rat. On this occasion, a small cage containing rat A was placed next to another cage containing rat B. The animals could only see and smell their rival without being able to fight but repeated their earlier responses. This is a clear illustration of a learned response, where stress

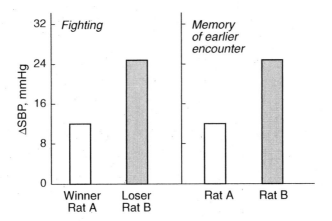

Figure 11.17. Left, changes in SBP of two rats after a short fight, in which the BP of the loser rose more than that of the winner. Right, the responses of the same two rats some weeks later were identical, when they recognized each other from their cages without being able to fight by, presumably, recalling the previous encounter. From Henry et al. (1995), after Fokkema and Koolhaas (1985), with permission of Raven Press, and Lippincott, Williams and Wilkins.

is experienced in the absence of behavioral conflict by recalling the event of the previous encounter.

In some losers there is little change in BP, but in others there is complete submission when confronted by a fierce antagonist, which is accompanied by a fall in SBP of 20–40 mmHg and a reduction in SNA (Adams and Blizard, 1987). It resembles events during the transition from the nonhypotensive to the hypotensive phases of hemorrhage (chapter 9). Perhaps forebrain mechanisms activate inhibitory slow transmitter neurons after complete defeat or submission, as suggested in figure 11.12.

Interpreting the Population Studies

The large variation in behavioral and BP responses after frequent violent fights suggests corresponding differences in the rat's perception of stress. One may conjecture that on the stress intensity-response curve of figure 11.14, the stresses seemed mild to the winners and extreme to the routed losers. In large colonies, the presence of many rivals creates uncertainties of life as in the lawless Wild West, and it is probably this middle group of subdominants that contributed to the greatest rises in BP. In the smaller population cages even the aggressive strains experienced less stress than in the larger population cages, even when BP increased.

Territorial and Sexual Stress: Role of Sex Chromosomes

Ely and colleagues (1997a, 1997b) used population cages housing 8 male and 8 female rats and measured their individual ambulatory BPs by telemetry at night when the rats were active. The strains examined were WKY, SHR, and two SHR-derived congenic strains: (1) SHR/y, which have the Y chromosome of SHR and the X chromosome and autosomes of WKY; (2) SHR/a, which have autosomes and the X chromosome of SHR and the Y chromosome of WKY. The males of each strain were classified into dominants and subordinates.

In all the SHR-derived strains, the SBP of the dominants was 15–25 mmHg higher than in the subordinates, with the higher BPs related to higher plasma NA levels (figure 11.18; table 11.5). In contrast, in WKY the dominants and submissives had similar SBP and NA levels and were below the corresponding groups of SHR.[5] Plasma corticosterone levels were greater in the subordinates of every strain.

Ely et al. also examined the responses to acute stress in the various groups, by placing an intruder from another strain in the cage for 1 hour. The largest BP rises occurred in the dominant SHR and SHR/y, while in their subordinates the BP rises were smaller than in the other two strains (figure 11.18). It suggests that the subordinates left the defense of the community to the dominants. In SHR/a and WKY, there was little difference in the BP responses between dominants and subordinates.

Comment

In the large mouse communities of aggressive strains, the rapid rises in average BP suggest that the male population consists of a significant proportion of fairly evenly matched rivals. The absence of a BP rise in the large BHR communities suggests greater variation in BP responses to the frequent violent fights between rats, with many

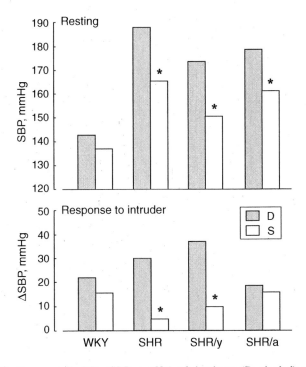

Figure 11.18. Top, systolic BPs (SBP, mmHg) of dominant (D, shaded) and subordinate (S, clear) rats of WKY, SHR, SHR/y, and SHR/a strains during normal nocturnal activity. Rats of a given strain lived in population cages holding eight animals. Bottom, peak changes in SBP during stress generated by placing an intruder from a different strain in cage for 1 hour. *$p < .01$ for significance of difference between dominant and subordinate rats of a given strain. Redrawn from Ely et al. (1997a).

of the animals showing rises and falls in BP. Both models simulate what happens in human populations, but only provide general clues about underlying mechanisms. The lesser range of stress intensities in the smaller populations reduce the likelihood that the animals will be overwhelmed by the stress. Indeed, in Ely's stable group of SHR, there appears to be a sense of cohesion in the animals' responses to an intruder.

Mental Challenges through Aversive Conditioning

Stress arising from territorial and sexual rivalry was overt in prehistoric times, but in modern societies it is less obvious and has become supplanted by mental stress (Charvat et al., 1964). Aversive operant conditioning attempts to simulate mental stress in animals. The stimulus is usually a mild electric shock, which the animal learns to avoid, reduce, or delay. Failure to do so adequately leads to punishment such as an additional electric shock, or to the withholding of an expected reward such as a food pellet or drop of fruit juice. The stress arises from fear of the shock or from the frustration about not receiving a reward; it is further enhanced by random uncertainties, which are features of many of the protocols.

Table 11.5. Mean Plasma Noradrenaline and Corticosterone Concentrations in Dominant and Subordinate Rats Belonging to SHR, SHR/y, SHR/a, and WKY Strains

Strain	Dominant	Subordinate	p
Plasma Noradrenaline (ng/ml)			
SHR	420	260	*
SHR/y	205	175	*
SHR/a	210	150	*
WKY	200	185	ns
Plasma Corticosterone (ng/ml)			
SHR	145	190	*
SHR/y	180	225	*
SHR/a	155	255	*
WKY	105	260	*

Note: SHR/a strain has Y chromosome of WKY and SHR's X chromosome and autosomes; SHR/y strain has Y chromosome of SHR and WKY's X chromosome and autosomes.
*$p \leq .05$ for significance of difference.

Source: Adapted from Ely et al. (1997a, 1997b).

In Sidman's avoidance conditioning, the animal first learns to associate a sound or light CS with an aversive UCS. It then has to respond to the CS in a particular way to avoid or delay the UCS. Sessions of several hours each day are repeated on most days of the week over a period of months. This results in gradual rises in BP of 20–30 mmHg in monkeys, with BP remaining raised between sessions (Forsyth, 1968; Herd et al., 1969; Henry et al., 1995). After the sessions are discontinued, BP returns to the starting value, except in a small proportion of animals in which hypertension persists.

Other protocols increase uncertainty. In the avoidance-avoidance paradigm, the rat receives a certain number of shocks if it fails to respond in time, but it also receives undeserved shocks when the answer is correct (Friedman and Dahl, 1975). Lawler et al. (1981) used this stress paradigm in normotensive BHR (figure 11.19). Baseline measurements were followed by a training period of 2 weeks consisting of sessions of 2 hours duration on 5 days per week: Each experimental rat (E-BHR) was placed in a special cage where it had to turn a wheel in response to a 1 kHz tone. One-quarter turn of the wheel delayed the next tone (and associated shock) by 10 seconds. If this was not done in time, the rat received five brief low-current electric shocks to the tail. This period was followed by 14 weeks of greater conflict. As before, the E-BHR rat received five shocks for failing to turn the wheel in time but also a single additional shock if the response was correct, increasing uncertainty. There were two control groups: (1) C_r rats for assessing the effect on BP of being placed in the test cage and hearing the tone without having to respond or receiving a shock; and (2) C_t rats, which remained in their holding cage and served as controls for time-related events.

During the conflict period, the BP increased gradually in E-BHR to an SBP ~40 mmHg above that of the time controls (figure 11.19). This developed despite improvement in the number of correct responses. The many tasks to be performed and the frequent extra shocks never gave the rat an opportunity to win.

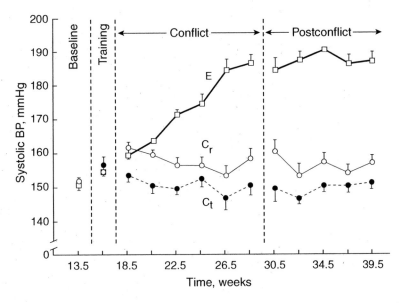

Figure 11.19. Mean systolic BP (mmHg) in BHR during baseline period, during training where they learned to respond to conditioned stimuli, conflict period of operant conditioning, and postconflict recovery period when test sessions had ceased. E, experimental rats (open squares, thick lines); C_r, controls for mild restraint and sound (open circles, fine lines); C_t, time controls (closed circles, dashed lines). Further discussion in text. From Lawler et al. (1981), with permission of *Hypertension*, American Heart Association, and Lippincott, Williams and Wilkins.

Most remarkably, after the sessions stopped the rats' BP remained high during the 9 weeks of observation following the end of the conditioning sessions. It suggests that during the conflict period there had been gradual synaptic strengthening along the pathway mediating the defense response.

In a second study, the findings in BHR were essentially similar (Lawler et al., 1984). In this study, the same conditioning protocol was applied to WKY. In the experimental rats, the rise in SBP during the training conflict and postconflict periods was about ~10 mmHg. It was similar to the rise observed in the C_r controls in the first series of BHR (figure 11.19), which had been subjected to the mild stress of being moved to another cage and listening to the CS. Thus, the threshold for eliciting the defense response is much greater in WKY than in BHR. Similar differences have been observed in conditioning experiments in SHR and WKY (Li et al., 1997).

In summary, the stress arising from avoidance-avoidance conditioning gives rise to persistent elevation in BP in BHR, suggesting sensitization of the defense pathway. In WKY the response is much smaller and conditioning does not cause sensitization.

Psychosocial and Mental Stress in Humans

Some types of chronic stress raise BP in virtually everyone, provided the stress is of sufficient intensity. What distinguishes persons developing EH from normotensives is that their defense pathway becomes sensitized, so that, in time, BP responds to stimulus intensities that have no effect in normal persons. This section briefly refers to examples where stress produces long-term changes in BP in everyone and other instances where only those susceptible to EH are affected, as discussed in chapter 4. The main part of this section considers the role of occupational stress in EH and that of socioeconomic factors and social support.

Chronic Stress and Sustained Elevation of BP

Recall three examples from chapter 4 in which exposure to fairly intense stress raised BP in virtually all members of the group. They included (1) soldiers engaged in a tank battle in North Africa (Graham, 1945); (2) prisoners moved into more crowded sleeping quarters (D'Atri and Ostfeld, 1975; D'Atri et al., 1981); and (3) Antarctic expedition members during enforced confinement indoors during the winter (Jennings et al., 1989; chapters 4 and 10). In these groups, the average rise in SBP ranged from 10 to 25 mmHg, with BP returning to normal when the stress was over.

Chronic stress has also been well recognized as a cause of elevation of BP in various migration studies in conjunction with dietary factors and obesity. The rise in BP is variable and only a proportion develop EH.

In the 30-year case control study of Timio et al. (1997) stress was identified as the main (if not the sole) factor responsible for the greater age-related rise in BP in laywomen compared to nuns (figure 4.13). Not all laywomen developed EH, and the slope of the age-BP relationship suggests that the proportion was similar to the average for women in Italy, that is, about 20% over the time of the study. Clearly, in this population EH develops in response to ordinary day-to-day stresses. It raises the question of what protects the nuns from similar stresses. Factors such as the well-ordered secure lifestyle and availability of social support may reduce their perception of stress intensity. In that case, the defense pathways may not become sensitized, so that BP rises only phasically during episodes of stress. Alternatively, because of their better lifestyle, sensitization of the defense pathway may be less pronounced, with the resulting rise in BP suppressed by the forebrain inhibitory systems and baroreflexes, as discussed earlier.

Recall that patients with Down syndrome were virtually EH-proof, with BPs significantly below those of various reference populations (figure 4.10). Their cognitive impairment may be a factor in their lower capacity to perceive stress (Morrison et al., 1996).

Occupational Stress and Raised BP

Two psychological models for quantifying stress are shown in figure 11.20. One model is due to Karasek and has proved useful in assessing cardiovascular risk in relation to occupational stress (Karasek et al., 1981, 1988). Persons in a highly demanding job, who have little control on how the tasks are to be done, are said to experience high job strain, exposing them to greater risk of developing myocardial infarction and other cardiovascular complications than persons free to decide how to perform the particular task.

The model at the bottom of figure 11.20 is the effort-distress model of Frankenhaeuser (1983), which examines (1) whether the mental effort to meet a particular challenge is high or low, and (2) whether the performance of the task gives

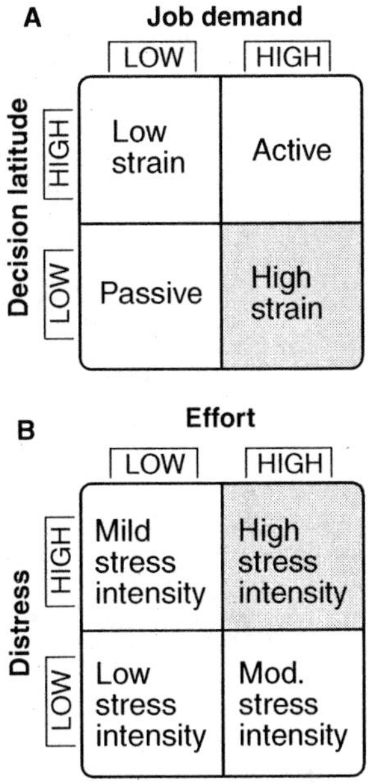

A   **Job demand**

	LOW	HIGH
HIGH (Decision latitude)	Low strain	Active
LOW	Passive	High strain

B   **Effort**

	LOW	HIGH
HIGH (Distress)	Mild stress intensity	High stress intensity
LOW	Low stress intensity	Mod. stress intensity

Figure 11.20. Diagram showing the four outcomes in the psychological demand-decision latitude model of Karasek for assessing occupational stress (A) and the more general effort-distress model of Frankenhaeuser (B). Adapted from Pickering (1994), with permission of Blackwell.

rise to a feeling of distress. If the challenge is great and the task causes distress, the level of stress is considered to be high and is associated with raised plasma cortisol and adrenaline but little change in SNA (Lundberg and Frankenhaeuser, 1980). On the other hand, if the effort is great but the subject feels able to cope, SNA is raised and hormone levels are normal, as in the rivals in animal populations (Lovallo et al., 1990). Thus the perception of stress intensity is related to the person's neural and hormonal responses, as in figure 11.14.

Decision latitude and *job demand* are not exactly equivalent to *distress* and *effort* in the two models. In the Karasek model, the range of stress is probably smaller, with the maximum perceived stress intensity corresponding to or just beyond the peak SNA response in figure 11.14.

The average SNA of those experiencing high job strain is usually raised, as assessed by urinary NA excretion (Pickering, 1994; Pickering et al., 1996). In a case control study of men recruited from businesses in New York, three times as many people with EH had high-strain jobs compared to normotensives (Schnall et al., 1990).[6] This led to another study in which about 20% of all subjects were in high-strain jobs, and their ambulatory SBPs and DBPs were significantly greater than in those in the other occupational categories (table 11.6; Schnall et al., 1992). Their BP remained higher during their activities at home and also while asleep.

The ambulatory BP of those with high-strain jobs increased with age, which was not the case in the other occupational categories. Moreover, regular high alcohol consumption by those with high-strain jobs further accentuated the age-related rise in BP. In contrast, high alcohol use was without effect on the BP of those experiencing less job strain (Schnall et al., 1992).

Table 11.6. Ambulatory Systolic and Diastolic BPs (SBP, DBP) in Four Occupational Groups Classified According to Job Demand and Decision Latitude (See Figure 11.20)

	Job Demand	
Scores	Low ($<$32)	High ($\geq$32)
Decision latitude		
High ($>$37)	Low strain SBP = 129 mmHg DBP = 83 mmHg ($n = 56$)	Active SBP = 132 mmHg DBP = 83 mmHg ($n = 60$)
Low ($\leq$37)	Passive SBP = 129 mmHg DBP = 82 mmHg ($n = 93$)	High strain SBP = 137 mmHg DBP = 85 mmHg ($n = 55$)*

*$p < 0.05$ compared to other groups.
Source: Schnall et al. (1992), with permission of *Hypertension*, American Heart Association, and Lippincott, Williams and Wilkins.

The anxieties associated with occupational stress not only affect alcohol consumption but also provide a stimulus to smoking. Epidemiological studies on the relationship between smoking and BP have been variable (for references, see Kaplan, 2002). However, Groppelli et al. (1992) found that ambulatory BP is raised when smokers are indulging their habit (figure 11.3; table 11.2).

Steptoe et al. (1999) related the BP responses of persons experiencing high and low job strain to their responses to acute stress tests in which the subject had varying control over the outcome. Thus, the subject had little decision latitude when performing a computerised color or word conflict test requiring rapid answers: In those with high job strain, the rise in BP was a few mmHg greater than in those with low job strain (figure 11.21). The other test was without time constraints and gave the subject time to think while completing various matrices with one of several choices provided; high and low job strain groups had identical BP responses.

Subsequently, Steptoe and Cropley (2000) used the stress test with little decision latitude to try to identify persons whose BP would increase after 1 year. They studied normotensive young adults experiencing low and high job demands, in whom SBPs

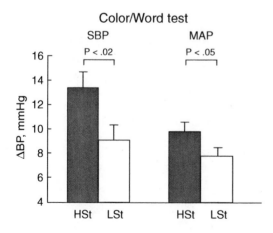

Figure 11.21. Ambulatory BP responses to a rapidly performed color-word test: Increases in ambulatory SBPs and MAPs (mmHg) were greater in schoolteachers in whom job strain was high (HSt) than in those in whom it was low (LSt). Baseline SBPs, DBPs, and MAPs were similar in both groups; bars, 1 SEM. From Steptoe et al. (1999), with permission of the *Journal of Hypertension* and Lippincott, Williams and Wilkins.

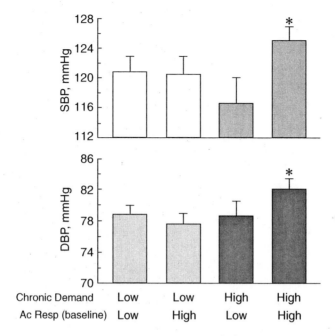

Figure 11.22. Average ambulatory SBPs and DBPs (mmHg) measured over working day in four groups, classified 1 year earlier on the basis of high or low job demands, and high or low cardiovascular responsiveness to stress test over which subject had no control. The high job demand group that was hyperresponsive at baseline was the only one with significant BP elevation after 1 year. From Steptoe and Cropley (2000), with permission of *Journal of Hypertension* and Lippincott, Williams and Wilkins.

and DBPs were similar at baseline. After 1 year, those with high job demands who were also hyperresponsive to acute stress had MAPs that were ~4 mmHg higher than in all the other groups (figure 11.22). The results support the idea that the defense pathways may be partially sensitized in the hyperresponders, so that repeated exposure to this type of stress raises BP gradually over the following 12 months. The rate of BP rise is in accord with estimates by Julius et al. (2004) for the rise in BP from high normal levels to those in established EH.

However, the question whether acute stress tests really differentiate persons with EH from normotensives has been controversial. One would expect that in a mixed population, persons with sensitized defense synapses would show greater rises in BP in response to acute stresses with low decision latitude. Yet such a correlation has been observed in only about half the studies (Weder et al., 1989; Fredrikson and Matthews, 1990; Julius et al., 1991; Pickering, 1994).

One factor that must have contributed to the variable findings is differences in the secretion of adrenaline, which in mild stress is often absent in normotensives but is a part of the response of persons with EH. As illustrated in relation to the Valsalva test, giving β-AR antagonists improves the correlation between stimulus and constrictor effect.

In conclusion, the job strain model helps to identify persons experiencing chronic occupational stress. Acute stress tests play a useful role in identifying long-term susceptibility to EH.

Socioeconomic Factors

Socioeconomic disadvantage correlates with BP in both developing and developed countries (Dressler, 1990; Pickering, 1994). In the United States, the BP of young adult African Americans is highest in those who strive through hard work and determination to make up for their social, economic, and educational disadvantages (James et al., 1983). Harburg and colleagues (Harburg, Erfurt, Chape et al., 1973; Harburg, Erfurt, Hauenstein et al., 1973) defined high- and low-stress neighborhoods of Detroit according to (1) socioeconomic factors such as income, home ownership, and education; and (2) social stability factors such as crime rate and state of marriage. The highest BPs were recorded in African Americans less than 40 years old, who lived in high-stress neighborhoods. Those living in low-stress neighborhoods had lower BPs, which were similar in blacks and whites.

Longitudinal studies demonstrate whether a particular factor persists or alters over a number of years, which strengthens any suggested association with BP. In one large American study of initially normotensive black and white men and women, the relationship between various socioeconomic factors and development of EH was examined in 3825 persons (age range 18–30 years on entry) on five occasions over a 10-year period (Matthews et al., 2002).[7] Over this time, there were 60 new cases of EH among whites (SBP $\geq$ 140, DBP $\geq$ 90 mmHg) and 195 cases in blacks, who were experiencing higher levels of stress. Continuing difficulty and the associated anxiety in paying for basic necessities were associated with increased incidence of EH and appeared to be more important than inadequacies in education.

Social Support

Factors that moderate some of the cardiovascular effects of stress include exercise and nonjudgmental social support provided by family and friends. Good support mechanisms have been estimated to reduce MAP by some 4–5 mmHg in those living in poor communities (Dressler, 1990; Christenfeld et al., 1997; Fontana et al., 1999). It suggests that social support provides a buffer against stress.

Owning a pet dog or cat is thought to have effects similar to social support (Friedmann and Thomas, 1995). This is illustrated by the results of a well-designed experimental study showing that pet ownership reduces the BP responses to acute stress (Allen et al., 2001). The subjects were 48 volunteers with previously untreated moderate hypertension (grade 2, SBP/DBP $\geq$ 160/100 mmHg). All were interested in stress reduction and had agreed to acquire a dog or cat if selected for the appropriate experimental group. Half the subjects were randomized into a group that subsequently acquired a pet, while the other half remained without a pet. All subjects were treated for 6 months with the ACE inhibitor lisinopril, which reduced their BPs to below 130/90 mmHg.

Before starting drug treatment, each person underwent a mental arithmetic test and made a speech: The responses in pet owners and those without a pet were identical

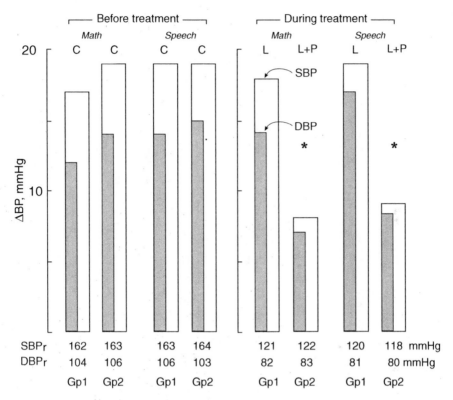

Figure 11.23. Left, in two groups of previously untreated patients with similar grade II EH, there were closely similar changes in ambulatory SBP and DBP during a mathematics test and when making a speech (Math, Speech); one group was to acquire a pet, but not the other. Right, after 6 months of treatment with lisinopril, resting BPs of both groups were identical. In the group that had acquired a pet (L+P), ΔSBP and ΔDBP during the stress test were about half the earlier value, while the responses were unchanged in the group on lisinopril alone but no pet (L). Clear bars, ΔSBP; shaded bars, ΔDBP; *$p < .001$ between baseline and treatment. Resting values before and during lisinopril at foot of each column. Redrawn after Allen et al. (2001).

(figure 11.23). After 6 months of lisinopril, the BP of both groups had fallen to the same resting values. In those without a pet, the BP responses to the stress tests were, as expected, similar to those before treatment (Dimsdale et al., 1992). However, those of the pet owners were reduced by about half, as were the tachycardia and renin responses (Allen et al., 2001).

The findings suggest that having a pet enhances a person's capacity to withstand stress. This concurs with the views of some social support theorists, who believe that the positive feelings generated by nonjudgmental support reduce stress (Cohen and Hoberman, 1983). Most pet owners lavish much affection on their pets, which is returned. It suggests that supportive cooperative relationships affect the stress threshold for raising BP.

A Hypothesis on How Psychosocial Stress Initiates EH

A rise in BP in response to chronic stress can be a normal phenomenon if the stress is of appropriate severity, for example, during the Antarctic winter. In such individuals, BP returns rapidly to normal when the stress stops, with little evidence of hyper-responsiveness to stressors, which is characteristic of persons with EH.

The brain recognizes the nature and intensity of a particular stressor (or a closely associated cue) through a neuronal network that extends from the thalamus to the sensory and prefrontal cortex, limbic regions, and the cerebellum. What matters most for long-term elevation of BP is the integration by the prefrontal cortex of the global stress intensity experienced as a result of the cumulative effects of individual episodes of stress over weeks or months (figure 11.24). The interpretation of this information depends on similar past experiences, genetic and dietary factors, the level of habitual exercise, and social support. The thalamocortical system communicates with the ANS through DA neurons affecting the hypothalamus and PAG, from which the autonomic effects on BP are mediated through fast transmitter target neurons to the sympathetic premotor and motoneurons. The emotional response to stress is expressed through the amygdala and is an important component of the overall response.

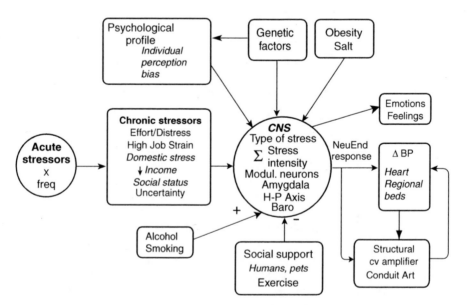

Figure 11.24. Chronic stress raises BP through repeated CNS activation. Persons genetically susceptible to EH tend to overestimate average stress intensity, but the main reason for their increased responsiveness is sensitization of defense pathway activated by stress. Increased alcohol consumption, smoking, and high salt intake accentuate the effects of stress, while exercise and social support antagonize its effects. Stress raises SNA (and BP) more in persons with EH than in normotensives, and the response is further enhanced by cardiovascular structural changes.

The hypothalamic defense area includes cell groups in DMHN, PVN, PAG, and other nuclei, which determine the pattern of vagal and spinal sympathetic motoneuron activity. The response to stress is one several variants of the defense response mediated through the hypothalamus.[8] Acute stress elicits elevation of cardiac SNA and rises in constrictor SNA in the major regulatory beds, on which adrenaline secretion is superimposed. The pathway from the hypothalamus to the spinal motoneurons is partly through direct monosynaptic connections and partly through hindbrain neurons, on which many other inputs converge, including those subserving baroreflexes.

The perception of stress has a large subjective component, as a result of which a given stressor is regarded as mild by some and severe by others, which results in corresponding differences of their autonomic responses (figure 11.14). This is partly due to differences in cognitive and affective capacities, which vary between individuals. At one extreme are patients with Down syndrome, who understimate stress intensity, which makes them virtually EH-proof (figure 4.10). In contrast, the personality of persons with EH results in their tendency to overestimate stress. The mechanism could be through mild sensory overload related to DA-induced gating of the sensory input from thalamus to the cerebral cortex (figure 11.13), which probably makes a small contribution to their neural hyperresponsiveness. However, the major factors that raise neural responsiveness are enhancement of synaptic transmission conveying information to some of the hypothalamic target neurons or more responsive receptors on some of these neurons.

In contrast to the minimal sensitization in normotensives subjected to episodic stress, the defense pathway is markedly hyperresponsive in persons with established EH. This is best assessed from constrictor SNA responses to a stressor (figure 11.9) or from the ratio of the slopes of the constrictor MAP-SNA relationship (figure 9.19).[9] In contrast, the more widely used hemodynamic estimates of hyperresponsiveness are difficult to quantify, partly because of uncertainty about R_1 vessel structural changes, and partly because of the role of adrenaline.

In EH, the rise in constrictor SNA is about 2–3 times that observed in normotensives (figure 11.9). However, the true increase in neural responsiveness of persons with EH is about 13 times the value observed in normotensives. It is normally masked mainly by the action of forebrain-mediated inhibition and to a lesser extent by baroreflexes. When the role of both are taken into account, the overall increase in neural responsiveness in EH could be as high as 15–20 times that of normotensives. The hyperresponsiveness applies to both SNA and adrenaline secretion. However, the threshold for eliciting the latter is somewhat greater, which is why it increases only phasically in EH (chapter 5).

Hypothalamic hyperresponsiveness could depend on the properties of the inhibitory or the excitatory modulatory interneurons in figure 11.12, and probably depends on both. The presence of a powerful inhibitory system explains why BP may take 5–10 years to rise to hypertensive levels in persons susceptible to EH. The inhibitory system appears to be linked to forebrain development and is more powerful in primates and particularly in humans than in subprimate species.

That genetic factors are important determinants of the hypothalamic hyperresponsiveness to stress is suggested by the cosegregation data discussed in chapter 3, which account for the differences in neural responsiveness between SHR and WKY

(Li et al., 1997), and BHR and WKY (Lawler et al., 1984). They also account for the strain specificity of the BP responses in other rodents to mental or physical stresses considered in this chapter. Nongenetic factors also play a role, for example, by accounting for the response differences between dominant and subordinate animals from genetically uniform SHR (figure 11.18). However, the BP and NA responses of dominant and subordinate SHR are greater than those of the corresponding dominant and subordinate animals in the WKY strain, suggesting that overall hypothalamic hyperresponsiveness is genetically determined. One may assume that this also applies to the autonomic response difference between persons with EH and normotensives.

The hypothesis is that genetic factors affect the threshold with which the DA (or 5-HT) slow transmitter neurons elicit the defense response. One method could involve strengthening of synaptic transmission between the DA neurons and hypothalamic premotor target neurons by inducing biochemical and structural changes in synaptic proteins similar to those in *Aplysia* (figure 8.7). Presumably after repeated stresses of similar intensities, more transmitter would be released or there would be more synaptic contacts in persons with EH than in normotensives. The threshold will be different on synapses with premotor target neurons subserving neural sympathetic responses than on those subserving adrenaline secretion.

We recall that the synaptic sensitization involves the cortical link with the hypothalamus. As Edelman has pointed out, an important attribute of the thalamocortical system is its capacity for rapid learning through synaptic sensitization, which is quite different from what happens at autonomic synapses subserving the baroreflex where sensitization is virtually unknown. In the majority of the population who are normotensive, this also applies to the corticohypothalamic interface, as judged by the rapid restoration of BP and autonomic changes at the end of a period of chronic stress. It seems reasonable to suggest that sensitization of synapses at this interface could be the result of regulation by a mutant gene with properties similar to those of thalamocortical synapses.

This seems more likely than a genetically determined increase in the reponsiveness of receptors on the target neurons on which DA (or 5-HT) act. Receptors are thought to exist in two conformations, an inactive R form and an active R* form (figure 11.25; Koch et al., 1996). When the agonist binds to R*, this results in an increase in the proportion of receptors in the R* conformation. Such changes occur when R is overexpressed, even without the agonist, as demonstrated in the myocardium of both transgenic mice and spontaneous mutants (Koch et al., 1996).

Even in persons with the EH genotype, hypertension does not develop except in the presence of appropriate environmental conditions. This is well illustrated in Timio et al.'s (1988, 1997) case control study on BP changes in Italian nuns and laywomen (figure 4.8). Another example is the much greater prevalence of EH in African Americans living in high-stress compared to low-stress neighborhoods (Harburg, Erfurt, Chape et al., 1973; Harburg, Erfurt, Hauenstein et al., 1973). One reason for not developing spontaneous hypertension is the relatively small number of high-BP genes in humans with EH. The corresponding animal model is the BHR, which has half the high BP genes of SHR and also only develops chronic hypertension in an adverse environment. In terms of the hypothesis proposed, the difference in resting BPs between animals with the BHR and SHR genotype could be largely

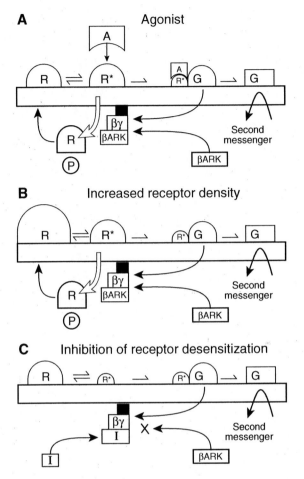

Figure 11.25. Receptors exist in R and R* conformations, with R* the active form. (A) The agonist (A) binds to R*, which causes further increase in proportion of R*; R* binds to the heterotrimetric G-protein (G), which dissociates into G_α-GTP and βγ subunits, which activate effector enzymes (e.g., adenylyl cyclase) and increase production of second messengers (e.g., cAMP). Binding of βγ-subunit to receptor allows translocation of βARK to the membrane compartment and phosphorylation (P) of R*. This interrupts the latter's interaction with G protein, which is termed desensitization. (B) A large increase in receptor density affects both R and R*, even without the agonist. Equilibrium favors R, but absolute concentration of R* may be greater than when agonist is present at lower receptor density. (C) The binding of an inhibitor (I) to βγ subunit prevents translocation of βARK, resulting in an effect similar to B, but at normal receptor density: R* does not become phosphorylated and continues to act on the G-protein. From Koch et al. (1996), with permission of *Circulation Research*, American Heart Association, and Lippincott, Williams and Wilkins.

due to differences in the degree of overexpression in DA receptors at strategic points of the defense pathway.

From the evidence presented, there seems little doubt that stress alone is capable of initiating EH. Of all the other major environmental causes of EH, a high dietary salt intake also acts through the defense pathway in salt-sensitive individuals, thus accentuating the elevation of BP caused by stress (chapter 12).

Last, seeking relief from stress-related negative emotions often results in greater consumption of alcohol. Similarly, food consumption is often raised in response to stress. High alcohol intake accentuates the rise in BP associated with high job strain, while obesity also has adverse effects (chapter 13). These are unsuccessful antistress measures that accentuate its adverse cardiovascular effects. The same applies to smoking, which increases SNA and BP and accentuates development of a number of complications of EH. As against those, the most successful physiological antidotes to EH are exercise training and social support.

12

Salt, Other Dietary Factors, and Blood Pressure

Lowering of the intake of salt for the treatment of hypertension was first employed by Ambard and Beaujard (1904) and by Allen (1925), who found improvement in some patients with hypertension and severe renal disease. Later, Kempner (1948) advocated a diet of fruit and rice of very low salt content and achieved a few successes in lowering BP in patients with severe hypertension. There were many more failures, but the results provided some encouragement in the days before antihypertensive drugs.

In 1961, Lewis Dahl suggested that EH would virtually disappear if dietary salt intake were reduced sufficiently. This was based on his epidemiological analysis, which was summarized in an illustration similar to figure 4.14. As discussed in chapter 4, the Dahl diagram overstates the effects of salt on BP. Nevertheless, there is now substantial evidence from the Intersalt study and clinical trials that a habitual high salt intake raises BP and that a low salt intake reduces it (Denton, 1982; Simpson, 2000). At times, physicians appear to forget the multifactorial nature of EH, with some believing that high salt is the overwhelmingly most important cause of EH, while this is anathema to others (Simpson, 2000). It is all too easy to stray into the realm of "the political science of salt" (Taubes, 1998). Sorting out this confusion requires an understanding of the main mechanisms through which dietary salt affects BP.

Body sodium is normally very tightly controlled through a large number of homeostatic mechanisms. These ensure that in healthy normotensive animals and humans, changing sodium intake has little effect on BP. Dahl also pioneered much important research on the cardiovascular effects of salt, including the development of rat strains that differ markedly in their salt sensitivity, that is, their BP responsiveness to salt. For example, the Dahl-S rat and most SHR substrains are extremely salt sensitive, while the Dahl-R and WKY rats are very salt-resistant (Dahl et al., 1962; Rapp, 1982; Oparil et al., 1988).[1] One mechanism by which a high salt intake raises BP in these animals has turned out to be through the action of the sodium ion on neurons that converge on the hypothalamic defense area (Leenen et al., 2002). This probably also plays a role in EH. Renal functional impairment is another important determinant of salt sensitivity.

Regulatory Mechanisms

Maintenance of body sodium balance during variation in sodium intake is normally dependent on modulation of renal mechanisms by the renin-angiotensin-aldosterone (RAA) system, by atrial natriuretic peptide (ANP), and by the baroreflexes. In special circumstances usually associated with renal dysfunction or severe constrictor hypertension, additional modulation occurs through the action of centrally and peripherally acting ouabain-like cardiotonic steroids.

Renal Mechanisms

The extent to which a sodium load is excreted depends on: (1) glomerular haemodynamics, (2) renal cortical and medullary blood flow, (3) renal tubular function, and (4) neurohumoral modulators of renal function.

The Pressure-Diuresis Function Curve

In a normal person, a change in dietary salt intake has a minimal effect on BP; hence the almost $90°$ slope of Guyton's MAP-sodium output curve (figure 12.1; Guyton, 1980; Hall and Granger, 1994). Guyton was the first to point out that BP sensitivity to salt increased considerably during either excessive activity or depression of the renin-angiotensin system (Guyton, 1980; Guyton et al., 1995). It suggests that dysfunction or a change in the balance in the various homeostatic factors increases salt sensitivity.

Under normal circumstances, the role of the neurohumoral modulators in maintaining constancy of plasma and body sodium is much greater than fluctuation of renal perfusion pressure. For example, in normal dogs fluctuations in renal perfusion pressure of -20 to $+10\%$ have little effect on resting BP (Seeliger et al., 2005). The pressure-diuresis mechanism thus plays only a small role in moment-to-moment adjustments of body sodium, but its role increases in the presence of renal functional impairment.

The factors that increase sodium sensitivity include a decrease in whole-kidney ultrafiltration coefficient (K_F) and an increase in tubular sodium reabsorption, or both (Kimura et al., 1994). The first occurs as a consequence of greater microcirculatory rarefaction, with reduction in the number of functioning glomeruli.

In Dahl salt-sensitive (S) rats, the availability of NO diminishes throughout the kidney, partly because of the limited supply of L-arginine and partly because of enhanced formation of reactive O_2 species (Cowley et al., 1995; Cowley and Roman, 1997; Ni et al., 1999). The reduction in NO compromises renal tubular function, particularly in the renal medulla. Normally the linear BP–blood flow relationship in the renal

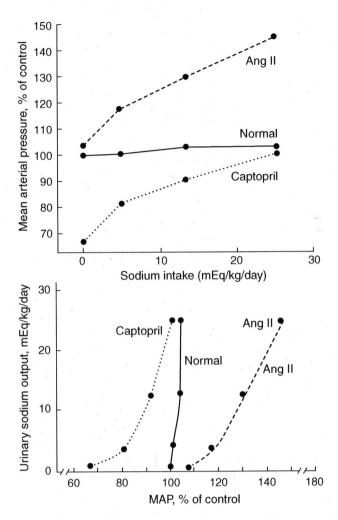

Figure 12.1. Bottom, relationship between MAP (mmHg) and urinary sodium output (mEq/kg/day) in normal dogs and in dogs infused with captopril or angiotensin II (Ang II). Top, the bottom graph has been replotted with sodium intake on abscissa and MAP on ordinate. Normally MAP is virtually independent of sodium intake, but becomes salt-sensitive when renin-angiotensin system activity is altered. From Guyton (1980), with permission of Raven Press and Lippincott, Williams and Wilkins.

medulla depends on high local NO production (figure 6.4), with the high blood flow reducing renal sodium reabsorption.[2] When medullary NO is reduced by local medullary infusion of L-NAME, sodium reabsorption increases, raising blood volume and BP and lowering urinary excretion of sodium (figure 12.2; Mattson et al., 1992, 1994). Similar changes occur in response to rises in medullary superoxide concentration (Majid and Nishiyama, 2002).

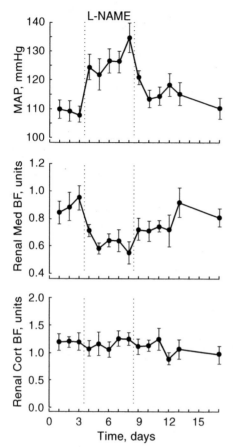

Figure 12.2. Effects of infusing the NOS inhibitor L-NAME into the renal medullary interstitium (between vertical lines) on mean arterial pressure (MAP, mmHg) and renal medullary and cortical blood flow (units) in conscious Sprague-Dawley rats. Blood flow measured by laser-Doppler flowmeters. From Cowley et al. (1995), with permission of *Hypertension*, American Heart Association, and Lippincott, Williams and Wilkins.

Tubular Mechanisms

BP sensitivity to salt depends on both Na^+ and Cl^- ions: Substituting HCO_3^- for Cl^- when salt load is raised does not cause a rise in BP (Luft et al., 1991). But $NaHCO_3$ also raises excretion of calcium, pointing to a role for Ca^{2+} in salt sensitivity. Another suggestion has been that augmented activity of the Na-K-2Cl cotransport mechanism accounts for an increase in salt sensitivity (Aviv et al., 2004).

In EH, the known defects in cellular sodium transport include (1) abnormalities in Na^+-Li^+ countertransport (Canessa et al., 1990), and (2) the nonmodulator response, with blunting of sodium excretion during high salt intake (Williams et al., 1992; chapter 3). Both appear to be genetically determined.

The operation of the Na^+-Li^+ countertransporter resembles that of the Na^+-H^+ exchanger: Overexpression of the latter in transgenic mice causes hypertension and reduction in urinary excretion of sodium and water (Kuro-o et al., 1995). Reduction in sodium excretion is often absent in EH but becomes apparent as renal blood flow heterogeneity increases (Roman, 1986).

Renin-Angiotensin-Aldosterone System

The RAA system helps maintain body sodium during changes in sodium intake (Sealey and Laragh, 1974; Laragh and Sealey, 1995). Aldosterone directly affects renal tubular sodium reabsorption, and its secretion is regulated by changes in plasma Ang II and K^+. Tubuloglomerular feedback signals from the macula densa region to the renin-secreting cells on the afferent and efferent arterioles occur in response to changes in tubular sodium and chloride composition, mainly in ΔCl^- (chapter 5). A fall in macula densa sodium chloride raises renal renin secretion, while a rise in sodium chloride concentration has the opposite effect (Schnermann and Briggs, 1992).

Increased renal renin release and local Ang II production alter afferent and efferent arteriolar tone. The above are also affected by changes in renal perfusion pressure, SNA, ANP secretion, and NO concentration.

In sodium depletion, elevation of renin production is mediated through the combined effects of baroreflexes, the renal barostat, and tubuloglomerular feedback (Davis and Freeman, 1976). The same mechanisms suppress renin production during sodium loading. Figure 12.3 indicates that the role of the RAA system on sodium reabsorption is substantially greater during sodium depletion than during sodium loading.[3]

Other accompaniments of sodium depletion include increases in renal and average NA spillover, indicating corresponding elevation in SNA (Watson et al., 1984; Friberg et al., 1990). PRA and Ang II levels rise, and Ang II may contribute to the increase in SNA through stimulation of AT_1 receptors on the area postrema and the other circumventricular organs (chapter 8). During sodium depletion, the brain renin-angiotensin system increases thirst and promotes intake of water and salt (Fitzsimons, 1994).

Atrial Natriuretic Peptide

ANP was discovered by de Bold (1982), who found granules containing the peptide in atrial and ventricular myocytes. ANP has potent natriuretic and diuretic properties, and its plasma concentration rises rapidly during acute elevation of the central blood volume (Ballermann and Zeidel, 1992; Brenner et al., 1990). An analogous peptide (brain natriuretic peptide, BNP) is located in the hypothalamus (Gutkowska et al., 1997). One of BNP's central actions is to antagonize some of the neural effects of salt-sensitive hypertension (Sakamoto et al., 1999). In rabbits, BNP reduces water and salt intake (Tarjan et al., 1988).

Resting plasma ANP is normal in mild EH, but it may rise in more severe grades of hypertension (Matsubara et al., 1989; Neyses et al., 1989). During exercise, it increases more in persons with EH than in normotensives, because their central blood volume is already raised at rest (figure 10.4).

Over the physiological range of plasma concentrations, most of the actions of ANP are on the kidney (Brenner et al., 1990; Ballermann and Zeidel, 1992). ANP dilates the afferent arteriole and constricts the efferent arteriole, increasing filtration fraction and glomerular filtration rate (GFR), which accounts for most of its diuretic

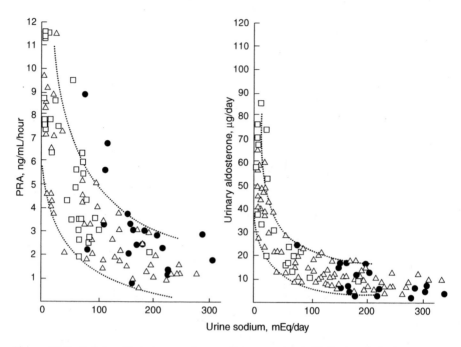

Figure 12.3. Relationship between urinary sodium excretion (mEq/day) and (1) plasma renin activity (PRA, ng/mL/hour, left), and (2) urinary excretion of aldosterone (μg/day, right). The triangles and squares are samples obtained under conditions of metabolic balance (2–3 samples per subject), while filled circles are random samples. Based on Brunner et al. (1972), with permission of *New England Journal of Medicine* and Massachusetts Medical Society.

and natriuretic actions (figure 12.4). This probably contributes to the well-known rapidity of excretion of an acute saline load in mild and moderate EH (Papper et al., 1960; Grim, Luft et al., 1979; Grim, Miller et al., 1979; Ulrych et al., 1971; Harshfield and Grim, 1997). ANP inhibits fluid reabsorption from the proximal tubule and sodium and water reabsorption in the medullary collecting ducts. Its renal cellular actions are mediated through stimulation of cyclic GMP in tubular cells.

In mice, genetic manipulation of ANP produces large long-term changes in BP. For example, 10-fold overexpression of the ANP gene in mice lowers BP by 20–30 mmHg below that of wild-type mice (Koh et al., 1993). Surprisingly, the overexpression of ANP has virtually no effect on water and sodium excretion, which suggests that these very high hormone levels have little physiological relevance. This is in accord with findings in rabbits in which ANP was raised to 10–30 times the normal resting value, which caused falls in MAP, CO, and atrial pressures, while sodium excretion remained unchanged (Woods et al., 1989).[4] The hemodynamic changes are due to venoconstriction causing loss of plasma from the circulation.

Conversely, after disrupting the gene for the ANP guanylyl cyclase-A receptor, the loss of ANP function produces chronic elevation of BP of ~20 mmHg on a normal salt diet (Lopez et al., 1995). Surprisingly, the BP in these mice was unaffected by salt loading.

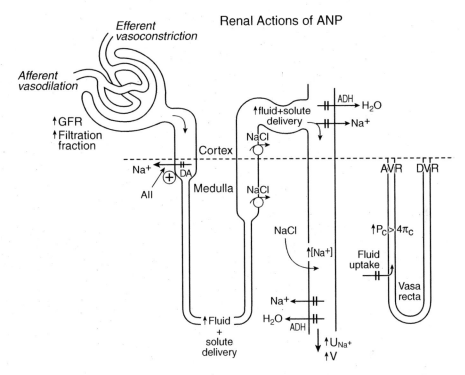

Figure 12.4. Atrial natriuretic peptide (ANP) at physiological concentrations causes afferent arteriolar dilation and efferent arteriolar constriction, increasing filtration fraction and glomerular filtration rate (GFR). In the proximal tubule, ANP inhibits Ang II-mediated reabsorption of fluid (AII), possibly in conjunction with dopamine (DA). ANP inhibits water and sodium reabsorption in medullary collecting ducts. This also occurs in response to a raised hydraulic pressure in the vasa recta. P_c, vasa recta capillary pressure; π_c, colloid osmotic pressure; AVR, DVR, ascending and descending vasa recta; ADH, antidiuretic hormone. From Ballermann and Zeidel (1992), with permission of Raven Press and Lippincott, Williams and Wilkins.

CNS Mechanisms: Salt Preference, Baroreflexes, Brain Ouabain System, and AVP

The brain has considerable influence on dietary salt consumption, because most individuals like the taste of salt. Baroreflexes respond to moderate alterations in salt loads. At high salt loads, endogenous ouabain (EO) neurons in the hypothalamus become activated in some individuals, as may posterior pituitary arginine vasopressin (AVP).

Salt Preference

In Japan and China, salt intake is often high, reflecting cultural traditions. Moving from a rural to an urban industrialized environment is generally accompanied by a greater salt intake (Denton, 1982; Beilin, 1994; Poulter and Sever, 1994).

Many cardiovascular effects of high salt are accentuated by reducing potassium intake (Tobian, 1991).

Dahl considered that the taste for salt was acquired in early life through consumption of salty foods. However, according to Denton (1982), innate genetic factors also play a role since all animals have a strong taste preference for salt. Persons with EH are said to have a greater craving for salt than normotensives (Schechter et al., 1973), but this has been disputed.

Baroreflexes

Sodium depletion evokes baroreflex-mediated rises in SNA in both normotensives and persons with EH, as assessed by average and renal NA spillover (Watson et al., 1984; Friberg et al., 1990). Conversely, salt loading elicits baroreflex-mediated reduction in SNA and renin release, which lower afferent arteriolar tone and promote diuresis. Normally these mechanisms are very effective, in conjunction with the RAA and ANP systems, in preventing changes in blood volume and body sodium. This is the reason why the BP of many laboratory animal species is highly unresponsive to salt loading. The buffering role of baroreflexes was examined in the Sprague-Dawley rat and the WKY (Osborn and Provo, 1992; Huang and Leenen, 1994). In both strains, the effects of salt loading were compared between animals with intact afferents and animals subjected to sinoaortic denervation (SAD) prior to salt loading (table 12.1).

After 4 weeks of marked salt loading, the MAP in intact rats had increased by ~ 6 mmHg, while the corresponding rise in SAD rats was 21 mmHg. In the Sprague-Dawley SAD rats the BP rise was relatively slow, which may have been due to the activity of the cardiopulmonary baroreceptors, which had not been denervated; changes in production of ANP and Ang II may also have contributed to the delay. Interestingly, SAD had no effect on the rise of BP in SHR, which is probably due to the readier access of the high sodium to their brain ouabain neurons.

Ryuazaki et al. (1991) compared the effects of high dietary salt intake on BP of rabbits that had been subjected (1) to SAD, (2) to removal of one kidney to lower

Table 12.1. Average Changes in Mean Arterial Pressure (ΔMAP, mmHg) in Two Normotensive and One Hypertensive Rat Strains in Which a Diet of Normal Salt Content Was Changed to a High-Salt Diet

	Days on HS (ΔMAP, mmHg)			
	Intact		SAD	
Strain	7–10	11–28	7–10	11–28
S-D[1]	4	5	10*	25*
WKY[2]		7		17*
SHR[2]		24*		21*

Note: ΔSBP; SAD, sinoaortic denervation; HS, high salt.
*p < .05 for difference from normal to high salt.

Source: [1]From Osborn and Provo (1992); [2]From Huang and Leenen (1994).

the capacity to excrete salt, and (3) to SAD and uninephrectomy. In the first two groups, there was little change in BP, whereas MAP and right atrial pressure increased in the SAD + uninephrectomy animals by, respectively, 15 mmHg and 2 mmHg (figure 12.5). In SAD + uninephrectomy animals, body sodium increased more than in the other groups. In addition, by the fourth day of salt loading, their plasma ANP, NA, and AVP were all raised (figure 12.6). The rise in BP was largely due to an increase in AVP, since IV infusion of a vascular AVP antagonist restored BP to normal (Ryuzaki et al., 1991).

We noted in chapter 9 that under normal laboratory conditions daytime BP and TPR are usually raised in SAD rabbits for several days after denervation (Korner, 1970; Blombery and Korner, 1979). This is consistent with the rises in plasma NA in the SAD and SAD + uninephrectomy groups prior to salt loading and the further increases following salt loading (figure 12.6). The raised SNA reduces vascular capacity, which together with the lower excretory capacity due to uninephrectomy tends to raise extracellular Na^+ concentration and osmolality, causing secretion of AVP.

Ang II and Salt Sensitivity

Krieger et al. (1990) found that a moderate increase in salt intake had little effect on BP of awake dogs, but when the same salt load was coadministered with a subpressor infusion of Ang II, MAP rose gradually by some 30 mmHg over the 7 days of the

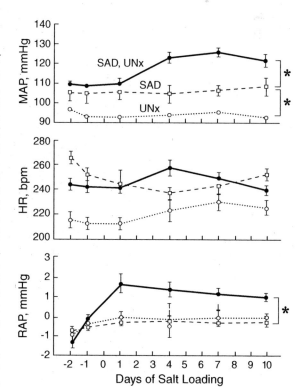

Figure 12.5. Responses of mean arterial pressure (MAP, mmHg), heart rate (HR, bpm, beats/min), and right atrial pressure (RAP, mmHg) in three groups of awake rabbits, before and after switching from 0.9% NaCl to 10% NaCl. The three groups were rabbits subjected to: (1) SAD alone (SAD, clear squares, dashed line); (2) removal of one kidney (UNx, clear circles, dotted line); (3) SAD plus UNx, black circles, solid line). Results are means ± 1 SEM; *p < .05, for difference between groups. After Ryuzaki et al. (1991), with permission of *Hypertension*, American Heart Association, and Lippincott, Williams and Wilkins.

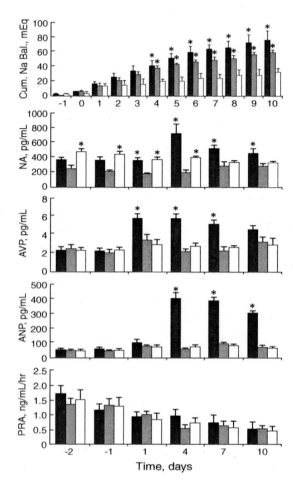

Figure 12.6. Effects in the three groups of rabbits referred to in figure 12.5 on (from top) cumulative sodium balance (mEq), plasma noradrenaline (NA, pg/mL), arginine vasopressin (AVP, pg/mL), atrial natriuretic peptide (ANP, pg/mL), and plasma renin activity (PRA, ng/mL/heart rate). Black bars, rabbits with SAD plus UNx; shaded bars, UNx alone; clear bars, SAD alone. From Ryuzaki et al. (1991), with permission of *Hypertension,* American Heart Association, and Lippincott, Williams and Wilkins.

observation period (figure 12.7). With the salt load alone, CO increased by about 8%, but the effect on BP was almost completely offset by a fall in TPR. With Ang II plus salt, a similar rise in CO (11%) was evoked, but now TPR rose steadily by 20% by day 7 of the high-salt period (figure 12.7). Clearly, this rise in TPR was the main hemodynamic determinant of the rise in BP in this group.

In another study, Krieger and Cowley (1990) focused on the role of blood volume on the response to coadminstration of Ang II plus salt. They compared the hemodynamic changes in normal dogs with those in other dogs in which total body weight was "clamped" at the low salt value. This was done by reducing the daily intake of water whenever the animal's body weight increased over a preceding period (Cowley et al., 1984).[5] Clamping body weight (and presumably total blood volume) prevented the rises in MAP, CO, and TPR that were induced by the same regimen in uncontrolled dogs (figure 12.8). Acordingly, the rises in MAP and TPR in the latter group were explained on the basis of long-term autoregulation, where the luxurious CO was said to trigger a sustained myogenic response. The reader will recall from chapter 2

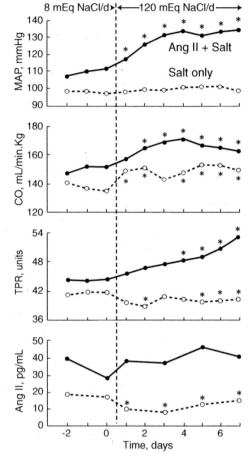

Figure 12.7. Effect of increasing sodium chloride intake from 8 mEq/day IV to 120 mEq/day IV, on mean arterial pressure (MAP, mmHg), cardiac output (CO, mL/min/kg body weight); total peripheral resistance (TPR, units), and plasma Ang II concentration (Ang II, pg/mL) in two groups of normal dogs. One group was infused with sodium chloride alone (dashed lines, open circles), while the other received a subpressor amount of Ang II (3 ng/kg/min) together with the saline solution (bold line, black circles). *$p < .05$ from last presalt day. Adapted from Krieger et al. (1990), with permission of *American Journal of Physiology* and American Physiological Society.

that Guyton and colleagues invoked long-term autoregulation to explain the late rise in TPR during salt loading on low-renal-mass hypertension, without appreciating the neural basis of the response (chapter 15).

However, Krieger et al. recognized that the explanation of the pressure rise in figure 12.7 was not consistent with that offered in figure 12.8 but made little attempt to resolve the discrepancy. The explanation of the "uncontrolled" experiments in figure 12.7 is in accord with the data discussed later in this chapter, in which an increase in constrictor factors raises BP sensitivity to salt, largely through sympathetic mechanisms. In contrast, clamping blood volume does not address the major hemodynamic effect associated with the interaction between Ang II and high salt.[6]

Cardiotonic Steroids

In the 1960s and 1970s, ouabain-like inhibitors of Na^+ K^+ ATPase were discovered in the plasma and urine of patients with renal disease and fluid retention

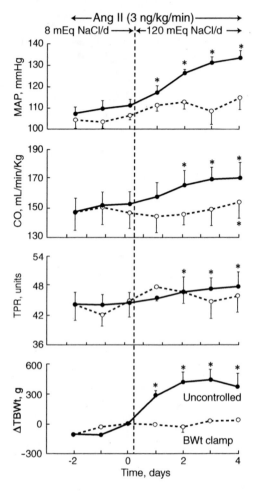

Figure 12.8. Effect of increasing sodium chloride intake from 8 mEq/day to 120 mEq/day IV, in two groups of dogs, both of which also received Ang II (3 ng/kg/min IV), on hemodynamic variables and plasma Ang II concentration (Ang II, pg/mL). In one group, body weight (BWt) was not controlled (solid line, black circles), while in the other body weight was clamped at the presalt value (dashed line, open circles). Adapted from Krieger and Cowley (1990), with permission of *American Journal of Physiology* and American Physiological Society.

(Hamlyn et al., 1996). This was confirmed in animals by Haddy and Overbeck (1976), who suggested that the enzyme inhibitors constricted resistance vessels and raised BP in response to volume expansion. Blaustein (1977) then proposed that the vasoconstriction was due to an initial increase in intracellular Na^+ of the VSM cells, which slowed the rate of efflux of calcium through the sodium-calcium exchanger. Therefore it was the increase in intracellular Ca^{2+} that caused VSM contraction (Blaustein, 1977).

Ouabain is part of a large family of digitalis-like cardiotonic steroids (Blaustein and Lederer, 1999). In patients with EH, plasma concentration of ouabain-like material is greater than in normotensives (Poston et al., 1981). It is produced endogenously, which led de Wardener and MacGregor (1980) to propose that in the presence of renal impairment an increase in EO-like material caused systemic vasoconstriction, raising BP and promoting sodium excretion through renal pressure-diuresis and reduction in tubular sodium reabsorption (Pitts, 1959; Alpern et al., 1992). The theory resembles

Guyton's theory of long-term BP control, except that long-term autoregulation has been replaced by oubain-mediated vasoconstriction.

All the early work on plasma and tissue EO was measured by bioassay. A specific radioimmunoassay only became available within the last 10–15 years. It soon became apparent that EO was synthesized solely in the hypothalamus and pituitary (de Wardener, 1996; Wang and Leenen, 2002). However, other cardiotonic steroids of different chemical structure were produced in the adrenal gland. Among them, marinobufagenin (MBG) appears to reduce BP in experimental salt-sensitive hypertension (Fedorova et al., 2000, 2001, 2005). MBG is a bufodienolide found in the skin gland venom of toads of the genus *Bufo*. Dried powdered toad skin was once used in Chinese and European folk medicine until it was replaced by the digitalis glycosides in the 19th and 20th centuries (Bowman and Rand, 1980).

Brain Ouabain Neurons

Activation of EO material in the brain raises SNA and BP in Dahl S rats and SHR and probably in a proportion of persons with EH. The EO material probably comes from slow transmitter neurons. The activation of brain ouabain by an increase in Na^+ was first suggested by Gotoh (1982), who found that cerebrospinal fluid (CSF) Na^+ concentration was greater in salt-sensitive than salt-resistant patients with EH. Over the whole group, CSF Na^+ and BP were linearly related.

Nakamura and Cowley (1989) observed that Na^+ concentration increased in the CSF of Dahl-S (S) rats after switching intake from low to high salt, while the same change had no effect in salt-resistant Dahl-R (R) rats. The difference was due to a greater sodium permeability of the blood-brain barrier in S than in R rats (Simchon et al., 1999). In both strains, the hypothalamic and pituitary tissue concentrations of EO were similar, and i.c.v. injection of a small volume of hypertonic NaCl evoked identical rises in BP in each strain, having bypassed the permeability barrier (figure 12.9).

Leenen and colleagues have worked out the central mechanism of the BP rise (Leenen et al., 2002). I.c.v. hypertonic NaCl raises BP, heart rate, and renal SNA in conscious Wistar rats. Exactly the same responses are evoked by i.c.v. injection of ouabain or extracts of brain EO. Both changes are prevented by pretreatment with a digoxin-specific antibody (figure 12.10; Huang et al., 1992). Thus, NaCl and EO mediate identical effects through a common central pathway.

An amiloride-sensitive gated Na^+ channel activates the central EO neurons, which release a transmitter with ouabain-like properties (figure 12.11; Huang and Leenen, 1996, 2002). The ouabain neurons stimulate downstream neurons, which release Ang II in the hypothalamus, raising SNA and BP.[7] The amiloride analogue benzamil blocks the activation of the Na^+ channel. Benzamil has no effect on the i.c.v. actions of EO and Ang II, suggesting that they act further downstream on the pathway that projects to the hypothalamic defense area. In S rats, an increase in salt load raises hypothalamic and pituitary EO and BP, and pretreatment with i.c.v. benzamil attenuates these changes (Wang and Leenen, 2002).

The ouabain neurons are probably close to the A3V3 region (Brody et al., 1983, 1991). The median preoptic nucleus is one source of these neurons (Budzikowski and Leenen, 1997). EO has been found in the brains of Wistar rats, S and R rats, SHR,

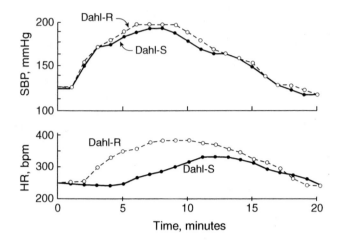

Figure 12.9. Time course of average changes in systolic BP (SBP, mmHg) and heart rate (HR, bpm) in 6-week-old Dahl-S and Dahl-R rats fed a low-salt diet (0.23% NaCl), following a 0.06 mL i.c.v. injection of 4.5 mol/L NaCl. From Simchon et al. (1999), with permission of *Hypertension*, American Heart Association, and Lippincott, Williams and Wilkins.

and the Milan hypertensive rats. In the latter strain, the brain has the endogenous enzymes required for EO synthesis (Murrell et al., 2005).

Peripheral Cardiotonic Steroids

One of the main steroids is MBG, which is synthesized in the adrenal cortex and inhibits $Na^+ K^+$ ATPase. Its role in relation to brain EO has been investigated in S rats, which were subjected to a sudden large sodium load of hypertonic NaCl administered intraperitoneally (Fedorova et al., 2000). Over a 3-hour observation period, plasma EO was transiently raised, which was followed by increasing rises of plasma MBG and BP and enhanced renal sodium excretion (figure 12.12; Fedorova et al., 2005). The high plasma EO was associated with an increase in plasma NA. The EO-related rise in sympathetic activity preceded and was probably responsible for the increase in production of MBG by the adrenal cortex.

Pretreatment with specific antibodies to MBG and ouabain abolished the elevation of BP and attenuated natriuresis and the activity of the renal sodium pump (Fedorova et al., 2005). Similar effects were observed after pretreatment with the AT_1 antagonist losartan. Fedorova et al. (2005) emphasized the natriuretic action of MBG in the salt-loaded S rat, but also considered that the steroid contributed directly to the high BP.

The mechanism underlying the diuretic action of ouabain remains unclear. Cardiotonic steroids consist of a sugar moiety, an unsaturated lactone ring, and a steroid moiety. The unsaturated lactone ring is required for the cardiac stimulation and VSM constriction, and may also contribute to the $Na^+ K^+$ ATPase-mediated transport of sodium from cells to plasma in the renal cortical collecting duct (Alpern et al., 1992).

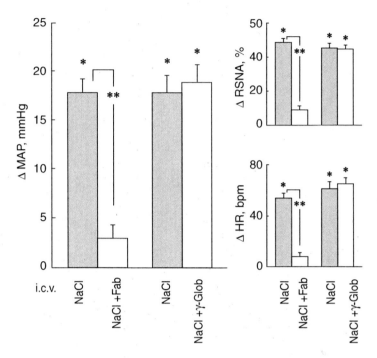

Figure 12.10. Peak changes (mean $\pm$ 1 SEM) in mean arterial pressure (ΔMAP, mmHg), renal sympathetic nerve activity (ΔRSNA, % resting), and heart rate (ΔHR, bpm) in Wistar rats after 10 minutes i.c.v. 0.3 M NaCl (3.8 μL/min); shaded bars, no pretreatment; clear bars, pretreatment with digoxin-specific antibody Fab fragments (Fab), or control (γ-globulin). An antagonist for cardiovascular actions of AVP was administered before hypertonic NaCl. There were 7–9 rats per group. I.c.v. ouabain or brain extracts with ouabain-like activity produced effects closely similar to those of hypertonic NaCl. After Huang et al. (1992), with permission of *Circulation Research*, American Heart Association, and Lippincott, Williams and Wilkins.

Figure 12.11. High CSF Na$^+$ binds to an amiloride-sensitive sodium channel, which activates brain endogenous ouabain (EO) neurons, which excite neurons releasing Ang II, which, in turn, stimulate defense area, causing an increase in SNA and BP, as discussed in text. After Huang and Leenen (2002), with permission of *Hypertension*, American Heart Association, and Lippincott, Williams and Wilkins.

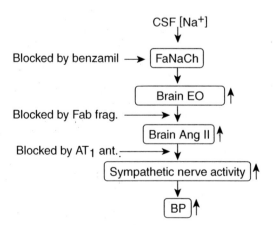

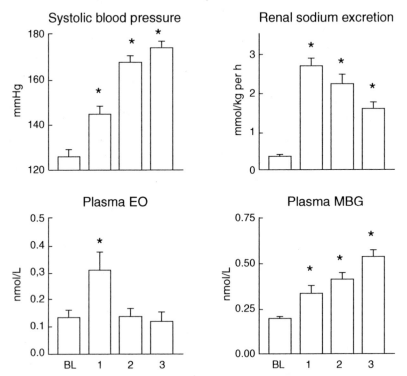

Figure 12.12. Effect of intraperitoneal injection of hypertonic NaCl on systolic blood pressure, renal sodium excretion, plasma endogenous ouabain (EO), and plasma marinobufagenin (MBG) of Dahl-S rats after. *$p < .05$ from baseline value (BL). Data from Fedorova et al. (2005).

Inhibition of this pump has only a modest diuretic effect. Many years ago, Pitts (1959) suggested that the steroid moiety of ouabain is probably a nonspecific aldosterone antagonist, which accentuates the diuretic response of the glycoside.

What then happens in the Dahl-S rat during salt loading? The brain EO mechanism tonically increases renal SNA and heart rate (Huang et al., 1994). A simultaneous increase in constrictor tone and cardiac support is important for maintaining chronically high BP (chapter 7). There is no obvious advantage in reinforcing EO-mediated neural vasoconstriction with more vasoconstriction through MBG, which would disturb the matching of cardiac and peripheral vascular performance. Possibly a lower concentration of MBG is required for its diuretic action, which probably depends on its aldosterone antagonist properties. This would provide a coordinated response, with brain EO the main source of elevation of SNA and MBG the natriuretic factor.

A Role for the Na+/Ca2+ Exchanger?

The use of very large salt loads in all the above studies makes it more difficult to differentiate the roles of central and peripheral cardiotonic steroids. This also applies to the experiments of Iwamoto et al. (2004) on the role of the Na^+/Ca^{2+} exchanger NCX1 in salt-sensitive rats, in which they used the molecule SEA0400, which blocks cellular entry of Ca^{2+}. Administration of the drug elicits sustained falls in BP in DOCA-salt hypertension and in salt-sensitive rat strains while on high salt but not on low salt; the drug had no effect in WKY rats on high salt. The conclusion was that the Na^+/Ca^{2+} exchanger is important in salt-sensitive hypertension. What is not yet known is whether it affects VSM contraction and whether it also acts on central EO neurons.

AVP

Elevation of plasma AVP has been reported in low-renin subjects with EH and raised SNA (Os et al., 1986; Bursztyn et al., 1990). However, plasma AVP is normal in most persons with EH. This is in accord with the finding that administration of a vascular AVP antagonist causes reduction in BP in only a small proportion of those with EH (Gavras and Gavras, 1995). It would seem that the central EO mechanism is engaged by smaller rises in brain sodium than required for AVP secretion. A lower threshold for elevation of SNA than for a rise in AVP was also noted during hemorrhage (Korner et al., 1990; Oliver et al., 1990).

Multiple Regulators or One Adaptive Controller?

It seems best to regard the various regulators as components of a single adaptive control system. Some components play a more prominent role when dietary sodium is low compared to when it is high, such as the RAA system (Hollenberg, 1980; Bonventre and Leaf, 1982). At any given level, two or more mechanisms are generally engaged. At low levels of sodium intake, body sodium is conserved through the actions of RAA and baroreflex systems on the kidney, while at high levels of sodium the effects of ANP, RAA, and baroreflexes try to maintain adequate excretion of body sodium. Under special circumstances, there is activation of EO neurons at high levels of salt intake. AVP increases when blood and tissue osmolality has increased substantially or during marked extracellular volume depletion in hemorrhage and dehydration. The renal transport mechanisms and the various neurohumoral modulators have probably developed in the course of evolution to maintain cellular and extracellular sodium concentrations within relatively narrow limits, despite the large range of dietary sodium.

Definitions of Human Salt Sensitivity and Salt Resistance

What clinicians want to know is the BP response to long-term changes in dietary sodium intake. Many of the answers have long been supplied by well-conducted clinical trials (chapter 4). Figure 12.13 illustrates the effects from a recent trial which shows that in persons on a typical U.S. diet, reducing salt intake from 8 g/day to 4 g/day alters SBP/DBP by 6.7/3.4 mmHg (Sacks et al., 2001). Similar results have been obtained in trials in the United Kingdom (MacGregor et al., 1989), in Australia

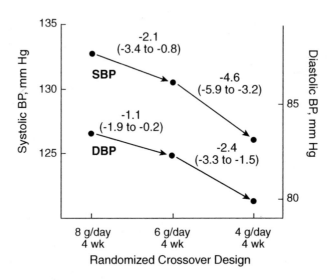

Figure 12.13. Average effects of varying dietary salt intake on systolic and diastolic BP in a randomized controlled trial with 412 participants, consuming a regular U.S. (i.e., Western) diet. Each dietary period was of 4 weeks duration. Data from Sacks et al. (2001), with permission of *New England Journal of Medicine* and Massachusets Medical Society.

(Australian National Health and Medical Research Council Trial, 1989), and in the Intersalt (1988) study. Hence, from the public health perspective we know that dietary salt intake should be reduced from current relatively high values. However, the average responses in all the trials mask a spectrum of individual BP responsiveness to a given change in salt load, raising the question as to the underlying factors involved.

We would like to know if BP increases predominantly through volume overload and elevation of CO, or whether there is also involvement of neural factors that raise constrictor tone. Unfortunately, salt sensitivity in human populations is less absolute than in the Dahl-S and Dahl-R rats, where all members of the S strain are salt-sensitive and all R rats are salt-resistant.

A test for salt sensitivity should identify subjects in whom a high sodium intake causes a substantial elevation in BP. Such a test is likely to have little merit if salt sensitivity really is continuously distributed in the population, like BP or body height. A model suggesting that salt sensitivity is probably more quantal is the chimpanzee study by Denton et al. (1995), in which salt intake was increased in steps from a very low to a very high value over a period of 84 months. In this study, 60% of the 13 animals turned out to be salt sensitive, while 40% were very salt resistant (chapter 4). Thus, salt sensitivity and salt resistance appear to be distinct entities in this primate population.

Clearly, in human studies protocols have to be much shorter, but their duration has to be sufficient to allow a rise in BP response to a salt load that differentiates salt-sensitive from salt-resistant individuals in a physiologically relevant manner. This is possible with only some of the protocols in current use.

Kawasaki et al. (1978) and Fujita et al. (1980) were the first to divide persons with EH into salt-sensitive or salt-resistant categories in a manner that meets the above objectives (table 12.2). After several days on low salt ($\sim$10 mmole sodium/day), each subject was switched to a high-salt diet for 7 days ($\sim$250 mmole sodium/day); potassium intake was increased to compensate for the K^+ loss due to high salt (table 4.2; Luft, Rankin et al., 1979; Tobian, 1991). If the difference in MAP between the last day on low salt and the last day on high salt ($\Delta MAP_{(LS-HS)}$) exceeded $\geq$10% of the initial value, a subject was deemed to be salt sensitive; otherwise he or she was regarded as salt resistant.

Some protocols differentiate salt-sensitive from salt-resistant persons on the basis of smaller $\Delta MAP_{(LS-HS)}$ after salt loading. On most salt loading protocols, it takes at least 5 days before $\Delta MAP_{(LS-HS)}$ exceeds the low salt value by 5% in a salt-sensitive person (Sullivan, 1991). It points to the advantage of protocols of at least 10–14 days duration and a $\Delta MAP_{(LS-HS)}$ of not less than 10 mmHg. With smaller $\Delta MAP_{(LS-HS)}$, the chance of misclassification increases (Grobbee, 1991), but, even more important, there is always doubt about whether the mechanisms activated in responders differ from those in nonresponders.

In some studies, salt sensitivity has been defined on the basis of BP response to salt depletion after an initial period of salt loading (Deter et al., 1997). If sufficient time has been allowed to establish a high salt baseline followed by an approximate equilibrium on low salt, the identification of salt-sensitive individuals should be the same as during salt loading. However, some of the very short salt depletion protocols based on

Table 12.2. Examples of Protocols for Determining Salt Sensitivity

Protocol Sequence	ΔMAP LS-HS	NT_{SS} (%)	HT_{SS} (%)	Reference[a]
109 mEqNa (7d), 9 mEqNa (7d), 240 mEq (7d)	>10%		50	Kawasaki et al., 1978
9 mEqNa (7d), 249 mEqNa (7d), 9 mEqNa (4d), 40 mg furosemide 3× (1d)	>10%		50	Fujita et al., 1980
Adlib (1d), 10 mEqNa (4d), adlib (2d) 200 mEqNa (4d)	>5%	15	29	Sullivan, 1980[b]
2 L normal saline (4h), 10 mEqNa, 40 mg furosemide 3× (1d)	−10 mmHg	26	51	Weinberger, 1986
220 mEqNa (7d), 20 mEqNa (7d)	−3 mmHg	46%		Sharma et al., 1989
20 mEqNa (9d), 200 mEq (10d)	>10 mmHg	[b]		Campese et al., 1991
170 mmolNa (7d), 50 mmolNa (7d), 340 mmol (7d)	>10%	[b]		Higashi et al., 1996

Note: ΔMAP LS-HS, difference in MAP between last day on low salt (LS) and last day on high salt (HS); mEqNa, mmol Na, mEq (or mmol) of sodium; d, day; NT_{SS}, % of salt-sensitive normotensives; HT_{SS}, % of salt-sensitive hypertensives; h, hour; d, day.

[a]Reference according to first author and year.

[b]Both salt-sensitive and salt-resistant subjects were investigated.

Source: Sullivan (1991).

a small $\Delta MAP_{(LS-HS)}$ probably provide insufficient discrimination between the groups (Grim, Miller et al., 1979; Weinberger et al., 1986; Harshfield and Grim, 1997).

Last, identifying salt-sensitive individuals in terms of their BP responses is only the first step. To obtain information about the underlying mechanisms requires additional variables.

Salt Sensitivity Is Enhanced in Hypertension

This section considers some of the characteristics of Dahl-S and Dahl-R rats, the effect of cellophane wrap hypertension on salt sensitivity, and some of the changes associated with salt sensitivity in persons with EH.

Dahl-S Rats and Salt-Sensitive SHR

Both S and SHR have a primarily neural type of hypertension, in which high BP develops even on a normal salt diet, with a high salt intake accentuating the response.

The Dahl-S and -R rats

The S rat develops high BP even on low salt by about 4–6 weeks of age (figure 12.14; Rapp, 1982). When placed on a high-salt diet soon after weaning, there is a large and rapid rise in BP with 100% mortality within 3–6 weeks. But if the switch to high salt is delayed until the age of 3–4 months, the rise in BP is smaller, as is the mortality.

Salt loading has no effect on BP of R rats; however, CO rises and TPR falls (Ganguli et al., 1979). In S rats, both CO and TPR increase during the first few days of salt loading.

The causes of S rat hypertension on normal salt include (1) elevation of SNA, which is of major importance; (2) increased secretion of 18-OH-DOC by the adrenal cortex, which accounts for 15–20% of the early rise in BP (chapter 3); and (3) primary impairment in renal tubular function (Rapp, 1982). The excess rise in BP on high salt is largely mediated through central EO neurons (Huang and Leenen, 1998).

The hypertension on both low- and high-salt diets is attenuated by neonatal chemical sympathectomy with IV 6-OHDA or guanethidine (Friedman et al., 1979; Goto et al., 1981; Mark et al., 1981).[8] Similarly, bilateral lesions of the PVN nucleus (Azar et al., 1981; Goto et al., 1981) or of the A3V3 regions (Brody and Johnson, 1980; Brody et al., 1991) attenuate the development of hypertension. There is also attenuation in response to regular treadmill exercise, provided this has started early in life (Shepherd et al., 1982). Structural R_1 vessel changes are present in the systemic vasculature with the usual properties (Mueller, 1983).

Renal Function

Isolated blood-perfused kidneys of S rats on high salt excrete less salt and water than kidneys of R rats perfused at the same BP (Tobian et al., 1978).[9] Persistent exposure to high salt causes renal damage by 8 weeks of age, with focal tubular collapse and

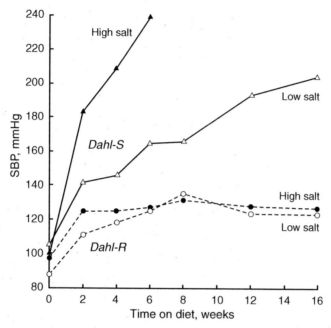

Figure 12.14. Time course of systolic BP (SBP, mmHg) in inbred Dahl-S (SS/Jr) and Dahl-R (SR/Jr) female rats after being placed on high (8% NaCl) and low (0.3% NaCl) salt after weaning at 30 days of age; $n = 10$ rats in each group. All S rats on high salt were dead after 8 weeks, while the others survived the 10-week observation period. From Rapp (1994), with permission of Elsevier.

dilation, together with scarring of the renal parenchyma. Micropuncture data indicate a greater prevalence of high glomerular pressures and hyperfiltration (Azar et al., 1977, 1978; Sands et al., 1992).

Roman (1986) examined renal function in two groups of 11–12-week-old S rats. In the low-salt group, the animals were maintained on low salt from birth. In the high-salt group, the rats received high salt for 5 weeks after weaning, which was followed by low salt for 2 weeks. In the high-salt group, the BPs and renal Vas Rs were higher than in the low-salt S rats, which, in turn, were greater than in R rats (table 12.3).

Perfusion was performed in the denervated kidneys with constant plasma levels of NA, AVP, aldosterone, and corticosterone. In each group, there was good myogenic autoregulation of renal blood flow at perfusion pressures between 100 and 150 mmHg, but GFR declined at the lower BPs (table 12.4). At all BPs, less water and sodium was excreted by the kidneys of the high-salt group than by any of the other groups. It suggests that the high-salt rats had not recovered from the exposure to high salt earlier in life. In low-salt S rats, excretion was also lower than in R rats, suggesting intrinsic tubuloglomerular dysfunction.

In S rats, a mutation in the $\alpha 1$-Na^+ K^+ ATPase increases the transport ratio of Na^+ to K^+ (Herrera and Ruiz-Opazo, 1990; Canessa et al., 1993). An analysis by Orosz

Table 12.3. Renal Hemodynamics in High-Salt Dahl-S Rats, Low-Salt Dahl-S Rats (S), and Dahl-R (R) Rats

Variable	High-Salt S	Low-Salt S	R
MAP, mmHg	158*	133*	123
Renal blood flow, mL/min/g KWt	4.5*	4.6*	5.4
Renal Vas R, units	35*	28.9*	22.8*
GFR, mL/min/g KWt	0.9	1.0	1.2
Kidney weight, g	1.7	1.5	1.5

Note: High-salt S rats were on 8% NaCl for 5 weeks from weaning followed by 2 weeks on low salt (0.3%); low-salt S rats and R rats were on low salt from weaning.
*$p < .05$ for difference from R rat. KWt, kidney weight.
At the perfusion study all groups had been on low salt for 2 weeks (see text).

Source: Adapted from Roman (1986).

and Hopfer (1996) has suggested that this increases renal sodium reabsorption (see Alpern et al., 1992). However, the magnitude of intrinsic tubular impairment in S rats is relatively small, and its effect on BP is related to the nephron heterogeneity that results from the high SNA and low NO.[10]

The high salt load reduces NO production, partly due to exhaustion of available substrate: When starting on a high-salt diet, simultaneous IV administration of L-arginine

Table 12.4. Findings in Isolated Perfused Denervated Kidney in Constant Neurohumoral Environment in Dahl-R Rats (R), Low-Salt Dahl-S Rats (LS-S), and High-Salt Dahl-S Rats (HS-S)

Renal PP (mmHg)	100	125	150
RBF			
R	4.7	5.3	5.3
LS-S	4.3	4.8	4.9
HS-S	3.5*	3.9*	4.2*
GFR			
R	1.2	1.2	1.2
LS-S	0.76*	1.0	1.0
HS-S	—	0.6*	0.95*
UV			
R	18	50	82
LS-S	12	30*	41*
HS-S	—	12*	28*
NaEx			
R	2	7.8	16.5
LS-S	1.8	4.0*	6.8
HS-S	—	0.9*	4.0

Note: Renal PP, renal perfusion pressure, mmHg; renal blood flow (RBF), glomerular filtration rate (GFR), urinary volume flow (UV) all in mL/min/g kidney weight; NaEx, sodium excretion μg/min/g kidney weight.
*$p < .05$ for difference from response of R rats.

Source: Adapted from Roman (1986).

attenuates or prevents the high BP (Patel et al., 1993). Indeed, medullary infusions of L-arginine diminish hypertension. This suggests that the diminished capacity of S kidneys to eliminate the excess salt through pressure diuresis and natriuresis is mainly due to reduction in medullary NO (Miyata and Cowley, 1999).

SHR and Salt Sensitivity

SHR hypertension is a largely neurogenic form of high BP (see chapter 16). Most SHR substrains are salt sensitive, but a few are highly salt resistant (Folkow and Ely, 1987; Oparil et al., 1988; Calhoun et al., 1994; DiBona, 1991; DiBona et al., 1996). It is not known whether the salt resistance is due to impermeability of the blood-brain barrier in the particular substrain.

In salt-sensitive SHR, the excess rise in BP on a high salt intake is largely due to an increase in SNA through brain EO neurons, and is reversed by blocking the amiloride-sensitive sodium channel with benzamil (figure 12.15; Huang et al., 1992). Even on a normal salt diet, the brain EO mechanism contributes to the elevation of BP. Recall that in these rats the rise in BP during salt loading is unaffected by SAD (table 12.2).

Renal Cellophane Wrap Hypertension

Renal cellophane wrapping induces gradual renal parenchymal compression due to pericapsular fibrosis (West et al., 1975; Fletcher et al., 1976; Korner, 1982;

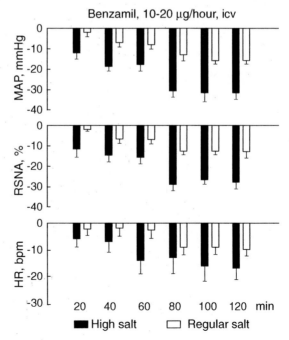

Figure 12.15. Effect of i.c.v. benzamil (10–20 µg/hour), which blocks the amiloride-sensitive Phe-Met-Arg-NH$_2$ sodium channel, on mean arterial pressure (MAP, mmHg), renal sympathetic nerve activity (RSNA, % of resting), and heart rate (HR, bpm) in salt-sensitive SHR on high salt (black rectangles) or regular salt (clear rectangles). After 60 minutes, all changes statistically significant. From Huang and Leenen (2002), with permission of *Hypertension*, American Heart Association, and Lippincott, Williams and Wilkins.

Denton et al., 1983; Denton and Anderson, 1985). It is a constrictor type of hypertension, the causes of which are discussed in chapter 15. In addition to the renal compression and elevation of renal Vas R, the causes include elevation of Ang II, a small increase in SNA, and widespread amplification of the systemic constrictor effects through R_1 vessel hypertrophy.

Korner, Oliver, and Casley (1980) compared the BP responsiveness to salt in wrapped and sham-operated rabbits. In each group, one kidney had been removed in half the animals at the time of operation, while the others retained both kidneys. The rabbits were on normal sodium for 6 weeks after operation and were then assigned to low-, normal-, or high-sodium diets of approximately 0.5, 5, or 50 mmol sodium/day, with tap water ad libitum.[11]

The sham-operated controls were very salt resistant, with $\Delta MAP_{(LS\text{-}HS)}$ averaging 2–3 mmHg in both one- and two-kidney subgroups (table 12.5). However, in wrapped rabbits $\Delta MAP_{(LS\text{-}HS)}$ averaged 15 mmHg, with the rise in MAP greater in those with only one kidney (17 vs. 12 mmHg). The greater salt sensitivity could result from greater nonuniformity of cerebral perfusion associated with R_1 vessel remodeling, where the microcirculatory blood vessels that are excessively perfused become more permeable to sodium, enhancing access to EO neurons through the blood brain barrier.

Table 12.5. Average Effects at the End of 2 Weeks on Low (L), Normal (N), and High (H) Dietary Salt Intake on Hemodynamic and Renal Variables in Sham-Operated and Renal Cellophane Wrapped Rabbits

Variable	Sham			Wrap		
	L	N	H	L	N	H
MAP, mmHg						
2K	88	89	90	126	133	138*
1K	87	90	90	118	132	135*
CO, mL/min						
2K	660	688	579	614	712	766*
1K	517	573	569	593	699	709*
Plasma Na$^+$, mmol/L	139	140	139	137.6	142.1	141.4
UV, mL/day	92	119	168*	96	84	129*
U Cr, mmol/d						
2K	0.98	1.02	0.90	0.86	0.85	0.80
1K	0.83	1.03	0.94	0.74	0.90	0.79
C_{CR}, mL/min						
2K	8.5	8.9	7.8	6.35	5.36	5.91
1K	4.8	6.1	5.3	3.38	4.81	4.20

Note: MAP, mean arterial pressure; CO, cardiac output; plasma Na$^+$, plasma sodium; UV, urinary volume; U Cr, urinary creatinine; C_{CR}, creatinine clearance; 2K, animals with both kidneys; 1K, animals with one kidney removed. *$p < .05$ for difference between low and high salt. For plasma renin values, see table 9.6.

Source: Korner, Oliver, and Casley (1980), and unpublished data.

The daily urine and sodium outputs of wrapped rabbits on high and normal salt were below those of normotensive controls, which suggests that their intake of sodium was smaller. This may have been due to the more pronounced depression of PRA and Ang II on high salt (table 9.6), lowering the input to the brain renin-angiotensin system that would normally result in drinking more water and eating more salt (Fitzsimons, 1994). In the wrapped animals, the increase in PRA on low salt was greater than in controls. In this series, the PRA level on normal salt was similar in wrapped and sham-operated groups, although in other series it had been raised during the first 4–6 weeks of hypertension (Denton and Anderson, 1985).

Despite being a constrictor hypertension, blood volume and CO were raised on high salt (Korner, Oliver, and Casley, 1980). This was due to a lower GFR, as suggested by the fall in creatinine clearance (see chapter 15). It is consistent with EO-induced renal vasoconstriction.

Salt Sensitivity in EH

Salt sensitivity is greater in lean and mildly overweight persons with EH than in those who are frankly obese.

Salt Sensitivity in Nonobese Persons with EH

Salt-sensitive and salt-resistant persons with established EH were selected on the basis of responses to salt-loading protocols where $\Delta MAP_{(LS-HS)} \geq 10$ mmHg after at least 6 days on high salt.[12] The subjects included in the four studies all had mild to moderate established EH: In two, the salt-sensitive and salt-resistant subjects were both Japanese; in one series, the salt-sensitive subjects were African Americans while the salt-resistant subjects were Caucasians; in the fourth study, all subjects were Caucasians (table 12.6). In all of them, the proportion of salt-sensitive subjects was approximately 40%. Clearly, salt-sensitive and salt-resistant phenotypes occur in all races, although there are racial differences in prevalence (Akinkugbe, 1985; Hall et al., 1985; Luft et al., 1985).

Fujita et al. (1990) studied the effects of salt loading on central hemodynamics. Average $\Delta MAP_{(LS-HS)}$ in salt-sensitive subjects was 15 mmHg, which was associated with a 20% rise in CO and a small fall in TPR. In the salt-resistant subjects, $\Delta MAP_{(LS-HS)}$ was 6 mmHg, and the small 10% rise in CO was largely offset by a fall in TPR. The most striking difference between the two groups was in the regional hemodynamic patterns. In salt-sensitive subjects, the defense response became manifest after switching to high salt, with forearm vasodilation and vasoconstriction in the hepatomesenteric and renal beds (figure 12.16). No such pattern developed in salt-resistant subjects.

The renal changes in salt-resistant subjects during salt loading included a decrease in renal Vas R, while salt-sensitive individuals developed renal vasoconstriction (Campese et al., 1991; Higashi et al., 1996). Campese et al. (1991) noted elevation in both afferent and efferent arterioles, with rises in filtration fraction and in estimated glomerular pressures (table 12.7). In the subjects studied by Higashi et al. (1996),

Table 12.6. Proportion of Salt-Sensitive Individuals in Four Groups of Subjects, as Discussed in Text

Total n	n, SS	%, SS	Reference
22	9	40	Fujita et al., 1990
26	11	42	Campese et al., 1991
23	10	43	Higashi et al., 1996
25	8	32	Koolen and Van Brummelen, 1984
96	38	40	*Total*

Note: n, number of subjects; n, SS, % SS: number and percentage of salt-sensitive subjects. In all series, $\Delta MAP_{LS-HS} \geq 10$ mmHg.

filtration fraction remained unchanged in salt-sensitive individuals but decreased in salt-resistant subjects (table 12.8).

Higashi et al. (1996) assessed the effect of dietary salt on renal NO production from the effect of a standard IV infusion of L-arginine on renal Vas R. In salt-resistant subjects, this elicited similar 13% falls in Vas R on high and low salt. In salt-sensitive subjects, the same 13% fall in Vas R occurred on low salt, but was lower (7%; $p < .001$) on high salt. The smaller Δrenal Vas R was accompanied by a smaller rise in plasma cGMP, suggesting that in this group the renal vasculature's capacity to produce NO was reduced.

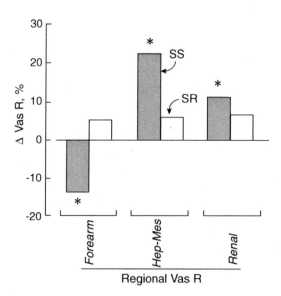

Figure 12.16. Regional Vas R changes after 7 days of salt loading in salt-sensitive (shaded bars) and salt-resistant (clear bars) subjects with mild to moderate EH. In salt-sensitive subjects, loading elicited defense response, while changes in salt-resistant subjects were not significant. From Fujita et al. (1990), with permission of *Hypertension*, American Heart Association, and Lippincott, Williams and Wilkins.

Table 12.7. Average Renal Hemodynamic Values in Salt-Sensitive and Salt-Resistant Patients with EH While on Low and High dietary Salt

Variable	SS (n = 11)		SR (n = 15)	
	Low Salt	High Salt	Low Salt	High Salt
MAP, mmHg	100	114	102	98
GFR[a]	102	107	97	100
RPF[a]	538	464*	482	534*
FF	19	23*	21	19
Ren Vas R, u	901	1238*	1026	954
R.Aff Vas R, u	460	571	432	452
R.Eff Vas R, u	440	667*	494	391
Est.Glom.P, mmHg	48	58*	58	52

Note: SS, salt sensitive; SR, salt resistant; GFR, glomerular filtration rate, mL/min; RPF, renal plasma flow, mL/min; FF, filtration fraction, Ren Vas R, renal vascular resistance; R.Aff Vas R, R.Eff Vas R, renal afferent and efferent arteriolar resis-tance; Est.Glom.P., estimated glomerular pressure, mmHg; u, units of vascular resistance.
[a]Expressed per 1.73 m^2 of body surface area; $*p < .05$ compared to low salt.

Source: Data from Campese et al. (1991), with permission of *Hypertension*, American Heart Association, and Lippincott, Williams and Wilkins.

In the fourth study, sympathetic function was assessed by examining plasma NA and NA spillover after 2 weeks on high and 2 weeks on low salt (Koolen and Van Brummelen, 1984). Following the change from normal to low salt, the rise in plasma NA was similar in salt-sensitive and salt-resistant subjects (figure 12.17).

During the first week after switching from low to high salt, plasma NA decreased significantly in both salt-sensitive and salt-resistant subjects (figure 12.17). However,

Table 12.8. Renal Hemodynamic Data in Salt-Sensitive and Salt-Resistant Patients with EH, While on Low and High Dietary Salt

Variable	SS (n = 10)		SR (n = 13)	
	Low Salt	High Salt	Low Salt	High Salt
MAP, mmHg	102	119*	103	105
GFR[a]	85	87	86	88
RPF[a]	568	617	587	676*
FF	14.7	13.6	14.6	12.9*
Ren Vas R, u	1050	1220	1020	940
PRA, ng AngI/mL/h	1.88	0.31*	2.46	0.38*
Ang II, pg/mL	39.3	20.2	30.9	18.1
P.Aldo, pg/mL	111	52.5	137	53

Note: Salt loading protocol in table 11.10.
[a]Expressed per 1.48 m^2 body surface area. PRA, plasma renin activity; Ang II, angiotensin II; P.Aldo, plasma aldosterone concentration. Other abbreviations as in table 12.7.

Source: Higashi et al. (1996), with permission of *Hypertension*, American Heart Association, and Lippincott, Williams and Wilkins.

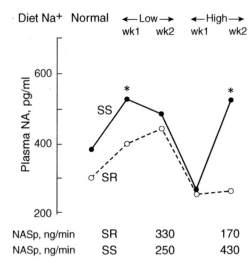

Figure 12.17. Plasma noradrenaline (NA) levels on normal, low (50–100 mmol/day) and high (300 mmol/day) sodium intake in salt-sensitive (SS) and salt-resistant (SR) subjects with mild to moderate EH. The order of the 2-week periods on low and high salt was allocated at random. NA spillover values at bottom were measured at end of period on low and high salt. From Koolen and Van Brummelen (1984), with permission of *Hypertension*, American Heart Association, and Lippincott, Williams and Wilkins.

in salt-sensitive persons it increased substantially during the second week on high salt. In addition, NA spillover at the end of the second week was greater than at the end of the low-salt phase. In contrast, in salt-resistant subjects plasma NA remained low, and average NA spillover declined from the value on low salt during the second week on high salt.

Thus, salt depletion initially evokes a rapid increase in SNA through baroreflexes, which minimize the reduction in BP in conjunction with reduction in RAA activity. This is more successful in salt-resistant than in salt-sensitive subjects. On the other hand, switching from low to high salt causes rises in BP in salt-sensitive subjects only, which is accompanied by a gradual rise in SNA, which is probably mediated through brain EO neurons that project to the defense area. Excitation of these neurons could be through increased sodium permeability of the blood-brain barrier or through renal ischemia in a challenged kidney, as discussed in chapter 15.

Salt Sensitivity in Obese Hypertensives

In obesity-related EH, the total and central blood volumes and the exchangeable Na^+ space are all greater than in lean hypertensives (chapter 13). Although renal SNA is raised, renal Vas R is lower than in lean hypertensives due the peripheral vasodilator action of insulin. PRA is raised and glomerular perfusion is not uniform.

Body sodium is closely linked to the raised fat mass, and in obese persons placed on a very low-calorie diet, the fall in BP is closely similar, whether sodium intake is low, normal, or high (Maxwell et al., 1977; Tuck, 1994). This is not so in obese adolescents, in whom the fall in BP on a low-calorie diet is somewhat greater when sodium intake is low compared to when it is high (Rocchini et al., 1989).

Obese individuals are thus fairly salt resistant (Tuck, 1994). The effect of altering dietary salt in obese persons in the absence of body weight reduction is not known. In animals, obesity produced by rapid overfeeding raises BP considerably

(Hall et al., 1992, 1993; West et al., 1992). Here too the independent effects of salt loading or depletion have not been determined.

Other Determinants of Salt Sensitivity

Three questions are considered below: (1) How does salt sensitivity affect the BP response to stress? (2) Why is salt sensitivity greater in human normotensives than in healthy animals? (3) Why is renin responsiveness to salt depletion and salt loading smaller in blacks than in whites?

Stress

A high-salt diet enhanced the BP responses to stress in a large study in male civil servants with normal BPs (Staessen et al., 1994). This suggests an interaction between EO neurons and the pathways subserving the hypothalamic defense response.

A related finding was that the BP responses to a stress test were greater in salt-sensitive than in matched salt-resistant normotensive men while on a normal salt diet (figure 12.18; Deter et al., 1997). Their salt sensitivity had been determined several months earlier. Here too the greater BP response is consistent with an enhanced defense response. A psychological questionnaire was performed at the time of the test, which indicated that the salt-sensitive men were more anxious, more irritated by their surroundings, and less able to contain anger than the salt-resistant subjects. These differences are similar to those that differentiate persons with EH from normotensives (chapter 11). From the BP findings and the psychological profile, it seems reasonable to conclude that salt sensitivity is a marker for the EH genotype.

The BP findings resemble the interaction between acute stress and dietary salt intake in BHR (figure 3.14, chapter 3). In BHR, the BP response to stress is slightly enhanced on a near-normal dietary salt intake (1% NaCl) and is greatly enhanced on high salt (8% NaCl), which also raises resting BP (Sanders and Lawler, 1992; Tucker and Hunt, 1993; DiBona et al., 1996; Huang and Leenen, 1998).

A high salt intake also increases BP responses during operant conditioning in Dahl-S rats (Friedman et al., 1979). Similar but smaller potentiation of BP responses has been observed in normotensive dogs and baboons (Anderson et al., 1983; Anderson, 1984; Turkkan and Goldstein, 1991).

Salt Sensitivity in Human Normotensives

In a normotensive population, the prevalence of salt sensitivity is smaller than in mild to moderate EH. The best available data suggests that the prevalence is close to 25–30% in normotensives, rising to 40–50% in those with mild to moderate established EH. The estimate of 25–30% is greater than that of less than 5% in healthy normotensive animals. It suggests that some members of the normotensive human population have features of the EH genotype.

Such a "pre-EH" group was identified by Harrap et al. (2000) in a survey in which the population was divided into four groups on the basis of their parental and personal

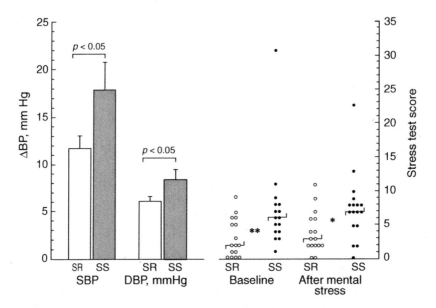

Figure 12.18. Left, systolic and diastolic BP responses (SBP, DBP, mmHg; means and SDs) to acute mental stress test in 16 salt-resistant (clear) and 16 salt-sensitive (shaded) normotensive subjects. Salt sensitivity and resistance determined several weeks earlier. Right, psychological scores of responses to EWL-60s questionnaire measured on two occasions before and after test. The psychological profile was different in salt-sensitive and salt-resistant subjects. From Deter et al. (1997), with permission of *Journal of Hypertension* and Lippincott, Williams and Wilkins.

BPs (Watt, 1986). Those with the highest personal and parental BPs had a lower exchangeable sodium space and plasma volume than the other groups and greater plasma renins, renal Vas Rs, and GFRs (table 12.9). Salt sensitivity was not determined, but the earlier experimental analysis suggests that these are some of the changes associated with increased salt sensitivity. Harrap et al. (2000) detected no polymorphisms in the genes for renin, angiotensin-converting enzyme, and angiotensinogen, which could have accounted for some of the differences in renal function.

Last, the absence of a rise in BP in salt-resistant subjects does not mean that the salt load is without effect. For example, during salt loading the rise in CO is often completely offset by a reduction in TPR (figure 12.19; Sullivan et al., 1980). It suggests highly efficient BP regulation due to the combined action of baroreflexes and ANP- and RAA-mediated hormonal changes. Even in salt-sensitive subjects, it is the effectiveness of these regulators that is responsible for the delay of several days before BP rises when some of the CNS mechanisms are engaged.

Racial Differences

Renin-angiotensin system responsiveness is significantly blunted in black compared to white subjects during both salt depletion and salt loading. This was observed after

Table 12.9. Blood Pressure, Renal and Volume Variables, Plasma Renins, and Body Weight in 100 Young Males and Females, Selected on the Basis of Their Personal and Parental BPs

Variable	Low Parental BP		High Parental BP	
	Low Personal BP	High Personal BP	Low Personal BP	High Personal BP
SBP	117	123	119	124
DBP	68	73	66	75
Exch.Na	41.0	38.8*	40.0	38.4*
Plasma vol	44.7	40.2*	40.9	39.2*
Pl.active renin	35.4	40.0*	38.0	47.6*
GFR	121	119	124**	138**
Ren pl.flow	611	597	611	621
Ren Vas R	83.4	89.5*	83.2	91.7*
Body weight	62.7	72.1*	66.4	69.5*
n	22	26	26	26

Note: SBP, DBP, systolic and diastolic BPs (mmHg); Exch.Na, exchangeable sodium (mmol/kg); Plasma vol, plasma volume (mL/kg); Pl.active renin, plasma active renin (mU/mL); GFR, glomerular filtration rate (mL/min/1.73 m²); Ren pl.flow, Renal plasma flow (mL/min/1.73 m²); Body weight (kg).
*$p < .02$ for personal BP from ANOVA; **$p < .02$ for parental BP from ANOVA.

Source: Harrap et al. (2000), with permission of *Hypertension*, American Heart Association, and Lippincott, Williams and Wilkins.

a furosemide-induced acute natriuresis (Kaplan et al., 1976) and also during several days of salt loading and salt depletion (Luft et al., 1977; Luft, Grim et al., 1979; Luft, Rankin et al., 1979). Whether this is genetically determined is uncertain.

Similar effects have been observed in black and white subjects with EH, who, after an initial period on high salt, were placed on a low-salt diet for 5 days (figure 12.20; He et al., 1998). In neither whites nor blacks was there a rise in BP during salt loading, but after 5 days on low salt, SBP and DBP fell considerably more in black subjects, in whom PRA and plasma Ang II rose less than in whites, while reduction in blood volume was similar in both. The greater fall in BP in the black subjects was explained on the basis of less Ang II-mediated systemic vasoconstriction than in whites. The lower responsiveness of the renin-angiotensin system in blacks resembles the nonmodulator pattern of Hollenberg and Williams (chapter 3). This also occurs in whites, so that the racial difference could simply reflect a difference in prevalence of this trait.

Last, the racial differences in responses to salt loading relate to differences in access and activation of central EO neurons. In S and SHR rats, the blood-brain barrier is very permeable to Na^+, contrasting with its marked impermeability in R and WKY rats. In humans there is probably a considerable range in sodium permeabilities related to both genetic and nongenetic factors. Among the latter is an increase in vascular permeability following local ischemic injury, which could increase production of vacular endothelial growth factor. The latter uncouples the intercellular junctions of endothelial cells, increasing permeability (Weiss and Cheresh, 2005). The increasing microcirculatory rarefaction and steal syndromes as

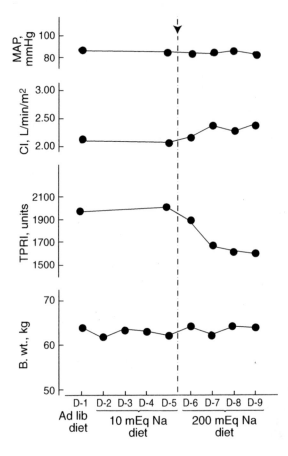

Figure 12.19. Average changes in mean arterial pressure (MAP, mmHg); cardiac index (CI, L/min/m^2); total peripheral resistance index (TPRI, units); body weight (B. wt., kg) in 10 normotensive subjects on low salt (10 mEq sodium/day) followed by 4 days on high salt (200 mEq sodium/day). From Sullivan et al. (1980), with permission of *Hypertension*, American Heart Association, and Lippincott, Williams and Wilkins.

EH becomes more severe bring about such ischemic changes in the brain. Other vascular growth factors of the angiopoietin family enhance focal apoptosis of endothelium, causing breakdown of the vascular barrier (Nag et al., 2005).

Other Dietary Factors and Their Relation to Salt

The rise in BP that is associated with migration from an "unacculturated" rural environment to a more sociologically complex "acculturated" urban environment has often been attributed to an increase in salt intake (Poulter and Sever, 1994). However, this is only one of several factors, including psychosocial stress and changes in other dietary constituents, which are summarized in figure 12.21.

In the urban environment, average calorie consumption is greater, hence the greater prevalence of obesity. The higher salt intake is associated with reduced consumption of potassium, while intake of refined carbohydrates, animal proteins, saturated fats, and dairy products are all greater than in the rural setting.

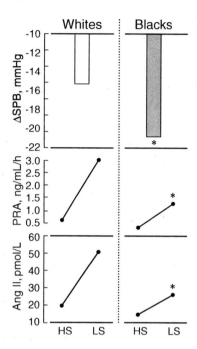

Figure 12.20. Changes in systolic BP (ΔSBP, mmHg), plasma renin activity (PRA, ng/mL/h), and plasma Ang II concentration (Ang II, pmol/L) in black and white subjects with EH after 5 days on low salt (LS, 50 mmol sodium/day) following 5 days on high salt (HS, 350 mmol sodium/day). *$p < .05$ for response differences between groups. From He et al. (1998), with permission of *Hypertension*, American Heart Association, and Lippincott, Williams and Wilkins.

Most of the effects on the acculturated side of figure 12.21 have adverse effects on health, while eating less red meat and more fish and fish oils containing ω3 fatty acids is generally beneficial (Beilin, 1994). Individually, each factor has only a small effect on BP, as a result of which their role has not always been taken very seriously. However, the effect on BP is quite appreciable in the framework of a dietary package in which several of the above factors have been altered. This was found with the DASH (Dietary Approaches to Stop Hypertension) study in the United States (Appel et al., 1997).

The DASH diet is rich in fruit, vegetables, and grain products and includes low-fat and fat-free dairy products, fish, legumes, poultry, and lean meat. On this diet, SBP/DBP were 6/3 mmHg below that of a matched group of subjects on a representative American diet of similar salt content. In a subsequent trial, the DASH investigators compared the effects on BP of the control and DASH diets at three levels of salt intake (table 12.10; Sacks et al., 2001; Greenland, 2001; Meneton et al., 2005). There was some interaction between salt intake and the DASH diet, but its major BP-lowering effect was largely independent of salt.

A switch from the control diet on 8 g salt per day to the DASH diet on 4 g salt per day reduces SBP/DBP on average by 10/4.5 mmHg. The changes are greater in hypertensives than in normotensives, greater in women than in men, and greater in African Americans than in other ethnic groups. Taken in conjunction with the BP-lowering effects of exercise and weight reduction, there is a substantial potential for nonpharmacological treatment of EH.

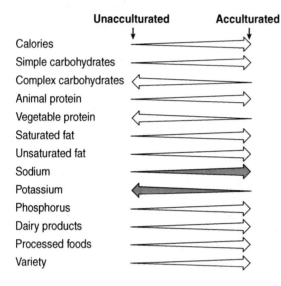

Figure 12.21. Typical dietary changes in persons migrating from a unacculturated rural to an acculturated urban environment. Adapted from McCarron et al. (1992), with permission of *Hypertension*, American Heart Association, and Lippincott, Williams and Wilkins.

How the DASH diet lowers BP is not known. Likely mechanisms include less production of reactive oxygen species, which may reduce vascular tone and diminish age-related fibrotic changes in the heart and conduit arteries (Hamilton et al., 2001; Dominiczak, 2005; Fuller and Young, 2005; Morris, 2005).

Role of Salt in the Pathogenesis of EH

The regulation of body sodium involves a large number of mechanisms, and their cooperative action ensures that changes in body sodium are relatively small during

Table 12.10. Comparison of Systolic and Diastolic BPs on a Regular Western Diet (R) and on the DASH (D; Dietary Approaches to Stop Hypertension) Diet

| | Salt Intake | | |
	8 g/day	6 g/day	4 g/day
SBP, mmHg			
R	132.6	130.5	125.9
D	127.0	125.7	124.0
DBP, mmHg			
R	83.0	81.9	79.5
D	80.1	79.5	78.5

Note: There were 412 participants, who were randomly assigned to either R or D diets, consuming the assigned diet at three levels of daily salt intake, allocated at random and each lasting 30 days.

Source: Sacks et al. (2001).

alterations in salt intake. The hormonal components of the control system modulate renal tubular function, while the neural mechanisms regulate renal hemodynamics, including GFR. At high dietary salt intake, the hypothalamic and peripheral cardiotonic steroids also become engaged in salt-sensitive individuals.

The action of the cardiotonic steroids in the CNS is a major factor in the excess elevation of BP on high salt in Dahl-S rats and salt-sensitive SHR. Both have a blood-brain barrier that is highly permeable to the sodium ion, which permits Na^+ to stimulate the EO neurons that project to the hypothalamic defense area. Their stimulation raises BP by elevating constrictor and cardiac SNA. The resulting high BP increases the level of systemic (and renal) vasoconstriction, which offsets any increase in salt excretion through the pressure-diuresis mechanism. The peripheral cardiotonic steroids, notably MBG, are probably more important in promoting diuresis.

In salt-sensitive humans, the sodium permeability of the blood-brain barrier appears to be of intermediate magnitude compared to the high permeability of S rats and the low permeability of R rats. In salt-sensitive individuals, a high-salt diet induces renal vasoconstriction, while plasma NA and average NA spillover increase, suggesting that EO neurons have become engaged. In subjects with high-renin EH, there may also be activation of central Ang II–producing neurons (figure 12.11). Last, in patients with long-standing severe EH with marked deterioration of renal function, high sodium loads readily accentuate renal ischemia, raising SNA through renal chemoreceptor-mediated input to the hypothalamic defense area (see chapter 15).

In normotensive salt-resistant individuals in whom all components of the control system are working, a corollary of the minimal changes in extracellular Na^+ and Cl^- concentrations is that the alterations in salt intake have very little effect on BP. This accounts for the almost complete salt resistance of healthy normotensive laboratory rats and rabbits. However, in the same animal, BP responsiveness to salt increases when renal mass is reduced, when the activity of the regulatory hormones is disturbed, or when baroreflex function is impaired. Salt sensitivity also increases in renal hypertension, reflecting the crucial importance of renal function. For example, in chronic renal cellophane wrap hypertension, all animals become salt sensitive. With moderate sodium loads, the rise in BP is largely due to elevation of CO, while with very high sodium loads it is due to increases in SNA and AVP (cf. figures 12.5, 12.6).

About 25% of human normotensive subjects are salt-sensitive in response to salt loading, indicating a much greater prevalence of salt sensitivity than in healthy animals. It suggests that a proportion of the human normotensive population has high-BP genes important in EH.

In mild to moderate EH, the prevalence of salt sensitivity increases to about 40%, with further rises occurring as EH becomes more severe. The increase in prevalence is associated with progressive elevation in renal Vas R, decline in GFR, greater nephron perfusion heterogeneity (figure 5.3), and reduction in renal NO. The cumulative effect of these changes is a reduction in renal capacity to excrete a salt load. The above changes represent the long-term effects of vasoconstriction on the kidney, which is associated with progressive reduction in functional renal mass and glomerular number, as discussed in chapter 15.

Many persons with EH also have genetically determined dysfunction of one or more renal tubular mechanisms involved in the transport of sodium, for example, the

Na^+/H^+ exchanger, the Na^+ K^+ ATPase, and the Na^+-K^+-$2Cl^-$ cotransporter. These mutations appear to have much smaller effects on BP than the very substantial effect that occurs in Liddle's syndrome and related types of monogenic hypertension. The reason for this is not clear: One possibility is that the renal dysfunction is partially compensated through other mechanisms, with the discrepancy becoming more evident when the number of functioning nephrons is low. This appears to be what happens in the Dahl-S rat when tubular dysfunction has a greater effect on salt sensitivity once the number of functioning nephrons has declined as a result of chronic renal vasoconstriction and the associated redistribution of blood flow.

During salt loading in the presence of renal impairment, blood volume and CO increase at least transiently, accounting for the early rise in BP. In addition, the systemic vasoconstriction associated with EH causes reduction of the capillary area, the extravascular tissue space, and total blood volume (chapter 5). On high salt, extracellular Na^+ concentration increases. At the same time a number of factors, including reduction in NO and local episodes of cerebral ischemia, make the blood-brain barrier more permeable to sodium, resulting in stimulation of EO neurons. There seems to be little stimulus for increasing AVP secretion by physiological the rises of Na^+ associated with a high salt intake. This resembles the difference in thresholds of the two mechanisms during hemorrhage (chapter 9).

The EO neurons in the diencephalon are tonically engaged in salt-sensitive persons with EH. This is suggested by the enhanced effect of stress on BP. Similar interactions have been observed in BHR. The important point is that it makes the EO neurons a normal part of the adaptive control system regulating sodium, rather than a mechanism of last resort.

This makes a strong case for reducing dietary salt intake in the routine management of EH. The International Society of Hypertension (ISH) recommends that the present intake of 9–12 g/day of salt should be reduced to 5–6 g/day. Indeed, it has been suggested that it be reduced to 3–4 g/day (Sacks et al., 2001; He and MacGregor, 2003). This may be going too far, since the associated large increases in aldosterone could cause excessive fibrosis in the myocardium and blood vessels (Weber et al., 1994; Nicoletti et al., 1995). Clearly, balancing the advantage of less neural drive with the disadvantage of more fibrosis is an area requiring further research. Hence, at the present time it may be best to aim at the 5–6 g/day target. This may also be more realistic, since most individuals still have an innate hunger for salt (Denton, 1982). Lowering the level of salt intake should be part of an overall dietary package that includes the DASH diet.

13

Normotensive and Hypertensive Obesity

The prevalence of obesity has increased over the last 50 years throughout the world, probably in response to greater affluence in many countries and a corresponding reduction in physical activity. There is talk of an obesity pandemic (Hill et al., 2003; Kopelman, 2000). In obese persons, there is a high probability of developing non-insulin-dependent diabetes mellitus (NIDDM, type 2 diabetes) together with coronary artery disease and EH. The combination of obesity, NIDDM, atherosclerosis, and EH is collectively known as syndrome X (Reaven, 1988, 1991, 1995). The reason for the association between obesity and EH is uncertain, and quite often one develops without the other.

A distinctive neural control system regulates energy balance. It includes a relatively straightforward feedback circuit that makes day-to-day adjustments of the balance between food intake and energy expenditure. Other components of the system determine longer term eating habits and physical activity. Like all areas of the CNS that deal with voluntary behavior, the operation of these other components is complex and has probably more to do with the development of obesity than the more automatic feedback mechanisms. Some of the hypothalamic neural mechanisms regulating energy balance influence BP but others do not. In about 50% of obese persons, BP is only a few millimeters of mercury above that of lean normotensives, and these are referred to in this chapter as having normotensive obesity. The other 50% of obese persons have considerably higher BPs than lean normotensives and are referred to in this book as having hypertensive obesity, that is, obesity plus EH.

The chapter begins with a brief review of the regulation of energy balance, including the sources of energy intake and expenditure and the CNS circuits involved. The latter include the forebrain mechanisms that sometimes override the strictures from the basic feedback circuits. This is followed by discussion of the hemodynamic and blood volume changes in obesity and the underlying hormonal and neural mechanisms. In gross obesity, free fatty acids become the preferred substrate for metabolic processes, while glucose transport is impaired (i.e., insulin resistance increases), resulting in NIDDM.

Obesity is associated with elevation of sympathetic neural activity (SNA). Some have regarded the development of hypertension in obesity as a failure of sympathetic control of energy balance (Bray and York, 1979; Bray et al., 1989). Another theory is that it is a by-product of the system's normal operation under conditions of excess food intake (Landsberg and Young, 1978; Landsberg, 2001). A third theory considers that stress is the underlying cause of both EH and obesity (Björntorp et al., 2000). The hypothesis suggested here is, broadly speaking, a variant of the last theory, that in some persons with EH the excessive food consumption is a stress-relieving response.

Definitions, Cardiovascular Risk, and Role of Genetic and Environmental Factors

Body mass index (BMI) is body weight in kilograms divided by the square of the height in centimeters. It correlates closely with densitometric estimates of body fat mass and is the most widely used clinical index for quantifying obesity (table 13.1; Kopelman, 2000). On BMI criteria, about 30% of U.S. adults were overweight in 1994 and 15–20% were obese (Kuczmarski et al., 1997). On current trends, it is envisaged that 40–50% of Americans will be frankly obese by 2008 and the trend in many other countries will be the same (Hill et al., 2003).

Another index is the waist/hip circumference ratio (W/H), which provides information about the sites of fat deposition (Kissebah et al., 1982; Kissebah and Krakower, 1994). The ratio is greater in men than in women and increases with age in each group. After allowing for age and sex, a high W/H ratio signifies greater abdominal fat deposition compared to deposition in the subcutaneous stores. Preferential deposition in the abdominal stores is called upper body obesity, while deposition in the limbs is known as lower body obesity. Overweight persons with a BMI of 28–29 kg/m^2 are at 5 to 10 times the risk of developing NIDDM than age-matched lean persons, and at 2 to 3 times the risk of developing coronary artery disease and EH (Kannel, 1991).

Table 13.1. World Health Organization (WHO) Classification of Excess Weight According to Body Mass Index (BMI; Body Weight, kg/[height, cm^2]) in Men and Women

BMI	WHO Class	Designation
<18.5	Underweight	Thin
25.0–29.9	Grade 1	Overweight
30–39.9	Grade 2	Obesity
>40 Obesity	Grade 3	Morbid

Source: Kopelman (2002), with permission of *Nature* and Macmillan Publishers, Ltd.

About 25% of the variance of body weight is attributable to genetic factors and 25–30% to cultural and shared environmental factors. The good news is that 45–50% of the variance is due to environmental and lifestyle factors, which makes obesity treatable (Bouchard and Perusse, 1988; Bouchard, 1993). The genetic inheritance is largely polygenic, except in rare individuals in whom obesity is due to a single gene defect.

Association between Obesity and EH

The Framingham data indicate that the chances of becoming overweight over a 10-year period are greater in those with EH than in those with normal BP (Kannel et al., 1967). A similar conclusion was reached in the Tecumseh study (Julius et al., 2000). In one analysis, 32-year-old subjects with mild EH were matched for age and sex with a group of normotensives. Both groups had been regularly examined from the age of 6 years onward. At that age, the BP was slightly higher in those who later developed EH than in normotensive controls, while body weight and skinfold thickness (another index of obesity) were similar in both groups. By 22 years of age, the BP, skinfold thickness, W/H ratio, and plasma insulin had all risen more in the future EH group, and these trends continued until the age of 32 years (Julius, Jamerson et al., 1990).

Another group was selected prospectively on the basis of being in the upper quintile of the BP distribution at 6 years of age. They were matched for age, sex, and skinfold thickness with other members of the same cohort. By 22 years of age, the rises in BMI and skinfold thickness were greater in those with the original elevation of BP (Julius et al., 2000).

Results from another investigation illustrate the association between family history for EH and gain in body weight. Here, healthy normotensive 25-year-old male offspring of hypertensive parents were matched for BP, age, and sex with offspring of normotensive parents (Allemann et al., 2001). Five years later, the resting BP was still the same in both groups, but body weight, BMI, and W/H had increased more in the children of hypertensive parents.

These examples suggest that a familial predisposition to EH is associated with a greater gain in body weight, which is often associated with impairment of glucose tolerance (Sharma and Grassi, 2001). This is also in accord with data from the countless series on various aspects of the clinical physiology of hypertension, in which lean subjects with EH are invariably 2–3 kg heavier than age- and sex-matched normotensives. It suggests a link between the mechanisms that elevate BP in EH and those that stimulate eating.

Energy Balance

In most adults, energy balance remains stable. When the balance becomes positive due to habitual overeating, the mechanisms by which the control system tries to restore body weight to the previous level include (1) consumption of less food; (2) an increase in physical activity; (3) an increase in metabolism through SNA-mediated adaptive thermogenesis; and (4) utilization of more fat in metabolic processes. The first two mechanisms require a psychological adjustment, that is, some intentional effort. If this is not forthcoming, the body utilizes the last two types of metabolic regulation.

Energy Intake and Expenditure

The intake of energy involves consumption of carbohydrate, fat, and proteins.[1] Energy expenditure is usually partitioned into several components: (1) basal metabolic rate (BMR), which includes energy for resting metabolism and maintenance processes, that is, the requirements for staying alive; (2) additional expenditure due to sport- and fitness-related exercise, which requires a continuous supply of ATP; and (3) adaptive thermogenesis (that is, heat production not related to ATP synthesis), which occurs due to an increase in SNA after a meal or in response to cold (Jequier and Tappy, 1999; Lowell and Spiegelman, 2000).

Energy balance becomes positive when energy intake exceeds energy output over days or weeks, when the resulting increase in body weight is mostly due to fat. Similarly, the loss of weight associated with negative energy balance is mostly due to reduction in the size of the fat stores.

Food-Related Energy Expenditure in Rodents and Humans

Young rodents have a special organ, brown adipose tissue (BAT), in which heat production increases through elevation of SNA after meals or in response to cold, which dissipates some of the excess energy. The brown appearance of BAT is due to the large number of mitochondria in its adipocytes, which contrasts with the smaller number in the white adipocytes in the other fat stores. BAT has a protein, UCP-1, which uncouples oxidative phosphorylation from ATP synthesis, so that an increase in SNA generates heat independently of work. Adult humans do not have any obvious BAT, and the postprandial rise in heat production is smaller than in rodents. Nevertheless, SNA also determines the postprandial and cold-related rises in heat production in humans, suggesting that their thermogenesis differs only quantitatively from that of rodents (Landsberg and Young, 1978, 1985; Landsberg, 2001).

It has long been a puzzle why, on closely similar diets, some people put on more weight than others. This was examined in healthy adults in whom body composition, energy intake, and expenditure were measured before and at the end of an 8-week period, during which 1000 kcal/day in excess of each person's maintenance requirements were consumed (Levine et al., 1999).[2] On average, 432 kcal/day were stored as fat and 531 kcal were dissipated through increased energy expenditure. However, weight gain varied considerably between different individuals, from 0.36 kg to 4.32 kg. At the end of the 8-week period, BMR had increased on average by 8% and food-related thermogenesis by 14%. Neither change in individual members of the group correlated closely with the corresponding increase in body fat (figure 13.1). However, there was a good inverse relationship between individual differences in the rise in body fat and the physical work due to nonexercise activity thermogenesis (NEAT), such as fidgeting and related spontaneous movements. The prominence of NEAT was due to the fact that the protocol did not allow sport-related exercise, in order to minimize the effects of variation in sporting prowess. The cumulative effect of NEAT-type muscle

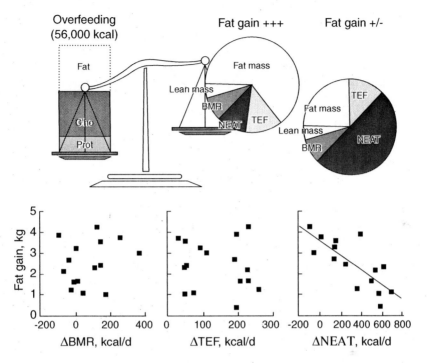

Figure 13.1. Top, results of 8 weeks of overfeeding by 1000 excess kilocalories per day, that is, a total of $8 \times 7 \times 1000 = 56,000$ kcal. In subjects in whom weight gain was greatest (fat gain +++), there were modest increases in basal metabolic rate (BMR), thermogenesis expended on food (TEF), and in nonexercise activity thermogenesis (NEAT). In those in whom there was little weight (fat gain +/−), this was largely due to NEAT-related energy expenditure. Bottom, data from individual subjects showing relationship between fat gain (kg) and ΔBMR (left), ΔTEF (middle), and ΔNEAT (right). Only the association between fat gain and ΔNEAT was statistically significant and accounted for ~60% of between-subject variation in weight gain. Adapted from Levine et al. (1999) and Ravussin (1999), with permission of *Nature* and MacMillan Publishers, Ltd.

movements on weight gain was surprisingly large and suggests that the fidgeters might normally have performed more recreational exercise than the nonfidgeters (Ravussin and Danforth, 1999).

Intake of Macronutrients and Metabolic Changes

The macronutrients are carbohydrate, proteins, and fat. In heavy drinkers, alcohol is sometimes considered separately as a fourth macronutrient.

Carbohydrate

Intake of carbohydrate stimulates release of insulin by the pancreas, which limits the rise in blood sugar by promoting glucose transport across cell membranes of insulin-sensitive tissues such as liver, skeletal muscle, and adipocytes.[3] In lean subjects, the process is efficient and rapid. In obesity, glucose transport is impaired and the pancreas compensates by secreting more insulin, which is responsible for the greater and more prolonged rise in plasma glucose than in lean subjects (figure 13.2). The changes are greater in upper than in lower body obesity. The extent to which the areas under the time–plasma glucose and insulin curves in figure 13.2 are greater than normal provides a measure of the degree of impairment in glucose transport, that is, in resistance to the action of insulin. As the compensatory capacity of the pancreas declines, NIDDM develops gradually (Kissebah et al., 1982; Kissebah and Krakower, 1994; Reaven, 1995).

Any glucose consumed in excess of metabolic need is transformed into glycogen in skeletal muscle and liver (Elliott and Elliott, 1997). However, the body's capacity to store glycogen is very limited, in contrast with its almost unlimited capacity to consume carbohydrate. Excess sugars are converted to fat, thereby utilizing some 25% of the energy content of the ingested carbohydrate (Jequier and Tappy, 1999).

Insulin secretion diminishes after a period of fasting when blood glucose concentration falls below resting. This is associated with raised secretion of the pancreatic hormone glucagon, which promotes breakdown of the hepatic glycogen stores to glucose. Liver glycogen provides the glucose used by most cells in the body, whereas breakdown of muscle glycogen is used solely for the muscle's own energy needs (Elliott and Elliott, 1997).

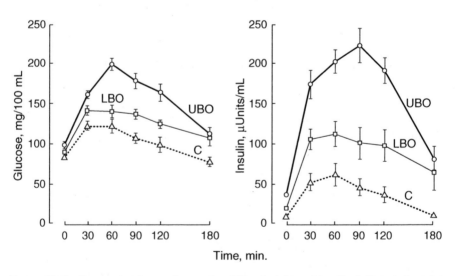

Figure 13.2. Changes in plasma glucose (mg/100 mL, left) and insulin (μUnits/mL, right) during standard glucose tolerance test in subjects with upper body obesity (UBO), lower body obesity (LBO), and lean controls (C). From Kissebah et al. (1982), with permission of *Physiological Reviews* and American Physiological Society.

Proteins

Dietary proteins are digested and absorbed as amino acids. They are used in tissues for the synthesis of proteins and peptides, and any excess is destroyed. The NH_2 groups are converted into urea and excreted by the kidney, while the carbon-hydrogen skeleton is converted to glycogen or fat.

Fat Storage and Mobilization

Following digestion, emulsification, and intestinal absorption, fat is transported through the lymphatics and bloodstream in the form of chylomicron particles (Elliott and Elliott, 1997). These consist of a core of neutral fat triacylglycerol and cholesterol esters surrounded by a shell of phospholipids, cholesterol, and proteins. In the capillaries, triacylglycerol is hydrolyzed by lipoprotein lipase, which allows it to pass through the wall as glycerol and free fatty acids (FFA). The expression of the enzyme differs in the various capillary beds, which accounts for the variation in FFA uptake by the different tissues. It is most plentiful in the capillaries perfusing adipocytes.[4]

Fat Stores

The abdominal depots include the mesenteric, perirenal, and pelvic fat, while the main peripheral stores are in the inguinal and gluteal regions and the subcutaneous tissue of the limbs and back (Jequier and Tappy, 1999; Kissebah and Krakower, 1994). In human adults, the fat is in the form of white adipose tissue. In adult rodents most fat is also stored this form, whereas in young rodents BAT is present in substantial amounts. BAT is also present in other young mammals.

   The body's fat stores are substantial even in lean individuals, in whom the fat stores suffice to supply 1 month's energy needs. In contrast, the glycogen stores are exhausted after 1 to 2 days without food (Levine et al., 1999).

   When energy balance is positive, FFA and glycerol become the preferred fuels in muscle and many other tissues. They are broken down from fat by hormone-sensitive lipase and by β_3-AR agonists and other lipolytic agents. Only the brain does not use FFA as a direct energy source and needs a continuous supply of glucose.

   In abdominal obesity, the susceptibility to lipolysis during elevation in SNA is greater in mesenteric than in peripheral adipocytes. Abdominal adipocytes have more β-ARs and fewer α-ARs than the peripheral fat cells. In addition, they release large amounts of FFA and triglycerides into the portal vein and liver, which stimulates hepatic formation of glucose (gluconeogenesis; Jequier and Tappy, 1999).

   With high rates of fat metabolism, more cholesterol is transported between liver and peripheral tissues in the form of different lipoproteins, increasing the risk of atherosclerosis.[5]

Central Control System Regulating Energy Balance

The sensing of information arising from the gastrointestinal tract and adipocytes occurs in the hypothalamus and NTS region. These signals elicit changes in eating behavior, autonomic activity, thermogenesis, and the level of arousal. A person may ignore (or suppress) the signals or respond to alternative stimuli.

Hypothalamus and Other Neuron Groups

Lesions of the ventromedial hypothalamus cause hyperphagia and obesity (Hetherington and Ranson, 1940; Le Magnen, 1983; Rosenzweig et al., 1996). Initially, food intake increases two- to threefold, but when after several weeks or months body weight has stabilized at a new high level, the food intake is often only slightly greater than before the lesion. It suggests that the control system responds to the usual afferent signals about a new set point, usually at lower gain (Schwartz et al., 1996). Lesions of the lateral hypothalamic area (LHA) are accompanied by the opposite response, with reduction in food and water intake until the attainment of a lower stable level of body weight (Anand and Brobeck, 1951).[6]

Kennedy (1953) was the first to propose that the hypothalamus influences eating by responding to inhibitory hormonal signals, which varied in proportion to the size of the fat stores. Experimental injection of insulin into glucose-sensitive hypothalamic areas lowered food consumption, leading Kennedy to think that insulin was the hormone in question. We now know that the hormone is leptin, the protein product of the *ob/ob* gene in adipocytes (Friedman and Halas, 1998).

The current consensus is that both leptin and insulin play a role in central regulation of energy balance. Rising leptin levels lower appetite and food consumption, while falling levels increase food intake. Targeted disruption of the *ob/ob* gene in adipocytes results in hyperphagia and obesity owing to plasma leptin deficiency (Woods et al., 1998; Schwartz et al., 2000). Hyperphagia also occurs after inactivation of the gene expressing hypothalamic leptin receptors. However, targeted destruction of the genes that express hypothalamic insulin receptor is accompanied by considerably milder obesity than that observed after inactivation of the *ob/ob* gene (Schwartz et al., 2000).[7]

During chronic overeating, the control system attempts to reduce food intake and to stimulate heat production and oxidation of various fuels. Weight loss has the reverse effect.

Plasma leptin acts on two populations of neurons in the arcuate nucleus (figure 13.3; Woods et al., 1998; Schwartz et al., 2000). The first is inhibited by high levels of leptin, causing release of two peptide transmitters, neuropeptide Y (NPY) and agouti-related peptide (AgRP). The second group of neurons is stimulated by high leptin concentrations, which increases production of proopiomelanocortin (POMC), the precursor of α-melanocortin-stimulating hormone (α-MSH), and a number of other peptides. Leptin also raises secretion of corticotropin-releasing hormone (CRH), which increases pituitary production of ACTH.

The neurons in the arcuate nucleus project to other hypothalamic nuclei, including PVN and the ventromedial and dorsomedial hypothalamic nuclei (VMH, DMH n; Fig.8.2) and neurons in the lateral hypothalamic and perifornical areas (LHA, PFA; figure 13.3; Elias et al., 2000; Elmquist, 2001; Marsh et al., 2003). Projections from LHA and PFA also engage a number of forebrain mechanisms.

Rises in leptin lower NPY and increase α-MSH concentration, reciprocally reinforcing each other to decrease appetite. AgRP acts on melanocortin receptors to

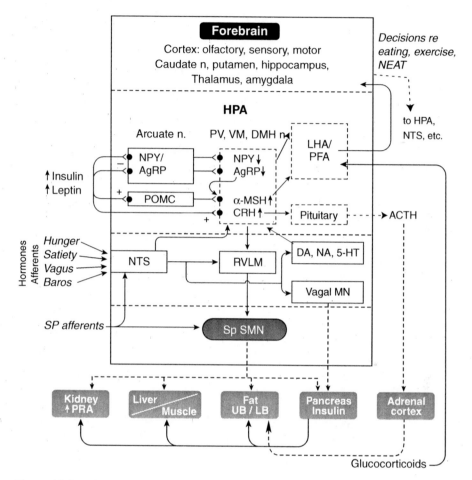

Figure 13.3. Diagram of control system regulating energy balance. Changes in plasma leptin and insulin affect neuron activity in arcuate nucleus (n), paraventricular (PV), ventromedial (VM), and dorsomedial (DM) hypothalamic nuclei (n). Transmitters released are (1) neuropeptide Y (NPY) and agouti-related peptide (AgRP); (2) α-melanocyte stimulating hormone (α-MSH), which derives from proopiomelanocortin (POMC); and (3) corticotropin-releasing hormone (CRH). Projections to forebrain, midbrain, and hindbrain regions go via lateral hypothalamic area (LHA) and perifornical area (PFA). Hunger/satiety hormones, vagal afferents from liver and gastrointestinal tract, and baroreceptor afferents project to NTS. DA, NA, and 5-HT neurons modulate target neuron responsiveness as discussed in text, including circuits mediating reward-related and addictive behavior. Effectors are at the bottom of the diagram. CRH increases glucocorticoid secretion, promoting upper-body obesity (UBO). Forebrain mechanisms may enhance or suppress activity in target neurons activated by leptin. RVLM, rostral ventrolateral medulla; MN, motoneuron; SpSMN, spinal sympathetic motoneuron.

antagonize the anorectic action of α-MSH. During weight loss, the fall in plasma leptin causes an increase in NPY and reduction in α-MSH, promoting eating and restoration of body weight. In obese individuals, the leptin-NPY and α-MSH-mediated feedback still operates during fluctuations in energy balance but at a lower sensitivity than when body weight is normal (Schwartz et al., 1996; Hansen et al., 2005). This is characteristic of an adaptive control system that has undergone a change in state. However, only the sensitivity for leptin-induced changes in food intake is reduced in obesity, while that for its cardiovascular actions remains unaltered (Mark et al., 2002).

In humans, mutations causing loss of function of the melanocortin receptor gene (MC4R) are associated with more binge eating and food-seeking behavior than in persons without these mutations (Branson et al., 2003; Farooqi et al., 2003).

Cortisol

High leptin also increases secretion of ACTH and adrenal glucocorticoids: Cortisol promotes increased abdominal obesity and often euphoria. In addition, glucocorticoid feedback to the hypothalamus antagonizes the actions of leptin. The absence of feedback in Addison's disease owing to the very low plasma cortisol may be the reason for the marked anorexia that occurs in this condition (Orth et al., 1992; Jequier and Tappy, 1999; Schwartz et al., 2000; Björntorp et al., 2000).

In a study on the effects of structured daily activity on cortisol secretion in 51-year-old men, about 10% found the experience stressful (Rosmond et al., 1998). Their daytime cortisol levels were greater than those who took the task in their stride (figure 13.4). The largest rises in cortisol occurred during the communal lunch period and were presumably due to stress arising from interactions with other people. The high cortisol promotes greater deposition of upper body fat in stress-related EH, while the euphoria may ameliorate some of the adverse feelings associated with stress.

Hunger/Satiety

Changes in fat stores depend on the size and frequency of individual meals and the associated signals about hunger and satiety (Le Magnen, 1983; Waldeck, 1983;

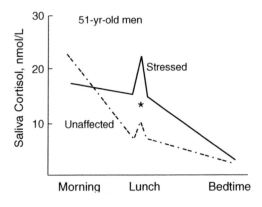

Figure 13.4. Saliva cortisol measured in morning, during lunch, and in the evening in 284 men aged 51 years engaged in structured activity around hospital. About 25% reported this experience as stressful, particularly during the communal lunch, whereas about two thirds found experience not challenging. In just under 10%, salivary cortisol was subnormal (not shown). Adapted from Björntorp et al (2000).

Woods et al., 1998; Schwartz, 2002). These are mediated through hormonal signals, through activity of vagal gastrointestinal afferents and segmental spinal afferents. Apart from leptin and insulin, the local hormones include (1) ghrelin, which is a hunger hormone that stimulates eating and is secreted by the stomach in anticipation of a meal (Schwartz, 2002); and (2) PYY_{3-36}, which inhibits eating for several hours and is secreted by intestinal and colonic cells (Batterham et al., 2002).

Forebrain and Subcortical Mechanisms

Some of the outputs from hypothalamus and NTS project to cortical and subcortical centers, which may influence and sometimes override the leptin-mediated feedback relating to the eating behavior (figure 13.3). In this regard, neurons in LHA are on the pathway for reward-seeking self-stimulation (figure 11.2), with connections to the orbitofrontal cortex (Le Magnen, 1983). Laboratory animals easily become addicted to freely offered tasty food, overriding the signals arising from the obesity-related peptides. Some humans also become addicted to eating, which initially gives comfort and relief from habitual anxiety and stress. Others simply enjoy the social companionship. Still others may resist the culinary temptations, partly due to insight about their body image or because they know about the adverse effects on health. Some persons are compulsive eaters, most of them without mutations of the melanocortin-4-receptor gene; it suggests that the brain can suppress obesity-related regulatory signals. Of course another important group is persons with restrictive eating disorders, who habitually override hunger signals and reduce food intake.

Monoaminergic and Peptidergic Neurons

Some of the molecules affecting eating behavior and energy expenditure are listed in table 13.2 (Schwartz et al., 2000). There may be some redundancy, with several

Table 13.2. Some Neuropeptides and Central Monoamines That Play a Role in the Regulation of Energy Balance and Appetite

Promoting Food Intake	Promoting Anorexia
Neuropeptide Y* (NPY)	α–Melanocortin stimulating hormone (α–MSH)*
Agouti-related peptide* (AGRP)	Corticotropin-releasing hormone (CRH)*
Melanocortin-concentrating hormone (MCH)	Thyroid-releasing hormone (TRH)*
Galanin	Cocaine and amphetamine regulated transcript (CART)*
Noradrenaline (NA)	Interleukin 1β (IL–1β)*
Dopamine (DA)	Serotonin (5–HT)

*Known to respond to leptin/insulin signals.

Source: Schwartz et al. (2000). with permission of *Nature* and Macmillan Publishers, Ltd.

transmitters subserving similar functions. For example, disruption of the NPY gene does not affect food intake, suggesting that other slow transmitter neurons compensate for its loss (Erickson et al., 1996).

The monoaminergic neurons affect eating behavior in response to stimuli that may complement or override the effects of adiposity-related signals (Oltmans, 1983; Salamone et al., 1993; chapter 11, this volume). Some NA and 5-HT neurons receive input from gastrointestinal afferents through the NTS, while DA neurons respond to anticipation of a reward such as food. Microinjecting NA or DA into the PVN increases food intake (Leibowitz et al., 1984). Experimental underfeeding lowers DA activity in substantia nigra neurons that project to the nucleus accumbens, which is part of the reward circuit (Pothos et al., 1995). Receiving a reward increases DA activity (Fiorillo et al., 2003) and stimulates eating. An increase in 5-HT neuron activity lowers food intake (Leibowitz and Alexander, 1998; Myers, 1978).

After i.c.v. 6-OHDA, the depletion of transmitter in DA and NA neurons is associated with substantial decreases in food and water intake and weight loss (figure 13.5; Korner, Oliver et al., 1978).[8] Eating is resumed after 2–3 days, but the pretreatment level of food intake is not reached for about 3 weeks. Thus, after depletion of DA and NA from the neuron terminals, it seems that the response to adiposity-related signals, which should elicit marked hyperphagia, is substantially impaired.

After destruction of 5-HT terminals, body weight also declines, with more gradual recovery than after destruction of CA terminals (figure 13.5; Head and Korner, 1982). This is not what would be expected from the results of PVN microinjections of 5-HT antagonists, which cause an increase in food consumption (Leibowitz and Alexander, 1998). Possibly, i.c.v. injection of 5,6-DHT exerts its action by lowering DA neuron activity, assuming that the series arrangement in figure 8.19 also applies to eating behavior.

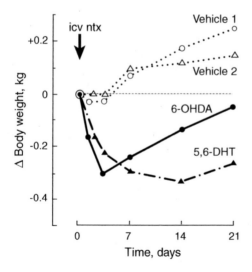

Figure 13.5. Effect on changes in body weight (kg) of i.c.v. injection (at arrow) of either 6-OHDA, 5,6-DHT, or vehicle for each neurotoxin, in awake rabbits. Body weights were similar in all groups at time of injection. Data from Korner et al. (1978b), and Head and Korner (1982).

Comment

This brief review has emphasized the adiposity-related feedback designed to maintain energy balance near normal levels. The change in system gain that occurs in stable obesity compared to its value during stable leanness is one pointer to the adaptive nature of the control system. Apart from interactions between the system-regulating energy balance and that regulating the circulation, there are additional levels of regulatory complexity associated with forebrain mechanisms that often modify the responses of the feedback circuits. They include psychosocial and cultural factors that influence eating behavior. Some components of these systems must be very old phylogenetically, as suggested by the recent analysis of feeding behavior in the nematode worm *Caenorhabditis elegans* (*C. elegans*), which is briefly considered below.

Stress and Feeding Behavior in *C. elegans*

Behavioral ecologists have long known that many organisms form social groups when encountering adverse circumstances (Wilson, 1975): (1) solitary locusts become gregarious in response to drought; and (2) birds of some species postpone mating to help their parents in the nest when nest sites are scarce (Sokolowski, 2002).

De Bono et al. have described two types of genetically determined feeding behavior in *C. elegans* (Coates and de Bono, 2002; de Bono et al., 2002). The worms normally feed on clumps of bacteria and, when presented with food, exhibit two types of behavior that depend on a single amino acid difference in NPR-1, the protein product of the *npr-1* gene, which is related to the NPY family.

The first variant is the solitary feeder, which forages alone and slows down and, on encountering food, separates from nearby worms. The other variant is the social feeder, which moves rapidly toward food in the company of other worms, so that the group eventually aggregates around the clumps of bacteria.

The sensors of adverse conditions (stress) in the external environment and celomic fluid are special transduction channels, which respond to pheromones. Two neurons, known as ASH and ADL, integrate the information and increase production of NPR-1 during stress, which suppresses social feeding. In contrast, inactivation of the gene from the ASH and ADL neurons transforms solitary feeders into social feeders.

Group feeding enhances the total amount of enzymes available for destroying the bacterial toxins, which are produced in amounts that can kill a single worm. Social eating thus has survival value, but the downside is that less food is available for each worm. The solitary feeder has more food but is at greater risk of being killed. De Bono has pointed out that, like NPR-1, mammalian NPY has a sedative action and decreases sensitivity to noxious stimuli.

Circulatory Effects of Obesity

The changes in hemodynamics and blood volume are similar in obese humans to those in obese animals. The effects of obesity depend on the actions of leptin and insulin and are similar in normotensive and hypertensive obesity. The higher BP in the latter condition is due to the major factors causing EH, including stress, salt, and obstructive sleep apnea (OSA). In normotensive obesity, the small magnitude of the rise in BP is due to partial masking of the central pressor action of leptin by the peripheral dilator action of insulin. In hypertensive obesity, the defense response is superimposed on the effects of normotensive obesity.

Hemodynamic and Blood Volume Changes in Obesity

The changes are similar in humans with chronic obesity and in animals in which obesity has been induced experimentally. The studies in humans are based on cross-sectional data in which the participants are in a metabolic steady state, whereas in animals steady-state conditions are often not fully attained after 4–5 weeks of overfeeding.

Normotensive and Hypertensive Obesity in Humans

Messerli et al. (1981) studied three groups of subjects who were lean, mildly obese, and markedly obese; each group included persons with normal BP, with mild EH, and with moderate to severe EH. The data in figure 13.6 illustrate four of the nine possible combinations of obesity and BP.

In the comparison of normotensive obese and lean individuals (NL → NO panel), MAP is only 6 mmHg greater in the obese group, while CO and blood volume are ~25% greater. TPR is markedly lower in the obese than in the lean normotensives, which suggests considerable peripheral vasodilation.

When lean persons with EH become obese (HL → HO panel), CO and blood volume both increase as in normotensive obesity and TPR is lower than in lean hypertensives. The MAP in obese hypertensives is only 6 mmHg greater than in lean hypertensives. On the other hand, when lean normotensives develop EH while remaining lean (NL → HL), CO remains normal and blood volume decreases, while MAP rises by ~25 mmHg due to elevation in TPR (chapter 5).

When lean persons simultaneously develop obesity plus EH, their BP becomes about 25 mmHg higher (NL → HO panel). CO and blood volume increase as in normotensive obesity, while (TPR between mild and severe hypertension increases, reaching a level well above that of obese normotensives.

Thus, obesity per se, that is, normotensive obesity, raises BP by only a few millimeters of mercury. It contrasts with the much larger rise in BP in the 50% of individuals with hypertensive obesity who are diagnosed as having EH.

Experimental Obesity in Animals

In dogs and rabbits on a high-fat diet, the hemodynamic and blood volume changes are similar to those in humans (Carroll et al., 1995; Hall et al., 1993; Hall, 2003b). The rises in MAP and heart rate in dogs, by 14 mmHg and 30 bpm respectively, are larger than in humans, which may simply reflect an absence of a steady state after a period of rapid elevation in body weight. Greater elevation in renin-angiotensin system activity may be an additional factor (table 13.3).

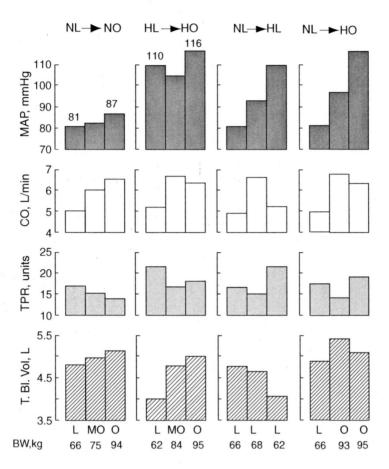

Figure 13.6. Hemodynamic and blood volume data in normotensive, mildly hypertensive, and more severely hypertensive subjects. Each group included lean (L), mildly obese (MO), and markedly obese (O) persons. MAP, mean arterial BP; CO, cardiac output; TPR, total peripheral resistance; T. Bl. Vol, total blood volume; N, normotensive; H, hypertensive. The body weight (BW,kg) at bottom is the mean of each group. Based on data in Messerli et al. (1981).

In the kidney, GFR and renal plasma flow are raised, while tubular sodium reabsorption has risen, accounting for the increase in extravascular volume (figure 13.7). Plasma glucose, insulin, and PRA are all substantially larger (table 13.3).

In dogs, the greater rise in MAP compared to humans is probably due to the more pronounced rate of development of obesity. It was associated with a 40% rise in CO compared to a 30% rise in humans. The renal vasodilation occurs despite a significant increase in renal SNA and increased renin-angiotensin system activity, the effects of which are masked by the peripheral vasodilator action of insulin.

Table 13.3. Changes in Cardiovascular, Hormonal, and Metabolic Variables and Body Weight in Conscious Dogs Studied before and after 1, 3, and 5 Weeks on a High-Fat Diet

| | Normal Diet | High-Fat Diet | | |
		1 Week	3 Weeks	5 Weeks
MAP, mmHg	83	83	94*	97*
HR, bpm	68	82*	96*	102*
CO, L/min	2.9	3.2	3.8*	4.1*
BWt, kg	24	26*	32*	35*
PIns, μU/ml	11.1	15*	38.5*	30.1*
PGluc, mg %	103	93	119*	121*
PRA, ng AngI/mL/h	0.46	0.90*	0.73*	1.10*
Aldosterone, units	2.7	3.8	3.1	3.7

Note: MAP, mean arterial pressure; HR, heart rate; CO, cardiac output; BWt, body weight; PIns, plasma insulin concentration; PGluc, plasma glucose concentration; PRA, plasma renin activity.
*$p < .05$ for difference from control on normal diet.

Source: Hall et al. (1993).

Role of Leptin, Insulin, and the Renin-Angiotensin System

Acute elevation of plasma leptin and insulin simulate conditions that take several days to develop in response to excess food intake and deposition of excess fat in the intact organism. At that time the most striking action of leptin is the elevation of SNA, while the hyperinsulinemia is causing widespread peripheral vasodilation. Elevation of renin occurs in response to the local vasodilator action of insulin and results in local formation of Ang II.

Actions of Leptin

Autonomic Changes.   During 3 hours of leptin infusion in rats, there is elevation in SNA in the outflows to BAT and to the kidney, with changes in the properties of the corresponding baroreflexes (figure 13.8; Hausberg et al., 2002). In the BAT baroreflex, leptin causes large shifts in both plateaus of the function curve, while SNA range and G_{av} remain unchanged. This is a "baroreflex-independent" shift (Korner, Shaw, Uther et al., 1973; Korner, 1979a; see chapter 10) and is in accord with a largely thermogenetic action of SNA on adipocytes. In humans, the rich sympathetic innervation on white adipocytes (Ferrannini, 1992; Rosell, 1984) probably subserves a similar function, but of smaller magnitude than in BAT.

In contrast, leptin affects the renal baroreflex properties mainly by increasing RSNA range and G_{av}, while the shift in the lower plateau is small. It suggests that leptin affects mainly the cardiovascular sympathetic outflow, with possibly a small BP-independent thermogenetic effect on renal fat (Haynes et al., 1999).

Circulatory and Hormonal Changes.   Following several days of IV (or intracarotid) administration of leptin, food intake fell by 60% in Sprague-Dawley rats, while MAP, heart rate, and renal Vas R increased by 8%, 7%, and 20% respectively

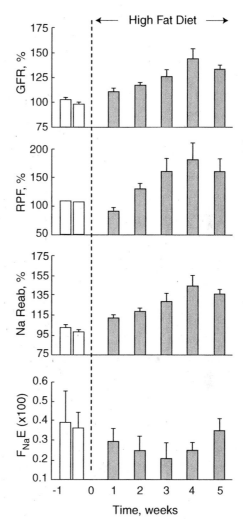

Figure 13.7. Effects of experimental obesity in conscious dogs on glomerular filtration rate (GFR), renal plasma flow (RPF), tubular sodium reabsorption (Na Reab), and fractional urinary sodium excretion ($F_{Na}E$); changes expressed as percentage of pretreatment control. Average control MAP 83 mmHg; after 2 and 5 weeks on high fat, MAPs were 87 and 97 mmHg, respectively. Adapted from Hall et al. (1993), with permission of *Hypertension*, American Heart Association, and Lippincott, Williams and Wilkins.

(Shek et al., 1998; Correia et al., 2001). Plasma glucose and insulin were also greatly reduced due to the fall in food intake, which is in accord with the major CNS action of leptin in increasing SNA to the fat depots (figure 13.8). Leptin also increases activity in some of the cardiovascular outflows, which accounts for the elevation in BP and heart rate; these changes do not occur in rats pretreated with α- and β-AR antagonists (Carlyle et al., 2002).

Chronic Leptin Deficiency. In leptin-deficient mice without a functioning *ob/ob* gene, NPY is raised, resulting in hyperphagia and obesity. NA turnover is reduced (Young and Landsberg, 1983) and resting MAP is about 14 mmHg below that of lean littermates from the parent strain (Mark et al., 1999). The *ob/ob* gene knockout mouse illustrates that obesity and hypertension are not always linked.

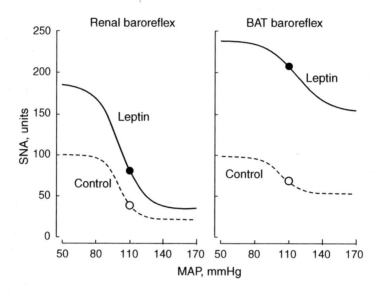

Figure 13.8. Baroreflex function curves from anesthetized rats, relating MAP to (left) renal sympathetic neural activity (RSNA, units) and (right) sympathetic neural activity to brown adipose tissue (BAT; SNA, units). Solid line, leptin infusion; dashed line, control; circle, resting value. After Hausberg et al. (2002), with permission of *Journal of Hypertension* and Lippincott, Williams and Wilkins.

Role of Hyperinsulinemia

After several days of insulin infusion in dogs, CO has increased markedly and TPR has fallen, which is similar to the corresponding changes in obesity, except that MAP falls slightly instead of rising (figure 13.9; Hall et al., 1992). The changes indicate pronounced peripheral vasodilation. The absence of a greater fall in BP is probably due to baroreflex influences and the effects of the raised Ang II (see below). In humans, similar changes have been evoked during acute euglycemic hyperinsulinemia (figure 13.10; Anderson, Hoffman et al., 1991; Baron et al., 1993).

Mechanisms likely to cause vasodilation include (1) raised endothelium-dependent NO production; (2) stimulation of the sodium/potassium ATPase pump; and (3) increased Ca^{2+} ATPase activity (Anderson and Mark, 1993). Ouabain abolishes the dilator response, suggesting that insulin stimulates the $Na^+ K^+$ ATPase to produce vasodilation (figure 13.11; Tack et al., 1996). The blood flow-related increase in NO undoubtedly plays an additional role.

The actions of insulin on the kidney simulate many of the renal effects of obesity (Hall et al., 1992). For example, insulin-induced vasodilation is mainly responsible for the rise in GFR, while increased tubular sodium reabsorption is partly due to the direct action of insulin on the proximal convoluted tubule (Baum, 1987; Kurokawa et al., 1992). The rise in PRA is a local response to afferent arteriolar vasodilation due to insulin (Ferrannini, 1995). The obesity-related elevation in SNA and the local actions of Ang II on efferent and afferent arteriolar tone limit the extent of renal vasodilation.

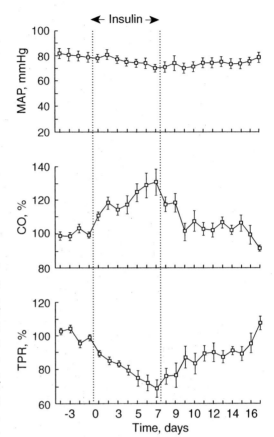

Figure 13.9. Effect of 7 days IV infusion of insulin (1 mU/kg/min) on mean arterial pressure (MAP, mmHg), cardiac output (CO, % of control), and total peripheral resistance (TPR, % of control) in conscious dogs. From Hall et al. (1992), based on Brands et al., (1991) with permission of *Hypertension*, American Heart Association, and Lippincott, Williams and Wilkins.

This contributes to enhanced glomerular perfusion nonuniformities, which is a factor tending to raise BP.

As NIDDM develops, renal nephropathy is accentuated (Dworkin and Brenner, 1992). A relative insulin deficiency develops in the glomeruli, which enhances the microalbuminuria, while the various lipid abnormalities accentuate the glomerulosclerosis (Kurokawa et al., 1992; Martinez-Maldonado et al., 1992). The end result is gradual loss of glomeruli and eventual renal failure (Dobrian et al., 2000).

Thus, the circulatory effects of obesity are to a large degree due to the peripheral vasodilator action of insulin, which also contributes to the elevation of blood volume. The simultaneously occurring CNS actions of leptin mainly subserve thermogenesis during transition from the lean to the obese state. Leptin also increases SNA in some of the cardiovascular outflows, for example, to the kidney. Its effect on G_{av} and SNA range may partially compensate for the dilator action of insulin. This also applies to Ang II, with elevation in PRA also a feature of human obesity (Grassi et al., 1995). However, the modest elevation in MAP is probably largely due to hydraulic feedback in the dilated vascular bed.

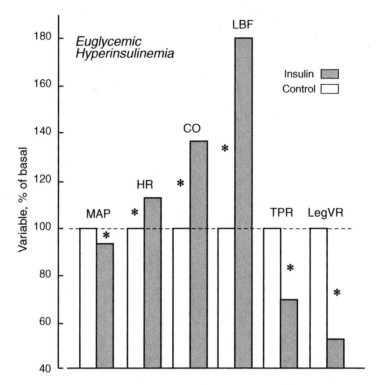

Figure 13.10. Effects of IV insulin (600 mU/m^2/min) given under euglycemic clamp conditions, on mean arterial pressure (MAP), heart rate (HR), cardiac output (CO), leg blood flow (LBF), total peripheral resistance (TPR), and leg vascular resistance (LegVR), all expressed as percentage of basal resting values in 19 subjects (BMI ≤27). *$p < .05$ for changes from resting, that is, Δ between white and shaded bars. Data from Baron et al. (1993).

Mechanisms Underlying Impairment of Glucose Transport

Insulin receptor signaling is abnormal in obesity. The impaired glucose transport leads to greater utilization of FFA and triglycerides for energy expenditure. Elevation of SNA, structural changes in R$_1$ vessels, and other microcirculatory factors may further impair glucose transport. In gross obesity, the number of adipocytes available for storage of fat becomes inadequate, further compounding the metabolic problems.

Role of Insulin Receptors

Glucose cannot penetrate the lipid bilayers of cellular membranes and requires transporter proteins to enter the cytoplasm, which are recruited by insulin signaling (Elliott and Elliott, 1997).[9] In contrast, FFA is freely soluble in cellular membranes and rapidly diffuses into cytoplasm. Hepatic FFA metabolism increases markedly in upper body obesity and stimulates glycogen breakdown and glucose production

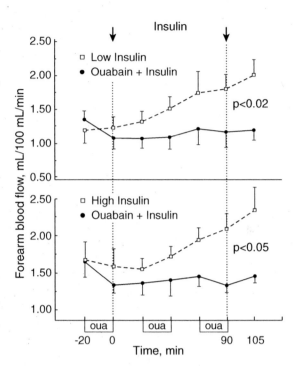

Figure 13.11. Time course of changes in human forearm blood flow (mL/100 mL/min) during IV insulin infusions given under euglycemic conditions. Insulin infused into the control arm (dashed line), while other arm (solid line) received insulin plus intraarterial ouabain to block Na,K-ATPase activity. Six subjects received low-dose insulin (430 pmol/m^2/min) and six others received high-dose insulin (860 pmol/m^2/min). From Tack et al. (1996), with permission of *Hypertension*, American Heart Association, and Lippincott, Williams and Wilkins.

(Jequier, 1993; Reaven, 1995). This accounts for the higher plasma concentration of FFA and the greater utilization of FFA over glucose in upper compared to lower body obesity.

In obesity, signaling through the insulin receptor becomes less efficient. This may be due to (1) factors that inhibit the action of insulin on different target cells (figure 13.12), thereby causing the pancreas to increase insulin secretion to compensate for this; and (2) major genetic structural defects in the insulin receptor, which is a tyrosine kinase transmembrane receptor; these defects are rare and are unrelated to insulin resistance in obesity (Kahn, 1995).

Insulin receptor inhibitors include the glycoproteins pp63 and PC-1, which prevent phosphorylation of insulin receptor substrate-1 and may play a minor role in adult obesity (Lienhard, 1994). A molecule of potential interest is Rad, a member of the Ras/GTPase superfamily, which plays a role in the translocation of glucose transporters. A factor that is produced in increased amounts by adipocytes in obesity is tumor necrosis factor α (TNF-α), which reduces insulin receptor tyrosine kinase activity in skeletal muscle and fat (Hotamisligil et al., 1994, 1996).

The expression of TNF-α by adipocytes is prevented by inactivation of the gene that encodes fatty acid binding protein aP2 (Hotamisligil et al., 1996). The homozygous mutants of this gene are metabolically normal: The animals become obese when offered a tasty diet but do not develop insulin resistance, in contrast to what happens in wild-type mice. It suggests that additional signals from adipocytes can impair glucose transport in obesity.

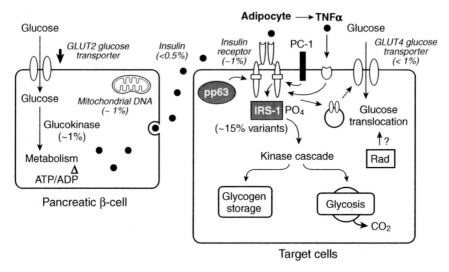

Figure 13.12. Some factors that give rise to non-insulin-dependent diabetes mellitus (NIDDM). NIDDM can results from insulin resistance at target cell (liver, muscle, fat) and from inadequate insulin production by pancreatic β-cells. Genetic defects account for a small percentage of NIDDM (i.e., number in parentheses). Another factor is downregulation of GLUT2 glucose transporter in β-cells. The action of insulin in target cells can be inhibited by PC-1, pp63, Rad (a Ras-related protein), and signals mediated by the TNF-α receptor. PC-1, pp63, and TNF-α reduce the insulin-receptor tyrosine kinase activity, while Rad acts intracellularly and affects translocation of GLUT4 transporter to the plasma membrane. From Kahn (1995), with permission of *Nature* and Macmillan Publishers, Ltd.

In the FIRKO (fat-specific insulin receptor knockout) mouse, the insulin receptor gene has been inactivated solely in adipose tissue (Blueher et al., 2003). The fat mass and body weight of these mutants are lower than in wild-type mice and they have normal glucose tolerance and a 25% longer life span (figure 13.13). The beneficial effects of fat-specific loss of insulin receptors contrast strikingly with the effects of generalized loss of insulin receptors, which are uniformly adverse, causing insulin resistance, obesity, severe diabetes, and reduction in life span (Kahn et al., 1992). A beneficial effect on health similar to that in the FIRKO mouse was described by Elsie Widdowson in the 1930s and 1940s in rats subjected to a lifetime of calorie restriction (McCance and Widdowson, 1974).

Differentiation and Growth of Adipocytes

As obesity increases, the fat stores expand through an increase in size of existing adipocytes and formation of new adipocytes from fibroblast-like preadipocytes. Differentiation of the latter is normally inhibited by several factors produced by mature adipocytes, including (1) mitogens and oncogenes, such as PDGF, EGF, and FGF; and (2) cytokines, such as TNF-α, IL-1, IL-6, TGF-β, and interferon-γ (Hu et al., 1996; Frühbeck, 2004). The inhibition is due to phosphorylation of peroxisome proliferator activated receptor γ, which is the dominant transcription factor in adipose tissue.

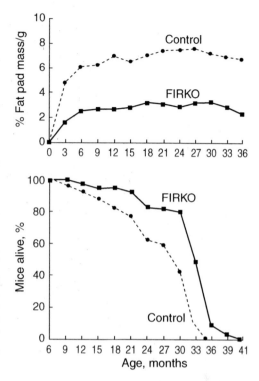

Figure 13.13. In the FIRKO mouse, there has been targeted disruption of insulin receptors in adipocytes, resulting in (top) less subcutaneous fat deposition than in wild-type controls, and (bottom) an increase in life span. From Blueher et al. (2003), with permission of American Association for the Advancement of Science.

Another inhibitor of differentiation is Ang II (Sharma et al., 2002). Adipocytes normally express Ang II-forming enzymes in amounts that are inversely related to insulin sensitivity (Gorzelniak et al., 2002; Janke et al., 2002). Ang II produced by large adipocytes is believed to inhibit differentiation of nearby preadipocytes (figure 13.14). If fat storage is inadequate, lipid is deposited as droplets in many tissues, including muscle, liver, and pancreas, causing further impairment of glucose transport (McGarry and Dobbins, 1999). Blockade of the renin-angiotensin system causes an increase in preadipocyte differentiation to new adipocytes. The new adipocytes are smaller and more responsive to insulin than the large adult adipocytes. Last, the incidence of type 2 diabetes is reduced by treating obese hypertensives with ACE inhibitors or AT_1 receptor antagonists.

Microcirculatory Factors

The state of the microcirculation in the skeletal muscle bed is a major factor contributing to the variation of glucose uptake between subjects. During administration of insulin, the large average vasodilator response (e.g., in figure 13.10) masks the considerable variation in individual responses. Baron et al. (1993) noted that glucose uptake was greatest in those with the widest cross-sectional area of the bed and was least in those with the narrowest cross-sectional area. They concluded that glucose uptake depended on the capillary area in contact with the skeletal muscle fibers.

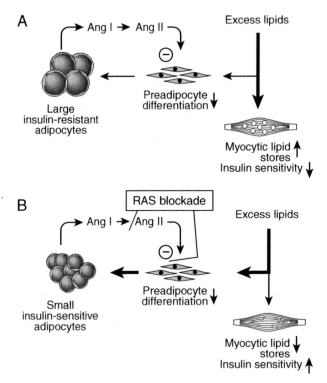

Figure 13.14. Diagrams show (A) that Ang II formed in relatively insulin-resistant large adipocytes inhibits differentiation of preadipocytes into mature adipocytes, so that excess lipid is stored in droplet form in skeletal muscle and other cells. (B) After blockade of the renin-angiotensin system, the preadipocytes differentiate into small insulin-sensitive adipocytes. From Sharma et al. (2002), with permission of *Hypertension*, American Heart Association, and Lippincott, Williams and Wilkins.

Rocchini et al. (1992) reached the same conclusion from the results obtained in 95 obese adolescents. They compared the results obtained during a standard glucose tolerance test with the magnitude of the dilator response during maximum reactive forearm hyperemia. The rise in plasma insulin was smallest in those with the lowest value of Vas R during maximum dilation (R_{min}), which corresponds to the widest average arteriolar diameter (figure 13.15). Moreover, they studied the effect of a 20-week weight reduction program, in which about two thirds of the subjects had lost weight. The extent of their improvement in glucose transport was directly related to the degree of fall in R_{min}.

Some of the factors that alter the size of the capillary bed in muscle include (1) alterations in SNA; (2) changes in endothelial or neural NO; and (3) vascular structural remodeling.

Sympathetic Activity

In resting skeletal muscle, blood flow per gram is low, so that neural vasoconstriction further increases the proportion of capillaries that are poorly perfused, limiting the interface available for diffusion of glucose. This explains the results of reflex elevation in sympathetic tone in the human forearm, which reduces insulin-mediated glucose uptake by about 20%, without affecting O_2 utilization (Jamerson et al., 1993).

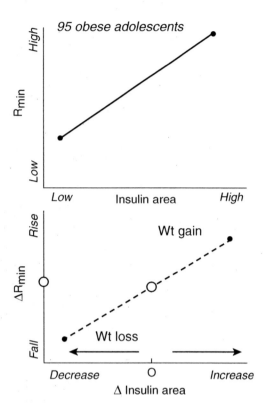

Figure 13.15. Results of glucose tolerance test performed in obese adolescents. Top, during reactive hyperemia, forearm R_{min} is directly related to area under the insulin time-concentration curve, so that the greater the insulin resistance, the greater R_{min}, which is a measure of R_1 vessel structural changes. Bottom, extent of variation in responses in the same subjects after 20-week low calorie diet. In those who lost weight, insulin area and R_{min} both decreased, while both increased in those unable to lose weight. Adapted from Rocchini et al. (1992).

Rocchini et al. (1999) studied the effects of clonidine on glucose transport in dogs on a high-fat diet. Although they gained as much weight as untreated controls, their glucose transport remained normal (figure 13.16) and they did not develop the characteristic circulatory and hormonal changes associated with obesity. Clonidine produces long-term reduction in SNA through stimulation of central α_2-AR in the hindbrain, which is more likely to have caused the above changes than the drug's effect on the parasympathetic nervous system (Shaw et al., 1971; Korner, West et al., 1974; Badoer et al., 1983).

Reduction of NO Availability

The high resting blood flows in obesity due to the hyperinsulinemia raises NO and makes microcirculatory perfusion more uniform (chapter 6). This explains the greater glucose uptake by skeletal muscle when R_{min} is low and flow rates are high (Baron, 1996). NOS inhibitors (or factors that inhibit NOS, e.g., glucocorticoids) have the opposite effect and reduce glucose uptake.

In rats on a high-fat diet for 16 months (i.e., for a large part of their life span), NO is reduced considerably compared with animals on a low-fat diet (Roberts et al., 2000). High-fat diets also raise prostanoids, vascular thromboxanes, and endothelin-1 (Traupe et al., 2002).

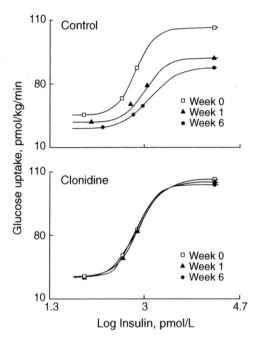

Figure 13.16. Top, effects of a high-fat diet on whole body insulin-mediated glucose uptake (M) over a wide range of steady-state insulin concentrations studied under euglycemic conditions: at times 0 (before diet) and after 1 and 6 weeks on diet. Note gradual reduction in glucose uptake on diet. Bottom, in dogs receiving clonidine (0.3 mg orally, 2×/day) on the same diet, glucose uptake remained unchanged. Body weight gain on high fat was 3.9 kg (17%) in dogs not receiving clonidine, and 4.2 kg (19%) while on clonidine. From Rocchini et al. (1999), with permission of *Hypertension*, American Heart Association, and Lippincott, Williams and Wilkins.

Structural Changes

Insulin and insulin-related growth factors promote hypertrophy and hyperplasia of VSM cells. However, in obese hypertensives the amplifier action of the R_1 vessels is less than that caused by similar changes in lean persons with EH. This is mainly due to the greater widening of their resting R_1 vessels, which reduces the mechanical advantage of the structural remodeling (see table 6.5).

Autonomic Mechanisms and Human Obesity

There is a considerable divergence of views about the role of the sympathetic nervous system in obesity (Grassi, 1999; Somers, 1999). Some have considered that obesity is due to inadequate sympathetically mediated thermogenesis (Bray and York, 1979; Bray et al., 1989). Others regard thermogenesis-related SNA in obesity as sufficient to raise BP to levels in EH (Landsberg and Young, 1978, 1985; Landsberg, 2001). A third view is that psychosocial stress is the cause of both obesity and EH (Björntorp, 1996; Björntorp et al., 2000).

What none of the theories has adequately allowed for is that the functional priorities of the sympathetic nervous system alter during the period of overeating before body weight becomes stable. This is illustrated below by considering the regulatory mechanisms after (1) the first large meal, before there has been significant accumulation of fat; (2) a 10-day period of overfeeding, when adaptive thermogenesis is high; and (3) during the new steady state in chronic normotensive and hypertensive obesity, when adaptive thermogenesis is nearly normal. Last, the SNA patterns in hypertensive and normotensive obesity have been compared with the patterns in lean normotensives and in lean persons with EH.

The Start of Overfeeding: Effects of a Large Meal

Esler and coworkers studied the effects of a rather gargantuan meal (Cox et al., 1995; Vaz et al., 1995):[10] MAP remained unaltered, while gastrointestinal, renal, and forearm blood flows all increased, with the latter rising in parallel with body O_2 consumption.

Plasma insulin levels peaked by about 30 minutes after the ingestion of food, with more gradual rises in SNA and body O_2 consumption (figure 13.17). The increases in renal and muscle SNA were greater than average NA spillover, while cardiac NA spillover and plasma adrenaline remained unchanged.

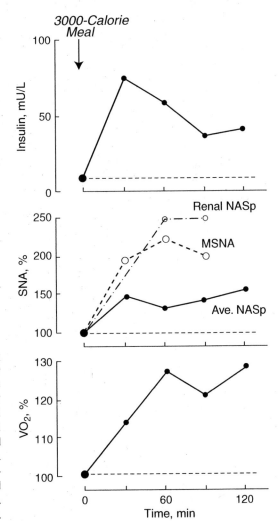

Figure 13.17. Effects of a high-calorie meal (consumed at arrow) on plasma insulin concentration (mU/L), sympathetic neural activity (SNA) including average and renal noradrenaline spillover (Ave, renal NASp), muscle SNA (MSNA), and body O_2 consumption (VO_2). SNA and VO_2 data expressed as percentage of preprandial control ($\equiv 100\%$). Based on Cox et al. (1995); Vaz et al. (1995).

The rise in SNA evoked by the meal moderates the substantial insulin-induced peripheral vasodilation and is most likely mediated through baroreflexes. Little fat accumulates over the first 2 hours since starting the meal, so that only some of the rise of SNA subserves adaptive thermogenesis.

It has been suggested that the central action of insulin accounts for much of the increase in SNA (Anderson et al., 1991; Baskin et al., 1987). However, it is more likely that baroreflexes are the dominant mechanism raising SNA and maintaining MAP. Gastrointestinal vasodilation is large, due partly to digestion and partly to the peripheral dilator action of insulin, and the arteriolar vasodilation is responsible for a large passive increase in regional blood volume because of the marked venous distensibility, which means drawing the extra blood volume from the low-pressure regions of the central thoracic compartment (chapter 5). This produces unloading of the cardiopulmonary baroreceptors despite absence of a significant fall in MAP.

Ten Days of Overeating

O'Dea et al. (1982) examined the metabolic and autonomic effects of three dietary regimens, each of 10 days duration, in 6 subjects.[11] The diets were (1) one that maintained body weight constant, (2) a high-energy diet in excess of metabolic requirements, and (3) a low-energy diet. Sodium intake was kept constant at 160 mmol/day on all diets.

Underfeeding caused a fall in body weight and slight decreases in average NA spillover and plasma triiodothyronine (T_3) concentration (figure 13.18). With overfeeding, the body weight increased by 2.5 kg and MAP rose by 4 mmHg, while total NA spillover and T_3 also increased. After 10 days of excess food intake there was a significant accumulation of fat, with rises in plasma leptin and insulin. The actions of leptin at this time subserved increased thermogenesis and vasoconstriction and cardiac support (figure 13.8), with T_3 also contributing to the greater metabolic heat production (Larsen and Ingbar, 1992). The rise in renal SNA helped to raise renal sodium and water reabsorption, contributing to the renal actions of insulin in raising extravascular fluid and blood volume. Overall this increases load on all the cardiopulmonary baroreceptors. Hence, the only excitatory source of SNA is through leptin, which slightly overcorrects the peripheral vasodilation.

Conditions during overfeeding in this experiment probably represent the time when thermogenesis is near maximal during development of obesity. Landsberg and Young's theory that the rise in SNA was sufficient to raise BP to levels in EH was largely based on NA turnover studies in BAT and LV (Landsberg, 2001). This overestimates the corresponding changes in human SNA of the outflows in fat, the peripheral tissues, and heart.

Chronic Changes in SNA Patterns in Normotensive and Hypertensive Obesity

The serial changes in average and renal NA spillover from the first large meal to chronic normotensive obesity are summarized in figure 13.19 (Esler, 1995; Rumantir et al., 1999; Vaz et al., 1997). In chronic obesity, average SNA has declined from the

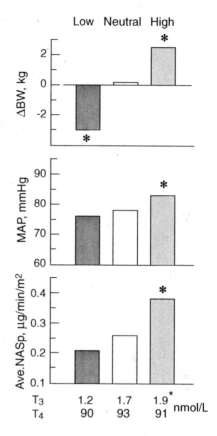

Figure 13.18. Change of body weight (ΔBW, kg) and values of mean arterial pressure (MAP, mmHg) and average noradrenaline spillover rate (Ave.NASp, μg/min/m^2) at the end of three 10-day periods on (1) a neutral diet; (2) a diet of 1000 kcal/m^2 BSA/day above maintenance requirements (high); (3) a 400 kcal/day diet (low). Numbers at bottom: plasma triiodothyronine and thyroxine levels (T_3, T_4, nmol/L). Data from O'Dea et al. (1982).

larger earlier values, which suggests that at the new body weight equilibrium SNA-mediated thermogenesis has decreased from the earlier peak.[12] Another factor is that the high cardiopulmonary load due to fluid retention causes some baroreflex-mediated inhibition of SNA.

However, renal SNA in chronic obesity is only slightly less than at the start of overeating. This could be an ongoing specific cardiovascular effect through the melanocortin pathway, even though food intake has fallen from the original peak (Mark et al., 2002). Another possibility is that increased stimulation of renal chemoreceptors may raise RSNA, as deterioration of renal function accelerates (chapter 15; Stella and Zanchetti, 1991; DiBona and Kopp, 1997).

Sympathetic Patterns in Lean Persons with EH Compared with Those in Hypertensive and Normotensive Obesity

Average, renal, and cardiac NA spillover are all greater in lean persons with EH than in lean normotensives (figure 13.20; chapter 5). In obese hypertensives, the SNA pattern is similar to that of lean persons with EH, except that in obese hypertensives the rises in SNA are smaller than the corresponding rises in lean hypertensives. The findings suggest (1) a common mechanism of pattern generation in both groups of hypertensives,

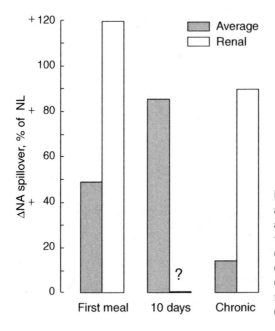

Figure 13.19. Mean change in average and renal NA spillover rates, as percentage of corresponding values in lean normotensives (NL), (1) at time of first large meal, (2) after 10 days of overeating, and (3) during chronic obesity. Data from O'Dea et al. (1982); Vaz et al. (1997); Rumantir et al. (1999).

and (2) modest inhibition of SNA through baroreflexes superimposed on this pattern in obese hypertensives. Engagement of baroreflexes is through the considerably higher cardiopulmonary load in hypertensive obesity. For example, even in normotensives with gross obesity (average BMI 40 kg/m^2), there is marked depression of the gain of muscle and cardiac baroreflexes (figure 13.21; Grassi et al., 1995), which has also been observed in very obese rats (Bunag and Barringer, 1988; Bunag et al., 1990). It seems reasonable to assume that in hypertensives in whom obesity is less gross (BMI ($\leq$30 kg/m^2)), there will also be significant depression of cardiac and constrictor baroreflexes.

Last, figure 13.20 indicates that at the same level of obesity the SNA patterns of obese hypertensives and obese normotensives are distinctive, suggesting different sources of sympathetic drive. In hypertensive obesity, the SNA pattern corresponds to that of the defense response, while in normotensive obesity cardiac SNA is depressed and average SNA is much lower. Only renal SNA is similar to that in hypertensive obesity.

Conclusions

In chronic normotensive obesity, the increase in average SNA is much smaller than during the phase of weight gain. It suggests that thermogenesis is no longer raised, which is consistent with the behavior of an adaptive control system operating about a new set point. In those with hypertensive obesity, the sympathetic outflow pattern resembles that of lean persons with EH, suggesting common underlying causes, including psychosocial stress and elevation in salt intake.

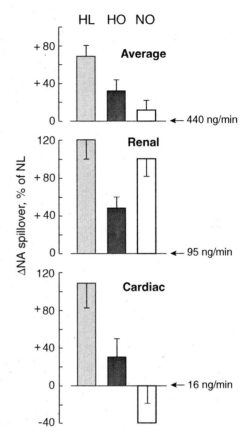

Figure 13.20. Average, renal, and cardiac NA spillover rates in lean hypertensives (HL, shaded), obese hypertensives (HO, black) and obese normotensives (NO, clear), expressed as percentage change from corresponding values of lean normotensives (NL); numbers on right indicate mean spillover in NL group. In HO subjects, SNA attenuated compared to HL group. Based on Rumantir et al. (1999).

Of course, the term *normotensive obesity* is a misnomer, since there is some elevation of BP over that of matched lean normotensives, even though it is small. The term is intended to indicate that the BP of persons with normotensive obesity is below the range of clinical hypertension.

Obesity and Its Relationship to EH

The system that normally regulates energy balance is an elaborate feedback system which maintains body weight (and fat content) close to the prevailing set point (figure 13.3). It responds to signals relating to hunger, satiety, and body fat mass, which evoke changes in food intake, heat production, substrate metabolism, and somatic motor activity. The signals engage neurons, many of them in the hypothalamus, which modulate the activity of target neurons subserving the above functions.

In the excitement of discoveries about the role of various hypothalamic neurons involved in day-to-day regulation of energy balance, it is sometimes forgotten that habitual eating behavior and food consumption primarily depend on other neuron groups. These are located in the cortex and forebrain and can modify or suppress the

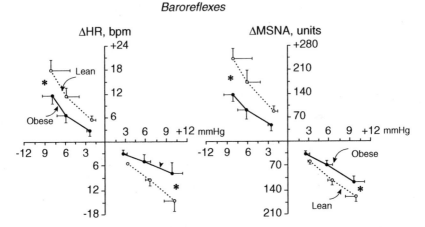

Figure 13.21. Left graphs relate ΔMAP from resting (mmHg) to Δ heart rate (beats/min, bpm) in lean (dotted line) and grossly obese (solid lines) normotensives; right graphs show corresponding function curve relating ΔMAP to ΔMSNA (arbitrary units). *$p < .05$. From Grassi et al. (1995), with permission of *Hypertension*, American Heart Association, and Lippincott, Williams and Wilkins.

adiposity-related feedback. Indeed, obesity would not exist without these extrahypothalamic mechanisms.

The system regulating energy balance has close links with the CNS cardiovascular pathways and with the systems regulating somatic motor activity and body temperature. One example of its direct cardiovascular linkage is the leptin-induced elevation of SNA in the renal constrictor outflow. However, adaptive thermogenesis has declined and average SNA is only slightly raised, making it unlikely that EH is the by-product of obesity-related thermogenesis (Landsberg, 2001). Similarly, the absence of much increased thermogenesis during chronic obesity is not a sign of control system failure but is a typical sign of a change in state of an adaptive control system.

The nature of the linkage between the system regulating energy balance in hypertensive obesity is distinct from that in normotensive obesity, as seen in their sympathetic output patterns (figure 13.20). Hence the hypothesis that the circulatory responses in hypertensive obesity are due to the factors that determine normotensive obesity plus those that give rise to EH; the latter include stress-related sensitization of the defense pathway and the CNS actions of high dietary salt (chapters 11, 12).

Epidemiological studies have suggested that genetic predisposition to EH increases the likelihood of becoming overweight or obese. This could be mediated through one or more neural mechanisms that are common to both systems. For example, increased activity of DA neurons raises BP through the defense pathway and causes an increase in food intake and body weight. The raised DA activity may also play a role in addictive overeating, probably in conjunction with other slow transmitter neurons such as orexins or enkephalins. The net result is suppression or attenuation of the feedback regulating energy balance. Such behavior is in accord with the hypothesis that eating relieves stress-related anxiety or is a reward for previous exertions (Kissebah and Krakower, 1994; Schultz et al., 1997; Fiorillo et al., 2003).

In the majority of persons with EH, the increase in body weight is 2–5 kg, suggesting that attenuation of the feedback is slight. Such persons may derive comfort from an occasional episode of overeating. However, most of the time they will have the behavioral attributes of persons with EH, such as anxiety, defensiveness, depression, and repressed anger (chapter 11). It suggests that relief from day-to-day stresses afforded by overeating is only transient, as occurs with many addictions.

The above hypothesis differs from that proposed by Björntorp et al. (2000), in which stress is regarded as the underlying cause of both EH and central obesity. Certainly, the associated increase in plasma cortisol promotes the accumulation of abdominal fat, which is the site of fat deposition in most persons with hypertensive obesity. However, cortisol is also part of the defense response and its increase is greater in lean than in obese hypertensives (figure 5.18; Filipovsky et al., 1996). EH predisposes to the development of obesity in a proportion of those with EH rather than the other way around, in view of the large proportion of obese normotensives. Moreover, the EH-related elevation of average SNA in hypertensive obesity accentuates insulin resistance and accelerates development of NIDDM (figure 13.20). In contrast, average SNA is near normal or only slightly raised in stable normotensive obesity.

Not all obese persons are stressed and anxious like those with hypertensive obesity. Obese normotensives are mostly good company and have a cheerful happy disposition, as was recognized by Shakespeare: "Let me have men about me that are fat, Sleek-headed men, and such as sleepe a-nights: Yon Cassius has a leane and hungry looke, He thinks too much: such men are dangerous" (*Julius Caesar*, Act I, Scene II). Falstaff is the prototype of an obese normotensive, who relishes the social side of eating and drinking, which has become a habit in which he often indulges. It is not an addiction, which implies complete dependence, but has become part of a preferred lifestyle. Probably these social attitudes develop in obese normotensives from an early age and may have a genetic basis. After all, even nematode worms include social eaters, while the worm equivalent of hypertensive obesity is a greedier solitary eater.

The circulatory effects of normotensive obesity are not complicated by the effects of EH. BP is only 6 mmHg above that of lean normotensives and is due to the elevation of CO and the constrictor effect of leptin and Ang II. The rise in BP is the result of hydraulic plus neural feedback, which overcorrects the generalized vasodilator action of insulin.

Obesity results from storage of excess fat in adipocytes, which is critically dependent on specific stimulation of insulin receptors of these cells. Selective disruption of the receptors on adipocytes prevents obesity and increases longevity, contrasting with the uniformly adverse effects on health of generalized impairment of insulin receptors.

In obesity, TNF-α and other autacoids are secreted by adipocytes, which depresses cellular glucose transport in other tissues. The resulting preferential utilization of FFA and glycerol as sources of energy might appear to be a desirable regulatory option for dissipating the excess fat. However, it places a great burden on the pancreas, which in the long term causes NIDDM and an enhanced risk of atherosclerosis and renal failure, which is greater in hypertensive than in normotensive obesity. The high CO and blood volume accelerate development of eccentric LVH.

Similar changes occur in persons with hypertensive obesity, except that the higher BP further raises cardiopulmonary load and the likelihood of developing cardiac failure. The increased constrictor drive causes further impairment of glucose transport and more renal and atherosclerotic complications than in those with normotensive obesity.

Although the effects of obesity plus EH are additive, the coexistence of the two conditions potentiates each factor's adverse effects on health. Hence, in the management of hypertensive obesity it is important to institute programs of weight reduction in combination with exercise (chapters 4, 11). Because of the links between the two conditions, a modest food intake and reasonable exercise should become a permanent part of the person's lifestyle.

14

Obstructive Sleep Apnea

Obstructive sleep apnea (OSA) is a primary respiratory disorder, to which obese persons are more susceptible than those who are lean. It gives rise to nocturnal hypertension and, in a proportion of subjects, also to daytime hypertension. In this chapter, some of the features of OSA and its clinical physiology are considered briefly, followed by a discussion of the mechanisms that contribute to the autonomic cardiovascular changes. The responses have features of the diving response of marine mammals and to arterial hypoxia of some terrestrial species. Both conserve O_2 and represent distinctive variants of the defense response from the "ready-for-action" variants of exercise and mental stress. The daytime rise in BP depends on repeated nocturnal arousals with unpleasant associations, not unlike the response to mental stress. However, the rise in BP is smaller than in stress-related EH, and the synaptic strengthening also appears to be of a different kind. Moreover, the diurnal elevation of BP affects both lean and obese people, whose BP may be normal or raised.

Epidemiological Links between Obesity, OSA, and Hypertension

OSA is defined as "a sleep disruption syndrome sufficient to cause symptoms, that is due to respiratory problems engendered by sleep itself" (Stradling, 1996, p. 2909). Various indices have been used to assess its severity, such as the apnea-hypopnea index (AHI), which indicates the total number of respiratory irregularities per hour of sleep. OSA affects about 4% of men and 2% of women (Young et al., 1993). About 40% of obese

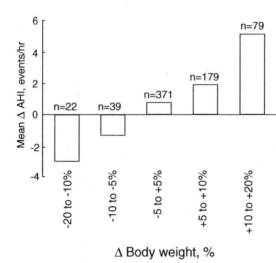

Figure 14.1. Relationship between recent change in body weight (% of baseline) and change in apnea-hypopnea index (Δ AHI, events/hour) in a prospective study among randomly selected Wisconsin residents; *n* is the number of persons in each category. From Peppard, Young, Palta, and Skatrud (2000), with permission of the *Journal of the American Medical Association.*

individuals have OSA, while about 70% of those with OSA are obese (Vgontzas et al., 1994; Caples et al., 2005). A recent weight gain is associated with increased prevalence and severity of OSA, while loss of weight diminishes the frequency of bouts of OSA (figure 14.1; Peppard, Young, Palta, and Skatrud, 2000).

About 30% of patients with OSA have both nocturnal and daytime hypertension. In the prospective Wisconsin Sleep Cohort Study, the initial severity of OSA was related to the chances of developing sustained daytime hypertension during the next 4 years (Peppard, Young, Palta, Dempsey et al., 2000). On current estimates, OSA affects about 5–10% of subjects regarded as having EH.

Cardiorespiratory and Autonomic Changes in OSA Patients

The respiratory obstruction in OSA affects the upper airway during sleep and is accompanied by specific respiratory and cardiovascular changes that are superimposed on the normal changes during the different phases of sleep. Two approaches have been used in animals to try to reproduce the hypertension associated with OSA: (1) simulation of the cyclic nocturnal respiratory changes, and (2) cyclic exposure for several weeks to severe arterial hypoxia without respiratory obstruction.

Mechanisms of Upper Airway Obstruction

The normal upper pharyngeal airway subserves two functions: (1) swallowing, in which the pharynx behaves like a floppy and collapsible muscular tube, similar to the esophagus; and (2) breathing, during which the pharynx is held open through active contraction of the pharyngeal dilator muscles (Stradling, 1996). During sleep there is reduction in the activity of these muscles, which results in pharyngeal narrowing in most individuals.

Many factors can cause pharyngeal airway obstruction and sleep disturbances. Because of the close relationship between obesity and OSA, it has been suggested that the threshold for apneic stimuli is reduced by a number of obesity-related peptide molecules (Considine et al., 1996); some molecules accentuate nocturnal narrowing of the airway by depressing the response of the pharyngeal dilator muscles (O'Donnell et al., 2000). In obese persons, deposition of excess fat in the upper airway may increase pharyngeal obstruction (Schwartz et al., 1991). Another possible mechanism is the deposition of fat droplets in the pharyngeal muscles when obesity is so severe that there are insufficient adipocytes to accommodate the excess fat (figure 13.14; Sharma et al., 2002). Droplet deposition in muscle will reduce contractile efficiency. Last, in gross obesity the Pickwickian syndrome may be present: This involves chronic hypopnea and arterial hypoxia at all times, with the poor ventilation providing a potential trigger for respiratory obstruction through nasopharyngeal stimulation.

Various factors causing central respiratory depression can also cause apnea, while secretions associated with snoring or nasal obstruction may raise BP by stimulating trigeminal afferents in the upper airway. Respiratory obstruction may occur due to tonsillar enlargement and pharyngeal tumors and in myopathies, such as Duchenne's muscular dystrophy.

It appears that bouts of nasopharyngeal obstruction may occur in obese individuals who may be either hypertensive or normotensive, as well as in lean persons who are either normotensive or have stress-related EH. Like the changes during and after exercise, OSA can affect everyone.

Respiration, Circulation, and MSNA during Sleep

Subjects with OSA are usually investigated in a sleep laboratory, where their cardiorespiratory responses are related to the phases of sleep, which are identified from the electroencephalographic (EEG) and electromyographic (EMG) patterns.

Normal Phases of Sleep

Sleep is normally subdivided into rapid eye movement (REM) and non-rapid eye movement (NREM) phases (Somers et al., 1993; Narkiewicz and Somers, 1997). During REM sleep, the subjects dream and their postural muscle tone diminishes. NREM sleep is subdivided into stages I through IV, with stages II and IV being the two longest periods.

During REM sleep, the EEG typically displays marked short increases in brain activity that occur at intervals of about 90 minutes (Hobson, 2005; Siegel, 2005). The BP, heart rate, and muscle sympathetic nerve activity (MSNA) all increase in association with bursts of raised postural muscle tone. An arousal stimulus such as a loud noise affects the EEG, causing further phasic increases in BP and MSNA. During the NREM phase, the levels of BP, heart rate, and MSNA decline gradually and reach their nadir during stage IV.

Cardiorespiratory and Autonomic Changes during OSA

Sleep in obese individuals with severe OSA (BMI range 32.4–52.8 kg/m^2) is punctuated by successive cycles of apnea. After complete apnea, the subject attempts to breathe despite closure or severe obstruction of the glottis, but eventually this subsides and is followed by frank hyperventilation (figure 14.2; Somers et al., 1995). About 20 seconds after the start of apnea, there are gradual rises in MSNA and BP, while heart rate decreases slightly. SaO_2 falls to 60–70% ($\equiv paO_2$ of 30–40 mmHg) and $paCO_2$ increases, which will cause an increase in arterial chemoreceptor discharge. This may be the reason for the sporadic attempts at inspiration against the closed airway (Müller's maneuver) that begin some 10–15 seconds after the start of apnea. As arterial chemoreceptor discharge gains strength, hyperventilation develops and is responsible for the large surges in BP and heart rate (figure 14.2), during which SBP/DBP may become as high as 260/110 mmHg. The hyperventilation-related elevation of CO pumps the blood into a partially constricted peripheral vasculature evoked during the preceding apnea (Guilleminault et al., 1986). The BP rise at the start of hyperventilation is responsible for inhibiting MSNA, which later increases gradually when the Müller maneuver commences while the subject is still apneic (figure 14.2). Both BP and MSNA are reduced by adequate nasal continuous positive airways pressure (nCPAP), which raises SaO_2.

Cardiac baroreflex sensitivity is depressed during sleep but returns to normal during the waking hours (Parati et al., 1997). In OSA patients, average BP and MSNA are greater during sleep than while awake (Somers et al., 1995). In awake subjects with OSA, MSNA is greater than in those without OSA (Narkiewicz et al., 1998).

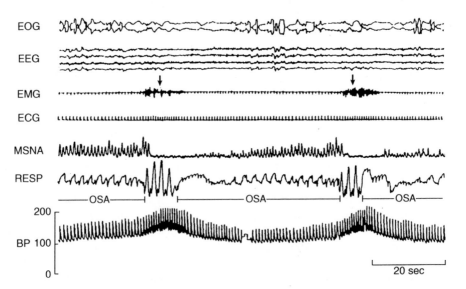

Figure 14.2. Recording (from above): electrooculogram (EOG), electroencephalogram (EEG), electromyogram (EMG), electrocardiogram (ECG), muscle sympathetic nerve activity (MSNA), respiration (RESP), and arterial blood pressure (BP, mmHg) during REM sleep in a patient with obstructive sleep apnea (OSA). Lines show duration of OSA cycles: initially apnea is complete, while subject attempts later to inspire against obstructed airway. Note large BP surge during hyperventilation, which corresponds to period of increased muscle tone (arrows on EMG), as part of arousal response. From Somers et al. (1995), with permission of *Journal of Clinical Investigation*.

Effective Treatment Lowers BP during Both Night and Day

Despite earlier doubts (Dimsdale et al., 2000; Wolk et al., 2003), nCPAP given at high enough airway pressure to abolish the apneas reduces the BP during sleep (Somers et al., 1995; Wolk et al., 2003).

In a placebo-controlled study in which subjects received treatment for about 9 weeks, one group (16 subjects) received effective nCPAP treatment at an airway pressure of about 9 cm H_2O (figure 14.3, top), while in the 16 placebo subjects, airway pressure was too low to prevent the apneas (figure 14.3, bottom; Becker et al., 2003). Ambulatory baseline BPs were similar in both groups, as was the frequency and magnitude of their episodes of nocturnal apnea-hypopnea (table 14.1). After 9 weeks, average 24-hour BP had been reduced by 11 mmHg (range 5–20 mmHg) in the treatment group, while the BP of placebo subjects was unchanged.

Simulation Studies in Animals

In one study, OSA was simulated in dogs and compared with the effects of repeated arousals in the absence of OSA. In another study, rats were exposed to cycles of severe arterial hypoxia without respiratory obstruction for several hours each day.

OSA in Dogs

OSA was induced for 5–12 weeks in four instrumented dogs (Brooks et al., 1997). Each dog had a tracheostomy with a permanent side hole through which an endotracheal

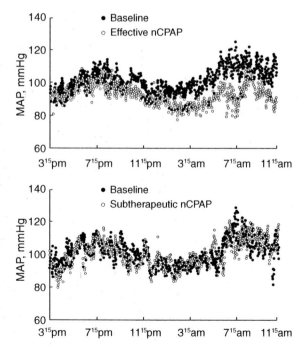

Figure 14.3. Top, Individual night and day ambulatory mean arterial pressure values (MAP, mmHg) at baseline prior to treatment (black circles) and in the same patients treated by applying effective continuous positive airway pressure (nCPAP, open circles) for several hours during the night. Bottom, results in a matched group of patients, showing MAPs at baseline (black circles) and while on treatment with subtherapeutic levels of nCPAP, which did not abolish apneas. From Becker et al. (2003), with permission of *Circulation*, American Heart Association, and Lippincott, Williams and Wilkins.

Table 14.1. Comparison of Average Ambulatory BPs, Apnea-Hypopnea Index (AHI) and Total Sleep Time (TST), and Other Variables in a Placebo-Controlled Trial of Nasal Continuous Positive Airway Pressure (nCPAP) in 32 Patients Randomly Allocated to Treatment (Rx) and Placebo Groups

	Baseline		End of Treatment	
Groups	Rx	Placebo	Rx	Placebo
Day MAP, mmHg	104	104	94	105
Night MAP, mmHg	96	94	86	95
Epworth Sleepiness Scale[a]	14.4	14.1	5.1	8.9
AHI, events/hour	62.5	65.0	3.4	33.4
Total sleep time, min	349	342	376	351
Age	54.4	52.3	–	–
BMI, kg/m^2	33.3	33.5	–	–
n Hypert/Total[b]	8/16	8/16	–	–

Note: [a]maximum score 24; [b]EH was diagnosed if SBP/DBP $\geq$ 160/90 mmHg, or patient was receiving antihypertensive treatment; BMI, body mass index; n Hypert/Total, proportion of hypertensives in group.

Source: Becker et al. (2003).

tube was inserted at night. A computer recognized that the dog had been asleep for a few seconds from the EEG pattern, which activated a valve that obstructed the airway until the animal was aroused; spontaneous breathing was then allowed to resume. The number of nocturnal apneic events was gradually increased, and after 4–7 weeks MAP had increased by 12 mmHg at night and by 17 mmHg during the day (figure 14.4). When the noctural sessions ended, the nighttime BPs returned to normal by the next night, whereas daytime BPs took several weeks to gradually recover, as at the start and end of exercise training (figure 10.15).

In another experiment, sleep was interrupted by frequently repeated acoustic stimuli without obstructing the airway: This raised nocturnal BP but not that during daytime. In contrast, sleep deprivation caused slight elevation of the daytime BP only (Kato, Phillips et al., 2000).

Periodic Hypoxia without Airway Obstruction

In this experiment, normotensive rats were placed in a special cage in which they were exposed to very low inspired O_2 concentration for a few seconds every 30 seconds for 7 h/day. This was done for up to 40 days, and at the end of each day's session they were returned to their holding cages (Lesske et al., 1997). The increase in body weight was smaller than in controls, but hematocrits and hemoglobins remained normal. Intraarterial BP was measured prior to hypoxia and 2 days after the last day of hypoxia: On both occasions, the animals were breathing room air, and paO_2 was normal.

BP had not altered from baseline after 20 days of intermittent hypoxia, but by day 30 there was a small rise (figure 14.5); this continued until day 35, when maximum elevation of MAP of 13 mmHg was reached (Fletcher et al., 1992; Lesske et al., 1997). In rats with carotid body denervation, exposure to similar cycles of arterial hypoxia caused no change in BP, indicating that stimulation of the arterial chemoreceptors had been responsible for the rise.

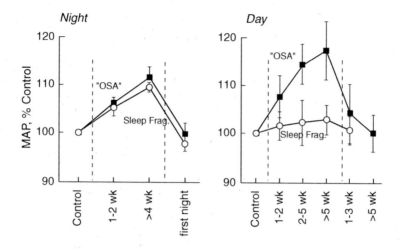

Figure 14.4. Average results in four dogs during simulated obstructive sleep apnea (OSA, black squares) and sleep fragmentation (Sleep Frag., open circles), showing nighttime (left) and daytime (right) MAPs (±SEMs), as percentage of initial baseline. The sleep fragmentation experiments were performed ~6 months after OSA period. Dashed vertical lines show duration of OSA or sleep fragmentation, which ranged from 5 to 14 weeks and 5 to 7.5 weeks in different dogs, hence the range of time values on abscissa. Data points are joined for ease of interpretation. Adapted from Brooks et al. (1997), with permission of *Journal of Clinical Investigation*.

Effects of Apnea and Arterial Hypoxia in Different Species

In each cycle of OSA, the cardiovascular response is initiated by apnea due to nasopharyngeal obstruction, which causes mild to moderate arterial hypoxia plus hypercapnia, increasing arterial chemoreceptor discharge until ventilation starts again. This section examines the circulatory effects of nasopharyngeal stimulation and of arterial hypoxia in several species to obtain insights into the mechanisms of human OSA. Some of the species variation in the circulatory responses to arterial hypoxia is due to differences in the extent to which respiration suppresses the arterial chemoreceptor-induced autonomic patterns emanating from the hypothalamus.

Nasopharyngeal Stimulation in Rabbits and Other Species

When seals and other diving mammals submerge in the water, they develop instant apnea together with marked reduction in heart rate and CO and widespread systemic vasoconstriction (Elsner et al., 1964; Scholander, 1964; Blix et al., 1975). This pattern is a variant of the defense response and is often maintained for many minutes during submersion. Blood flow is very low in every bed except the brain, myocardium, and active muscles, in which it remains normal or high, allowing the animal to remain alert while swimming underwater.

A quasi-diving response can be elicited in rabbits by stimulating the nasal mucosa with a puff of cigarette smoke or formalin vapor. This evokes apnea in expiration,

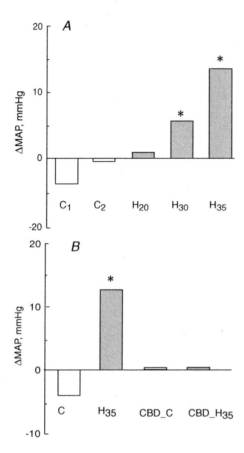

Figure 14.5. (A) Average changes from initial baseline in mean arterial pressure (ΔMAP, mmHg) measured 2 days after end of hypoxia sessions in (1) two groups of control rats (C_1, breathing room air; C_2, receiving compressed air in special chamber); (2) rats subjected to cycles of severe hypoxia for 7 hours/day for 20, 30, and 35 days (H_{20}, H_{30}, H_{35}). (B) ΔMAPs 2 days after completing 35 days of the following: (1) control, breathing air (C); (2) cycles of severe hypoxia (H_{35}); (3) rats breathing air with denervated carotid bodies prior to baseline measurements (CBD, C); (4) CBD rats subjected to standard cycles of severe hypoxia (CBD, H_{35}). *$p < .05$ for difference from baseline. Adapted from Lesske et al. (1997), with permission of *Journal of Hypertension* and Lippincott, Williams and Wilkins.

marked reduction in heart rate and CO, and a small rise in MAP (figure 14.6; White et al., 1974). There is marked reduction in blood flow and elevation in Vas R in the gastrointestinal, renal, and limb beds, while cerebral and coronary blood flows are well maintained (McRitchie, 1973; White and McRitchie, 1973; White et al., 1974). The apnea lasts 10–15 seconds, during which paO_2 falls to 40–50 mmHg, $paCO_2$ increases by 3–5 mmHg, and the animals become immobile until breathing is resumed.

The main afferents for the nasopharyngeal reflex are (1) trigeminal nociceptors, stimulation of which initiates apnea and autonomic changes; (2) lung inflation receptor activity, which is reduced to near zero during apnea; this enhances vasoconstriction and bradycardia initiated by trigeminal stimulation;[1] (3) olfactory receptors, which increase the duration of apnea; and (4) arterial chemoreceptors, which contribute to the cardiovascular effects and eventually terminate the apnea by stimulating respiration (McRitchie and White, 1974).

Role of Suprapontine and Bulbospinal Centers in Rabbits

The role of suprapontine and bulbospinal centers was investigated by comparing responses to nasopharyngeal stimulation using a puff of cigarette smoke in intact,

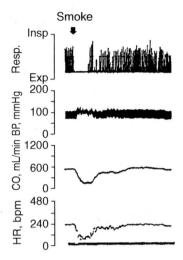

Figure 14.6. Record in awake rabbit of (from top): respiration (Resp), ear artery BP (mmHg), cardiac output (CO, mL/min), heart rate (HR, bpm). A puff of smoke blown at the nostrils (at arrow) elicits apnea in expiration, a small rise in BP (mmHg), and substantial falls in CO and HR. Adapted from White et al. (1974).

thalamic, and pontine rabbits (figure 14.7). In intact rabbits, this elicited apnea, brady-cardia, and mesenteric vasoconstriction, and the response was virtually identical in thalamic animals. In pontine rabbits, the apnea was of similar magnitude, but vasocon-striction and bradycardia were smaller (White et al., 1975).

The effects of apnea without prior smoke stimulation of the trigeminal afferents were also examined while the animals were ventilated artificially.[2] The circulatory changes in both intact and thalamic animals were similar to the effects of smoke-induced apnea in spontaneously breathing animals (figure 14.7, right). It suggests that loss of the normal inhibitory input from the lung inflation receptors makes a major contribu-tion to the cardiovascular response (see below). In pontine rabbits, the circulatory changes were smaller than in intact animals. White et al. (1975) also studied the effects of smoke inhalation without apnea while the animals were ventilated artifi-cially. This caused a somewhat greater rise in BP, but bradycardia and systemic vaso-constriction were similar to that observed in the spontaneously breathing preparations.

After prior denervation of the carotid sinus and aortic nerves, the apnea time was prolonged considerably, but bradycardia and vasoconstriction were markedly attenu-ated in all preparations (White et al., 1975). This was due not only to the loss of arterial chemoreceptors but also to interactions with input from the baroreceptors, which play an integral part in the circulatory response, as noted in relation to exercise (figures 10.11, 10.14).

In summary, interactions between projections from the various afferents probably influence cardiovascular neurons at all levels of the neuraxis. This allows brainstem mechanisms to compensate partially for the loss of higher centers.

Responses in Other Species

Blowing smoke on the nostrils of dogs elicits about half the bradycardia evoked in rabbits, while the same stimulus only elicits slight apnea or cardiovascular changes in monkeys and humans (White and McRitchie, 1973). In humans, more pronounced

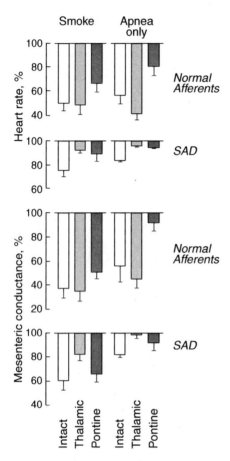

Figure 14.7. Nasopharyngeal reflex responses in intact (clear bars), thalamic (light shaded bars), and pontine rabbits (dark shaded bars). Left, peak effect of a puff of cigarette smoke on heart rate and mesenteric vascular conductance. Right, effect of a 15-second period of apnea in animals artificially ventilated at resting minute volumes. The tests were performed in 12 rabbits (4 for each preparation) with normal afferents and in 12 rabbits with sinoaortic denervation (SAD) performed 7–10 days earlier. Adapted from White et al. (1975), with permission of *American Journal of Physiology* and American Physiological Society.

bradycardia and forearm vasoconstriction are evoked when breath-holding is combined with facial immersion (Elsner and Scholander, 1965; Elsner and Gooden, 1983). Here, the increased facial and nasopharyngeal afferent activity potentiates the effects of arterial chemoreceptor stimulation (Daly, 1986). In professional human divers, a brief rise in heart rate quickly changes to a fall of about 50% of resting as the dive proceeds, presumably through similar potentiation (Scholander et al., 1962; Irving, 1963; Scholander, 1964).

Cardiorespiratory Regulation in Arterial Hypoxia

The respiratory responses to arterial hypoxia are similar in most mammalian species. However, their circulatory and autonomic responses differ considerably, particularly during severe arterial hypoxia (Korner, 1959, 1971b, 1979a). In some species, including rabbits and rats, the autonomic responses depend mainly on the magnitude of afferent activity of the lung inflation receptors relative to that of the arterial chemoreceptors. However, in primates the intrinsic activity of the respiratory centers plays a major additional role.

Responses to Arterial Hypoxia in Rabbits

The experiment involved measuring the respiratory and circulatory effects of breathing gas mixtures of low inspired O_2 composition for about 25 minutes in awake rabbits. The gas mixture remained constant in a given experiment, but different animals were exposed to varying degrees of hypoxia ranging from mild to severe reduction in paO_2 (Chalmers et al., 1967b; Korner and Uther, 1970).

Respiratory minute volume begins to rise at a paO_2 of ~50 mmHg and continues to increase until a maximum is reached at paO_2 35–30 mmHg. Ventilation declines at still lower paO_2 due to slight respiratory depression associated with hypocapnia (figure 14.8; Chalmers et al., 1967b; Korner and Uther, 1970). The autonomic effects of hypoxia on heart rate and TPR (aHR, aTPR) were estimated from the response differences in animals with intact effectors and animals subjected to total autonomic blockade (TAB; figure 14.9; Korner et al., 1969; Korner and Uther, 1969, 1970).[3]

In mild hypoxia, there was an increase in aHR and a slight rise in aTPR, both of which were due to elevation of SNA. Severe hypoxia elicited a marked fall in aHR and substantial elevation in aTPR, with both changes greatest at the start of hypoxia;

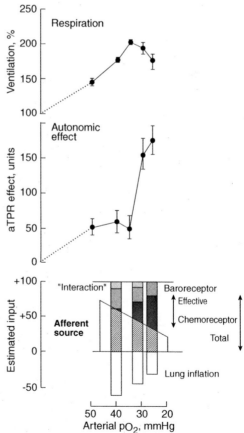

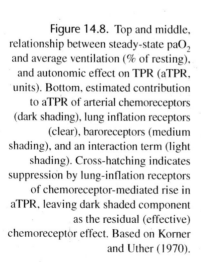

Figure 14.8. Top and middle, relationship between steady-state paO_2 and average ventilation (% of resting), and autonomic effect on TPR (aTPR, units). Bottom, estimated contribution to aTPR of arterial chemoreceptors (dark shading), lung inflation receptors (clear), baroreceptors (medium shading), and an interaction term (light shading). Cross-hatching indicates suppression by lung-inflation receptors of chemoreceptor-mediated rise in aTPR, leaving dark shaded component as the residual (effective) chemoreceptor effect. Based on Korner and Uther (1970).

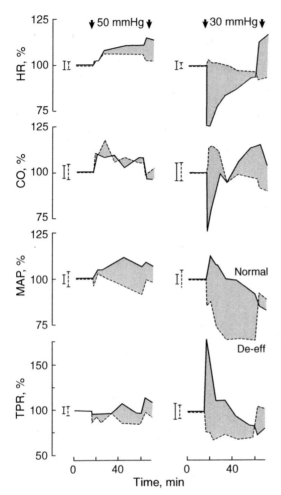

Figure 14.9. Average circulatory changes in awake rabbits with normal autonomic effector function (Normal, solid lines) and rabbits with total autonomic blockade (De-eff, dashed lines). The animals were exposed (between arrows) to mild hypoxia (left, paO$_2$ 50 mmHg) and to severe hypoxia (right, paO$_2$ 30 mmHg). Heart rate (HR), cardiac output (CO), mean arterial pressure (MAP), and total peripheral resistance (TPR), all expressed as percentage of baseline. The autonomic effects on heart rate and TPR (aHR, aTPR) are shaded areas between responses of normal and de-efferented animals. From Korner and Uther (1970).

the bradycardia was mainly due to vagal excitation, but there was also inhibition of cardiac SNA (Korner, 1965b; Chalmers et al., 1967b; Korner, Shaw, West et al., 1973).

The rise in respiration is entirely due to stimulation of the arterial chemoreceptors (Chalmers et al., 1967b). As the lung inflation receptor activity increases in proportion to the rise in ventilation, cardiac SNA increases correspondingly, but chemoreceptor-mediated vagal excitation and systemic vasoconstriction are suppressed (figure 14.10; Daly and Hazzledine, 1963; Daly and Scott, 1963; Daly et al., 1967; Crocker et al., 1968; Daly and Robinson, 1968; Korner, Shaw, West et al., 1973; Daly, 1986).

The top two panels of figure 14.8 show the reciprocal changes in average respiratory minute volume and aTPR at different levels of hypoxia. The lowest panel gives an estimate of the contribution to the aTPR response of the arterial chemoreceptors, lung inflation receptors, and arterial baroreceptors (Korner and Uther, 1970).[4] The arterial chemoreceptor-mediated systemic vasoconstriction is suppressed by the activity of the lung inflation receptors up to the respiratory maximum; the slight elevation in

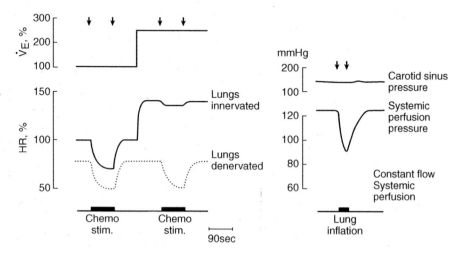

Figure 14.10. Left, stimulation of isolated carotid chemoreceptors with hypoxic + hypercapnic blood at two levels of ventilation (V_E, % resting) in a dog with normally innervated lungs (solid lines) and after section of pulmonary vagi (dotted lines). Right, effect of lung inflation (between arrows) on systemic BP in dog in which systemic circulation was perfused at constant flow while carotid sinus BP remained constant. From Korner (1971b) based on Daly and Hazzledine (1963, left), and Daly and Robinson (1968, right), with permission of *Physiological Reviews* and American Physiological Society.

aTPR is a baroreflex response to the dilator effect of peripheral tissue hypoxia. Beyond the maximum lung inflation, receptor activity declines, while arterial chemoreceptor discharge increases dramatically (Hornbein et al., 1961; Paintal, 1973; Fukuda et al., 1986). Hence, in severe hypoxia the arterial chemoreceptors become the prime mover in the elevation of aTPR and bradycardia (Korner, 1965b; Scott, 1966; Chalmers et al., 1967b; Korner and Uther, 1970; Carmody and Scott, 1974).

Not all the actions of the arterial chemoreceptors on the vagal and constrictor motoneurons are direct. Their raised activity alters the properties of the baroreflexes, increasing gain and range of constrictor baroreflexes (figure 14.11). Depression of the cardiac SNA baroreflex and facilitation of the vagal baroreflex are responsible for the bradycardia (Korner, Shaw, West et al., 1973; Iriki et al., 1977a, 1977b; Iriki and Korner, 1979; Iriki and Kozawa, 1983). The enhancement of constrictor baroreflexes contributes to the elevation of BP, while cardiac baroreflex depression moderates this response (see chapter 10). The two opposing trends are probably the reason for the smaller increase in BP in OSA than during exercise or psychosocial stress, in which both cardiac and constrictor reflexes are enhanced. In apnea-arterial hypoxia, some of the cardiac depression is due to activation of BP-independent autonomic motoneurons (figure 10.10), which further reduces the effect of the constrictor reflexes on BP.

The tachycardia response in mild hypoxia is due to an increase in cardiac SNA resulting from increased lung inflation receptor activity. This is largely mediated through BP-independent heart rate neurons as assessed from the plateau shifts in the reflex function curve (figure 14.12; Korner, Shaw, West et al., 1973). In severe hypoxia,

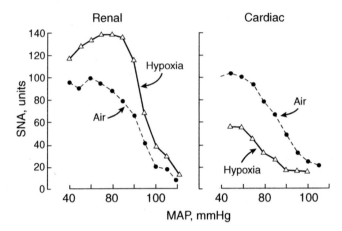

Figure 14.11. Average baroreflex function curves relating sympathetic neural activity (SNA, units) to mean arterial pressure (MAP, mmHg), obtained from 6 anesthetized rabbits in which ventilation artificially maintained constant. Curves obtained while breathing room air (circles, dashed lines) and severe arterial hypoxia (paO$_2$ ~30 mmHg, triangles, solid lines). Left, renal SNA is enhanced during arterial hypoxia at a given MAP, while (right) cardiac SNA is depressed. After Iriki et al. (1977a), with permission of *European Journal of Physiology* (Pflüger's Archiv) and Springer Verlag.

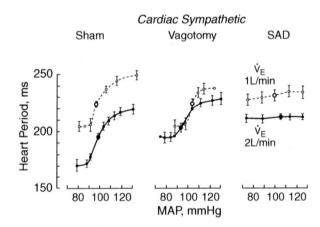

Figure 14.12. Effect of changing ventilation (V$_E$) from 1 L/min to 2 L/min on MAP-sympathetic heart period reflex in (left) 5 sham-operated rabbits with all afferents intact, (middle) 5 vagotomized rabbits, and (right) 4 rabbits with sinoaortic denervation (SAD). From Korner, Shaw, West et al. (1973), with permission of *Circulation Research*, American Heart Association, and Lippincott, Williams and Wilkins.

the marked initial bradycardia also has a large BP-independent component due to the sudden increase in arterial chemoreceptor activity; in addition, the vagal component of the cardiac baroreflex is facilitated. Recall from chapter 8 that the latter depends on the integrity of the A_1 and A_2 NA neurons.

Role of Suprapontine and Bulbospinal Mechanisms in Rabbits

The responses were examined at three levels of arterial paO_2 of approximately 50, 40, and 30 mmHg in (1) sham-operated rabbits with intact CNS; (2) rhinencephalic animals without neocortex; (3) thalamic rabbits without forebrain; and (4) pontine animals subjected to infracollicular decerebration (Korner et al., 1969; Uther et al., 1970; Korner and Uther, 1975).[5]

In all preparations, the respiratory minute volume rose to a maximum within seconds of the onset of hypoxia and settled at a slightly lower plateau within the first few minutes. The increases in intact and rhinencephalic animals were virtually identical (table 14.2), while in thalamic animals, the resting minute volume of which was increased, the responses were smaller and were unrelated to the severity of hypoxia (Korner et al., 1969). In pontine rabbits, the rise in ventilation was greater than in intact and rhinencephalic animals, due to the metabolic acidosis that develops during hypoxia in this preparation.

In all three suprapontine preparations, the increases in aTPR were greater than in pontine rabbits (figure 14.13). During spontaneous respiration there were small aTPR response differences between intact, rhinencephalic, and thalamic animals, which were greatly reduced by constant artificial ventilation. It suggests that they were due to differences in the breathing patterns of the various preparations (Korner et al., 1969).

The aHR response in intact rabbits is biphasic, with mild hypoxia eliciting tachycardia, while moderate and severe hypoxia evoke bradycardia (figure 14.14). In contrast, in rhinencephalic and thalamic animals there is bradycardia at all levels of hypoxia. It suggests that in the intact animal increased lung inflation receptor activity suppresses

Table 14.2. Respiratory Response to Three Grades of Severity of Arterial Hypoxia in Various Neurological Rabbit Preparations

Preparation	paO_2 50 mmHg	paO_2 40 mmHg	paO_2 30 mmHg
Intact CNS	146 ± 4.9%	179 ± 3.2%	194 ± 5.8%
De-efferented	147 ± 2.7%	187 ± 8.1	170 ± 7.3%
Rhinencephalic	129 ± 3.8%	174 ± 6.3%	180 ± 2.4%
Thalamic[a]	135 ± 2.6%	123 ± 3.4%	138 ± 3.7%
Pontine	139 ± 3.2%	207 ± 6.1%[b]	218 ± 8.6[b]

Note: Results are means ± SEMs; [a]response significantly smaller than in other preparations by 1-way ANOVA; [b]response greater than corresponding responses with intact CNS.

Source: Adapted from Korner et al. (1969), with permission of *Circulation Research*, American Heart Association, and Lippincott, Williams and Wilkins.

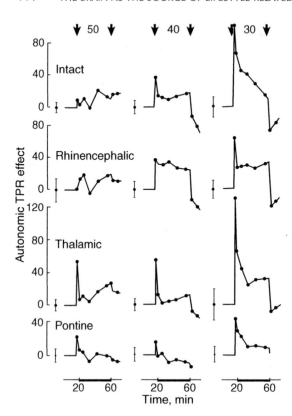

Figure 14.13. Effect of mild, moderate, and severe arterial hypoxia (paO$_2$ 50, 40, 30 mmHg, between arrows) on autonomic TPR effect in intact, rhinencephalic, thalamic, and pontine preparations. From Korner et al. (1969), with permission of *Circulation Research*, American Heart Association, and Lippincott, Williams and Wilkins.

chemoreceptor-induced bradycardia through a loop via the neocortex, which affects heart rate premotor neurons in the hypothalamus.

Thus, during mild hypoxia the aHR response of intact rabbits is an attenuated form of the high cardiac SNA of pontine rabbits. Their bradycardia response during severe hypoxia is close to that of thalamic rabbits, indicating that the vagal excitation and cardiac sympathetic inhibition is due to chemoreceptor-induced changes in hypothalamic heart rate neuron activity. In pontine rabbits, tachycardia is mediated through cardiac SNA and rises with severity of hypoxia.

Peripheral Autonomic Patterns.   The peripheral autonomic patterns were studied at paO$_2$ ~30 mmHg in intact, thalamic, and pontine rabbits (Uther et al., 1970; Korner, 1980a). In animals with intact CNS, there was sympathetically mediated renal and gastrointestinal vasoconstriction, but vasodilation in the skeletal muscle bed (figure 14.15). The vasodilation was due to adrenaline, which masked α-AR-mediated neural constriction, as evident from the responses of previously adrenalectomized rabbits (figure 14.16; Fukuda and Kobayashi, 1961; Chalmers et al., 1966; Uther et al., 1970). The peripheral autonomic pattern in intact animals resembles the classic defense response, except for the marked ear skin vasodilation that is part of the O$_2$ conservation mechanism (see below; Chalmers and Korner, 1966).

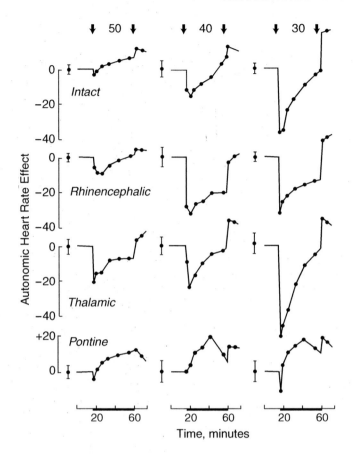

Figure 14.14. Effect of mild, moderate, and severe arterial hypoxia (paO_2 50, 40, and 30 mmHg, between arrows) on autonomic effect on heart rate in intact, rhinencephalic, thalamic, and pontine preparations. From Korner et al. (1969), with permission of *Circulation Research*, American Heart Association, and Lippincott, Williams and Wilkins.

In thalamic animals, the changes in BP and aVas R in gastrointestinal, renal, and ear skin beds were the same as in intact animals, but there was vasoconstriction in the skeletal muscle bed rather than vasodilation. This was not affected by adrenalectomy, suggesting that thalamic rabbits do not secrete adrenaline during arterial hypoxia.

In pontine rabbits, the BP response was similar to that in intact animals (Korner et al., 1969; Korner and Uther, 1969; Uther et al., 1970). However, there was minimal renal vasoconstriction while gastrointestinal vasoconstriction was about half the normal response (figure 14.15). In the muscle bed the response was biphasic with an initial fall in aVas R followed by a rise. This can be accounted for by a progressive increase in plasma adrenaline (figure 5.4; Fukuda and Kobayashi, 1961). This gives rise to acidosis, which is prevented by pretreatment with β-AR antagonists or by adrenalectomy (figure 14.16) (Chalmers et al., 1966; Uther et al., 1970; Korner, 1980a).

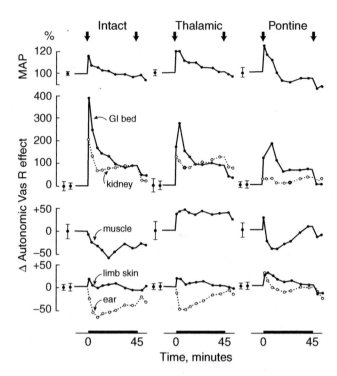

Figure 14.15. Time course of mean arterial pressure (MAP) and autonomic changes in Vas R in gastrointestinal, renal, hindquarter muscle, hindquarter skin, and ear skin beds during severe arterial hypoxia (paO$_2$ ~30 mmHg, between arrows) in intact, thalamic, and pontine rabbits. Changes during and after hypoxia expressed as percentage of baseline breathing room air. From Korner (1971a).

Significance of Cardiorespiratory Response

Wild rabbits often encounter a low-O$_2$ environment in their burrows, which they may have to endure for prolonged periods if there is a predator at the entrance. Hence, the cardiovascular pattern is a variant of the classic defense response, with emphasis on O$_2$ conservation rather than on fighting an adversary. The bradycardia reduces cardiac work and myocardial O$_2$ consumption, while the large ear skin vasodilation causes rapid reduction of body temperature, a lowering metabolism, and less demand for O$_2$ (Korner, 1965b; Chalmers and Korner, 1966). The remaining peripheral autonomic vascular pattern resembles that of the classic defense response.

Responses in Other Subprimate and Primate Species

In dogs, cats, and monkeys, even very severe arterial hypoxia always evokes tachycardia and variable peripheral changes when the animals are breathing spontaneously (Korner, 1959, 1971b; Comroe and Mortimer, 1964; Korner, Reynoldson et al., 1979). In dogs, it is possible to elicit bradycardia beyond the animal's respiratory maximum, which is similar to the rabbit's response to severe hypoxia (Cross et al., 1963).

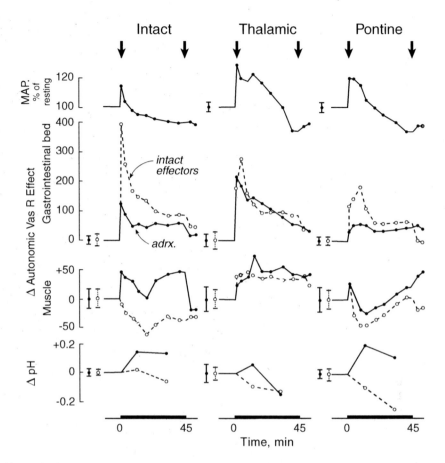

Figure 14.16. Responses to severe arterial hypoxia (paO$_2$ ~30 mmHg, between arrows) of autonomic component of Vas R in gastrointestinal and muscle beds and arterial pH of intact, thalamic, and pontine rabbits. Responses studied include changes with intact autonomic effectors (dashed lines) and in animals subjected to adrenalectomy 2 weeks earlier, maintained on fixed steroids (solid lines). From Korner, 1971a.

However, this does not occur in conscious monkeys in which the respiratory maximum is well below paO$_2$ 30 mmHg (White et al., 1972, 1973; Brown, 1973). At paO$_2$ 40 and 30 mmHg, the respiratory response is similar to that of rabbits, but heart rate increases and TPR falls, with the level of TPR similar to the responses of hypoxic rabbits subjected to autonomic blockade (figure 14.17; Korner et al., 1967).[6] Brief exposures to paO$_2$ values as low as 20–25 mmHg have not evoked bradycardia or a rise in TPR (White, personal communication). Thus, circulatory regulation in monkeys is mediated mainly through a large increase in cardiac SNA, while regulation of tissue perfusion is mediated through local regulators of the peripheral circulation (chapter 6). Such data as is available suggests that this also applies to the effects of acute hypoxia in humans (Korner, 1959; Pugh, 1964).

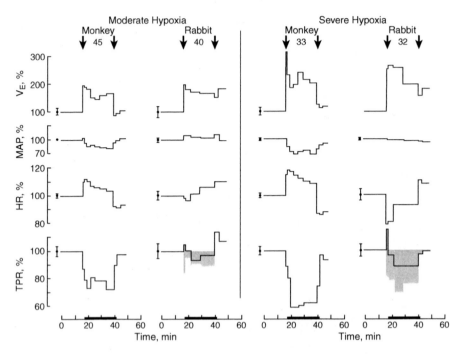

Figure 14.17. Left, average effects (% of resting) of moderate hypoxia (paO$_2$ 45 mmHg, between arrows) on respiratory minute volume (V$_E$), mean arterial pressure (MAP), heart rate (HR), and total peripheral resistance (TPR) in 6 conscious monkeys and 5 rabbits. Right, responses to severe hypoxia (paO$_2$ 32 mmHg) in 4 monkeys and 4 rabbits. The shading indicates TPR responses of rabbits during autonomic blockade. Adapted from White et al. (1972, 1973).

Nasopharyngeal-Arterial Chemoreceptor Interactions

Many insights into the nature of the interactions between inputs arising from the arterial chemoreceptors, lung inflation receptors, and nasopharyngeal receptors have been obtained through the work of Michael Daly and colleagues, as noted earlier in this chapter (Daly, 1986).

In anesthetized dogs and cats, stimulation of the arterial chemoreceptors under conditions of constant artificial ventilation evokes bradycardia and vasoconstriction. The responses are greater when ventilation is low rather than high, which reflects the inhibitory actions of lung inflation receptor activity on heart rate and vasomotor neurons (figure 14.10). In spontaneously breathing monkeys, these chemoreceptor responses only become manifest at very low paO$_2$, indicating that their threshold is much greater than in rabbits.

Brief bilateral carotid body stimulation with cyanide in spontaneously breathing anesthetized monkeys increases ventilation and mostly evokes slight bradycardia and vasoconstriction (figure 14.18A; Daly et al., 1978b). With more prolonged chemoreceptor stimulation, the larger respiratory response evokes tachycardia but little change in femoral Vas R. However, stimulation of the arterial chemoreceptors in the

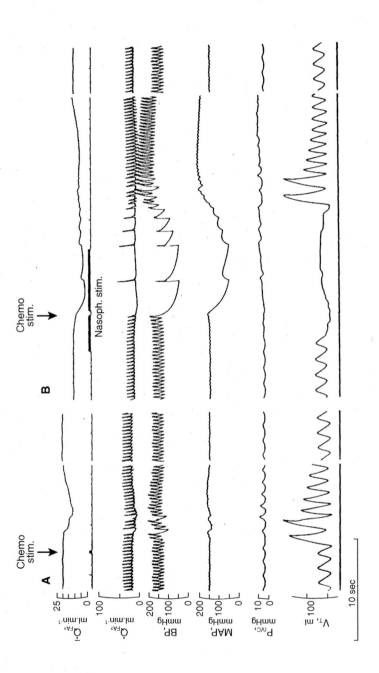

Figure 14.18. (A) effects of carotid body stimulation with 0.05 mL of NaCN into each carotid artery (at arrow) on femoral blood flow (Q, mL/min), pulsatile and mean arterial (BP, MAP, mmHg), inferior vena caval pressure (P_{IVC}, mmHg), and tidal respiratory volume (V_T, mL) in anesthetized monkey, showing hyperventilation, transient bradycardia, and femoral vasoconstriction. (B) Continuous signal stimulation of nasopharynx, which induced apnea but had little circulatory effect; at arrow, bilateral injection of 0.05 mL of NaCN elicited marked bradycardia and vasoconstriction. Note systemic BP surge when ventilation resumed. From Daly et al. (1978b), with permission of *American Journal of Physiology* and American Physiological Society.

presence of nasopharyngeally induced apnea evokes substantial bradycardia and vasoconstriction.[7] Moreover, the hyperventilation that follows the apnea is accompanied by a large rise in BP (figure 14.18B; Daly et al., 1978a). This resembles the BP surge of patients with OSA (figure 14.2).

Thus, the combination of activity of the respiratory center and lung inflation receptors completely inhibits chemoreceptor-mediated bradycardia and vasoconstriction in monkeys, so that complete cessation of respiratory effort is crucial for eliciting these responses.

O₂-Conserving Variant Forms of the Defense Response

The autonomic effects of nasopharyngeal stimulation and arterial hypoxia also conserve O_2, which has major survival value in particular environments. In marine mammals and diving birds, the stimulation of trigeminal afferents during submersion provides the trigger for the apnea, marked systemic vasoconstriction and reduction in CO. The response conserves O_2 everywhere except in the brain and myocardium (Elsner et al., 1964; Elsner and Scholander, 1965; White and McRitchie, 1973; White et al., 1974; Elsner and Gooden, 1983). The diving response allows the animal to remain submerged for 2–5 minutes and often much longer. Diving may allow escape from a predator or provide the means of surprising a quarry when foraging for food. Under these circumstances, there is vasoconstriction in the kidney, gut, and skin but not in brain, heart, and active muscles.

The nasopharyngeal reflex in rabbits is a response similar to the above but of much briefer duration. This reflex is minimal in subhuman primates and humans, unless reinforced by other excitatory inputs. For these species, the risk to their sophisticated brain is too great to make the diving response anything except a priority of last resort. That this is well founded is seen in patients with OSA, in whom symptoms such as daytime sleepiness are a handicap for social intercourse.

Similar priorities apply to the autonomic response to arterial hypoxia, which is about making the most of a limited O_2 supply. In rabbits and rodents the threshold for eliciting O_2-conserving arterial chemoreceptor reflexes is lower than in primates, in which it has become a last resort option when respiration is suppressed. Fortunately, the effect is transient in OSA, but its cumulative effects should not be underestimated. It resembles life at high altitudes (Korner, 1959; Pugh, 1964).

A Schema for Cardiorespiratory Control in OSA

The schema in figure 14.19 assumes that the CNS pathways mediating the effects of the arterial chemoreceptors, nasopharyngeal receptors, and baroreceptors are similar in the various mammalian species but that response differences between them are due to variation in the thresholds at which their excitatory actions are suppressed by the activity of the lung inflation receptors and respiratory center.

The inhibition occurs through the neocortical inhibitory system, which suppresses the hypothalamic neurons responsible for pronounced bradycardia and systemic vasoconstriction. This involves comparisons of the relative magnitude of the activity of

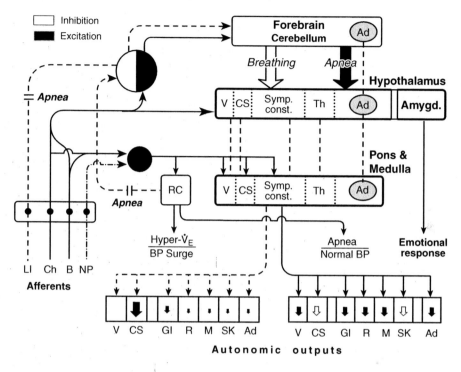

Figure 14.19. Suggested mechanisms determining autonomic responses in OSA. Forebrain, in conjunction with cerebellum, compares relative magnitude of inhibitory and excitatory inputs. Main inhibitory inputs are lung inflation receptors (LI) and respiratory center (RC), and main excitatory inputs are arterial chemoreceptors (Ch) and nasopharyngeal receptors (NP). When (LI + RC) > (Ch + NP), forebrain inhibits hypothalamic centers, while Ch, NP, and baroreceptors (B) evoke attenuated response through bulbospinal centers. If (Ch + NP) > (LI + RC), hypothalamic excitation generates autonomic pattern on the lower right (black arrows, excitation; clear arrows, inhibition). V, vagus; CS, cardiac SNA; SNA in gastrointestinal (GI), renal (R), skeletal muscle (M), and skin (SK) outflows; Ad, adrenaline. Apnea responses are similar or greater, but without rise in adrenaline. Patients with OSA have this pattern during (apnea + hypoxia + hypercapnia), while during hyperventilation they switch to pattern on lower left, with high cardiac SNA but only slight constrictor SNA. The rise in BP is due to high cardiac SNA and CO before vascular tone is back to normal. Aversive feelings accompany arousal at the end of apnea.

the lung inflation receptors and respiratory center on the one hand, and that of the arterial chemoreceptors on the other. It is a comparison not unlike that between central command and muscle chemoreceptors performed by the cerebellum during exercise. We may speculate that the cerebellum makes similar comparisons of receptor activity during the apnea-arterial hypoxia-hyperventilation sequence, with the outcome conveyed to the hypothalamus and baroreflex centers in the hindbrain through 5-HT and NA modulatory neurons.

In rabbits, the inhibitory system is weak: Marked stimulation of the arterial chemoreceptors excites the hypothalamus even during spontaneous respiration. In contrast, in primates the hypothalamic neurons remain inhibited except during apnea and strong stimulation of the arterial chemoreceptors and nasopharyngeal receptors.

Arterial Hypoxia

In mild hypoxia, the neocortical mechanisms linked to respiration suppress excitability of hypothalamic neurons, which generate bradycardia and the peripheral sympathetic defense pattern. In rabbits, the hypothalamic activity is suppressed as long as lung inflation receptor activity exceeds that of the arterial chemoreceptors, with the autonomic pattern as on the bottom left of figure 14.19. When lung inflation afferent activity declines and arterial chemoreceptor discharge rises markedly, the pattern is as on the bottom right of figure 14.19, owing to excitation of the hypothalamus.

Thus the ratio of lung inflation receptor activity to arterial chemoreceptor activity determines the autonomic pattern in rabbits. In primates, the intrinsic activity of the respiratory center is crucial (Korner, 1979a). As long as there remains any residual respiratory activity, hypothalamic excitation of constrictor SNA is suppressed with the autonomic response consisting mainly of hyperventilation-induced elevation in cardiac SNA (figure 14.17). The responses on the lower right of figure 14.19 require complete cessation of respiration during arterial chemoreceptor and nasopharyngeal stimulation.

Apnea and Nasopharyngeal Stimulation

In rabbits, similar autonomic responses are evoked by (1) nasopharyngeally induced apnea, (2) passive apnea without nasopharyngeal stimulation, and (3) nasopharyngeal stimulation without apnea. This suggests that the responses due to loss of respiratory activity or strong trigeminal nociceptor stimulation alone can virtually substitute for the full response in the spontaneously breathing animal. This is not the case in primates (figure 14.18A): Apnea, arterial chemoreceptor stimulation, and nasopharyngeal stimulation are all necessary to elicit the pattern on the lower right of figure 14.19.

Responses in OSA

Bradycardia and elevation of MSNA develop after the phase of complete apnea, as the patient tries to inspire against a closed glottis (figure 14.2). The inputs at this time include the arterial chemoreceptors, probably respiratory skeletal muscle chemoreceptors that increase their discharge during the Müller maneuver as in exercise, and trigeminal nasopharyngeal nociceptors. Once hyperventilation begins, there is a rapid switch to tachycardia and inhibition of constrictor SNA; Vas R falls more gradually owing to the slow response time of vascular smooth muscle. The high CO is the result of the large hyperventilation-induced increase in cardiac SNA together with mechanically induced elevation of blood flow, with the raised perfusion of the partially constricted vasculature responsible for the large surge in BP.

Thus, during each OSA cycle the initial autonomic pattern on the bottom right of figure 14.19 switches to that on the bottom left. The first is the response to cutting off the tissues' O_2 supply associated with apnea, while the second is the response associated with its restoration after the nasopharyngeal obstruction has lifted.

Relationship between OSA and Essential Hypertension

From the preceding section, the nocturnal elevation of BP in OSA is due to tachycardia and elevation of CO, which alternates with bradycardia and vasoconstriction. It is the postapneic phase that is responsible for the nocturnal elevation of BP. These are all very basic responses for the defense of the organism O_2 supply. They are elicited in anyone with nasopharyngeal obstruction and not just in those genetically susceptible to EH.

The cause of the obstruction remains unknown. However, its key role is evident from the dramatic way in which nCPAP abolishes apnea and hypertension. Obesity, including normotensive and hypertensive obesity, predisposes to OSA. Adiposity-related peptides and an increase in nasopharyngeal fat may both play causal roles in the obstruction, in view of the beneficial effects of weight reduction. However, OSA also occurs in 30% of patients who are lean, including some who are normotensive and some who have stress-and-salt-related EH. It has been suggested that a fault of neural regulation is responsible for the low tone of the nasopharyngeal dilator muscles during sleep (Saper et al., 2005). As a result, many factors could accentuate the underlying obstruction.

Experimental Approaches

Cyclically induced nocturnal tracheal obstruction in dogs reproduces both nighttime and daytime hypertension. The frequent cycles of simulated OSA each night were clearly sufficient to cause not only nocturnal but diurnal hypertension in all the animals in which there probably was no genetic predisposition to EH.

The nocturnal hypertension is of modest degree, yet it simulates exactly that of patients. The modest nature of the BP rise is because the syndrome elicits the O_2-conserving variant of the defense response, where cardiac depression reduces the effects of vasoconstriction. The instant recovery on discontinuing the simulated OSA suggests that the nighttime hypertension is largely a response to the exigencies of the moment, without obvious synaptic strengthening.

In the dogs, all animals developed diurnal hypertension in response to frequent bouts of respiratory obstruction, presumably associated with unpleasant emotions, as in other types of stress. The uniform rise in daytime BP may have been related to the severity of the nighttime episodes. The more gradual recovery at the end of the experiment suggests that the synaptic changes were functional, without growth of new synaptic contacts.

In OSA patients, the magnitude of the diurnal rise in BP is similar to that at night. It is observed in only about half the patients, suggesting that the average severity of attacks of apnea-hypopnea may have been less pronounced than in dogs. However, institution of nCPAP caused rapid recovery in daytime hypertension, suggesting that any strengthening of synaptic transmission was functional and relatively small.

In rats, too, each cycle of severe arterial hypoxia raises BP through the pattern on the lower right of figure 14.19; it takes three weeks of intermittent stimulation before the BP exceeds baseline values under normoxic conditions (figure 14.5), when the enhanced hypothalamic responsiveness has increased sufficiently. The poststimulus rise in BP suggests that the aversive conditioning caused some strengthening of synaptic transmission, similar to that in human OSA.

Relationship between OSA and Stress-Related EH

As noted in chapter 11, the rises in BP and MSNA evoked by arterial hypoxia are greater in persons with EH than in normotensives, with the difference much enhanced when cortical inhibition of the hypothalamus is removed by voluntary apnea (figure 11.9; Somers et al., 1988). Trzebski et al. (1982) had noted a greater BP responsiveness to arterial hypoxia in persons with EH, following earlier observations in SHR (Trzebski et al., 1975; Fukuda et al., 1986). The point is that many hypothalamic neurons that respond to arterial hypoxia also respond to mental stress. When these neurons have become sensitized in the course of developing EH, they are hyperresponsive to both stimuli.

In OSA, the nocturnal rise in BP is mainly caused by the high CO due to the hyperventilation that follows vasoconstriction due to apnea-arterial hypoxia. The hypertension is thus related indirectly to defense pathway activity. Daytime activation of the pathway is due to functional synaptic sensitization, but the rise in BP is smaller than in stress-and-salt related EH or in hypertensive obesity, which is probably due to the disparate nocturnal changes in cardiac baroreflex and sympathetic constrictor baroreflex properties (figure 14.11). In addition, the diminished awareness of the aversive stimuli at night may contribute to the smaller increase in daytime BP.

Because of its primarily respiratory origins, OSA is often regarded as a secondary form of hypertension rather than an EH syndrome (Kaplan, 2002). This is true, and it should probably be classified in this way. The reason for considering it in this book is that the cardiovascular changes are a variant of the defense response. However, it clearly differs from the "getting-ready-for-action" variants, which give rise to the bulk of EH.

OSA is probably the only type of high BP that is a response to a general impairment of tissue perfusion from an early stage, as originally postulated by Irving Page. Treatment with nCPAP addresses the prime cause of the cardiovascular dysfunction and has been remarkably successful. A proportion of OSA patient also have hypertensive obesity and stress-related EH in lean persons. Determining the true cause of the respiratory disturbance in OSA must await further research. In the meantime, it is best regarded as a secondary type of hypertension.

PART VII

CAUSES AND MECHANISMS OF RENAL AND SHR HYPERTENSION

15

More About the Kidney in Hypertension

The kidney makes a major hemodynamic contribution to EH, and this chapter addresses the question whether the kidney is the source of EH or its victim. Although the kidney plays a highly significant role in the elevation of BP in either case, the answer has major implications for prevention and treatment.

The notion that EH could be due to a genetic renal fault stems from the results of renal transplantation in genetically hypertensive rats (Bianchi et al., 1974; Dahl et al., 1974). A renal graft from a hypertensive donor raises the BP of a normotensive recipient, while grafting a normotensive donor kidney into a hypertensive recipient causes a fall in BP. Hence Dahl's famous dictum, "Blood pressure travels with the kidney." Most authorities still consider this as cast-iron evidence of a genetic or developmental renal fault (e.g., Guyton, 1980; de Wardener, 1990; Cowley, 1992). However, other factors are also involved, for example, structurally remodeled arterioles transplanted in the graft.

In severe long-standing EH, the nephron numbers are reduced, and one hypothesis has been that this is a consequence of fetal stress during development (Brenner et al., 1988; Zandi-Nejad et al., 2006). This factor is undoubtedly of potential importance, but the epidemiological evidence considered in chapter 4 suggests that it accounts for only a small proportion of subjects with EH. In the majority of persons with severe EH, the low nephron number is a consequence of long-standing chronic vasoconstriction and associated rarefaction of the renal microcirculation.

The remainder of this chapter considers the intrarenal and systemic effects of several types of renal hypertension in humans and experimental animals. Human renovascular hypertension (RenVH) was at one time regarded as the quintessential pressor hormone-mediated nonneural type of chronic high BP. There is no doubt that

Ang II is important in pathogenesis, probably more for its intrarenal actions than for its role as a systemic pressor hormone. However, there is now good evidence that sympathetic neural activity (SNA) is raised in RenVH and also in renal failure due to other causes. The common requirement is severe underlying renal ischemia, which increases the activity of renal chemoreceptors and raises BP through the hypothalamus. The only nonneural type of renal hypertension considered here is primary aldosteronism, where the action of aldosterone on an otherwise normal kidney gives rise to pure volume overload and some reduction in SNA. Some of the monogenic types of hypertension also fall into this category (chapter 3).

Our understanding of the mechanisms of renal hypertension is largely based on animal models. Three types of RenVH are considered in this chapter: (1) one kidney, one clip (1K-1C) hypertension; (2) two kidneys, one clip (2K-1C) hypertension; and (3) Page cellophane wrap hypertension. All are constrictor types of high BP and are associated with considerable renal ischemia. Low-renal-mass hypertension is a prototype of renal failure to which ischemia is readily superadded if the few nephrons left are made to work harder by subjecting them to a moderate salt load or a high protein intake. The last part of the chapter compares the above four types of renal hypertension, relates them to the renal changes in EH, and addresses the question why there has been so much uncertainty about the effects on BP of the associated renal tubular transport abnormalities known to occur in this disorder.

Interpreting Renal Transplantation Experiments

The first experimental renal transplants in relation to hypertension were performed in the Milan hypertensive rat, the Dahl S rat, and later in the SHR and their corresponding normotensive controls (Bianchi et al., 1974; Dahl et al., 1974; Dahl and Heine, 1975; Rettig and Schmitt, 1994; Rettig and Grisk, 2005).

Transplantation in SHR

Graft rejection was common in the early studies, which biases interpretation of the results (Rettig and Schmitt, 1994; Rettig and Grisk, 2005). Since all immunosuppressive drug regimens are hypertensinogenic, their use is inappropriate in experiments on the pathogenesis of hypertension. Rettig overcame the rejection problem by using borderline hypertensive rats (BHR) as recipients; BHR have a single copy of each parent's allele, so that they do not reject kidneys from either SHR or WKY.[1]

Transplanting a WKY kidney into a BHR recipient produces no change in the recipient's BP, while grafting an SHR kidney causes a rise in BP (Kawabe et al., 1979; Rettig et al., 1990). The rise has been assumed to be due to a defect in tubular function but could also be due to structural narrowing of the R_1 vessels in the graft. Such narrowing is present in 4-week-old SHR (chapters 6, 16; Gattone et al., 1983; Smeda et al., 1988; Skov et al., 1994; Kett et al., 1995).[2] For technical reasons, the great majority of renal transplants have been performed in 9–15-week-old rats except for a small number of transplants performed on 5–6 week-old-rats.[3] Therefore the donor kidney always includes stenotic R_1 vessels, which become more stenotic after transplantation.

Indeed, Rettig's own experiments have provided strong support for the role of structural factors (Rettig et al., 1990). After 3 months of 2K-1C hypertension in WKY, the untouched kidney was grafted into a normotensive WKY and the resulting elevation of BP was assumed to be due to the marked structural vascular changes present in the donor kidney.

Another transplantation study that illustrates the role of structure was performed in an experiment in which the donors and recipients were SHR littermates and transplantation was performed at 15 weeks of age (Smallegange et al., 2003). Half the animals of each group had been treated with the ACE inhibitor enalapril between the ages of 4 and 13 weeks, while no drug was given to the others. As discussed in chapter 16, enalapril interferes with vascular development during the neonatal period, which causes permanent widening of the R1 vasculature of SHR (Korner and Bobik, 1995).

The four posttransplant groups consisted of animals with (1) untreated donor kidneys grafted into untreated recipients (U_{donor}, U_{recip}); (2) enalapril-treated donor kidneys grafted into untreated recipients (T_{donor}, U_{recip}); (3) U_{donor} kidneys grafted into T_{recip}; and (4) T_{donor} kidneys grafted into T_{recip}. In each animal, mean arterial pressure (MAP) was measured continuously over 24 hours from day 36 to day 50 after the operation (table 15.1).

The highest BP in U_{donor}, U_{recip} rats was 35 mmHg above that of T_{donor}, U_{recip}, in which the renal R_1 vessels were permanently widened (Korner and Bobik, 1995). Of the other two groups in table 15.1, the BP of U_{donor}, T_{recip} rats was 13 mmHg higher than that of T_{donor}, T_{recip}, suggesting that the vasculature of the recipient also affects the response.

Sexual BP dimorphism is another example where the recipient rather than the donor determines the BP after renal transplantation. The BP of male SHR is considerably greater than in females (chapter 16). Accordingly, Harrap et al. (1992) examined whether the difference was due to genes affecting renal function. Transplanting male SHR kidneys into female SHR and vice versa had no effect on the recipient's BP.

Table 15.1. Average Mean Arterial Pressures (MAP, mmHg) in Four Combinations of Renal Transplants and Recipients in 15-Week-Old SHR

Group	MAP
Untreated donor → untreated recipient	148 mmHg
Treated donor → untreated recipient	113 mmHg
	ΔMAP 35 mmHg
Untreated donor → treated recipient	138 mmHg
Treated donor → treated recipient	125 mmHg
	ΔMAP 13 mmHg

Note: Treatment consisted of enalapril 25 mg/kg/day in drinking water from 4 to 13 weeks of age; MAP measured continuously through a pressure transducer implanted at 11 weeks of age. MAP for each combination was the average MAP between days 36 to 50 after transplantation.

Source: Smallegange et al. (2003).

Transplantation in Dahl Rats

In Dahl's original transplant experiments and most subsequent studies, the rats were maintained on a normal salt intake (~0.4% NaCl) after transplantion (Dahl et al., 1974; Dahl and Heine, 1975). BP increased in R rats that had received an S kidney and fell in S rats given an R kidney.

Morgan et al. (1990) recognized the need to examine the responses to high dietary salt in the transplanted rats. After first confirming Dahl's findings on a normal salt intake (table 15.2), another experiment was performed in which the animals were switched to a high-salt diet (8% NaCl) after transplantation. This elicited rises in BP in all groups, except in R recipients given an R kidney. Surprisingly, the BP rise in S recipients with an R kidney was similar to that in S recipients given an S kidney.

The large BP rise in S recipients with an R kidney indicates an extrarenal source of the hypertension (Leenen et al., 2002), for example, elevation in SNA through central endogenous ouabain (EO) neurons (figure 12.10), through which cardiac and nonrenal constrictor SNA must be raised. Last, an S kidney grafted into an R recipient includes not only abnormalities in tubular transport mechanisms but also narrowing of R_1 vessel arterioles (Mueller, 1983).

Transplantation in EH

Curtis et al. (1983) performed some of the early human transplantation studies: They grafted kidneys from normotensive donors into six patients with severe EH and pronounced nephropathy and retinopathy. Their BP fell dramatically, and the transplant cured their hypertension over a 4.5-year-period of follow-up. However, the same result would be expected in the BP of patients with primary renal failure. One cannot make an etiological interpretation based on end-stage renal disease.

In other renal transplants, performed largely for renal failure, it was found that postoperative BP was greater in patients with grafts from donors with EH or a family history of EH, compared to that of normotensive donors without such a history (Guidi et al., 1985, 1996). All patients received immunosuppressive drugs, which makes it difficult to draw conclusions about the etiological role of the kidney.

Table 15.2. Mean Arterial Pressures (MAP ± SEM, mmHg) in Renal Grafts Transplanted between Dahl R (R) and Dahl S (S) Rats When on a Normal (0.4% NaCl) or High (8.0% NaCl) Salt Diet

Transplant		MAP (mmHg)	
Recipient	Donor	Normal Salt	High Salt
R	R	96 ± 3	103 ± 2
R	S	108 ± 4	145 ± 5
S	R	99 ± 2	151 ± 7
S	S	119 ± 3	160 ± 5

Source: Data from Morgan et al. (1990), with permission of *Hypertension*, American Heart Association, and Lippincott, Williams and Wilkins.

Comment

For a time, the results of renal transplantation in genetic rat hypertension did suggest that the kidney was the source of the high BP. They still point to a major role for the kidney in genetic rat hypertension and probably in EH. However, it is clear that other factors also play a role, including some of nongenetic origin. To their credit, this has been recognized by Rettig and Grisk (2005). Like so many approaches, renal transplantation has not provided the hoped-for unequivocal answers about the etiology of primary hypertension.

Are Low Nephron Numbers a Consequence or a Cause of EH?

Nephron numbers are reduced in established EH. One well-designed study by Keller et al. (2003) used two groups of subjects, aged 35 to 59 years, who had died suddenly in accidents. One group had a clear medical history of severe EH, including LVH and R_1 vessel changes,[4] while the second group consisted of normotensive controls matched for sex, age, height, and weight with the subjects with EH. State-of-the-art stereological methods were used to estimate each subject's total number of glomeruli and average glomerular volume (Kett and Bertram, 2004).

In persons with EH, the median number of glomeruli and the glomerular volume are, respectively, 49% and 2.35 times that of controls. This was thought to be in agreement with a hypothesis by Brenner et al. (1988) that the low number was a consequence of fetal stress during development. The theory was based on the data of Moore (1931), who had observed a four- to sixfold range of nephron numbers in autopsies performed on young normal subjects (Mackenzie et al., 1995). Brenner speculated that diastolic BPs were likely to be greater in those with low nephron numbers, resulting in EH. However, Moore may have overestimated the variation in glomerular numbers due to the limitations of the counting methods then available. Similar variation in glomerular numbers has been observed in more recent studies with state-of-the-art methods (Nyengaard and Bendtsen, 1992; Hoy et al., 2003; Hughson et al., 2003). In these studies, the subjects were considerably more heterogenous than in the study of Keller et al. (2003), with large differences in age, sex, and racial factors. Clearly, for a hypothesis about the role of fetal factors in EH, matched groups of young adults are required, with the study of Keller et al. (2003) representing the maximum allowable age range. They observed only a 2.5-fold range of variation of total glomerular number in normotensives and a 1.8-fold range in persons with EH (figure 15.1).

In Barker's theory of the fetal stress origin of adult cardiovascular disease, low birth weight was used as a marker of fetal stress. Recall from chapter 4 that this factor accounted for only a small proportion of adult cases of EH. A recent extension of Barker's theory has been that fetal stress increases the formation of a "survival phenotype" in which development of the brain and reproductive organs is favored over that of the viscera and kidney (Gluckman and Hanson, 2005).

One test of the theory involved genetic manipulation of renal development by disrupting the gene for glial cell line–derived neurotrophic factor (GDNF). Absence of this

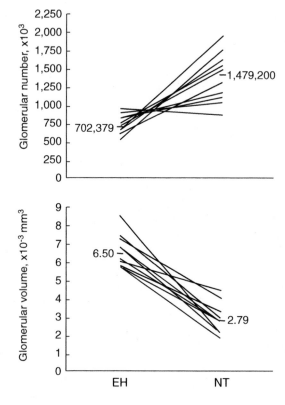

Figure 15.1. Total number of glomeruli in kidneys of 10 subjects with known severe EH and 10 matched normotensives (top) and the corresponding mean glomerular volumes. The numbers refer to the median values of each group. From Keller et al. (2003), with permission of the *New England Journal of Medicine* and Massachusetts Medical Society.

factor proved lethal in homozygotes, but in heterozygous GDNF mice the number of nephrons was 30% below that of wild-type littermates (Cullen-McEwen et al., 2003). The first BP measurement was not made until 14 months of age, when it was 18 mmHg above that of wild-type mice; glomerular filtration rate (GFR), renal blood flow (RBF), and daily renal sodium and potassium excretion were similar in both groups. The rise in BP in these old rats is definite but small compared to that of persons with EH. Nor do the GDNF mice show the renal hemodynamic changes of established EH (figure 5.3).

In other experimental studies, the interventions have included marked impairment of the placental blood supply or injections of cortisol: The BP rises soon after birth without the temporal delay to adult life that occurs in EH. This also applies to experiments in which removal of one kidney within 24 hours of birth causes elevation of BP by 8 and 18 mmHg at 8 and 20 weeks of age, and an increase in salt sensitivity (Woods et al., 2001). All these experiments indicate that the renal mass is a determinant of BP, but they do not indicate that early reduction in mass is a factor in EH and other types of primary hypertension.

The alternative hypothesis that the decline in glomerular numbers is a consequence of the elevation of BP is supported by findings in two studies in SHR. Kett et al. (1996) found that glomerular numbers in 10-week-old rats were the same as in age-matched WKY. In contrast, Skov et al. (1994) studied 12-week-old SHR in which nephron numbers were 20% lower than in WKY. The timing of the first study is about 1 week from the end of the phase of rapid BP rise, while that of the second study is 3 weeks later. Taken together, the two studies suggest that SHR are born with normal nephron numbers but that some decrease begins soon after the first substantial BP rise and associated structural changes and rarefaction. In SHR, BP continues to increase until about 24 weeks of age, over which time renal function deteriorates further (Arendshorst and Beierwaltes, 1979).

The idea that renal function is normal at the start of EH and deteriorates as EH progresses is supported by results of a radiological study performed over 30 years ago (Hollenberg et al., 1969a, 1969b). The purpose was to screen potential donors for renal transplantation. It involved examining the distal interlobar and arcuate arteries and the origins of the interlobular branches, which are often the site of arterial lesions in patients with EH (Bell, 1950; Corcoran et al., 1948). Table 15.3 shows the basis for grading the radioangiographic abnormalities, while table 15.4 shows their relationship to RBF measured by the ^{133}Xe indicator washout technique (Thorburn et al., 1963).

No arterial lesions were observed in the younger subjects with mild to moderate EH, in whom mean RBF and creatinine clearance ($\equiv$GFR) were normal (table 15.4). As the severity of EH increased, RBF and GFR were increasingly depressed and the number of arterial lesions increased. In very severe EH, the start of the renal cortical vessels was hard to visualize, renal renin secretion was raised, and the nephrons in the outer cortical layers were poorly perfused (figure 15.2),[5] as judged from the fast exponential component of the indicator disappearance curve.

Thus the following sequence of changes may be envisaged: At the start of EH renal blood flow, Vas R, GFR, and, by inference, glomerular numbers are all normal. Over time, the increase in renal SNA leads to progressive functional rarefaction and reduction in the number of well-perfused nephrons. As R_1 vessel structural changes develop and availability of NO declines, renal microcirculatory rarefaction increases, with increasing permanent nephron closure (chapter 6). However, the number of glomerular remnants that can be distinguished is small (Keller et al., 2003), suggesting that the nephron closure rapidly results in apoptosis.

Table 15.3. Grading of Renal Arterial Lesions in Distal Interlobar and Arcuate Arteries and Their Initial Branches

Grade	Arterial Abnormality
0	All arteries visible; no irregularity or filling defect; smooth tapering of vessels from inner to outer cortex, as in healthy normotensives
I	Slight irregularity and tortuosity in <20% of vessels; normal cortical tapering, but no stenosis or filling defects
II	Tortuosity and irregularity in ~50% of vessels, cortical tapering normal; scattered filling defects in ~10% of vessels
III	All vessels visible, but ~25% of cortical branches not identifiable; tapering in distal vessels abrupt ("stepladder" appearance)
IV	Very few cortical branches visible; most arcuate arteries abnormal and frequent filling defects; very abnormal cortical tapering; slow transit of contrast medium

Source: Hollenberg et al. (1969a).

Table 15.4. Average Renal Blood Flow, Creatinine Clearance, and Clinic BP in a Group of Healthy Normotensives and Another with EH

Group	Age, yr (n)	Mean RBF (mL/100 g/min)	C_{Creat} (mL/min)	Clin.SBP/DBP (mmHg)
Healthy NT	[a](36)	338	—	<130/85
EH, RV 0	29, (12)	342	116	151/100
EH, RV I	39, (10)	318	105	154/104
EH, RV II	44, (19)	307*	101	170/110*
EH, RV III	51, (19)	247*	75*	177/116*
EH, RV, IV	37, (6)	117*	26*	195/120*

Note: NT, normotensive; EH, essential hypertensive; RV 0 to IV grading of appearance of renal distal interlobar and arcuate vessels (table 15.3); n, number of subjects; RBF, renal blood flow (mL/100 g tissue/min); Clin.SBP/DBP, clinic systolic and diastolic BPs (mmHg); C_{Creat}, creatinine clearance. [a]Age range from 23 to 69 years.
*$p < .01$ difference from NT group.
Grading according to angiographic abnormalities in distal interlobar and arcuate arteries.

Source: Hollenberg et al. (1969a), with permission.

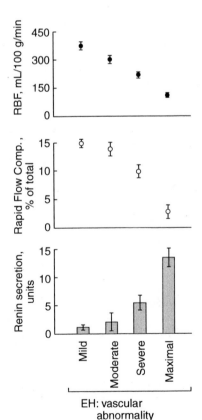

Figure 15.2. Patients with EH grouped according to severity of angiographic abnormalities (see table 15.3). In the most severe grades mean RBF is greatly reduced, due to impairment of rapid flow component of the indicator disappearance curve, which suggests some functional shutdown of outer cortical nephrons. After Hollenberg et al. (1969b), with permission of the *American Journal of Medicine* and Elsevier.

Human Renal Hypertension

This section considers clinical and pathophysiological aspects of RenVH, volume overload hypertension, and malignant hypertension. As to the underlying mechanisms, as Derx and Schalenkamp (1994) have pithily expressed it: "If essential hypertension is a disease of theories, then renovascular hypertension is a disease of experiment" (p. 237). In other words, current understanding of underlying mechanisms is largely based on analysis of the various animal models.

Renovascular Hypertension

RenVH is caused by renal artery obstruction and accounts for about 4% of adult high BP (Wilkinson, 1994; Pickering and Mann, 1995). However, not everyone with renal artery stenosis has high BP, nor does correction of the stenosis always lower BP. Hence a practical definition of RenVH is that it is hypertension due to renal artery obstruction that is cured or improved by surgical or angioplastic amelioration of the stenosis.

In Western countries, atherosclerotic plaques are responsible for renal artery stenosis in about two thirds of patients. They are more common in older subjects, in whom the obstruction gradually increases over time. In the remaining, mostly younger, patients, the stenosis is due to congenital fibromuscular dysplasia. A common type is medial fibroplasia, in which short stretches of fibrosis along the vessel are separated by dilated segments, giving a radiological "string of beads" appearance (Wilkinson, 1994). In Asian and African countries, RenVH is often caused by Takayasu's arteritis, which is a disorder of uncertain etiology. It may be an autoimmune disease in which the stenosis is due to obstruction caused by inflammatory changes in the wall of the artery.

Renal artery stenosis may be unilateral or bilateral. In unilateral stenosis, plasma (and blood) volumes are often normal, PRA is raised, and ACE inhibitors usually lower BP (Pickering and Mann, 1995). In bilateral stenosis, plasma volume and PRA may be normal or raised, with considerable variation between patients. In both types of RenVH, treatment with ACE inhibitors often causes deterioration of renal function, suggesting that angiotensin II (Ang II) participates in intrarenal regulation. High Ang II may raise plasma aldosterone and promote sodium reabsorption. What happens to blood volume depends on dietary sodium intake, the degree of systemic vasoconstriction, the actions of aldosterone, and BP-mediated pressure diuresis.

Renal function is always compromised in severe RenVH. Long-term prognosis is poor, with high morbidity and mortality due to stroke, renal failure, and cardiac failure. Hunt et al. (1978) found that 73% of patients treated with antihypertensive drugs died over a follow-up period of 7–14 years, contrasting with a 30% mortality in patients treated surgically.

Until recently, the role of the sympathetic nervous system in RenVH has tended to be ignored. We now know that SNA is generally raised in RenVH and in the high BP associated with renal failure.

Volume Overload Hypertension

Primary aldosteronism causes volume overload due to the action of aldosterone on an initially normal kidney. Volume overload also accompanies long-standing severe renal disease in which there has been gross reduction in nephron numbers, greatly reducing the kidney's capacity to excrete sodium chloride. This occurs not only in primarily renal hypertension, but also in long-standing severe EH.

Primary Aldosteronism

In hypertension due to an aldosterone-producing tumor, the increase in hormone levels results in greater tubular reabsorption of sodium and water. An illustration of the sequential hemodynamic and blood volume changes during its development comes from a study in 12 patients with discrete adrenal adenomas, whose BPs had been well controlled on spironolactone (Schalekamp et al., 1985). In order to attempt a permanent cure, it had been decided to remove the tumors surgically. This required discontinuing spironolactone for several weeks before the operation, thus providing an opportunity to study spontaneous redevelopment of the hypertension.

In the six younger patients, CO and blood volume increased and remained high without a significant rise in TPR (figure 15.3, right). The slight bradycardia suggests a baroreflex response to the increasing cardiopulmonary load. The high CO is in response to the greater rise in blood volume, which is in accord with the predictions of Guyton's model before the invention of long-term autoregulation, as discussed in chapter 2.

In the six older patients, CO also rose for the first 2–3 weeks of redevelopment of hypertension, followed later by a more definite rise in TPR than in the younger patients (figure 15.3, left). The rise in TPR is unlikely to be due to an increase in SNA since in primary aldosteronism plasma sodium concentration and osmolality are normal and muscle sympathetic nerve activity (MSNA) is about 20% below that of normotensive controls (Miyajima et al., 1991). One mechanism to explain the rise in TPR in the older patients is reduction in renal NO due to high renal papillary blood flow. There may also have been more pronounced structural changes due to the greater duration of the hypertension, which would also be accentuated by lower renal papillary NO.

Similar variation in CO and TPR responses has been observed in animals with experimental mineralocorticoid hypertension (Bravo et al., 1977). The underlying mechanisms have not been determined, but variation in renal NO production and in the extent of the structural changes could also explain the response differences.

Volume Overload in Severe Renal Disease

McGrath et al. (1977) studied 15 patients with severe renal disease (age range 23–56 years), who had been managed on a chronic dialysis regimen. Their renal failure was due to a range of etiological factors, including chronic glomerulonephritis, chronic pyelonephritis, analgesic nephropathy, and severe glomerulosclerosis. All the patients had the kidneys in place; 11 were hypertensive and 4 had normal BPs. All had moderate

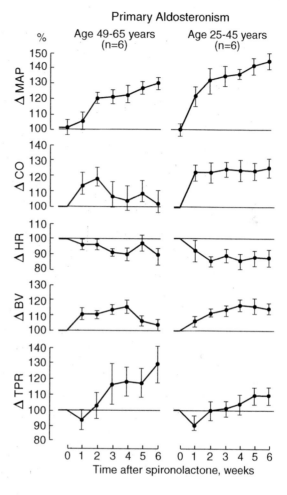

Figure 15.3. Changes during redevelopment of hypertension in primary aldosteronism after discontinuing spironolactone at time 0 in (from top) mean arterial pressure (ΔMAP), cardiac output (ΔCO), heart rate (ΔHR), blood volume (ΔBV), and total peripheral resistance (ΔTPR; all as % of baseline). Left, data from 6 patients aged 49–65 years and (right) from 6 patients aged 25–45 years. Adapted from Schalekamp et al. (1985), with permission of *Journal of Hypertension* and Lippincott, Williams and Wilkins.

anemia with a hematocrit of about 20%, which was a common complication in dialysis patients in the 1970s.

The dialysis regimen remained fixed throughout the 4-week study period, during which patients' sodium intake was 10 mmol/day for 2 weeks and 100 mmol/day for 2 weeks. On the high sodium intake the hypertensive subjects' extracellular sodium and blood volumes were greater than on low sodium (figure 15.4). Similarly, their CO, right atrial pressure, and heart rates all rose on high sodium, but TPR remained the same on both levels of sodium. The responses of the normotensive subjects were closely similar.

The hemodynamic effects of total autonomic blockade (TAB) were investigated on each sodium intake. In the hypertensive group, there was marked reduction in MAP and TPR, with the latter falling by 35%, which was the same on low and high sodium. However, TAB had no effect on the TPR of the normotensive subjects with renal failure. The results suggest that in the hypertensive subjects with renal failure

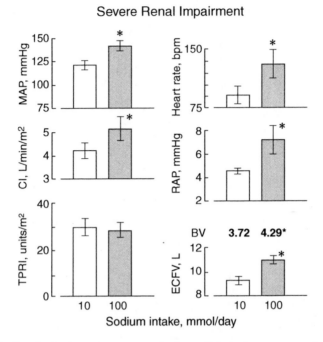

Figure 15.4. Results in six patients on regular hemodialysis for severe renal impairment, showing effects of two levels of dietary sodium on mean arterial pressure (MAP, mmHg), cardiac index (CI, L/min/m^2), total peripheral resistance index (TPRI, units/m^2), heart rate (bpm, beats/min), right atrial pressure (RAP, mmHg), and extracellular fluid and blood volumes (ECFV, BV, L). Diet was either 10 mmol/day (clear), or 100 mmol/day (shaded), with each diet maintained for 2 weeks. *$p < .05$ for difference between diets. From McGrath et al. (1977), with permission of *Kidney International* and Nature Publishing Group.

there was an increase in average resting SNA, which was the same on the two levels of sodium.

Coleman et al. (1970) had studied another group of chronic hemodialysis patients, whose kidneys had been removed earlier to treat their severe hypertension. Elevation of sodium intake in these anephric patients caused an initial elevation of CO, followed by a rise in TPR after about 10–14 days. The latter change was attributed to long-term autoregulation in response to volume overload. However, as discussed in chapter 2, long-term autoregulation has turned out to be something of a will-o'-the-wisp, and Coleman et al. undertook no further analysis of the mechanisms causing the rise in TPR.

The conditions under which SNA increases in renal failure and RenVH are discussed later in this chapter.

Malignant Hypertension

Malignant hypertension is defined as very severe high BP, which is rapidly fatal in the absence of treatment. Its features were originally described by Volhard and Fahr

(1914) as a condition of severe hypertension in which renal function became severely impaired and progressed rapidly to renal failure. They noted many vascular lesions in the kidney, including fibrinoid arteriolar necrosis and proliferation of the intima in the small arteries. The vascular lesions were widespread throughout the body, including the brain and retina: Characteristic clinical signs are papilledema, retinal hemorrhages, and exudates, which carry an ominous prognosis (Keith et al., 1939).

Up to the 1950s and 1960s, malignant hypertension was common, but today it is seen considerably less frequently, probably reflecting the better management of hypertension by primary care physicians (Lee and Adamson, 1978; Kincaid-Smith, 1985). Kincaid-Smith found that in 20% of patients with malignant hypertension, the malignant phase followed a period of benign EH, while in about 50% of patients it progressed from relatively stable RenVH and hypertension due to parenchymal renal disease.

The great importance of renal involvement in the malignant phase was first recognized by Wilson and Byrom (1939) in experimental animals. In both animals and patients, PRA and plasma Ang II are raised, while aldosterone secretion is high (Laragh et al., 1960; Barraclough, 1966). In malignant hypertension, blood volume is low and body sodium is often depleted despite the high aldosterone (Möhring et al., 1976; Kincaid-Smith, 1980).

Rapid loss of nephrons is never uniform, with closure of some nephrons associated with marked hyperfiltration in the nephrons that are still being perfused. As BP continues to rise, the kidney behaves almost like an open-ended tube, through which increasing amounts of water and sodium are being lost. Neurohumoral activity rises rapidly, so that there is intense systemic vasoconstriction with marked functional rarefaction in many vascular beds. This rapidly leads to one or more complications of hypertension, including cardiac failure, stroke, intravascular thrombosis, and permanent organ damage.

The critical feature appears to be the rapidity and magnitude of the renal deterioration. Remarkably, many patients respond dramatically to antihypertensive drugs. Indeed, the treatment of malignant hypertension with ganglionic blocking and vasodilators was one of the truly dramatic therapeutic success stories of the 1950s (Smirk, 1957; Harrington et al., 1959). Today, the therapeutic armamentarium is larger, and many drugs are successful in reversing malignant hypertension. The beneficial effect of lowering BP has convinced many that it was the high BP per se that caused malignant hypertension (Pickering, 1968). However, it is more likely that the malignant phase is mostly due to rapid, extensive renal deterioration (see below).

The Kidney and Sympathetic Neural Activity

An increase in renal SNA or in pressor hormone concentration affects the blood flow of different nephrons in a nonuniform manner, which sets the scene for the gradual deterioration of renal function. In EH, the brain is the initial source of elevation of systemic SNA. However, in renal hypertension elevation of SNA arises from the kidney: It is a sign of significant renal ischemia, and the resulting rise in BP is an attempt to improve renal perfusion.

Renal Vasoconstriction Is Not Uniform

The renal sympathetic nerves terminate on the afferent and efferent arterioles, the renin-producing cells, and the glomeruli and tubules (DiBona and Kopp, 1997). There are some differences in the profiles of transmitters released at the different terminals, though the functional significance of these differences remains to be determined (Luff et al., 1991, 1992; Denton et al., 2004). However, we know some of the reasons why raising SNA does not cause uniform vasoconstriction (Sands et al., 1992). First, the outer cortical afferent arterioles are more densely innervated than those of the inner cortex. In addition, the interlobular arteries taper on their way to the outer cortex, so that the outer afferent arteriolar BP is lower and the vessels are narrower. Accordingly, constrictor stimuli produce considerably greater narrowing of the afferent arterioles in the outer cortex than in those of the inner cortex (Aukland, 1989), which may result in shunting more blood flow through the latter vessels (figure 15.5).

Hence, a moderate increase in renal SNA reduces outer cortical blood flow, while that to the inner cortex usually increases (Pomerantz et al., 1968; Sands et al., 1992; Eppel et al., 2004). Moreover, hyperfiltration of inner cortical nephrons may partly compensate for the low GFR in outer glomeruli. At high levels of renal SNA, the perfusion of all nephrons decreases. The decline in average RBF is greater than in GFR, since the greater constrictor action of Ang II or SNA on the efferent arterioles results in elevation of filtration fraction (FF). Recall from chapter 5 that this is exactly what occurs in EH as the BP gradually rises (figure 5.3).

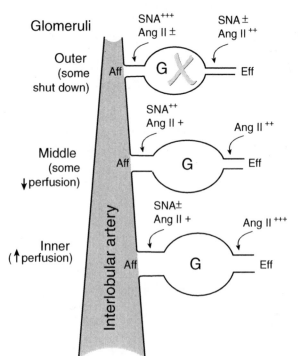

Figure 15.5. Because of the taper of the outer glomeruli, an increase in sympathetic neural activity (SNA) causes a greater vascular narrowing and pressure drop in the outer than the inner preglomerular vessels. This is further accentuated by the greater postglomerular elevation in Vas R due to locally produced Ang II.

A second type of nonuniformity in EH relates to the differential effects on renal vascular tone and renin release. SNA is raised in mild to moderate EH and, with the VSM cells on the resistance arterioles close to the renin-producing cells, it has been surprising that renal Vas R is raised, while PRA decreases in a high proportion of subjects (figure 5.17). SNA raises Vas R through stimulation of α-ARs on VSM cells, while β-AR stimulation of renin-producing cells increases renin secretion. The threshold for SNA-induced elevation of Vas R appears to be well below that for renin secretion, as observed in the response to hemorrhage (Oliver et al., 1990). Therefore the fall in renin production in mild to moderate EH has little to do with baroreflexes but is probably a local action of the high renal BP on the renin-producing cells. However, when SNA is high, renal Vas R and renin production increase simultaneously, as occurs in high-renin EH.

In RenVH, the redistribution of renal blood flow is greater than in EH and is due to the intrarenal actions of both Ang II and renal SNA. The elevation of SNA is a marker of renal ischemia. In EH too, a renal component may be added to the primarily CNS component as hypertension causes renal functional impairment.

Elevation of SNA in Renal Hypertension

Miyajima et al. (1991) were the first to observe that MSNA was markedly raised in patients with RenVH when compared to controls on the same dietary sodium intake. This was due to renal ischemia, since MSNA declined after successful angioplasty, which also lowered BP, PRA, and plasma Ang II.

Similarly, Johansson et al. (1999) found that MSNA was 65% greater in RenVH than in matched normotensives, while average body NA spillover was about twice as great (figure 15.6). Cardiac NA spillover was raised by a similar amount (Petersson et al., 2002).

MSNA is often very high in renal failure, and the kidney appears to be the major afferent source (Converse et al., 1992; Augustyniak et al., 2002). This is suggested by the contrasting levels of resting MSNA in two patients with chronic renal failure on regular hemodialysis (figure 15.7). In one patient with both kidneys in place MSNA was markedly raised, while in the other patient, whose hypertension had been treated with bilateral nephrectomy, MSNA was normal.

Renal Afferent Mechanisms

The kidney has both renal mechanoreceptors and renal chemoreceptors (Stella and Zanchetti, 1991; DiBona and Kopp, 1997). The mechanoreceptors respond to local changes in renal vascular, tubular, and ureteric pressures (Aström and Crafoord, 1968; Beacham and Kunze, 1969; Uchida et al., 1971). One type of renal chemoreceptor responds to moderate changes in urinary composition, while the other responds to local ischemia (Recordati et al., 1978, 1980).

Renal Reflexes

A change in renal pressures or urinary chemical composition in one kidney elicits a segmental reno-renal reflex. An increase in ipsilateral afferent activity in the affected

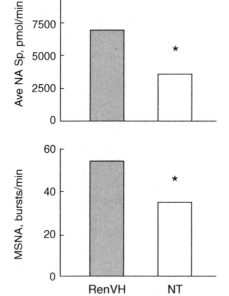

Figure 15.6. Average (total) NA spillover rate (pmol/min) and muscle sympathetic nerve activity (MSNA, bursts/min) in 65 patients with RenVH (shading) and 15 healthy normotensives (NT, clear). *$p < .01$ for Δ between groups. After Johansson et al. (1999), with permission of *Circulation*, American Heart Association, and Lippincott, Williams and Wilkins.

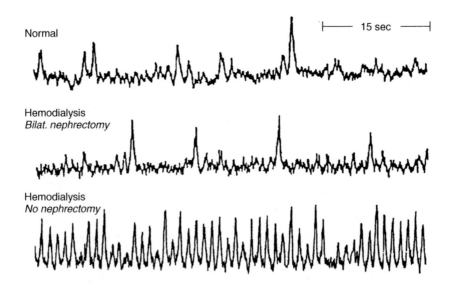

Figure 15.7. Recording of muscle sympathetic nerve activity (MSNA) in (top) a normal subject, (middle) in an anephric patient with renal failure on regular hemodialysis, and (bottom) in another renal failure patient on regular hemodialysis with kidneys in situ. The difference in MSNA between the patients suggests that the failing kidney is the source of elevation of SNA. From Converse et al. (1992), with permission of *New England Journal of Medicine* and Massachusetts Medical Society.

kidney inhibits contralateral renal SNA, thereby increasing urine flow and sodium excretion, equalizing excretory behavior in the two kidneys (Di Bona and Kopp, 1997). The reflexes are suppressed in 2K-1C and SHR hypertension (Kopp et al., 1987; Kopp and Buckley-Bleier, 1989).

Severe renal ischemia stimulates renal chemoreceptors, probably through increased production of adenosine (Katholi and Woods, 1987). This elicits substantial elevation in SNA and BP. The renal chemoreceptors function predominantly as an emergency mechanism (Winternitz and Oparil, 1982; Winternitz et al., 1982; Faber and Brody, 1985). However, their effect is manifest during transient lower body ischemia in the renal sympathetic baroreflex as the hypertensive reversal response (figure 9.18; Dorward et al., 1985). The response is normally largely inhibited by baroreflexes; its magnitude increases dramatically after sinoaortic plus cardiac baroreceptor denervation and in severe renal ischemia. Other tissue chemoreceptors also play an important role in circulatory control: The skeletal muscle chemoreceptors are important during exercise; cardiac chemoreceptors are excited by localized myocardial ischemia and raise BP to improve the regional blood supply (James et al., 1975). Renal chemoreceptors raise BP to improve blood flow in the ischemic organ and moderate accumulation of sodium in the body through pressure diuresis.

That the renal afferent nerves are actively involved in the rise of BP in RenVH was convincingly demonstrated by sectioning the dorsal root afferents in segments T8 to L2 on the side of the clip (figure 15.8; Wyss et al., 1986). After 4–5 weeks' hypertension, the rise in BP of the rhizotomized 1K-1C rats was attenuated by about 50% compared to that of 1K-1C rats with intact afferents. The BP was still well above the level of unclipped unrhizotomized controls, indicating that SNA was only one factor responsible for the raised BP (see below).

Similarly, in rats with low-renal-mass hypertension, after removal of 5/6 of the renal mass, bilateral dorsal root rhizotomy attenuates the hypertension by about 60% (figure 15.9; Campese and Kogosov, 1995). Here too BP remains significantly above the level of the control group, indicating that other factors contributed to the hypertension. An earlier study by Liard (1981) suggested that the response during salt loading is mediated through the hypothalamic defense area (figure 15.10). The vasoconstriction affects mainly the renal and splanchnic beds, while the skeletal muscle bed is dilated on day 1 of salt loading and is only slightly raised on subsequent days.

Parenthetically, low-renal-mass hypertension was used by Coleman and Guyton (1969) to illustrate the importance of renal impairment in the elevation of BP during increased intake of salt. The early rise in CO was due to an increase in blood volume, while the late rise in TPR, which we now know to be neurally mediated, was thought at the time to be due to long-term autoregulation.

The renal sensory nerves synapse in the spinal cord, from which they project to the NTS via slow transmitter neurons to the hypothalamic defense area. It has been suggested that NA neurons located in the A6 (locus coeruleus, LC) region convey information about renal ischemia from NTS to the hypothalamic nuclei (Winternitz et al., 1982; Wyss et al., 1986; Campese and Kogosov, 1995). There is no doubt that the NA neurons are activated by the renal afferents, but the rise in their activity probably occurs in response to the elevation of BP. This is suggested from the analysis of NA neuron function in chapter 8, where the NA LC neurons moderate the rise in BP.

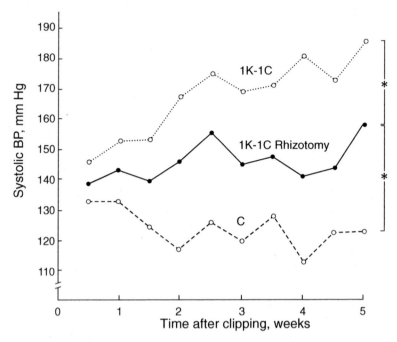

Figure 15.8. Mean systolic BP (mmHg) measured in Sprague-Dawley rats over 5 weeks after clipping. Top, animals with one kidney, one clip (1K-1C) hypertension; middle, animals subjected to unilateral dorsal spinal rhizotomy from spinal segments T8 to L2, 7 days before clipping; lower, uninephrectomized unclipped controls (C). *$p < .05$ for difference between groups. From Wyss et al. (1982), with permission of *American Journal of Physiology* and American Physiological Society.

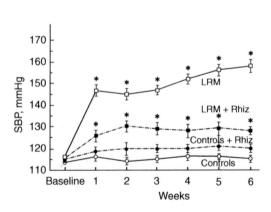

Figure 15.9. Time course of systolic blood pressure (SBP, mmHg) in (from top) (1) rats with low renal mass (LRM) after removing 5/6 of kidney mass; (2) LRM rats subjected to bilateral dorsal spinal rhizotomy from spinal segments T10 to L2 (LRM + Rhiz) prior to removal of renal mass; (3) normal rats subjected to bilateral rhizotomy (Control + Rhiz); (4) normal rats (Controls). Adapted from Campese and Kogosov (1995), with permission of *Hypertension*, American Heart Association, and Lippincott, Williams and Wilkins.

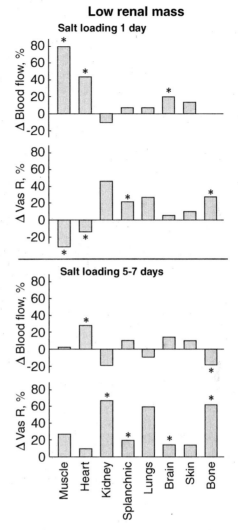

Figure 15.10. Effects of salt loading on regional blood flows and Vas Rs in dogs with low renal mass; beds indicated at bottom of graph. Top, after 24 hours of salt loading; bottom, after 5–7 days of salt loading. Blood flows and Vas Rs expressed as percentage of means of dogs not loaded with salt. On day 1, MAP was 27 mmHg above control; on days 5–7, MAP had risen to 35 mmHg. From Liard (1981), with permission of *American Journal of Physiology* and American Physiological Society.

The actual renal ischemia-induced hypothalamic excitation is probably mediated through DA neurons or another group of slow transmitter neurons other than NA neurons. The finding that NA turnover increases in the LC and the posterior and lateral hypothalamus is in accord with a baroreflex-mediated action, as is the abolition of the response by bilateral rhizotomy.

Experimental Renal Hypertension

The three types of RenVH considered here include Goldblatt one kidney, one clip (1K-1C) and two kidney, one clip (2K-1C) hypertension and cellophane wrap hypertension. In 1K-1C hypertension, only half the normal number of nephrons is initially present, while animals with 2K-1C hypertension have the full complement thanks to the untouched kidney. In renal cellophane wrap hypertension, the pericapsular fibrosis compresses the kidney slowly but relentlessly. The longer the time after operation, the lower the functional renal mass.

In the earlier studies, renal artery narrowing did not always result in hypertension because the narrowing was inadequate. This was overcome by (1) developing accurately machined renal artery clips for use in small animals (Ruzicka and Leenen, 1994), and (2) by monitoring the effects of stenosis on RBF or MAP (Lupu et al., 1972).

One Kidney, One Clip Hypertension

Our group at the Baker Institute wished to know why milder grades of renal artery stenosis did not produce some degree of chronic hypertension. This involved observing the renal and systemic changes at different degrees of narrowing. In most other studies, narrowing of the renal artery had continued until long-term elevation of BP had been achieved.

Acute Renal Hemodynamic Changes

Experiments were performed in awake uninephrectomized dogs, instrumented with a Doppler flowmeter and inflatable cuff around the renal artery and indwelling catheters for measuring systemic and distal renal arterial BP (Anderson, Johnston, and Korner, 1979; Anderson, Korner, and Johnston, 1979). To induce renal artery stenosis, fluid was injected into the perivascular cuff so as to reduce MAP distal to the stenosis ($RMAP_{distal}$) to either 60, 40, or 20 mmHg. The cuff tubing was then clamped and the hemodynamic changes observed for the next 30–60 minutes without further cuff adjustments.

After lowering $RMAP_{distal}$ to 40 mmHg, the systemic MAP increased by only a few mmHg (figure 15.11, left). Initially, there was a large pressure gradient across the stenosis and vasodilation (reduction of Vas R) of the renal vascular bed. After 2–3 minutes $RMAP_{distal}$ and Vas R began to recover, and by 30 minutes the MAP gradient and the "ohmic" stenosis resistance had fallen substantially from their initial high values.[6]

Restoration of $RMAP_{distal}$ was due to Ang II-mediated intrarenal vasoconstriction. When endogenous formation of Ang II was prevented by infusing the ACE inhibitor teprotide, both $RMAP_{distal}$ and renal Vas R remained low (figure 15.11, middle). Moreover, infusing Ang II into the distal renal artery in the presence of teprotide restored normal recovery of $RMAP_{distal}$ (figure 15.11, right).

The initial reduction in $RMAP_{distal}$ results in renal tissue hypoxia and a lowering of renal Vas R. The vasodilation is quickly masked by Ang II-mediated intrarenal vasoconstriction. With milder stenosis (lowering $RMAP_{distal}$ to 60 mmHg), there is better temporal separation of the dilator and constrictor effects but even smaller

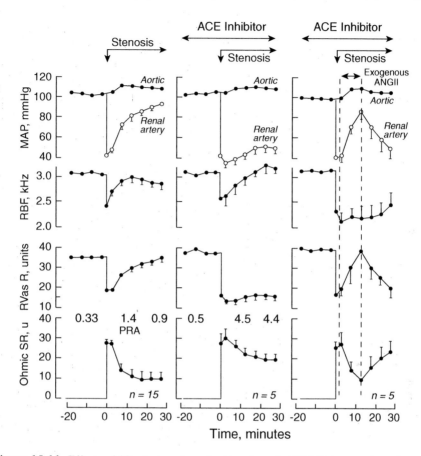

Figure 15.11. Effects of 30 minutes of renal artery stenosis (1K-1C) in conscious dogs, in which distal renal artery BP was rapidly lowered to 40 mmHg with occluder cuff, with tubing then clamped. Left, normal response, showing effects on aortic and renal artery MAP (mmHg), renal blood flow (RBF, kHz), renal vascular resistance (RVas R, units) and Ohmic stenosis resistance (SR, units). Middle, stenosis induced during infusion of ACE inhibitor teprotide into renal artery. Right, soon after inducing stenosis during intraarterial teprotide, Ang II was infused into distal renal artery (between vertical lines) simulating normal restoration of renal artery BP and distal Vas R. n, number of dogs. From Korner (1982).

systemic changes (Anderson, Johnston, and Korner, 1979; Anderson, Korner, Angus et al., 1981).

Greater narrowing of the renal artery by lowering $RMAP_{distal}$ to 20 mmHg gives rise to systemic hypertension (figure 15.12, A; Anderson, Johnston, and Korner, 1979; Anderson, Korner, and Johnston, 1979). MAP had risen by 25 mmHg after one hour's stenosis, but this had declined to 8 mmHg after 3 days and had almost disappeared by the end of the week.

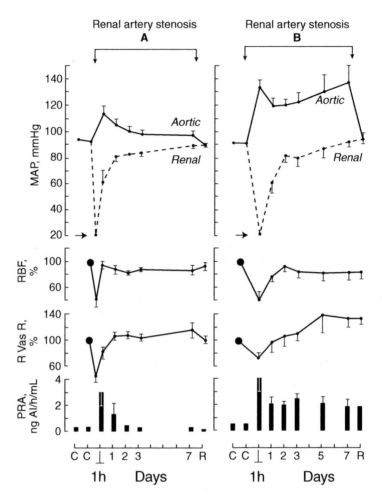

Figure 15.12. Average effect on aortic and distal renal MAP (mmHg), renal blood flow (RBF, % of control), renal Vas R (% of control), and PRA (ng Ang/hour/mL) of 7 days of stenosis (1K-1C) after lowering distal renal artery pressure to 20 mmHg: (A) by a single rapid inflation (5 dogs); (B) by relowering renal BP to 20 mmHg four times over 1 hour by additional cuff inflations, and then maintaining the clamp until day 7 (6 dogs). C, control day; 1h, at the end of the first hour of stenosis; 1 . . . 7, days of stenosis; R, recovery. From Anderson, Johnston, and Korner (1979), with permission of *Hypertension,* American Heart Association, and Lippincott, Williams and Wilkins.

Hydraulic Properties of Arterial Stenosis

The resistance to blood flow is determined (1) by the percentage narrowing of the arterial diameter; (2) by the upstream BP, the pressure gradient across the stenosis, and the degree of turbulent blood flow; and (3) by the tone of the distal vascular bed (May et al., 1963; Gould and Lipscomb, 1974; Berguer and Hwang, 1974; Young et al., 1975, 1977; Gould, 1980; Santamore and Walinsky, 1980; Santamore et al., 1980, 1981; O'Rourke, 1982b; Santamore and Bove, 1985; Henrich, 1992).

Marked turbulence is common in stenosis, increasing resistance to blood flow and markedly depressing RBF (figure 15.13; Gould, 1980; O'Rourke, 1982b; Fung, 1984). Turbulence is responsible for the depression of RBF when the renal artery is first narrowed (figure 15.11, left). The true stenosis resistance is underestimated considerably by calculating it in accordance with Ohm's law, which applies only to laminar flow. Indeed, soon after the publication of the paper by Anderson, Korner, and Johnston (1979), we were asked by Huisman and De Zeeuw (1985) to explain how RBF could increase after about 5 minutes while distal renal Vas R was also increasing. In our reply, we did not adequately discuss the changes in the degree of turbulence that occurred during stenosis as a result of the intrarenal action of Ang II (Anderson and Korner, 1985). It is high at the start of stenosis but has declined considerably by 30 minutes. This is due to Ang II-mediated restoration of $RMAP_{distal}$, which reduces the stenosis gradient. It is the reduction in turbulence that is responsible for the rise in RBF. This is predicted by the stenosis model of Santamore and Bove (1985), who found that increasing distal Vas R paradoxically raised blood flow.

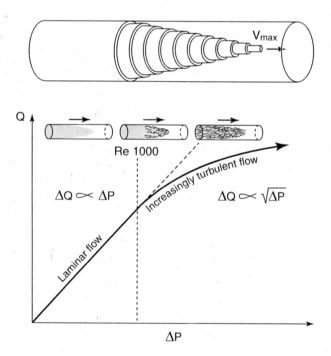

Figure 15.13. Top, diagram of laminar flow in a tube, wth low velocity near wall and maximum velocity in the center. The retarding force that slows the fluid near the wall is the product of the viscosity and the velocity gradient. After Milnor (1982). Bottom, relationship between pressure gradient (ΔP) and flow (Q) in a rigid tube during laminar (streamline) flow; turbulence develops as flow velocity increases above the Reynolds number of ~1000; Q becomes a function of $(\Delta P)^{0.5}$ rather than of ΔP as in laminar flow. From Folkow and Neil (1971).

Figure 15.14 summarizes the sequence of circulatory changes. Early on, the fall in $RMAP_{distal}$ and associated vasodilation increase renin release and Ang II production. Some renin spills over into the systemic circulation, increasing plasma Ang II and raising systemic BP slightly. Locally formed renal Ang II constricts the renal bed and restores renal Vas R and $RMAP_{distal}$. This increases nephron perfusion heterogeneity, reducing perfusion of outer nephrons and increasing that of inner nephrons. The rise in renal Vas R is partly through direct vasoconstriction and partly through greater power dissipation in the inner glomeruli, in which perfusion is increased (Borders and Granger, 1986).[7] Restoration of $RMAP_{distal}$ reduces systemic renin spillover, while PRA, plasma Ang II, and systemic BP return to baseline. It also diminishes turbulence across the stenosis, allowing RBF to recover partially. After 30–60 minutes, renal function is almost restored. The price is marked reduction of perfusion in

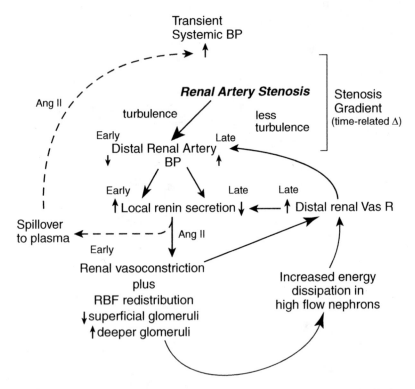

Figure 15.14. Sequence of renal changes after induction of arterial stenosis. Early renal vasodilation lowers distal renal BP and flow and raises renin secretion, some of which spills over into the systemic circulation. Local Ang II constricts distal renal afferent and efferent arterioles, raising Vas R and distal renal MAP, and causes redistribution of blood flow. At equilibrium, distal renal BP and Vas R are almost restored in mild and moderate stenosis, with renin production and systemic MAP also back to normal. In severe stenosis, the systemic hypertension and intrarenal changes help to reduce reduction in distal renal MAP; PRA and plasma Ang II remain high for several days.

5–10% of outer cortical glomeruli for the duration of stenosis. This has minimal effects in view of the kidney's enormous functional reserve.

The kidney is the only bed in which stenosis activates an inbuilt vasoconstrictor mechanism, Ang II, which encapsulates the ischemia in a small part of the organ by redistributing its blood flow. By contrast, after stenosis of a major coronary artery, distal vasodilation, low perfusion pressure, and ischemia are sustained until the stenosis is relieved.

The Concept of Critical Arterial Stenosis

The critical level of stenosis is the percentage of narrowing required to bring about reduction in BP or blood flow distal to the stenosis. Vascular surgeons have long known that less arterial narrowing is necessary to lower BP (or flow) in a dilated distal bed than in one that is constricted (figure 15.15; Anderson and Korner, 1980; Santamore and Walinsky, 1980; Santamore et al., 1980). In a dilated bed the critical level of stenosis is about 50%; when tone is normal it is about 70%; during vasoconstriction it is 80–90%.

The critical stenosis concept explains the findings in vivo where renal vascular tone was altered by brief intraarterial infusions of dilator or constrictor drugs at the time of applying the stenosis: In all experiments, RMAP$_{distal}$ was lowered to an identical value (40 mmHg) at the different levels of baseline tone (Anderson and Korner, 1980). In the constricted bed, the restoration of RMAP$_{distal}$ was slower, and the rises of systemic MAP and PRA were greater than in the dilated bed (table 15.5).

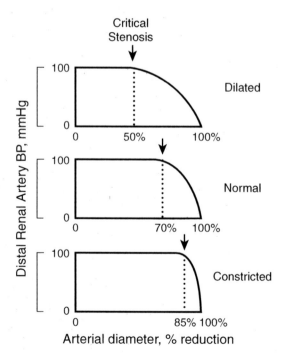

Figure 15.15. The level of critical stenosis is the percentage of narrowing beyond which distal artery BP (or blood flow) falls. It depends on the tone of the distal bed: In a dilated bed, narrowing is less than in a constricted bed. Arrow indicates approximate critical level at the various levels of tone. The renal vasculature is unique in that local production of renin and Ang II can modify the level of critical stenosis. After Anderson and Woods (1987), with permission of *Kidney International* and Nature Publishing Group.

Table 15.5. Systemic MAP and PRA Responses to Renal Artery Stenosis Induced by Rapidly Lowering Distal MAP to 40 mmHg in Conscious Dogs

I.r.a infusion[a]	Δ Renal Vas R When Inducing Stenosis	Systemic ΔMAP (mmHg)	PRA (ng Ang I/h/mL)
Ac.Choline	↓	4.3 ± 3.3	0.3 ± 0.2
0.9% NaCl	No Δ	11.3 ± 3.3	1.2 ± 0.4
Methoxamine	↑	29 ± 3.3	5.1 ± 1.4
Ang II	↑	26 ± 3.8	4.0 ± 0.7

[a]Infusions were started 2–3 minutes before inducing stenosis and were turned off 1 minute after clamping the perivascular balloon. ΔMAP, change from prestenosis value.

Tone of distal bed was altered briefly by renal artery infusions of vasoactive drugs when stenosis was induced.

Source: Anderson and Korner (1980).

Sustained Benign Hypertension

Lowering $RMAP_{distal}$ to 20 mmHg gives rise to only about 2 days of systemic hypertension (figure 15.12, A). In order to produce permanent hypertension, Anderson, Johnston, and Korner (1979) had to lower $RMAP_{distal}$ four times to 20 mmHg during the first hour, which raised systemic MAP by ~35 mmHg (figure 15.12, B). With each relowering of $RMAP_{distal}$, the renal bed becomes increasingly constricted due to additional renal renin release and Ang II production. Hence the stenosis is increased progressively as the critical threshold in figure 15.14 shifts to the right with more pronounced constriction of the distal bed.

For the first few days after 1K-1C stenosis, giving angiotensin antagonists or ACE inhibitors restores systemic MAP to control (Brunner et al., 1971; Ayers et al., 1974; Miller et al., 1975). After 10–14 days these drugs no longer lower BP, as PRA and plasma Ang II return to normal despite sustained elevation of BP. Hence, 1K-1C hypertension has been said to have renin-dependent and renin-independent phases (Barger, 1979). However, this applies only when the salt intake is normal or high. On a low salt intake, PRA and Ang II remain raised and RenVH remains renin dependent (Freeman et al., 1977; Gavras et al., 1979; Rocchini and Barger, 1979; Stephens et al., 1979).

Contribution of Stenosis Resistance

Goldblatt et al. (1934) rejected the idea that the tight arterial stenosis contributed to the elevation in TPR and BP. This was because they were unable to produce hypertension by creating stenosis of arteries supplying nonrenal beds. Accordingly, Ang II was regarded as the sole initiator of the high BP for the next 50–60 years (Barger, 1979).

Goldblatt's discovery was made before the days of ready availability of suitable arterial flowmeters (Kolin, 1936; Milnor, 1982). We now know that in both 1K-1C and 2K-1C hypertension, renal artery stenosis contributes to the rise in TPR ($\equiv \downarrow$ TPC). In moderate 1K-1C hypertension, this amounts to about 25% of the overall rise in TPR (Anderson, Korner, Angus et al., 1981).

Blood Volume

1K-1C hypertension is a constrictor type of hypertension, so that a reduction in total blood volume would be expected (see chapter 5). However, on a normal salt diet, total blood volume is either little altered or slightly raised, suggesting that renal function is more impaired than in EH (Anderson, Korner and Johnston, 1979; Barger, 1979; Woods et al., 1986).

Stenosis During ACE Inhibition

Miller et al. (1975) induced stenosis during administration of an ACE inhibitor and found that there was no increase in BP. Accordingly, they concluded that Ang II was an essential trigger for developing 1K-1C hypertension. At that time, they did not appreciate the influence of the tone of the distal renal vascular bed on the level of critical stenosis.

Selig et al. (1983) developed a method for narrowing the renal artery independently of the bed's vascular tone. They measured the volume of saline in the cuff sufficient to completely occlude the renal artery and then induced stenosis by inflating the perivascular balloon with a constant fraction of that volume, say 90%. Now the induction of stenosis elicited hypertension in the presence of the ACE inhibitor enalapril (table 15.6; Selig et al., 1983; Anderson et al., 1984; Woods et al., 1986). The rise in

Table 15.6. Average Aortic and Renal BPs, Renal Blood Flows, and GFR in Conscious Dogs before and for 2 Weeks during (1) Renal Artery Stenosis Alone and (2) Identical Renal Artery Stenosis Induced in the Presence of the ACE Inhibitor Enalapril

Variable	Control	Renal Artery Stenosis		
		1 & 2 d	7 d	14 d
Aortic MAP, mmHg	100	128	118	119
Renal MAP, mmHg	100	66	89	92
RBF, mL/min	400	325	380	400
GFR, mL/min	42	24	34	38
FF (GFR/RPF), %	0.161	0.117	—	0.153

Variable	Enalapril Only	Renal Artery Stenosis + Enalapril		
		1 & 2 d	7 d	14 d
Aortic MAP, mmHg	92	101	114	111
Renal MAP, mmHg	88	43	54	89
RBF, mL/min	430	325	420	395
GFR, mL/min	45	8	25	22
FF (GFR/RPF), %	0.159	0.035	—	.081

Note: The 1 and 2 d values are the average over days 1 and 2. Prestenosis PRA in dogs not treated with enalapril averaged 0.33 ng/mL/h, rising to 4.34 by days 1 and 2, but back to 0.5 ng/m/h by 14 days, with corresponding changes in plasma Ang II. The latter remained unchanged in the presence of enalapril.

Source: Selig et al. (1983), Woods et al. (1986), and Anderson and Woods (1987).

MAP was attenuated by about 15–20% over the first 2 days, but after 2 weeks the BP had risen by a similar amount as in untreated animals. However, in the presence of enalapril GFR remained about 40% below that of untreated animals (table 15.6).

The findings suggest that in the absence of the Ang II, greater than normal renal chemoreceptor-mediated elevation of SNA substitutes for the early systemic pressor action of Ang II. Elevation of SNA normally accounts for part of the elevation of BP in 1K-1C hypertension, so that the greater ischemia will increase activity of the renal chemoreceptors (figure 15.8; Wyss et al., 1982). However, SNA is not an adequate substitute for the hormone's postglomerular constrictor action, and in the absence of Ang II, GFR and FF remain below the values of animals with intact effectors.

Benign and Malignant RenVH

Dzau et al. (1981) induced RenVH hypertension in dogs by maintaining a large gradient across the stenosis (figure 15.16, left). The high BP was associated with marked reduction in RBF and elevation of plasma volume, suggesting that stenosis was more severe than in figure 15.12. However, the changes were reversed completely by

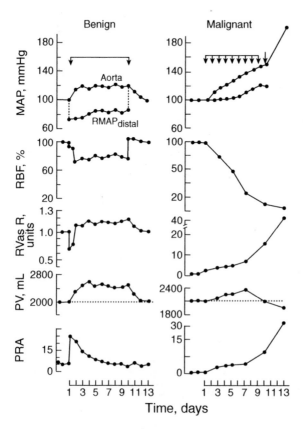

Figure 15.16. Left, effects of benign hypertension on aortic and renal MAP (mmHg), renal blood flow (RBF, %), renal Vas R (units), plasma volume (PV, mL), and plasma renin activity (PRA, ng Ang I/mL/h). The arterial narrowing was very severe, as discussed in text. Right, further progressive narrowing of the renal artery by a small amount each day produced malignant hypertension, following exhaustion of compensatory mechanisms and substantial renal ischemia. From Dzau et al. (1981), with permission of *Hypertension*, American Heart Association, and Lippincott, Williams and Wilkins.

deflating the perivascular cuff at the end of the experiment. The property of reversibility is responsible for the label of benign hypertension despite its severity.

In other dogs severe hypertension was induced as just described, but on every subsequent day $RMAP_{distal}$ was lowered by a few mmHg below the level to which it had risen after the intrarenal vascular adjustments of the previous day. This gave rise to malignant hypertension, with progressive decline in RBF, elevation in renal Vas R, and a decline in plasma volume (figure 15.15, right). By day 8 of the experiment, RBF had fallen by more than 80%.

Thus, in malignant hypertension more and more nephrons are closed down every day, as intrarenal vasoconstriction keeps increasing. By day 7, about 70–80% of nephrons have closed down, and over the next 2–3 days very few nephrons remain well perfused.

The rise in PRA over the first few days is relatively small, which is in accord with virtual shutdown of blood supply to a large proportion of outer cortical renin-producing cells. The renin entering the systemic circulation comes from the still reasonably perfused inner cortical glomeruli. However, from day 7 onward the blood supply of the inner nephrons also diminishes, causing a dramatic rise in PRA in order to maintain filtration through a rapidly diminishing number of glomeruli.

The initial elevation of plasma volume is smaller than in severe benign hypertension, but the volume declines from about day 7 onward, as urine output and sodium excretion increase and the animals' health deteriorates rapidly. Postmortem findings include widespread fibrinoid necrosis of blood vessels in every organ.

Similar loss of water and sodium has been described in other animal models of malignant hypertension; replacement of these losses often improves the animals' health (Möhring et al., 1976). Other systemic changes associated with malignant hypertension include reduction in endothelial NO, greater platelet adhesiveness, and increased capillary permeability. Intravascular thrombosis is common in the kidney and other regional beds. The ever-increasing recruitment of constrictor mechanisms (Ang II, SNA, local constrictor autocoids) and reduction in dilator autocoids (e.g., NO) provides positive feedback that rapidly destroys the kidney in the attempt to maintain some urine flow. In most other organs there is also widespread microcirculatory rarefaction.

Overview of Causes of 1K-1C Hypertension

The renal artery stenosis resistance is the initiating factor of RenVH. Narrowing of the renal artery diameter by 70–80% does not cause hypertension, because the Ang II-mediated intrarenal vasoconstriction compensates almost completely for the hemodynamic perturbations. As a result, the renal ischemia becomes localized to only a small proportion of outer cortical nephrons.

Sustained moderate to severe benign RenVH occurs when the renal artery diameter is narrowed by about 90%. Ang II again raises $RMAP_{distal}$, but the steady-state MAP gradient across the stenosis remains substantial together with significant turbulence. The high systemic MAP helps to limit the fall in RBF and to maintain urine flow.

In moderate RenVH, 20–30% of the rise in TPR is due to stenosis resistance (figure 15.17). For the first 7–10 days of stenosis, Ang II accounts for 60–70% of

Ren VH-1K-1C

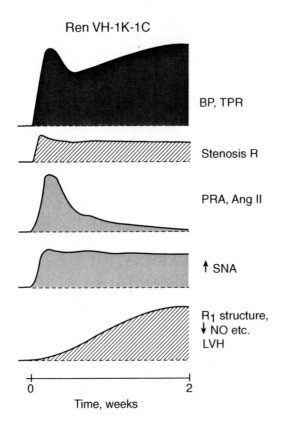

BP, TPR

Stenosis R

PRA, Ang II

↑ SNA

R₁ structure,
↓ NO etc.
LVH

0   2

Time, weeks

Figure 15.17. Causes of chronic elevation in MAP and TPR (black) in 1K-1C Goldblatt hypertension include the stenosis resistance R, the constrictor action of Ang II and of sympathetic neural activity (SNA), and cardiovascular structural and functional changes.

the additional rise in TPR and renal ischemia-induced elevation of SNA accounts for 30–40%. The raised SNA affects predominantly preglomerular renal Vas R, so that the ongoing maintenance of GFR and elevation of FF is largely due to the constrictor action of Ang II on efferent arterioles.

Cardiac and vascular hypertrophy start soon after BP begins to rise, and this is enhanced by the raised systemic Ang II. In severe RenVH the vascular amplification factor is about 2.0, so that during the chronic phase the remodeled vasculature enhances TPR by an amount equivalent to the earlier pressor action of Ang II. This factor contributes to the decline of systemic Ang II from its early high value, but its intrarenal action remains ongoing. The raised SNA and changes in local autacoids such as the decline in NO, account for 30–40% of the elevation of TPR. Blood volume changes associated with fluid retention contribute minimally to the hypertension.

Goldblatt Two Kidney, One Clip Hypertension

Before the clip is applied, 2K-1C hypertension has a normal complement of nephrons. The stenotic kidney is subjected to renal ischemia as in 1K-1C hypertension, while the initial changes in the untouched kidney are largely due to the production of more renin and Ang II by the stenotic kidney. Later on, the R_1 vessel structural amplifier and the decrease in renal NO accentuate the initial constrictor effects.

2K-1C RenVH is more difficult to induce experimentally than 1K-1C hypertension (Goldblatt, 1937, 1964; Ebihara and Grollman, 1968). Indeed, it was widely regarded as a transient type of high BP for many years. The lack of permanence was due to inadequate narrowing of the renal artery: Lupu et al. (1972) were the first to show that sustained hypertension invariably occurred in dogs if RBF was monitored during narrowing of the renal artery and was reduced by about 50–80%.[8] They also found that once hypertension had developed it was almost always cured by surgical removal of the stenotic kidney.

Systemic and Renal Hemodynamic Changes

When perivascular occluders are used in awake dogs, sustained hypertension usually requires more pronounced narrowing of the renal artery than is required in 1K-1C RenVH and even then, the elevation of BP is often smaller (Anderson, Ramsey, and Takata, 1990).[9] In the series in figure 15.18, MAP rose by an average of 13 ± 3 mmHg above baseline over the 25 days of stenosis, while in control dogs over the same period there was a small decline in MAP (-6 ± 2 mmHg). In the hypertensive dogs, CO remained unchanged and the rise in MAP was entirely due to a fall in TPC ($\uparrow$ in TPR).

In the stenotic kidney, the gradient across the stenosis was 30–35 mmHg for much of the time (figure 15.18). Initially, RBF was reduced by about 30%, settling later at 15% below the level before stenosis. The change suggests a moderate degree of renal ischemia, affecting mostly the outer cortical nephrons. Ang II was the chief determinant of the intrarenal vasoconstriction, which was abolished by IV captopril, unmasking the stenosis-induced renal vasodilation (figure 15.19). The ohmic stenosis resistance was maximal in the first few days after stenosis and then settled to a lower stable level; the corresponding rise in RBF suggests that the turbulence across the stenosis had declined.

In the untouched kidney, RBF fell by an average of about 20%, while renal Vas R was raised due to the action of Ang II (figure 15.18). The latter was demonstrated by infusing captopril, which caused renal vasodilation (figure 15.19).

On day 20 of stenosis, the paraamino hippurate clearance method was used to measure the combined RBF of both kidneys in order to determine the renal contribution to the fall in TPC (Anderson, Ramsey, and Takata, 1990). The fall in total renal conductance accounted for about one third of the fall in TPC (figure 15.20), with the contribution of stenotic:nonstenotic kidney to the overall change in renal Vas R in the ratio of 2:1.[10]

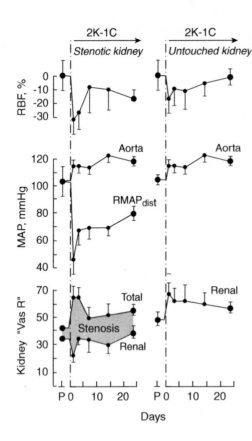

Figure 15.18. Responses of stenotic kidney and untouched kidney in 2K-1C hypertension in dogs. Variables (from above): renal blood flow (RBF, % of prestenotic value, P), aortic and distal renal MAP (mmHg), kidney vascular resistance (units), including total and renal, with the shaded difference due to stenosis resistance. After Anderson, Ramsey, and Takata (1990), with permission of *Hypertension*, American Heart Association, and Lippincott, Williams and Wilkins.

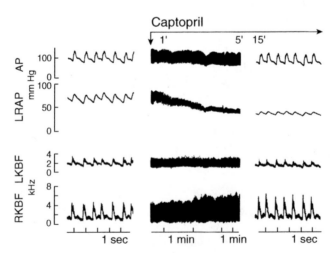

Figure 15.19. Recording obtained in awake dog showing effect of IV captopril on aortic and left stenotic renal artery pressures (AP, LRAP, mmHg) and left and right kidney blood flows (LKBF, RKBF, kHz). Note fall in LRAP with little change in blood flow in stenotic kidney and marked rise in blood flow in nonstenotic kidney. From Anderson, Ramsey, and Takata (1990), with permission of *Hypertension,* American Heart Association, and Lippincott, Williams and Wilkins.

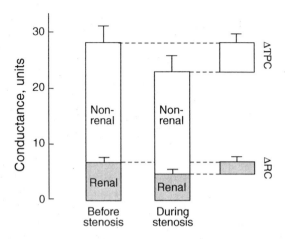

Figure 15.20. Bar graphs showing total and renal vascular conductances (TPC, RC, units) of both kidneys before and during 2K-1C renal artery stenosis. Renal vasoconstriction accounted for about one third of the fall in TPC. From Anderson, Ramsey and Takata (1990), with permission of *Hypertension*, American Heart Association, and Lippincott, Williams and Wilkins.

After induction of stenosis, PRA increased, reaching a maximum by day 3 and then declining slowly to reach close to normal levels by the end of the observation period. Atrial natriuretic peptide (ANP) increased over the first few days and then remained raised in response to elevation of venous pressure and central blood volume (Anderson, Ramsey, and Takata, 1990). The diuretic action of -ANP prevented a rise in total blood volume despite considerable renal functional impairment. However, plasma AVP concentration was unchanged throughout stenosis.

Causes of 2K-1C RenVH

One quarter to one third of the fall in TPC is due to overall renal vasoconstriction in the two kidneys (figure 15.20). The greater constriction in the stenotic kidney causes more redistribution of RBF than in the nonstenotic kidney, resulting in sufficient ischemia to raise SNA.

The remaining 75% of the fall in TPC is due to systemic vasoconstriction of the nonrenal vascular beds (figure 15.20). Early on, this is due to the systemic vasoconstrictor action of plasma Ang II and elevation in SNA. Later on, local reduction in NO and other dilator autacoids and elevation of several constrictor autacoids further enhances the vasoconstriction. All these factors are amplified by structural R_1 vessel changes that develop rapidly in the course of hypertension.

Cellophane Wrap Hypertension

Irvine Page first used cellophane wrap hypertension as a method for reliably producing severe hypertension (Page, 1939; Graef and Page, 1940). The cellophane induces renal capsular fibrosis, which encases and compresses the kidney, raising renal tissue pressure (Brace et al., 1974; Denton, 1989). The lowering of transmural BP in pre- and postglomerular blood vessels reduces RBF, indicating that wrap hypertension is another type of RenVH.

The renal compression is due to the slow contracture of fibrous tissue. The gradual changes are responsible for the very high BPs that develop: 1 month after wrapping, average BP rises are 30–40 mmHg (Ferrario et al., 1970; West and Korner, 1974; West, Angus, and Korner, 1975; Fletcher et al., 1976; Takata et al., 1988) and further rises of 10–20 mmHg occurred in experiments of 2–3 months duration (Korner, Oliver, and Casley, 1980; Blake, 1983; Denton and Anderson, 1985). These high BPs can be maintained because of the very substantial development of LV hypertrophy that is associated with wrap hypertension (chapter 7).

Wrap hypertension is a constrictor type of high BP due to elevation in TPR (figure 15.21; Fletcher et al., 1976).The chronic reduction in CO observed in this particular study has not been observed in later studies in another strain of rabbits (Korner, Oliver, and Caseley, 1980; Blake, 1983; Takata et al., 1988).

In some of the earlier studies, there was doubt whether the renin-angiotensin system played a role in wrap hypertension (Campbell et al., 1973; Fletcher et al., 1976). Subsequent investigations by Warwick Anderson, Kate Denton, and their collaborators have shown that the action of Ang II is similar to its role in renal artery stenosis.

From 4 to 8 weeks after wrapping the kidneys, RBF was often 50–60% of that in sham-operated rabbits (Denton et al., 1983; Denton and Anderson, 1985; Takata

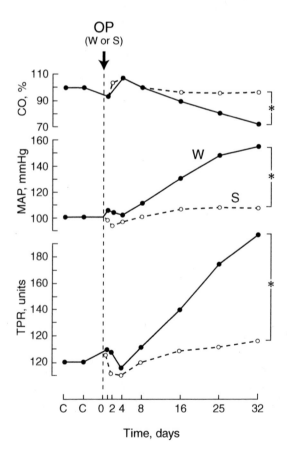

Figure 15.21. Average changes in cardiac output (CO, KHz Doppler shift, % of control), mean arterial pressure (MAP, mmHg), and total peripheral resistance (TPR, units) in renal cellophane wrapped (W, solid lines) or sham-operated (S, interrupted lines) rabbits. The early small rise in CO during the first week after operation was similar in both groups. *$p < 0.05$ for difference between groups. From Fletcher et al., 1976, with permission of *Circulation Research*, American Heart Association, and Lippincott, Williams and Wilkins.

et al., 1988). In addition, the renal paraamino hippurate extraction ratio (E_{PAH}) was depressed, pointing to enhanced nonuniformity of nephron perfusion (Stokes and Korner, 1964; Reubi et al., 1978).

Denton and Anderson (1985) investigated the role of Ang II in the systemic and renal responses by suppressing formation of Ang II in one group of wrapped and sham-operated rabbits and comparing their responses with those of corresponding groups of untreated animals.[11]

In the absence of Ang II, the rise in MAP due to wrapping was attenuated by about 50%, while the decline in GFR was more pronounced than in the corresponding group of untreated rabbits (figure 15.22). A more detailed analysis of the renal changes was performed in additional rabbits 4 weeks after wrapping or sham-operation, in which EPAH and filtration fraction (= inulin extraction ratio) were also measured (table 15.7). In the absence of Ang II, the rise in Vas R due to wrapping was nearly twice that of sham-operated animals, and RBF was 31% lower than in the latter group. In wrapped rabbits with intact effectors, both changes were considerably larger: In the wrapped rabbits, renal Vas R was 4.6 times that of sham-operated animals, while RBF was 60% below the level of the latter. However, in the untreated wrapped rabbits, FF was better maintained than in wrapped enalapril-treated animals.

The above results indicate that in intact wrapped rabbits the pressor action of Ang II is responsible for about half the rise in MAP (and presumably in TPR). Moreover, the renal vasoconstriction is a major component of the hypertension. Some of the renal actions of Ang II are postglomerular and account for the better maintenance of GFR and FF.

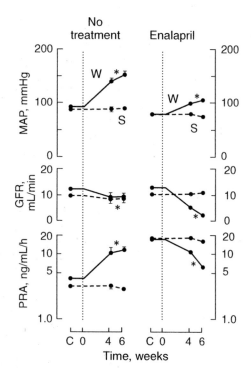

Figure 15.22. Mean arterial pressure (MAP, mmHg), glomerular filtration rate (GFR), and plasma renin activity (PRA, ng/mL/h) before (C) and over 6 weeks after operation in two groups of cellophane wrapped (W, solid lines) and sham-operated (S, dashed lines) rabbits. One group received enalapril throughout, while the other received no treatment. From Denton and Anderson (1985), with permission of *Hypertension*, American Heart Association, and Lippincott, Williams and Wilkins.

Table 15.7. Measurements Made 4 Weeks after Either Cellophane Wrapping or Sham Operation in One Group of Rabbits Treated with Enalapril (5 μg/kg/h IV) Given Continuously by Minipump for Several Days before Operation and for 4 Weeks Afterward

Variable	Group	Wrap	Sham
RBF, mL/min	Enal	64	93
	Untr	31.6	79
FF, %	Enal	8.8	12.1
	Untr	16.8	17.0
Ren Vas R, u	Enal	1.9	0.8
	Untr	5.5	1.2
E_{PAH}, %	Enal	51	93
	Untr	63	84

Note: Enal, enalapril-treated (8 wrapped, 6 sham rabbits); Untr, untreated rabbits (5 wrapped, 5 sham); RBF, renal blood flow; FF, filtration fraction (inulin extraction ratio); Ren Vas R, renal vascular resistance, units; E_{PAH}, para-amino hippurate extraction ratio, %.

Source: Denton and Anderson (1985).

The rise in MAP and renal Vas R in enalapril-treated wrapped rabbits is most likely due to the elevation in SNA that occurs in response to renal ischemia. The rise is probably greater than in intact wrapped animals in view of the greater fall in E_{PAH}, which suggests more pronounced ischemia (table 15.7, and see below). However, in intact wrapped rabbits the fall in E_{PAH} is also substantial, suggesting that SNA also contributes to their hypertension. That elevation of SNA contributes to the rise in TPR in wrap hypertension was demonstrated by Chalmers et al. (1974), who found that i.c.v. 6-OHDA attenuated the hypertension by about 50% (figure 15.23; Chalmers et al., 1974; Chalmers, 1975). The underlying renal ischemia stimulates renal chemoreceptors, which raise SNA through the hypothalamic defense area through excitation of DA and not NA neurons (chapter 8). Other evidence that SNA is raised in wrapped rabbits includes (1) elevation of NA turnover in the LV (Snell et al., 1986); and (2) clonidine-induced inhibition of cardiac SNA required higher doses in wrapped compared to sham-operated animals (Korner, Oliver et al., 1974).

The difference in renal E_{PAH} between wrapped and sham-operated rabbits provides a measure of the extent of the redistribution of RBF (Reubi et al., 1978); factors such as tissue hypoxia have been found to have little effect on E_{PAH} (Stokes and Korner, 1964). In intact wrapped rabbits, about 30% more blood is shunted away from the renal tubules than in sham-operated animals (table 15.7). In enalapril-treated wrapped rabbits, the figure is considerably greater, with about 80% more blood shunted away from the tubules than in the corresponding group of sham-operated rabbits. The difference illustrates the importance of the intrarenal action of Ang II in maximizing the proportion of functional nephrons. However, the considerable shunting that occurs in wrapped animals with intact effectors indicates the magnitude of the renal capsular compression forces. In many outer cortical glomeruli perfusion is very poor, while some of the inner cortical glomeruli are perfused at greater than normal rates, but not sufficiently to normalize RBF.

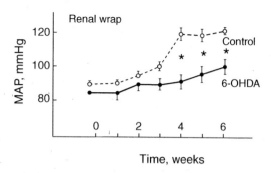

Figure 15.23. Mean arterial pressure (MAP, mmHg) during development of renal cellophane wrap hypertension in awake rabbits: One group received i.c.v. 6-OHDA (solid line) or vehicle (control, dashed line) shortly before the operation. From Chalmers et al. (1974), with permission of *Journal of Physiology* (London) and Blackwell.

Additional support for poorer glomerular perfusion after wrapping in the absence of Ang II comes from the PRA data in figure 15.22. The administration of enalapril raised the preoperative PRA to four to five times the level of animals with intact effectors. This is a well-known effect that is largely due to interruption of Ang II-related feedback to renin-secreting cells (Ayers et al., 1974, 1977; Davis and Freeman, 1976). After wrapping, PRA gradually declined by about 65% as hypertension developed. The high preoperative PRA can be regarded as a marker of the number of renin-secreting cells, suggesting that the decline in PRA is an indicator of underperfusion of renin-secreting cells due to renal compression. In contrast, in intact wrapped rabbits, PRA increased threefold as hypertension developed (figure 15.22, left). This is an indicator of Ang II formation, which contributes to the normal elevation of TPR and renal Vas R.

In summary, renal wrap hypertension is a slowly developing type of RenVH that inexorably leads to renal failure. The elevation of BP is mediated through rises in Ang II and SNA and to alterations in local autacoids. Ang II plays an important role in the elevation of renal Vas R and in the maintenance of GFR and FF. The amplifier action of the cardiovascular hypertrophy becomes increasingly important in the maintenance of high BP and is one factor contributing to the eventual return of Ang II toward normal from the high value shown in figure 15.22 (left; see below).

Renal Antihypertensive Humoral Mechanisms

Renal NO is now known to be an important renal autacoid (chapters 6,12). The question considered in this section is whether the putative renal hormone medullipin, discovered several years before NO, is also of physiological significance.

Grollman was the first to propose that the kidney produced an antihypertensive hormone with a counterregulatory action to the effects of Ang II and other pressor factors (Grollman et al., 1949; Grollman, 1951). Subsequently, Muirhead suggested that the interstitial cells of the renal medulla released the depressor hormone medullipin (Muirhead et al., 1977; Muirhead, 1991, 1994). On the basis of much experimental work, Muirhead hypothesized that the medullary interstitial cells secreted a prohormone medullipin 1, which, after release into the circulation, was converted into the active hormone medullipin 2 by the liver, eliciting systemic vasodilation, diuresis, and natriuresis.

Medullipin was thought to be responsible for the rapid fall in BP that occurred when the renal artery was unclipped in chronic 1K-1C hypertension. Removal of the clip causes a sudden rise in renal BP and increased formation of medullipin. The fall in BP could be prevented by prior chemical medullectomy with 2,bromoethylamine hydrobromide (BEA), which destroys the renal medulla and papilla following its IV administration (Swales et al., 1986, 1987).

Karlström et al. (1988) developed a method in which a rat kidney was perfused with blood at raised BP. When the venous effluent was injected into another rat, it elicited a fall in BP, which was thought to be due to medullipin release. A similar technique was employed by Christy et al. (1991) in which an extracorporeal circuit was used for high-pressure perfusion of one kidney and its outflow returned to the same animal's systemic circulation. Unfortunately, the renal perfusion at high BP also raises RBF. This increases renal NO production, making it difficult to distinguish the effects of medullipin from those of NO.

Raising BP in the perfused kidney evokes a fall in systemic BP and increases excretion of sodium and water (figure 15.24). The threshold for eliciting these responses is just above the animals' resting BP (Thomas et al., 1994). The responses were unaffected by autonomic ganglionic blockade, renal denervation, or ACE inhibition (Christy et al., 1993). The vasodepressor response was abolished by BEA-induced chemical medullectomy, but diuresis and natriuresis were little affected.

Nitric Oxide

Ang II directly affects renal afferent and efferent arteriolar tone (Navar et al., 1996). In addition, Ang II increases local NO production through its action on endothelial AT_1 receptors (Patzak et al., 2005). The effect is greater on the afferent than on the efferent arteriole, so that NO moderates Ang II-mediated preglomerular constriction. Recall from chapter 6 that, in contrast to the flow-related component, receptor-mediated endothelial production of NO is relatively unimpaired in hypertension. Hence, by reducing the Ang II-mediated preglomerular constriction, the hormone's constrictor action on the efferent arteriole may achieve greater prominence in the maintenance of a high FF in EH and RenVH.

When sodium load is high, both GFR and renal tubular flow increase: The ability to excrete adequate amounts of sodium and water depends on maintaining high renal medullary blood flow. In turn, this requires high rates of synthesis of NO to offset the myogenic response in renal medullary arterioles (figure 6.4). When flow-related NO production is impaired, the excretion of sodium and water fall and reabsorption increases, raising BP (figure 12.2; Mattson et al., 1992, 1994; Cowley et al., 1995; Majid and Nishiyama, 2002). Evans et al. (1995) used Christy et al.'s (1991) extracorporeal perfusion apparatus to investigate the role of NO on urinary flow and sodium and water excretion over a wide range of perfusion pressures. In intact rabbits, sodium excretion, urine flow, and water excretion increased in proportion to the elevation of perfusion pressure (figure 15.25). In the presence of a NOS inhibitor, the responses were attenuated. Clearly, in the intact animal NO synthesis is important for

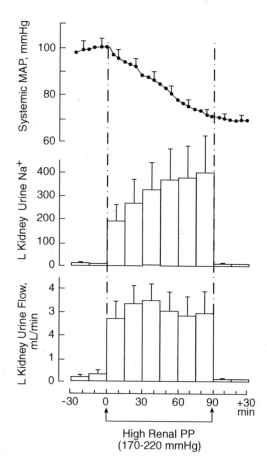

Figure 15.24. Left kidney of anesthetized dogs was perfused at high perfusion pressures (PP, 170–220 mmHg) during blockade of renin-angiotensin system and autonomic nervous system. Note progressive fall in systemic mean arterial pressure (MAP, mmHg) and increase in the perfused kidney's Na$^+$ excretion (μM/min) and urine flow (mL/min). From Christy et al. (1991), with permission of *Hypertension*, American Heart Association, and Lippincott, Williams and Wilkins.

producing an adequate diuresis and natriuresis, apart from direct actions of NO on some of the tubular transport mechanisms (Evans et al., 2005).

Thus the part played by NO in renal salt and water excretion is similar to the effects attributed to medullipin. Many of the renal actions of high-pressure perfusion are due to flow-related increase in NO production. In the absence of molecular identification of medullipin, one cannot differentiate its putative effects from those of NO. Muirhead's work indicates that a distinctive vasodepressor compound is produced by the renal interstitial cells. Indeed, rare medullipin-producing tumors that lower BP have been identified (Muirhead, 1994). But on current evidence, its physiological role seems doubtful.

The Kidney in Renal and Essential Hypertension

RenVH, like EH, is a constrictor type of hypertension, but soon after the initiation of the hypertension there are marked differences between them in the degree of renal

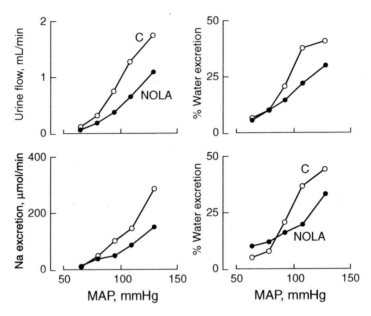

Figure 15.25. Effects of varying renal perfusion pressure in rabbits, on urine flow (mL/min), Na excretion (μmol/min), fractional water excretion (%), and fractional Na excretion, in animals given either vehicle (C, open circles), or the NOS inhibitor N^G-nitro-L-arginine (NOLA, 20 mg/g IV). From Evans et al. (1995) with permission of *Clinical and Experimental Pharmacology and Physiology* and Blackwell.

involvement. Over time, nephron numbers decline more rapidly in RenVH than in EH. When renal deterioration is very rapid in RenVH, malignant hypertension is common. If the deterioration is more gradual, the outcome is often renal failure. The analysis of the mechanisms underlying the three types of RenVH considered in this chapter, together with low-renal-mass hypertension, provides some insight into why clinical RenVH has a relatively poor prognosis.

As renal impairment increases, the high BP appears to be initially due to volume overload. From these very abnormal renal models, Guyton postulated that all hypertension started with volume overload, which, as already noted in chapter 5, is not the case in EH. Pure volume overload occurs in primary aldosteronism and in a number of rare monogenic types of hypertension in which there are major tubular transport abnormalities or excess secretion of adrenal mineralocorticoids or glucocorticoids. The likelihood that similar abnormalities in tubular ionic transport contribute to the elevation of BP in EH has become an article of faith since Dahl's first renal transplantation study. However, it appears that the effect of the genetically determined transport abnormalities on BP in EH and other types of neural hypertension is relatively minor compared to the hemodynamic effects on the kidney. Moreover, these vascular effects tend to accentuate the effects of the tubular abnormalities.

High BP and Renal Function during RenVH

The three experimental models of RenVH considered in this chapter are 1K-1C, 2K-1C, and renal wrap hypertension. In all of them, similar mechanisms contribute to the elevation of BP. All are reversible by removing the initial renal causes of the high BP, provided the duration of the hypertension has not been too long.[12] These models provide insight into the mechanisms that raise BP in human RenVH and of the sequence of systemic and renal changes that eventually give rise to stable hypertension.

In order to raise BP by producing renal artery stenosis, the arterial narrowing has to be substantial. This produces falls in RMAP$_{distal}$ and RBF and gives rise to hypoxic vasodilation of the renal bed. In turn, renal renin secretion and Ang II formation are raised and spill over into the systemic circulation, in addition to their renal actions. The systemic effects of Ang II include (1) systemic vasoconstriction, which raises TPR and MAP; and (2) promotion of cardiovascular hypertrophy. In addition, the tight stenosis itself accounts for some 15–30% of the rise in TPR.[13]

Within the kidney, Ang II constricts the afferent and efferent arterioles, which partially restores RMAP$_{distal}$ and RBF and masks the underlying renal vasodilation. Heterogeneity of RBF is accentuated: There is decreased perfusion of outer cortical nephrons and either little change or an increase in the perfusion of the inner cortical nephrons, which contributes to the elevation of renal Vas R. The resulting focal renal ischemia increases activity of the renal chemoreceptors, raising SNA through the hypothalamic defense area. The rise in SNA not only raises MAP but causes some further accentuation of renal perfusion heterogeneity. The systemic effects of the high SNA, in conjunction with the effects of the vascular structural amplifier, gradually replace the systemic constrictor actions of Ang II. The high BP improves renal perfusion, restoring renin production to close to normal. From then on, the hemodynamic effects of Ang II are almost exclusively intrarenal.

In severe 1K-1C hypertension, the estimated proportion of well-perfused nephrons is quite small (figure 15.26), which is in accord with micropuncture data showing reduction in the renal ultrafiltration coefficient (Gabbai et al., 1987). Under these conditions, sodium balance often becomes positive (Swales and Thurston, 1977; Thurston, 1994). It explains why blood volume is either normal or slightly raised, instead of being about 10–20% below normal as would be expected in a constrictor hypertension of this severity (chapter 5).

In 2K-1C hypertension, the mechanisms that raise and maintain high BP are closely similar. However, narrowing of the renal artery has to be greater than in 1K-1C hypertension, while the early vasoconstriction in the untouched kidney also develops rapidly. Here too the initial rise in BP results from systemic vasoconstriction due to Ang II, elevation of SNA, and the development of cardiovascular structural changes, all of which also affect the untouched kidney. In the stenotic kidney, both the high BP and the renal actions of Ang II help maintain renal function. In 2K-1C hypertension, the proportion of well-perfused nephrons is greater than in 1K-1C hypertension, most of them in the untouched kidney (figure 15.26). This results in a net loss of body sodium in which the action of ANP also plays a role. The negative body sodium balance (Miksche et al., 1970; Swales et al., 1972; Thurston, 1994) accounts for the

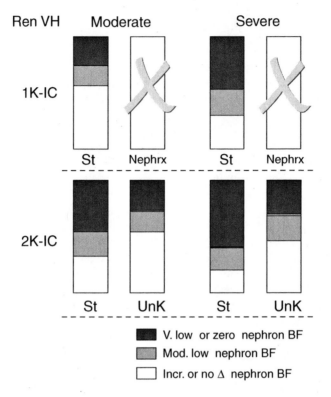

Figure 15.26. Cartoons illustrating redistribution of intrarenal blood flow in moderate and severe 1K-1C and 2K-1C renovascular hypertension. St, stenotic kidney; Nephrx, nephrectomy; UnK, untouched kidney. Black bars, very low or zero blood flow; shaded bars, moderately low blood flow; clear bars, unchanged or raised blood flow.

longer period of renin dependence in this type of RenVH (Swales and Thurston, 1977; Gavras et al., 1979).

Cellophane wrap hypertension develops more gradually, with the BP taking at least 6 weeks to reach a stable high BP. During this time PRA and plasma Ang II levels rise, but once hypertension has become stable, plasma Ang II returns toward normal. As in 1K-1C RenVH, its intrarenal role continues to be important, while elevation of SNA and structural changes account increasingly for the maintenance of systemic hypertension. Blood volume is close to normal (table 9.3). The renin-secreting cells respond to alterations in dietary sodium, except that the PRA responses are more pronounced than normal to rises and falls of dietary salt (table 12.5). It suggests more intense feedback from the tubules to the macula densa of the considerably smaller number of functioning nephrons. When the wrapped animals are on a high-salt diet, the rise in BP is largely due to an increase in blood volume in this constrictor type of hypertension. It suggests that although the kidney is unable to excrete the sodium load, there is no increase in the degree of renal ischemia or activation of brain EO neurons, which would have raised TPR.

Severe chronic wrap hypertension is a good model of serious renal functional impairment eventually resulting in renal failure. Here too the postglomerular actions of Ang II help maintain GFR to cope with a normal dietary salt intake. The Guyton low-renal-mass model is a model of renal failure, in which 85% of the renal mass has been amputated. BP remains normal when salt intake is low, but on 0.9% NaCl, BP rises dramatically (figure 2.14). The initial rise in BP is simply due to volume over-load. However, the extra workload on the few remaining nephrons causes very marked renal ischemia, raising TPR and further increasing MAP (figure 2.15; Langston et al., 1963). This is due to elevation in SNA (Campese and Kogosov, 1995), which is probably of the same magnitude as in human renal failure (figure 15.7). The elevation of SNA transforms the volume hypertension into a constrictor hyper-tension. At this level of renal function, this is a mechanism of last resort that causes further reduction in nephron numbers.

Renal Involvement in EH

As discussed earlier, in the vast majority of patients that develop EH, nephron num-ber and renal function are initially normal. From the epidemiological findings in chapter 4, reduction in nephron number due to fetal stress affects at best only a small proportion of adults with EH.

In EH, the primary mechanism for raising BP is unrelated to renal pathology but is evoked by lifestyle changes including stress, high salt intake, obesity, and several other factors. In genetically susceptible individuals, SNA is raised in all major con-strictor outflows, including that to the kidney. Successful nonpharmacological thera-peutic measures relate to lifestyle interventions including regular submaximal exercise, reduction in salt intake, other dietary measures, and body weight reduction, which lower SNA, thereby indirectly improving renal function.

Because of the constrictor nature of the hypertension, blood volume is reduced and PRA is normal or depressed in the majority of subjects, with only a relatively small proportion belonging to the high-renin group (figure 5.17). In mild and moderate EH, the high renal SNA causes some degree of nephron ischemia through the mechanism illustrated in figure 15.5, but the proportion of poorly perfused nephrons is consider-ably smaller than in moderate 1K-1C RenVH (figure 15.26). As BP gradually rises in EH, GFR is well maintained due to preponderant postglomerular vasoconstriction, as in RenVH. Presumably in the low-renin subjects there is some increase in intrarenal renin and Ang II sufficient to constrict the efferent arterioles. Alternatively, an increase in postglomerular SNA raises efferent arteriolar Vas R more than afferent arteriolar Vas R, simply because the former vessel is narrower (Denton et al., 2000). Last, since in mild and moderate EH there is a high proportion of well-perfused glomeruli, the blood volume remains low, which is commensurate with the reduction in microcircu-latory and venous capacity (chapter 5). This, in association with a raised central volume, is also the reason why acute salt loads are excreted relatively rapidly (Ulrych et al., 1971).

As BP increases further, the associated renal changes are shown schematically in figure 5.3. The time from mild to severe EH ranges from 10 to 20 years. The rise in BP is slower than in RenVH because of the smaller magnitude of the structural changes (e.g., vascular amplification factor 1.3 in EH vs. 2.0 in RenVH), the less rapid decline in renal NO, and the slightly smaller elevation in SNA. However, after a long period of severe EH, the nephron numbers and regions of focal ischemia are not very different from those in RenVH.

The fall in nephron numbers and renal functional deterioration in EH may be accelerated by sporadic events that damage the kidney. For example, during the 1950s and 1960s, excessive consumption of analgesics containing phenacetin was common in Australia, particularly in women (Kincaid-Smith, 1969). They were encouraged by advertisements proclaiming that when things got out of hand it was good to "have a cup of tea, a Bex and a good lie down."[14]

As discussed in chapters 3 and 12, EH, SHR, and Dahl-S rats all have some genetically determined abnormalities in renal tubular ion transport causing slower excretion of sodium and water. In the Dahl-S rat, salt excretion by the isolated perfused kidney is lower on high dietary salt than on low salt (table 12.4), which is at least partly due to differences in hypertension before the experiment. Moreover, the reduction in salt excretion was greatly ameliorated by renal medullary infusion of L-arginine, which points to the role of medullary NO in salt excretion. It suggests that the role of the tubular abnormality is smaller than the long-term hemodynamic effects on the kidney. This probably also applies to EH; otherwise blood volume would be raised, rather than low.

In conclusion, renal nephropathy is not the initiator of EH and develops more gradually than in RenVH. In renal hypertension, the rate of progression to renal failure or malignant hypertension is at least 3–5 times that in benign EH, in which the renal circulation is a major contributor to the rise in BP in EH throughout its natural history.

16

SHR Hypertension and Its Causes

SHR hypertension is a neurogenic type of genetic hypertension that develops in most environments (Okamoto and Aoki, 1963; Okamoto, 1969). This suggests that the rats possess sufficient appropriate high BP genes to develop hypertension soon after birth. These genes have been diluted in the borderline hypertensive rat (BHR), the hybrid between SHR and WKY, in which the environment has to reinforce the animal's genetic makeup to raise the responsiveness of the defense pathway (figure 3.15).

One advantage of working with inbred hypertensive and normotensive strains is that they permit reproducible timing of key events affecting BP. Accordingly, the focus in this chapter is on timing and magnitude of the sympathoadrenal and cardiovascular structural changes, both of which have independent roles in initiation of high BP in SHR. The CNS hyperresponsiveness is a lifelong attribute, while the greater responsiveness of the SHR's immature cardiac and vascular myocytes set the scene for the rapid development of the cardiovascular amplifier properties that raise BP and TPR from about 4–6 weeks of age onward. From about 5–6 months of age, the chronic constriction due to the structural and local functional changes accelerates the deterioration of organ function and lowers the expectation of life.

The immature VSM cells of SHR secrete more nerve growth factor (NGF) than those of WKY. This increases postganglionic innervation to the R_1 vessels, which accentuates the changes due to their hypothalamic hyperresponsiveness. The latter is further reinforced by the high levels of testosterone in male SHR, whereby their BP increases considerably more in males than in females.

The important role of the sympathetic nervous system in SHR is evident from the effects of sympathoadrenal inactivation in neonatal life, which completely prevents the hypertension. Neonatal inactivation of the renin-angiotensin system is almost as effective in preventing hypertension but operates through different mechanisms.

Output Patterns

Raised sympathoadrenal activity and structural changes in SHR contribute to the elevation of BP through most of the first year of life.

Resting Hemodynamics and Blood Volume

In all rodents, the cardiovascular system is very immature at birth: SBP is only 20–25 mmHg, rising by 50–60 mmHg during the first 3–4 weeks of life (Young, 1963; Dawes, 1968; Thornburg and Morton, 1994). It suggests that in rats much cardiovascular differentiation is only completed after birth.

There has been controversy whether BP in SHR is raised at birth. In some studies, average BPs were 3–5 mmHg greater in SHR than in WKY, while in other series there was no difference (Bruno et al., 1979; Gray, 1982, 1984; Lee, 1985; Lee et al., 1987; Adams et al., 1989). It is probably best not to overinterpret such small ΔBPs at a time of very rapid developmental change. It is only from 4–6 weeks of age onward that ΔBP$_{\text{SHR-WKY}}$ differ reliably between the two strains (figure 16.1).

During neonatal life, thyroid hormone activity is high and contributes to the raised body metabolism and cardiac index (CI) in all mammals (Rudolph, 1985; Fisher, 1992). In SHR, the rise in CI is greater than in WKY and accounts for much of the early elevation of BP (figure 16.2; Smith and Hutchins, 1979). After the age of 6–7 weeks, elevation of TPR accounts for much of the hypertension, with the rise continuing to increase as the animals get older.

By 5 weeks the defense pattern has been established, with renal vasoconstriction, skeletal muscle vasodilation, and elevation of heart rate (figure 16.3;

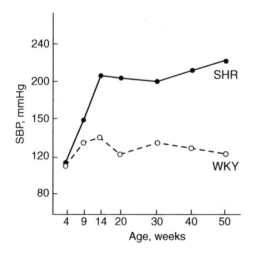

Figure 16.1. Age-systolic blood pressure (SBP, mmHg) relationship in SHR and WKY, during the first year of life. From Adams et al. (1989), with permission of *Hypertension*, American Heart Association, and Lippincott, Williams and Wilkins.

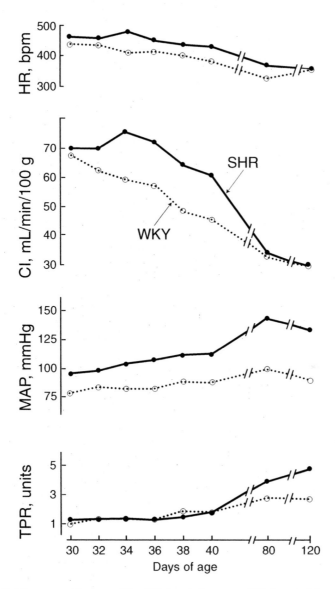

Figure 16.2. Time course from age 30 to 120 days in heart rate (HR, beats/min), cardiac index (CI, mL/min/100 g body weight), mean arterial pressure (MAP, mmHg), and TPR (units) in SHR (dark circles, solid lines) and WKY (clear circles, dotted lines). In SHR, HR and MAP raised throughout ($p < .05$); CI raised up to ~6 weeks of age and TPR from 8–10 weeks onward. Data from Smith and Hutchins (1979), with permission of *Hypertension*, American Heart Association, and Lippincott, Williams and Wilkins.

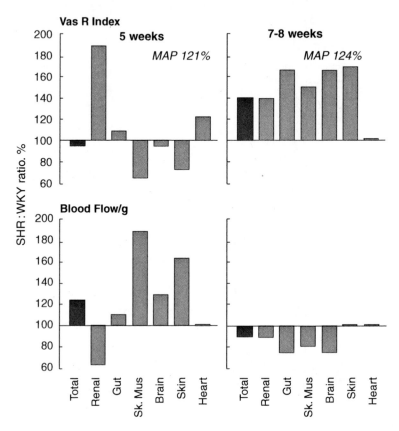

Figure 16.3. Regional Vas R and blood flows in SHR at 5 and 7–8 weeks of age, expressed as percentage of corresponding values in WKY. Blood flows were obtained with radioactive microsphere method; organs shown on abscissa. Data from Evenwel et al. (1983).

Evenwel et al., 1983). The muscle vasodilation is only transient and by 7–8 weeks of age vasoconstriction is present in most systemic vascular beds due to the relatively marked rise of plasma adrenaline in addition to the elevation of SNA (see below).

Blood Volume

At 5 weeks of age, the blood volume is greater in SHR than in WKY and is associated with slight sodium retention. However, by the age of 7–8 weeks the blood and plasma volumes have declined and are below those of WKY (Evenwel et al., 1983; Harrap, 1986). The fall in total blood volume is a consequence of vasoconstrictor-induced reduction in venous capacity in gastrointestinal and skin beds, while central blood volume has increased owing to the systemic vasoconstriction (chapter 5). The rapid BP rise marks a large increase in cardiopulmonary load, which corresponds to the first development of the vagal deficit of the cardiac baroreflex (figure 9.7; Head and Adams, 1988).

Neuroendocrine Changes

The neuroendocrine changes include sympathoadrenal changes, alterations in adrenal cortical hormones, and some of the related CNS mechanisms. As noted in chapter 3, cosegregation studies suggest that the raised resting SNA of SHR and the responses to acute stress are genetically determined (figures 3.10, 3.11).

Neonatal Period

In the embryo, the adrenal medulla, chromaffin tissue, and autonomic ganglia originate from migrating neural crest cells (Le Douarin, 1986; Jacobson, 1991; Walker, 1994). The CNS neurons in the SHR hypothalamus are already hyperresponsive in the neonatal period, and the immaturity of their VSM cells essentially limits the extent of vasoconstriction. However, the VSM cells secrete large amounts of NGF, which promote maturation of neurons in the sympathetic ganglia and growth of their axons toward the vasculature and heart (Thoenen and Barde, 1980; Levi-Montcalcini, 1987). The excess number of axons that make synaptic contact with the resistance vessels has received the evocative name of hypernoradrenergic innervation, with the implication that it could be a cause or even the sole cause of SHR hypertension (Head, 1989, 1991; Zettler et al., 1991).[1]

During the first 2–3 weeks of life, before the sympathetic nerves are fully functional, adrenal catecholamines (CAs) circulate in plasma of both SHR and WKY. By 5–7 weeks of age, plasma adrenaline is greater in SHR than in WKY, and this difference continues in older rats (table 16.1; Pak, 1981; Jablonskis and Howe, 1994).

The sympathetic nerves elicit constrictor responses from about 3–4 weeks of age. At that time, the concentrations of noradrenaline (NA) and neuropeptide Y (NPY) in the terminals are greater in SHR than in WKY (Dhital et al., 1988; Fan et al., 1995). The co-release of these transmitters enhances constriction in at least some vascular beds (Potter, 1988; Angus et al., 1995).

Age-Related Changes in Regional NA Turnover

At 4 weeks of age, sympathetic nerve activity (SNA) in renal, splanchnic, and cardiac nerves is greater in SHR than in WKY (Yamori, 1975; Thorén and Ricksten, 1979; DiBona et al., 1996). An indicator of this is the NA turnover in renal and LV tissue, which is greater in SHR from 4 to 14 weeks of age (figure 16.4; Adams et al., 1989).

Table 16.1. Plasma Adrenaline Concentrations in Young and Older SHR and WKY

Age	SHR	WKY
5–7 weeks	220 pg/mL*	120 pg/mL
7–9 months	275 pg/mL*	85 pg/mL

*$p < .05$ for difference between strain.

Source: Jablonskis and Howe (1994).

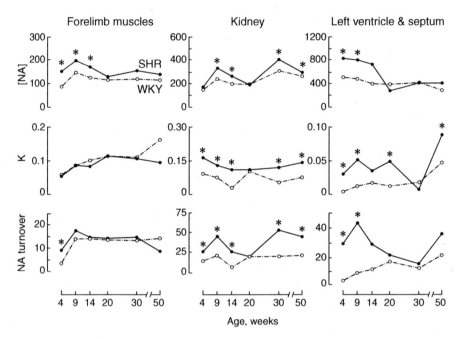

Figure 16.4. From top, tissue NA concentration (NA); fractional NA rate constant (K), and NA turnover (ng/g/hour) in forelimb skeletal muscles, kidney, and left ventricle including septum of SHR and WKY aged 4 to 50 weeks. *$p < .05$ for difference between strains. From Adams et al. (1989), with permission of *Hypertension*, American Heart Association, and Lippincott, Williams and Wilkins.

These between-strain differences appear to diminish between 20 and 30 weeks but then increase again to the earlier values, possibly in response to deteriorating organ function. Splanchnic vasoconstriction parallels the renal changes and the reduction of venous capacity and associated blood volume changes (chapter 5).

NA turnover in skeletal muscle in SHR exceeds that of WKY until about 9 weeks of age, but after that the differences between the strains are small. The muscle vasodilation in 5-week-old SHR (figure 16.3) is due to adrenaline-mediated β-AR stimulation, which masks the SNA-mediated α-AR vasoconstriction. The subsequent vasoconstriction may be due to the rise in plasma adrenaline from the low levels in younger rats. At these raised concentrations, the affinity of adrenaline for α-ARs is high, so that the SNA-mediated constriction is reinforced.

Adrenal Cortical Hormones

The adrenal steroids participate in a coordinated hypothalamopituitary response, in which the rise in corticotrophin-releasing hormone (CRH) increases ACTH production (Fisher and Brown, 1983; Hashimoto et al., 1989).

In very young SHR, mineralocorticoid secretion (19-noraldosterone) is enhanced transiently, which accounts for the early sodium retention (Takeda, Miyamori, et al., 1995). The main rat glucocorticoid is corticosterone, and its secretion is already high in young SHR (Sowers et al., 1981; Hausler et al., 1983, 1984; Hattori et al., 1986; Hashimoto et al., 1989). It suppresses activity of eNOS, resulting in attenuation of flow-related production of NO (chapter 6; Suzuki et al., 1996).

CNS Mechanisms

In normal mammals, cortical neurons are involved in the perception of stress, including those of the prefrontal cortex, which transmit information to the hypothalamus and amygdala through dopaminergic (DA) neurons (chapters 8, 11). In SHR, the DA neuron activity sensitizes the defense pathway during the first few weeks of life, with the sensitization probably dependent on the presence of the appropriate genes. Destruction of the DA neurons markedly attenuates the development of hypertension (figure 8.21; Haeusler et al., 1972; Haeusler, 1976; Van den Buuse, Versteeg, and De Jong, 1984).

Eilam et al. (1991) grafted hypothalamic tissue from SHR embryos into young WKY rats, which caused a ~30% increase in BP (figure 16.5). BP also rose after hypothalamic grafts from WKY embryos, but ΔBP was smaller and more transient, suggesting that SHR have more excitable hypothalamic neurons than WKY.

In SHR, the high postganglionic SNA is mostly due to raised CNS activity (Mills et al., 1989; Chan et al., 1991; Chalmers et al., 1994; Minson et al., 1996). It has been suggested that the hypernoradrenergic innervation reinforces vasoconstriction directly

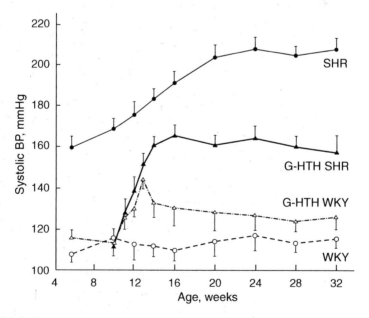

Figure 16.5. Top and bottom graphs show relationship between age and systolic BP in SHR and WKY (means, 1 SEM). Other graphs show effects in WKY: (1) embryonic SHR hypothalamic graft (G-HTH-SHR) in WKY; (2) embryonic WKY hypothalamic graft (G-HTH-WKY); and (3) control WKY. From Eilam et al. (1991), with permission of *Journal of Neuroscience* and Neuroscience Society.

(Longhurst et al., 1986; Head, 1989, 1991). One estimate of the overall rise in BP through a closely related mechanism comes from a cosegregation study in an F_2 population in which there was an 8 mmHg difference in MAP of SHR homozygotes for the NGF genotype and the corresponding homozygotes of normotensive rats (figure 16.6; Kapuscinski et al., 1996). The greater innervation could cause more direct constriction, but its main action may be to stimulate early R_1 vessel remodeling and help establish the amplifier properties in advance of the elevation of BP.

Thus, the early rise in adrenal catecholamines in young SHR is followed soon afterward by an increase in SNA. Adrenal cortical activity also rises early in response to elevation of CRH (Hashimoto et al., 1989; Fisher and Brown, 1983). The latter depends on the activity of proopiomelanocortin (POMC) neurons, which also regulate the production of β-lipotropin and β-endorphin.[2]

Behavior, Stress, and Salt Intake

In a normal environment, SHR are usually hypertensive and hyperactive, but the latter trait does not appear necessary for developing hypertension. This is suggested by the attributes of two additional inbred strains derived from SHR and WKY. One of these, the WKA rat, is normotensive and hyperactive, while the other, the WHT rat, is hypertensive but not hyperactive (Hendley et al., 1988; Knardahl and Hendley, 1990; Hendley and Ohlsson, 1991). In both hypertensive strains (SHR and WHT), the concentrations of NPY and NA at their sympathetic terminals are greater than in the two normotensive strains (WKY and WKA; Fan et al., 1995; Ralevic and Burnstock, 1995). These results have been taken to imply that independent genetic factors determine the levels of sympathoadrenal and somatic motor activity.

However, as noted in chapter 10, whether or not hyperactivity in SHR has a long-term effect on resting BP depends entirely on the level of habitual exercise. In view

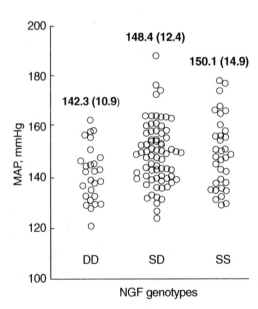

Figure 16.6. Mean arterial pressures (MAP, mmHg) in an F_2 population derived from SHR and Donryu rats, grouped according to NGF genotype (DD, SD, SS), where SS and DD are homozygotes and SD is the heterozygote. Numbers are means and standard deviations. From Kapuscinski et al. (1996), with permission *Journal of Hypertension* and Lippincott, Williams and Wilkins.

of the nonlinear relationship between work and resting BP, the amount of exercise-related diurnal activity may be too small to raise it.

The increases in BP and SNA in response to acute stress are greater in SHR than in WKY (figure 9.20; Lundin and Thorén, 1982; DiBona, 1991; Folkow, 1993). Reducing the level of chronic stress by housing SHR in individual cages is associated with lower resting BPs than when the cages contained 3–4 other rats (figure 16.7; Hallbäck, 1975).

Recall from chapter 12 that BP is increased by a high-salt diet in most SHR substrains through ouabain neurons that project to the defense area. However, some substrains are salt resistant (Folkow and Ely, 1987; Oparil et al., 1988; Huang et al., 1992; Calhoun et al., 1994). The mechanism could be due to a low permeability to the sodium ion of their blood-brain barrier, as in Dahl R rats (figure 12.9; Simchon et al., 1999).

Sexual Dimorphism of Blood Pressure

A BP difference between males and females (ΔBP_{m-f}) is found in both SHR and WKY, but its magnitude is greater in SHR and is genetically linked to their Y chromosomes (Ely and Turner, 1990). Accordingly, BP is higher in young adult male F_2 rats with an SHR grandfather than in animals with a WKY grandfather.[3] A similar sexual BP dimorphism occurs in SHR.SP (Davidson et al., 1995; Kreutz et al., 1996).

However, BP of both sets of F_1 males (i.e., SHR males × WKY females; WKY males × SHR females) is greater than in male WKY, which suggests that ΔBP_{m-f} is also affected by autosomal genes. This was confirmed by Turner et al. (1991) in two consomic strains: (1) the SHR/a strain, in which the Y chromosome of WKY replaced that of SHR while retaining the latter's X chromosome and autosomes; and

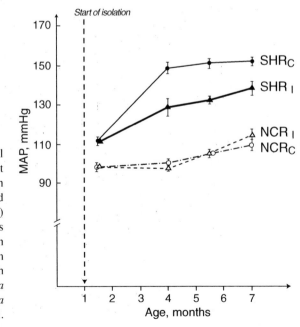

Figure 16.7. Mean arterial pressure (MAP, mmHg) at different ages (months) in control SHR (SHR$_c$) and normotensive rats (NCR$_c$) and in corresponding rats subjected to social isolation (SHR$_I$, NCR$_I$). From Hallbäck (1975), with permission of *Acta Physiologica Scandinavica* and Blackwell.

(2) the SHR/y strain, in which the Y chromosome of SHR is retained, while the X chromosome and autosomes have been replaced by those of WKY. Each set of genes on the Y chromosome and autosomes accounts for about half of ΔBP_{m-f} of SHR (figure 16.8).

Plasma testosterone rises earlier in SHR/y than in WKY, and the rise is greater and more prolonged (Ely et al., 1994). Hence, the genes on the Y chromosome of SHR must accelerate the onset of puberty. In contrast, the testosterone levels in male SHR/a lag behind those of SHR, suggesting that their higher BP is due to other factors (Iams and Wexler, 1979; Ganten et al., 1989; Ely et al., 1994).

Plasma NA in SHR/y and SHR/a are also raised, much as in SHR, suggesting that the elevation in SNA is similar in all strains (Ely et al., 1997b). The genes on the SHR's Y chromosome could raise SNA either directly or by promoting more aggressive behavior, as observed in some mouse strains by Henry and colleagues (chapter 11).

Structural Changes in the Heart and Vasculature

SHR have cardiovascular hypertrophy from an early age. Concentric LVH is present until about 6 months of age, after which eccentric LVH often develops. Over time, the resistance and conduit arteries both become less distensible.

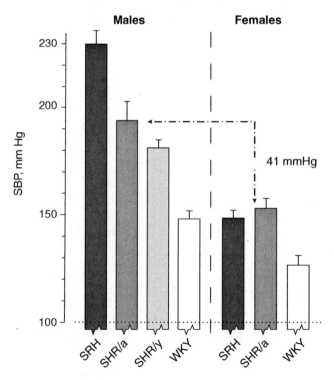

Figure 16.8. Average systolic BPs (SBP, mmHg) in adult male and female SHR and WKY, and two consomic strains SHR/y and SHR/a, as described in text. Data from Turner et al. (1991).

Heart

The resting heart rate is higher in SHR than in WKY through much of their life. This is due to (1) elevation of the intrinsic rate of the atrial pacemaker (Dyke et al., 1989), (2) the raised cardiac SNA, and (3) reduction in vagal activity from about 9 weeks of age due to rising cardiopulmonary load (Head and Adams, 1988).

At birth, the ratios of left and right ventricular weight to body weight (LV/BW, RV/BW) are greater in SHR than in WKY, despite the minimal BP difference between the strains (Hallbäck-Nordlander, 1980). The hypertrophy is due to stimulation of the immature cardiac myocytes by circulating CAs and high levels of insulin-like growth factors (Smolich et al., 1989; Robinson, 1996).

In both strains, the LV/BW ratio declines during the first 8–9 weeks of life, when body growth exceeds that of the heart (figure 16.9). WKY reach their definitive adult LV/BW ratio by about 10 weeks of age, but in SHR the ratio increases over several months as BP continues to rise slowly (Adams et al., 1989; Korner et al., 1993).

Thus, in neonatal SHR the slight degree of LVH is largely due to factors unrelated to BP, while the subsequent hypertrophy is largely due to the increasing hypertension.

Cosegregation Studies.   Tanase et al. (1982) examined 10-week-old male rats of 23 inbred strains to determine the extent to which genetic factors affect absolute and relative heart weights (HW, HW/BW). In 20 normotensive strains, a considerable fraction of the variance of HW and HW/BW was due to genetic factors unrelated to BP.

Another study was in a segregating population bred from two F_1 populations, each derived from one hypertensive and one normotensive strain (M520 × SHR.SP; SHR × WKY). In the F_2 rats, the relationship between BP and HW/BW accounted for a small but statistically significant fraction of the variance in HW/BW. One reason for the small magnitude may have been that in hypertension most of the load falls on the LV rather than on the heart as a whole.

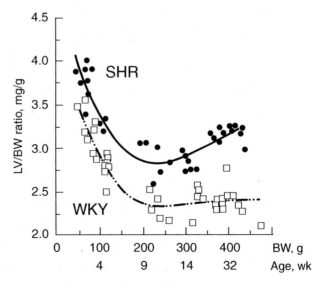

Figure 16.9. Relationship between age (weeks) and left ventricle weight/body weight (g, LV/BW) ratio in SHR (black circles, solid line) and WKY (open squares, dot-dash line). From Korner et al. (1993), with permission of *Hypertension*, American Heart Association, and Lippincott, Williams and Wilkins.

The only cosegregation study available for examining the association between BP and the LV/BW ratio was derived from SHR.SP and WKY (Davidson et al., 1995; Dominiczak et al., 1996). It was performed in 16–18-week-old male F$_2$ rats, which had received 1% salt in their drinking water for 2 weeks before the experiment. One group of rats was descended from an SHR grandfather, while the other had a WKY grandfather (figure 16.10, top and middle). Only in the first group was the association between BP and LV/BW statistically significant. Moreover, when BP-LV/BW data was pooled from both populations, the relationship was the same as in the first

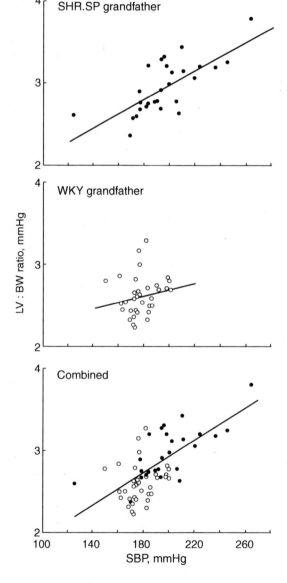

Figure 16.10. Cosegregation analysis in 16–18-week-old F$_2$ rats, derived from SHR.SP and WKY and given extra salt for several days. Note systolic BP (SBP, mmHg) significantly related to LV/BW ratio in rats with SHR.SP grandfather (top), but not in those with WKY grandfather (middle); (bottom) shows that after pooling the data the relationship resembles that in the top panel. I am most grateful to Professor Anna Dominiczak for providing the individual data points on which the calculations are based.

population (figure 16.10, bottom). Probably the greater variation in neuroendocrine activity in the F_2 rats with an SHR grandfather increases the range of their resting BPs and may thus be indirectly responsible for the variation in LVH.

Vasculature

The properties of the VSM cells have been studied in cell culture, while vascular resistance properties have been examined in both isolated R_1 vessels and in perfused vascular beds.

When fully differentiated VSM cells are placed in culture, they rapidly revert to the synthetic phenotype, in which cell metabolism and synthesis of proteins is high and susceptibility to mitogens is greater than when the cells are contractile (Chamley-Campbell et al., 1979; Scott-Burden et al., 1989; Bobik et al., 1994). In cells derived from SHR, the replication rate is about 20% more rapid than in those derived from WKY (Yamori et al., 1981, 1984; Owens, 1987). Moreover, their G_1 and S phases are of shorter duration (Yamori et al., 1984; Hadrava et al., 1992; Bacakova and Mares, 1995; Hamet et al., 1998).

In-culture stimulation of the α-ARs induces more growth in VSM cells derived from SHR than in cells derived from WKY (Simpson et al., 1982; Simpson, 1985; Korner et al., 1989; Bobik et al., 1990; Long et al., 1991). In addition, cells derived from SHR secrete more NGF (Tuttle et al., 1995). All these changes simulate the early changes in immature VSM cells in vivo, which are largely BP independent.

Under in vivo conditions, the between-strain differences are smaller than in culture (Schwartz et al., 1990). At 4 weeks of age, lumen of the resistance vessel in SHR is 2–3% narrower than in WKY, and by 20–24 weeks of age this difference has increased to 5–6%. Since Vas R is proportional to $1/r_i^4$, the small amount of narrowing has substantial hemodynamic consequences, as discussed in chapter 6.

R_1 Resistance Vessels

In mesenteric resistance arteries of 4-week-old SHR studied under standardized conditions in the isometric myograph, r_i was narrower and the ratio of media thickness to r_i (m/r_i) was greater than in WKY (Mulvany and Halpern, 1977; Warshaw et al., 1979; Dyke, 1989; Angus et al., 1990; Mulvany and Aalkjaer, 1990).

The responses of these vessels to field stimulation of the sympathetic nerves varied over the age range of 4 to 50 weeks. In a vessel of given geometry, the force developed depends on the amount of transmitter released, the rate of its removal by the reuptake pump, and the extent of α_2-AR-mediated autoinhibitory feedback (chapter 5; Dyke, 1989; Angus et al., 1990). After blocking the last two processes, the open-loop responses of each strain were about double those observed under closed-loop conditions (figure 16.11). The isometric tension developed was smallest in 4-week-old SHR and WKY, which is consistent with the VSM cells' relative immaturity at that time. It reached a maximum by about 9 weeks of age. From 9 to 50 weeks, the ratio of maximum tension developed in SHR:WKY vessels was 1.52 (open loop) and 1.41 (closed loop), reflecting the structural remodeling of SHR vessels. Under open-loop conditions, maximum tension tended to decline in SHR between 14 and 50 weeks of age, probably due to reduction in vascular distensibility.

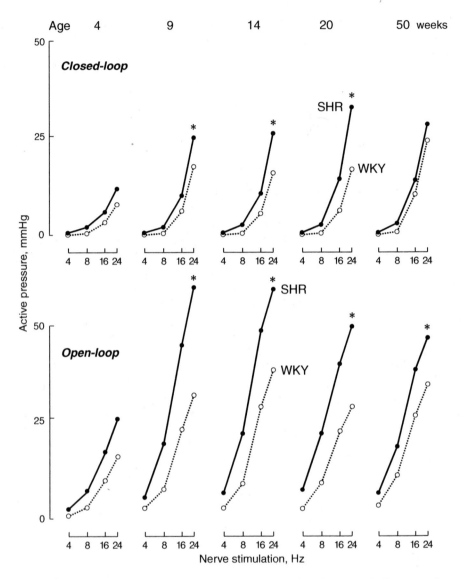

Figure 16.11. Average force (active pressure, mmHg) generated in isometrically contracting small mesenteric arteries during graded field stimulation of sympathetic nerves (Hz); SHR, black circles; WKY, open circles. Top, normal closed-loop conditions at terminal. Bottom, open-loop conditions after blocking NA reuptake and prejunctional α_2-ARs. Stimulus strength adjusted to make maximum $\equiv$ to about 30% of maximum tension evoked by exogenous NA. *p for $\Delta_{SHR\text{-}WKY} < .05$. Data from Dyke (1989).

The threshold ($\equiv EC_{50}$) for the contractile responses was lower in SHR than in WKY, with the difference greatest under open-loop conditions. It may be due to intrinsic differences in membrane properties between the strains (Postnov and Orlov, 1985) or to a greater number of α_1-ARs associated with the hypernoradrenergic innervation.

Hindquarter Bed

In the constant-flow perfused isolated hindquarter bed, R_{min}, R_{max}, and S were all greater in SHR than in WKY throughout the first year of life (figure 16.12; Adams et al., 1989). At 4 weeks of age, the between-strain differences in R_{min} and R_{max} were about half of those at 20 and 30 weeks of age. From 9 weeks onward, the ratio of slopes of SHR:WKY was 1.59, close to that in isolated resistance vessels.

Determinants of High TPR and BP in Vivo

Between 1 and 3 weeks of age, the VSM cells in vivo are mostly in the synthetic phenotype (figure 16.13; Woolgar and Scott, 1989; Miano et al., 1994; Price et al., 1994). When the VSM cells are still immature, the raised plasma CAs cause increased vascular narrowing in R_1 vessels of SHR. When the VSM cells become contractile by 5–6 weeks of age, the already established remodeling allows immediate enhancement of Vas R responses to constrictor stimuli.

The main determinants of the differences in regional Vas R and TPR between SHR and WKY are shown in table 16.2. They include differences in sympathoadrenal activity, vascular geometry, and changes in local concentrations of autacoids. The enhanced constriction in SHR R_1 vessels increases rarefaction downstream, reducing the capillary area for blood-tissue exchange.

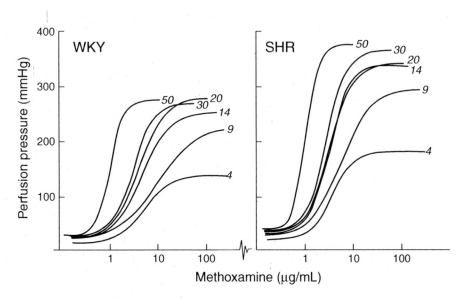

Figure 16.12. Relationship between log methoxamine concentration (μg/mL perfusate) and perfusion pressure (mmHg, $\equiv$ Vas R) over age range 4–50 weeks (label on each curve) in isolated SHR and WKY hindquarter bed perfused at constant flow with electrolyte-dextran solution. From Adams et al. (1989), with permission of *Hypertension*, American Heart Association, and Lippincott, Williams and Wilkins.

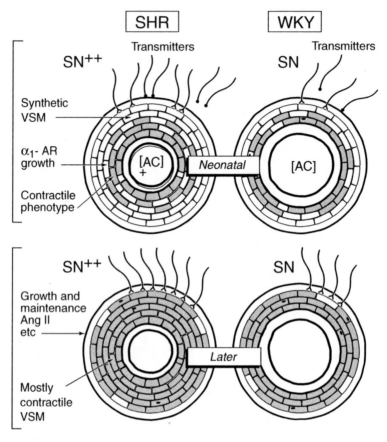

Figure 16.13. Cartoon of resistance vessel cross-section of SHR and WKY rats aged 1–4 weeks (top) and 9–12 weeks (bottom). In young rats, most VSM cells are immature (clear outline) rather than contractile (shaded outline). After 4–5 weeks, the great majority of VSM cells have become contractile. Young SHR have more cell layers due to inward growth of immature VSM cells, which narrows lumen. Sympathetic innervation density is greater in SHR. In young rats, AC (adrenal catecholamines) are an important stimulant to inward growth.

Cosegregation Studies

In the synthetic phenotype, the difference in cell cycle duration between SHR and WKY is probably genetically determined. However, in vivo analysis of the relationship between BP and vascular geometry in segregating populations have given variable results (chapter 3). A positive association was noted in a segregating male F_2 population, in which the internal radius (r_i) of the renal afferent arteriole at 7 weeks of age was closely related to the BP at 23 weeks (figure 3.11; Norrelund et al., 1994). At 7 weeks, the VSM cells have only recently become contractile and the vessel geometry is largely due to the CA-induced growth during the preceding neonatal period, which is related to the subsequent rise in BP.

Table 16.2. Local Circulatory Factors Contributing to Difference in TPR (or BP) between SHR and WKY

Factor	SHR	WKY
SNA	++	+
Adrenal CA	++	0
Local Ang II	+	0
Const. autacoids	+	0
Dilator autacoids	−	− −
$\Delta TPR_{SHR-WKY} = R_1$ Amplifier $\times \Delta$(N-H + Local) + Rarefaction		

Note: SNA, sympathetic neural activity; Adrenal CA, adrenal catecholamines; Ang II, local Ang II; Const. autacoids, e.g., superoxide ions; Dilator autacoids, e.g., NO. Excess of constrictor plus reduction in dilator factors equals 7+ units. Assuming a structural amplification $\times 1.4$ and a 16% rise in TPR due to rarefaction. $\Delta TPR_{SHR-WKY}$ is 11.4 units (chapter 6).

In contrast, the relationship between m/r_i ratio and BP in mesenteric R_1 vessels of 14–16-week-old F_2 rats was not statistically significant (Mulvany and Korsgaard, 1983). This suggests that the structural changes are not inherited. The result was also interpreted as indicating that they play no role in the rise in BP (Mulvany, 1988). The latter conclusion is not justified. The cosegregation test examines inheritance of the structural changes, but not their physiological properties. The remodeled vessels still amplify constrictor stimuli, as discussed in chapter 6.

Can these disparate findings be reconciled? One possibility is that the m/r_i ratio is less useful as a descriptive parameter of structural changes than wall thickness $(w)/r_i$ or r_i alone. Another is that in 7-week-old renal R_1 vessels, vessel narrowing is mostly due to preceding growth of immature VSM cells and is an important component of future vascular geometry in the small afferent arterioles. The size of mesenteric R_1 vessels from older rats is larger: They probably also experienced BP-independent growth when the animals were younger. Subsequent superposition of further BP-related hypertrophy may have been reduced by other factors such as greater tissue hypoxia, obscuring the relationship with BP.

Prevention and Attenuation of SHR Hypertension

Inactivation of the sympathoadrenal system early in life prevents development of SHR hypertension and vascular and LV structural changes. Long-term inactivation of the renin-angiotensin system in young rats attenuates the hypertension nearly as effectively.

Neonatal Sympathectomy

The first immunological and chemical sympathectomies were performed some 30 years ago, using NGF antiserum or 6-OHDA (Folkow et al., 1972; Cutiletta et al., 1977; Oparil and Cutiletta, 1979). Later, treatment with guanethidine for several weeks was added to the regimen (Burnstock et al., 1971). These methods attenuated SHR hypertension by 40–60% (e.g., Lee et al., 1987). This was widely interpreted as indicating that the sympathetic nervous system was only one of several initiators of SHR hypertension.

What had been overlooked was the role of the adrenal medulla. All the above treatments have no effect on its secretions, which had been known for several years (Brodie et al., 1966; Korner et al., 1967). Indeed, after destruction of the sympathetic nerve terminals, adrenal medullary NA concentration increases (table 16.3). It took some years before the inadequacy of neural sympathectomy alone was recognized (Lee, Borkowski et al., 1991; Korner, Bobik, Oddie, and Friberg, 1992, 1993).

In a preliminary study in 4-week-old SHR and WKY, the hindquarter vascular resistance properties were compared under the following conditions: (1) in untreated rats; (2) in rats treated with NGF antiserum plus daily guanethidine; and (3) in rats receiving the preceding treatment plus the α_1-AR antagonist prazosin, to eliminate the effects of adrenal CAs on vascular growth (Korner, Bobik, Oddie, and Friberg, 1992, 1993).

Hindquarter R_{min} was used as an index of internal R_1 vessel radius (r_i; chapter 6). In the group in which only the neural terminals had been destroyed, ΔR_{min} between SHR and WKY was greater than in untreated controls (figure 16.14), indicating a narrowing of r_i in SHR due to more growth stimulation by adrenal CAs. However, ΔR_{min} between the strains was abolished by neural sympathectomy plus prazosin.[4]

The dose of prazosin employed in the above experiment was large and retarded body growth. Hence in the main series the treated SHR and WKY received the same NGF regimen as before, plus 8 weeks of treatment with guanethidine to reduce regrowth of the postganglionic sympathetic nerves. They also received a lower dose of prazosin, which was administered only between the ages of 3 to 6 weeks (Korner et al., 1993).

This regimen prevented the development of SHR hypertension, while the BP of WKY was unaffected (figure 16.15). It also prevented the development of vascular structural changes, as assessed from the hindquarter resistance properties at 21 and 35 weeks of age, which remained close to those in WKY (figure 16.16). Similarly, it prevented an increase in LV/BW ratio.

Table 16.3. Mean Adrenal NA Concentration ± s.e.m. (ng/g) in 4-Week-Old SHR and WKY Rats under Control Conditions, after Neural Sympathectomy and after Sympathectomy + Prazosin

Group	SHR	WKY
Control (n)	110 ± 8.0 (14)	88 ± 6.3* (16)
Sympathectomy	159 ± 13.0[+] (6)	131 ± 16.0[+] (6)
Symp$_x$ + prazosin	201 ± 20 (7)	193 ± 7.5[++] (7)

Note: n, number of rats, in parentheses.

*$p < .05$ SHR v. WKY; [+]$p < .05$, Symp$_X$ v. control, within strains; [++]$p < .05$, (Symp$_X$ + prazosin) v. Symp$_X$, within strains.

Source: Korner et al. (1993).

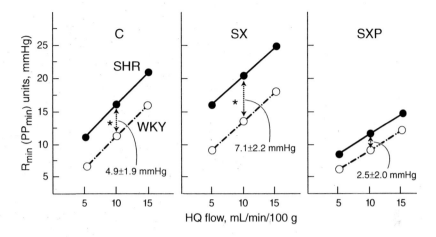

Figure 16.14. Relationship between HQ perfusate flow (mL/min/100 g HQ) and R_{min} ($\equiv$minimum perfusion pressure, PP_{min}) in fully dilated isolated HQ bed in three groups of 4-week-old SHR and WKY: untreated controls (C, left), after neural sympathectomy (SX, middle), and after neural sympathectomy + prazosin (SXP, right). Numbers are means ± SEMs of change. Intercepts between SHR and WKY. *$p < .05$. Based on data from Korner et al. (1993).

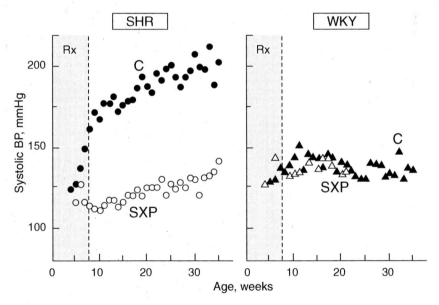

Figure 16.15. Relationship between age (weeks) and systolic BP (mmHg) in SHR (left) and WKY rats (right); C, control; SXP, sympathectomy + prazosin. Shaded area is treatment period (R_x). Observations made only until 21 weeks of age in SXP-treated WKY rats, but to 35 weeks in all other groups. From Korner et al. (1993), with permission of *Blood Pressure* and Taylor and Francis.

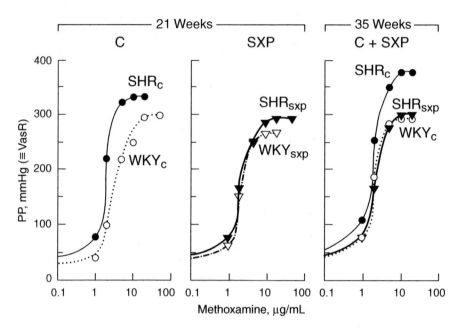

Figure 16.16. Relationship between log dose of methoxamine (μg/mL) and perfusion pressure (PP, mmHg) in isolated hindquarter bed perfused at constant flow in 21- and 35-week-old SHR and WKY. Groups were untreated controls (SHR$_c$, WKY$_c$), rats previously treated by sympathectomy + prazosin (SXP) rats (SHR$_{sxp}$, WKY$_{sxp}$), which abolished differences between the strains. From Korner et al. (1993), with permission of *Hypertension*, American Heart Association, and Lippincott, Williams and Wilkins.

Similar findings were obtained by Lee, Borkowski et al, (1991), who had treated the animals with NGF antiserum, guanethidine, and neonatal adrenal medullectomy. This prevented the hypertension and the development of mesenteric R$_1$ vessel structural changes.

Giving an α$_1$-AR antagonist alone attenuates hypertension by about 50%, which is similar to the effects of antagonizing the neural changes alone (McCarty and Lee, 1996). The same attenuation occurred after a single injection of NGF antiserum given to 3-week-old SHR (Brock et al., 1996).

An alternative approach was to induce development of a hypernoradrenergic innervation by injecting young WKY with NGF. This caused an increase in postganglionic sympathetic fibers but had no effect on BP (Zettler et al., 1991). It suggests that the elevation of BP is largely determined by the central sympathetic drive, rather than by the excess postganglionic innervation, which has a significant but small effect (figure 16.6).

In conclusion, SHR hypertension is prevented completely by combined neural sympathectomy and inactivation of adrenal CA secretion. The rise in plasma adrenaline and the hypernoradrenergic innervation contribute to inward growth of immature R$_1$ vessels, thereby enhancing the power of the vascular amplifier independently of BP.[5]

Long-Term Inhibition of Renin-Angiotensin System

Apart from its role as a pressor hormone and a CNS transmitter, Ang II is important in normal renal and cardiovascular development (Ganten et al., 1975; Phillips, 1987, 2000; Ekblom, 1992; Friberg et al., 1994; Guron and Friberg, 2000).

Many investigators found that long-term attenuation of hypertension results from several weeks of treatment of SHR with an ACE inhibitor or an AT_1 receptor antagonist, started soon after weaning (Guidicelli et al., 1980; Richer et al., 1982; Harrap et al., 1986, 1990; Christensen et al., 1989; Korner et al., 1989; Adams et al., 1990; Lee, Berecek et al., 1991; Mulvany et al., 1991; Oddie et al., 1992; Wu and Berecek, 1993; Thybo et al., 1994; Korner and Bobik, 1995; Notoya et al., 1996). The extent of the attenuation is a function of the duration of preceding treatment, with the SBP on average 20% below untreated controls after 5 weeks treatment starting at 4 weeks of age, and 80% below controls after 16 weeks of treatment (Adams et al., 1990; Korner and Bobik, 1995).

Figure 16.17 shows the effects on body weight and SBP of enalapril given between the ages of 4 and 20 weeks to SHR and WKY (Korner and Bobik, 1995). During treatment, the SBP was depressed well below each strain's normal value without treatment. On stopping the drug, SBP rose more rapidly in SHR than in WKY, but 15 weeks later the BP of previously treated SHR was well below that of untreated SHR, while that of previously treated WKY had caught up with the SBP of untreated WKY.

Korner and Bobik (1995) estimated the effects of enalapril on vascular structure from the changes in resistance properties from the vascular wall model in chapter 6. Immediately after stopping the drug, r_i of the R_1 resistance vessels of each strain was wider and the wall was thinner than in the corresponding untreated controls (figure 16.18). This is in good agreement with morphological data from similar studies (Notoya et al., 1996). In addition, ACE inhibitors and AT_1 antagonists increase vascular distensibility by reducing collagen in the wall (Simon et al., 1993; Albaladejo et al., 1994; Barenbrock et al., 1994).

Although enalapril widens the R_1 vessels of both SHR and WKY, the relative magnitude of their vascular geometry is not greatly altered; that is, r_i of treated SHR is narrower than in WKY, while wall thickness $(w)/r_i$ ratio is greater. Hence the R_1 vessels of treated SHR still enhance Vas R compared to vessels of previously treated WKY. This accounts for the greater rise in BP in SHR immediately after stopping treatment. But 15 weeks later, the R_1 vessels of previously treated SHR are still wider and their walls are thinner than in untreated SHR, suggesting that suppressing Ang II formation in childhood and adolescence produced virtually permanent vascular remodeling (figure 16.18). In contrast, the vessels of previously previously treated WKY are virtually normal.

Korner and Bobik (1995) suggested that Ang II plays a role in normal vascular development in both SHR and WKY and also contributes to the structural remodeling in SHR. The remodeling is mediated through both BP-independent and BP-dependent mechanisms. In SHR, the first is important in the early vascular narrowing of immature VSM cells, while the BP-related changes occur in contractile VSM cells during the gradual rise in BP. In WKY, the first mechanism plays a minimal role, while the second contributes to normal vascular development.

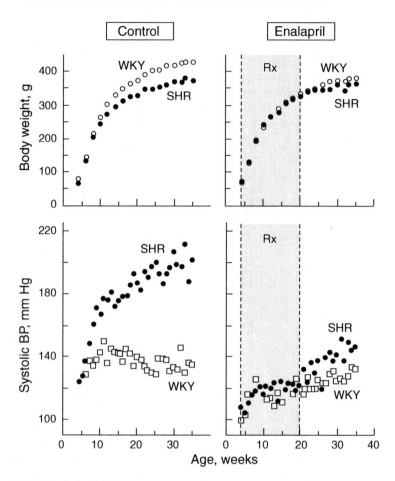

Figure 16.17. Relationship between age (weeks) and body weight (top; g), and systolic BP (mmHg; bottom). Left, control SHR and WKY; right, SHR and WKY treated with enalapril (25 mg/kg/day) from 4 to 20 weeks (shaded area, Rx) in which measurements were continued for another 15 weeks. From Korner and Bobik (1995), with permission of *Hypertension*, American Heart Association, and Lippincott, Williams and Wilkins.

Last, enalapril also attenuated the age-related changes in LV/BW ratio of both SHR and WKY. In SHR, this prevented the development of LVH long after the drug had been withdrawn, while in WKY the ratio had returned to the normal range (Korner and Bobik, 1995).

Still Earlier Start of Treatment

Wu and Berecek (1993) treated SHR with captopril throughout pregnancy and lactation and continued to treat the pups for a further 2 months after weaning. The MAP and body weight of the treated animals remained below corresponding values of untreated SHR for several months after stopping the drugs. More remarkably, the

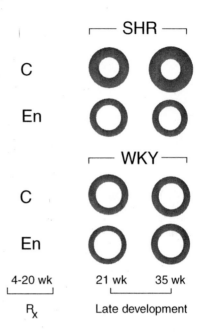

Figure 16.18. Estimated cross-sectional wall dimensions in hindquarter R_1 vessels of 21- and 35-week-old SHR and WKY, including controls (C); rats treated with enalapril (En) between 4 and 20 weeks of age. In control SHR, w/r_i ratio increases between age 21 and 35 weeks as BP increases, with little change in either variable in control WKY. After enalapril, lumen is wider and walls thinner in both strains, compared to 21-week-old controls. By 35 weeks, WKY vessels are close to normal, while most earlier changes have persisted in SHR, in which BP rise was greatly attenuated. Based on Korner and Bobik (1995), with permission of *Hypertension*, American Heart Association, and Lippincott, Williams and Wilkins.

hypertension was attenuated in a second generation of offspring of the previously treated SHR. It suggests that in young rats the ACE inhibitor moves readily across the blood-brain and blood-gonadal barriers.

Raizada et al. (2000) prevented the effects of Ang II more specifically. A single intracardiac injection of full-length antisense cDNA for the AT_1 receptor was administered to 5-day-old SHR.[6] This completely prevented development of hypertension in SHR but caused no changes in WKY (figure 16.19). In SHR, the renal artery was markedly wider and its wall was thinner than in control rats (Reaves et al., 1999). This is similar to the R_1 vessel remodeling after prolonged ACE inhibitor treatment (figure 16.18).

The antisense cDNA also affects the parental germ line of SHR (figure 16.19). These almost Lamarckian effects were probably due to permanent changes in mRNA translation, which were more stable over two generations than the effects of captopril.

The Koletsky Obese SHR

The Koletsky obese SHR was derived from the mating of an SHR female with a normotensive Sprague-Dawley male (Koletsky, 1975; Yamori, 1994). The obesity is due to a mutation of the leptin receptor gene, similar to that in normotensive obese Zucker rats (Bray and York, 1979; Yen et al., 1977). The Koletsky rat's hypertension is a model for human hypertensive obesity.

At 3–6 months of age, the body weight of Koletsky SHR is about double that of lean SHR, and their daily food intake is still greater (Ernsberger et al., 1993; Koletsky

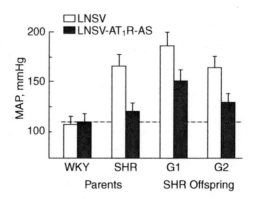

Figure 16.19. Average mean arterial BP (mmHg) in 120-day-old parent SHR and WKY and in first and second generation of SHR offspring (G1, G2). At age of 5 days, rats received intracardial injection of retroviral vector alone (open rectangle; LNSV for *l*ong terminal repeats, *n*eomycin selection, *s*imian *v*irus promoter) or virus containing AT$_1$ receptor-antisense (black rectangle, LNSV-AT$_1$R-AS). From Reaves et al. (1999), with permission of *Circulation Research*, American Heart Association, and Lippincott, Williams and Wilkins.

and Ernsberger, 1992). The obesity gives rise to NIDMM, with hyperinsulinemia, hyperglycemia, glycosuria, and lipid abnormalities. The resting MAP of Koletsky rats is 15 mmHg below that of SHR, which suggests a preponderance of insulin-mediated peripheral vasodilation over CNS-mediated vasoconstriction due to leptin, other adiposity peptides, and a sensitized defense pathway (chapter 13). Urinary glucocorticoids are raised, which is a marker of reduced NO availability.

Koletsky rats have marked renal nephropathy, with microalbuminuria, renal glomerular sclerosis, and reduction in glomerular number. Their cardiopulmonary load is greater than in lean SHR, and it will be interesting to compare the sympathetic outflow patterns in the two strains (cf. figure 13.20, HL vs. HO).

Renal Hypertension in SHR

The factors that initiate SHR hypertension and 2K-1C renovascular hypertension are distinctive, so that the induction of renovascular hypertension (RenVH) in SHR might cause additive increases in BP and in cardiovascular structural changes. In turn, the latter will accelerate vasoconstrictor-induced rarefaction and organ damage and the likelihood of developing cardiac failure.

Dilley et al. (1994) induced two kidney, one clip (2K-1C) renovascular hypertension (RenVH) in 6-week-old SHR and WKY, and compared their BP and structural responses over an 8-week period with the corresponding changes in control SHR and WKY. The rise in BP was smaller in 2K-1C SHR than in 2K-1C WKY, although the BP reached nearly the same level in each strain (figure 16.20).

In both strains, RenVH markedly increased the medial mass of mesenteric R$_1$ vessels (table 16.4). In SHR, this was about twice that in vessels of age-matched control SHR.

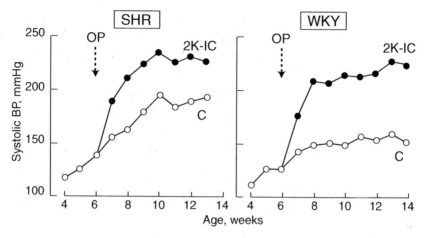

Figure 16.20. Average systolic BP (mmHg) between 4 and 14 weeks of age in SHR and WKY, which were subjected at 6 weeks of age to either two kidneys, 1 clip (2K-1C) hypertension or sham operation (C, controls). Left, results in SHR; right, results in WKY. From Dilley et al. (1994), with permission of *Hypertension*, American Heart Association, and Lippincott, Williams and Wilkins.

However, in both groups of SHR medial mass reached a maximum at 10 weeks, which tended to decline from the latter value by 14 weeks of age. The decline is consistent with changes associated with eutrophic vascular remodeling, where an initial period of inward VSM growth is followed by reduction in the outer vascular radius (r_o; figure 6.17). In eutrophic remodeling, the mechanical advantage of hypertrophy is maintained, as indicated in the hindquarter perfusion data in table 16.4.

In the heart, the superposition of RenVH on SHR hypertension caused a large increase in LV/BW ratio by 14 weeks of age; LV/BW was 83% above that of control SHR and 140% above that of control WKY. The increase in ratio provides a measure of myocyte volume enlargement and suggests that LVH was well above Linzbach's critical value of ~70% (chapter 7). The animals had LV failure, which caused right ventricular hypertrophy in 2K-1C SHR; the RV/BW ratio was about 60% greater than in control SHR and WKY.

In WKY with RenVH, the medial mass increased between 10 and 14 weeks of age and the lumen narrowed, suggesting VSM cell hypertrophy with inward growth, rather than eutrophic remodeling (figure 6.17). Changes in hinquarter resistance properties were similar to those of control SHR. The increase in LV/BW ratio was slightly greater than in control SHR, but RV/BW was normal.

Thus, when RenVH is superimposed on SHR hypertension the rise in BP is smaller than would be expected, owing to the development of LV failure with eccentric hypertrophy. In addition, the large degree of LVH strains the coronary blood supply's capacity to meet the extra work requirementsof the myocardium. However, the superposition of RenVH on SHR hypertension increases cardiac and vascular structure in an almost additive manner.

Table 16.4. Left and Right Ventricle Weight to Body Weight Ratios, Media Cross-Section in Mesenteric R_1 Vessel and Perfusion Pressures at Full Dilation, and Maximum Constriction in Constant Flow-Perfused Isolated Hindquarter of Control SHR and WKY and of Rats of Each Strain with 2K-1C Renovascular Hypertension

Variable	Age	SHR_c	SHR-2K1C	WKY_c	WKY-2K1C
LV/BW	10	3.0 ± 0.08	4.6 ± 0.09*	2.6 ± 0.05	3.7 ± 0.08*
	14	2.9 ± 0.05	5.3 ± 0.25*	2.2 ± 0.05	3.5 ± 0.20*
RV/BW	10	0.68 ± 0.03	0.74 ± 0.10	0.66 ± 0.02	0.70 ± 0.02
	14	0.63 ± 0.02	1.01 ± 0.1*	0.65 ± 0.02	0.69 ± 0.04
R_1 Media	10	19.3 ± 1.6	41.3 ± 2.7*	16.2 ± 0.9	16.8 ± 1.7
	14	15.9 ± 1.5	29.8 ± 4.4*	11.5 ± 1.0	21.4 ± 1.6*
PP_{min}	10	26.0 ± 0.8	31.3 ± 1.0*	24.9 ± 0.9	28.1 ± 0.9*
	14	31.1 ± 0.6	34.3 ± 2.1	26.9 ± 1.1	32.7 ± 1.2*
PP_{max}	10	338 ± 7	377 ± 15*	283 ± 4	313 ± 14*
	14	339 ± 9	435 ± 6*	297 ± 7	370 ± 7*

Note: LV/BW, RV/BW, left and right ventricle weight/body weight ratios (mg/g); R_1 media, medial cross-section of large resistance arteriole μm^2; PP_{min}, PP_{max}, perfusion pressures at full dilation and maximum constriction in isolated hindquarter perfused at constant flow (i.e., $\equiv R_{min}$, R_{max}); SHR_c, WKY_c, control SHR, WKY; SHR-2K1C; WKY-2K1C; rats with 2 kidney-1 clip renovascular hypertension. Age, weeks; numerical values are means ± s.e.m.
*$p < .05$, for Δ control vs. 2K-1C within strains.

Source: Dilley et al. (1994).

BP Genetics

Reference was made in chapter 3 to the methods of identifying high-BP quantitative trait loci (QTLs) on various chromosomes of genetic hypertensive rats. At least 12 QTLs influencing BP have been identified in SHR and SHR.SP (Dominiczak et al., 1998, 2000; Hamet et al., 1998; Rapp, 2000). Each QTL may include several BP genes, many of which remain to be identified. Some high-BP genes are known to affect neural regulation, for example, the NPY gene, the DA receptor gene, and genes relating to other central transmitters and receptors, brain ANP and brain AT_1 receptors, and Ang II.

The effects of a gene on BP depend on the animal's overall genetic background. Rapp et al. (1994) studied the effects of various renin alleles on BP in a number of F_2 populations on a high salt diet. In deriving each population, rats of the salt sensitive SS/Jr strain (which provide the *s* renin allele) had been crossed with an inbred normotensive or hypertensive strain and subsequently intercrossed. Seven F_2 comparisons were made and in all of them, the homozygotes for *s* had a higher BP than the contrasting homozygotes. ΔBP between *s* and *r* (which comes from the salt-resistant SR/Jr rats) was 24 mmHg and was the only ΔBP of unequivocal statistical significance. The other ΔBPs were small and variable, which was thought to be due to differences in genetic background. It suggests that it may be preferable to focus on genetic differences between specific strains rather than ignoring the role of these background differences.

A component of the renin-angiotensin system is likely to play a role in the progression of SS/Jr hypertension, but may also be involved in its initiation. Other genes probably also affect the progression of hypertension and its complications. These are often a consequence of rarefaction and changes in concentration of tissue autacoids, including NO, superoxides, and various prostaglandins (Sohal and Weindruch, 1996; Lee et al., 1999; Morris, 2005).

Cosegregation Studies in SHR

Relationships have been established in F_2 or backcross populations between BP and a number of trait differences between SHR and WKY or other normotensive strains. The traits include resting SNA; greater SNA (and BP) responsiveness during acute stress; the transmitter profile for NA and NPY at the vascular sympathetic terminals; sexual BP dimorphism; BP sensitivity to salt; increased responsiveness to arterial hypoxia; a more rapid cell cycle in VSM cells in the synthetic phenotype and their greater susceptibility to mitogens; enhanced growth in immature cardiac myocytes; increased secretion of glucocorticoids; and several components of the renin-angiotensin system.

The above list is by no means complete. A significant relationship increases the likelihood that genetic factors are important factors in a particular trait difference.

The Pathogenesis of SHR Hypertension

SHR hypertension is initiated soon after birth, which results in a lifelong hyperresponsiveness of the hypothalamopituitary axis (figure 16.21). In addition, the immature R_1 vessel VSM cells are more susceptible to growth, which results in the initiation of vascular structural changes independently of the elevation of BP. Later the rise in BP contributes to the development of the structural changes.

CNS Hyperresponsiveness

Hyperresponsiveness affects hypothalamic defense area neurons and the amygdala, with the DA neurons playing a key role in sensitizing these pathways, which results in permanent hypertension. Acute transmitter release elicits the defense response (figures 8.13, 8.21) while destruction of DA neurons in young animals attenuates or prevents the rise in BP. Since the hyperresponsiveness develops without specific environmental changes, it suggests that the genes determining DA neuron numbers, or receptor properties, or formation of synaptic proteins must be expressed sufficiently to bring about sensitization without external stimuli. Sensitization lowers the response threshold, so that the sympathoadrenal changes occur in a virtually normal environment.

Inputs other than those related to stress that converge on the hypothalamic defense area include central endogenous ouabain (EO) neurons, the arterial chemoreceptors, and various other tissue chemoreceptors including those from skeletal muscle and kidney. Last, bouts of moderate exercise training have a desensitizing effect on defense area neurons, lowering resting SNA and BP between training sessions.

Hormonal changes mediated through the pituitary and adrenal cortex are also prominent. An early transient increase in mineralocorticoids is followed by a rise in CRH, which is responsible for secretion of ACTH and adrenal glucocorticoids, which affect production of NO. In males, testosterone is also raised and may increase aggressive behavior.

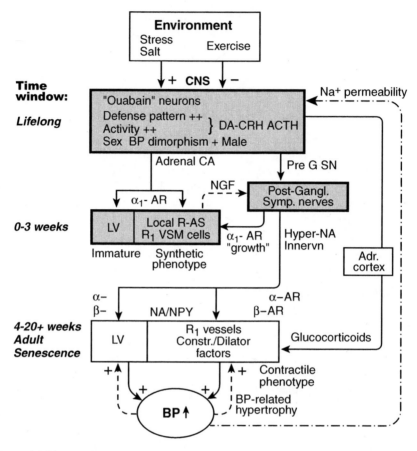

Figure 16.21. SHR hypertension is caused by lifelong hyperresponsivess of hypothalamic defense area and pituitary mediated through raised activity of dopaminergic (DA) neurons, corticotrophin-releasing hormone (CRH), and adrenal corticotrophic hormone (ACTH). In males, androgens contribute to BP rise. From birth to ~3 weeks of age, VSM cells are mostly immature (synthetic phenotype), with a shorter cell cycle and greater susceptibility to α_1-AR-induced proliferation and increased NGF secretion, which increase narrowing in R_1 vessels. Later, rise in BP accentuates LV hypertrophy and causes further structural changes in R_1 vessels. BP-related increase in sodium permeability accentuates neural drive through defense area.

Properties of Immature VSM Cells and Cardiac Myocytes in Neonatal SHR

The VSM cells are very immature from birth up to 3–4 weeks of age, while immaturity of cardiac myocytes is of shorter duration. The VSM cells have a shorter cell cycle in SHR than in WKY and are more responsive to mitogens, including CAs and Ang II. The early rise in plasma adrenaline stimulates VSM cell growth, narrowing r_i and increasing the w/r_i ratio of R_1 vessels, which results in BP-independent cardiovascular remodeling when the proportion of contractile VSM cells is low.

The immature VSM cells of SHR secrete more NGF than WKY cells, and the resulting hypernoradrenergic innervation may complement the effects of adrenaline in early development. Parenthetically, the growth properties of the immature VSM cells explain why narrowing of R_1 vessels in SHR is so pronounced at the time of renal transplantation.

Last, the growth of immature LV cardiac myocytes of SHR is also susceptible to stimulation by circulating CAs acting on α-ARs, and by local growth factors. As a result, BP-independent LVH has developed at the time of birth and during the neonatal period. This sets the scene for the later BP-related development of concentric LVH, allowing the heart to cope with the rising afterload from 4–5 weeks onward.

Natural History

SHR hypertension is a constrictor type of high BP, which is initiated through the mechanisms just considered. The early R_1 vessel narrowing and LVH ensure that BP rises rapidly at about 5 weeks of age, as soon as cardiovascular differentiation nears completion. By 7–8 weeks, sympathoadrenal activity is maximal and generalized vasoconstriction has developed, with the rather high plasma adrenaline concentrations reinforcing SNA-mediated constriction.

By then, the structural R_1 vessel amplifier and glucocorticoid-induced reduction of NO further enhance the vasoconstriction. This produces increasing rarefaction, with reduction in capillary area available for blood-tissue exchange and in total blood volume. However, central blood volume and cardiopulmonary load remain high, with the vagal deficit of the cardiac baroreflex a marker of the latter. With reduction in extracellular sodium space, tissue Na^+ tends to rise readily, raising EO neuron input to the defense area.

From about 12–15 weeks, signs of organ damage become manifest, including loss of nephron number and development of eccentric LVH. However, renal and cardiac functional reserves are large and evidence of functional impairment only becomes obvious from about 30 weeks of age. Mortality exceeds that of WKY from about 7 months of age onward. By 21 months, only about 20% of male rats of a given SHR cohort remain alive, compared to about 70–80% of WKY. Antihypertensive treatment from about 3 months onward greatly reduces SHR mortality (Weiss, 1974; Fleckenstein et al., 1987; Knorr et al., 1991).[7]

Two Therapeutic Models for Prevention

Elimination of sympathoadrenal activity during the neonatal period prevents SHR hypertension and the associated structural changes, which suggests that high sympathoadrenal activity is preeminent as initiator of the high BP. Parenthetically, after effective sympathoadrenal inactivation the structural cardiovascular properties of SHR are the same as in WKY, indicating that the latter provide a satisfactory baseline for assessing SHR responses.

In the second model, inactivation of the renin-angiotensin system attenuates SHR hypertension almost as effectively as sympathoadrenalectomy, with the most dramatic outcome following early administration of antisense cDNA for the AT_1 receptor. This and treatment with ACE inhibitors widens R_1 vessels and conduit arteries, causing thinning of their vascular walls and reduction in LV/BW ratio. These changes also occur in WKY, suggesting that the renin-angiotensin system plays a general role in cardiovascular development. However, adult WKY overcome the earlier retardation of development, while in SHR the changes are permanent, suggesting some difference in the expression of the genes regulating the development of the structure of the heart and blood vessels.

The widening of the R_1 vessels after treatment greatly reduces the amplification of Vas R (Korner and Angus, 1992). However, there should be no effect on the hypothalamic neural responsiveness. Hence, the remarkable long-term attenuation of the hypertension (figure 16.17) suggests that treatment may also have suppressed activity of neurons that release Ang II and project to the hypothalamic defense area (figure 12.11).

Future Challenges

In SHR, the defense pathway is sensitized in early postnatal life, while early remodeling of immature R_1 vessels proceeds independently. The DA neurons play a critical role in the sensitization process, and the resulting strengthening of synaptic transmission has been assumed to involve mechanisms resembling those in *Aplysia*. In SHR, environmental reinforcement is not required for the development of high BP. However, in BHR, which have only half the high-BP genes of SHR, exposure to an adverse environment (e.g., chronic stress, high salt) is required for the animals to become hypertensive. In turn, the WKY strain does not develop sustained high BP at all, even in an adverse environment (figure 3.14).

A useful starting point for developing ideas about hypothalamic hyperresponsiveness in EH is to examine some of the factors responsible for the differences in stress threshold of the defense pathways in SHR, BHR, and WKY. These could depend on (1) differences in the number of their DA neurons projecting to the hypothalamus; (2) mutations or conformational changes in DA receptors on hypothalamic neurons, whereby they become excited at minimal levels of agonist (Koch et al., 1996); (3) differences in regulatory proteins such as DARP-32 in the neurons of some of the strains (chapter 8); (4) varying disinhibition of forebrain inhibitory pathways to the hypothalamus; and (5) varying release of CRH. Nor do we know whether sensitization affects mainly synapses on the hypothalamic neurons such as PVN or DMHN, or whether synaptic transmission is also strengthened on some of the cortical sensory circuits (figure 11.13), memory circuits, and the amygdala. Other slow transmitter neurons project to the defense area (e.g., NA, 5-HT, Ang II, and ouabain neurons), some reinforcing the synaptic effects of DA, while others have a moderating effect on BP through baroreflexes.

SHR hypertension is a variant of normal development. This makes it likely that the initial organization of an important pathway such as that subserving the defense response will depend on signals from developmental genes, where one or more mutations could have substantial effects on its properties (Nüsslein-Volhard and Wieschaus, 1980; Gehring and Hiromi, 1986; Wolpert, 1998).

The other independent initiating factor of SHR hypertension is excess growth of immature vascular and cardiac myocytes and their greater susceptibility to mitogens. Here too, the determinants of the differences in myocyte properties between SHR,

BHR, and WKY and how they affect R_1 vessels are of interest. Possibly a battery of recombinant inbred strains may help sort this out (Pravenec et al., 1989; Kurtz et al., 1994).

Concluding Remarks

A considerable amount has been learned about the chief causes of SHR hypertension from a "low-resolution" analysis of the control system, as summarized in figure 16.21. This sets the scene for a new phase for extending our understanding of the cellular processes that determine sensitization and remodeling.

PART VIII

SYNTHESIS

17

Two Syndromes of Essential Hypertension

The key to better understanding of the pathogenesis of EH has been to take a less introspective position on how the ANS regulates the circulation, by reassessing how it responds to the world around us. Accordingly, the chapter begins with a brief review of the variants of the defense response and sensitization of the defense pathway that initiates EH.

EH includes at least two syndromes: (1) stress-and-salt-related EH (SSR-EH) in relatively lean persons, and (2) hypertensive obesity. The cardiovascular effects of OSA are best regarded as responses secondary to a respiratory disorder (chapter 14).

In both syndromes, the defense pathway becomes sensitized in persons of the appropriate genetic background through a number of lifestyle and environmental factors. In each syndrome, mild EH is due to stress-related elevation of sympathetic neural activity (SNA), with some additional increase in SNA due to salt or obesity. Later the two syndromes differ mainly in the nonneural factors that contribute to the elevation of BP. SSR-EH remains a constrictor hypertension throughout its course, while hypertensive obesity is a volume overload hypertension.

Some of the insights gained into the pathogenesis of EH have implications for prevention and treatment. The adoption of a healthier lifestyle at an early age specifically addresses the initiating causes and mechanisms of EH in each syndrome. This can be achieved through appropriate nonpharmacological interventions, which could prevent EH at least potentially. Current approach to treatment of established EH is based on lowering BP by means of antihypertensive drugs, which has greatly reduced mortality and morbidity. Nonpharmacological treatment has played a small and somewhat haphazard role in treatment. Therefore it would seem reasonable to examine whether more deliberate use of nonpharmacological measures in conjunction with drugs would provide additional benefit. It would make treatment more specific. It is most likely to benefit young and middle-aged persons with EH.

Central Autonomic Regulation and the Initiation of EH

The central neural apparatus regulating the circulation has many of the properties of man-made adaptive control systems. Alterations in the system's internal state are signaled through baroreceptors, respiratory receptors, tissue chemoreceptors, and others, each with a limited but highly specific information content. Our knowledge about the world around us comes largely through the thalamocortical system, which rapidly recognizes and categorizes persons, objects, and scenes. The thalamocortical system has a major role in the perception of mental stress through a network that involves neuron groups in different parts of the brain (figures 11.1, 11.10). Stress elicits a variant of the autonomic defense response, together with emotional and somatic motor responses.

In the ANS, the repertoire of effector patterns is small. During disturbances, a particular afferent input profile alters the activity of premotor neurons (e.g., in RVLM and hypothalamus), which mostly influence motoneuron activity through the release of fast transmitters. In turn, the responsiveness of the premotor or motoneurons is influenced by modulatory neurons that release slow transmitters (chapter 8). In the ANS, the slow transmitter neurons carry afferent information from various brain regions to particular autonomic target neurons. The evoked ANS responses are mostly short-lasting reflex changes, but they also include long-lasting tonic effects such as occur in EH.

One example of tonic modulation is the vagal heart rate deficit, which is a baroreflex response to chronic elevation of cardiopulmonary load. It contributes to the high resting heart rate and, more important, prevents excessive slowing of heart rate during rises in BP. It is the result of signals from the arterial, cardiac, and pulmonary baroreceptors, which increase 5-HT neuron activity and inhibit some of the vagal motoneurons (figure 9.12). Synapses along this pathway do not become sensitized, and a lowering of cardiopulmonary load rapidly restores vagal function.

Circulatory disturbances also affect the properties of constrictor baroreflexes. On assuming the upright posture or in nonhypotensive hemorrhage, there is concordant unloading of low-threshold arterial and atrial receptors, which greatly increases the gain and range of sympathetic baroreflexes. If postural hypotension develops or in more severe hemorrhage, cardiac filling becomes inadequate and signals from the left ventricle (LV) increase the activity of modulatory opiate neurons, thereby inhibiting SNA and causing a large sudden fall in BP (figures 9.18, 9.21). This represents a major change in the state of the control system: Circulatory control through the ANS is suspended and taken over by pressor hormones and regional myogenic and metabolic regulators until cardiac filling is again adequate.

The variants of the defense response are all generated through hypothalamic neuron groups that help the organism to cope with a range of challenges. They are highly effective acute responses. In EH they become chronic responses, when much of the advantage is quickly lost.

Variants of the Acute Defense Response

The three variants of the hypothalamic defense response are (1) the "ready-for-action" responses, (2) the O_2 conservation responses, and (3) responses evoked by marked local ischemia.

The Ready-for-Action Variants

Ready-for-action variants include the autonomic responses to exercise and mental stress.

In heavy exercise, there is widespread sympathetic vasoconstriction, cardiac stimulation, and abolition of vagal tone. The pattern is initiated by cortical command neurons, with the cerebellum adjusting the latter's motor program in the light of feedback from muscle chemoreceptors. Baroreflex properties are also affected (figure 10.17). Exercise training produces long-term falls in BP between bouts (figure 10.13). If the sedentary lifestyle is resumed, BP gradually increases again (figure 10.15).

The response to mental stress consists of elevation in BP due to rises of SNA in the cardiac, renal, gastrointestinal, muscle, and skin outflows and an increase in plasma adrenaline. This causes cardiac stimulation and vasoconstriction in renal, gastrointestinal, and skin beds. However, there is vasodilation in the muscle bed, in which adrenaline-mediated vasodilation masks the neural vasoconstriction. Cardiac and constrictor sympathetic baroreflexes are enhanced, as in exercise.

The O_2 Conservation Variants

O_2 conservation occurs in diving mammals and birds: Stimulation of trigeminal afferents triggers bradycardia and marked vasoconstriction in all beds except those supplying the brain, myocardium, and active skeletal muscle. A similar pattern is evoked in burrowing animals in response to nasopharyngeal stimulation by noxious vapors.

Under appropriate conditions, strong stimulation of arterial chemoreceptors excites hypothalamic neurons: The result is bradycardia as in the diving response, and peripheral sympathoadrenal changes similar to those during mental stress (figures 14.1–14.16). The association of cardiac depression and peripheral vasoconstriction accounts for the smaller rise in BP compared to the ready-for-action variants.

In spontaneously breathing rabbits and rats, the above effects are manifest during arterial hypoxia severe enough to cause slight respiratory depression (figure 14.8). However, in primates the hypothalamic excitation evoked by the arterial chemoreceptors is suppressed completely by a neocortical inhibitory system geared to respiration (figure 14.17). They only become manifest when the arterial chemoreceptors are stimulated during apnea. The hyperventilation that follows the apnea elicits a large rise in BP and suppression of bradycardia and vasoconstriction (figure 14.18).

In severe OSA, each nocturnal cycle resembles the above response: The BP surge induced by hyperventilation follows the apnea (figure 14.2). Daytime elevation of BP is probably a conditional response to the repeated nocturnal arousals at the end of each cycle.

The Tissue Ischemia Variant

This variant arises through marked tissue ischemia in skeletal muscle (chapter 10), myocardium (James et al., 1975), and kidney (chapter 15). Each elicits rises in BP and in cardiac and constrictor SNA. The changes are maintained for the duration of the ischemia (Miyajima et al., 1991).

Sensitization of the Defense Pathway

Mental stress elicits the classic ready-for-action variant of the defense response through the DA neuron link between cortex and hypothalamus. The raised DA neuron activity increases BP by raising SNA in the sympathetic outflows to the heart and to the renal, gastrointestinal, skin, and muscle beds. Muscle vasoconstriction is present most of the time, but becomes masked periodically by adrenaline-mediated vasodilation (figure 5.4).

An acute stressor elicits this pattern in everyone, but in normotensives it subsides rapidly when the stress is over. During chronic stress the defense pattern may be maintained for weeks or months, often through conditional cues linked to the original stress (figure 11.11). But once the stress is over, the autonomic pattern subsides rapidly and does not outlast the stimulus.

However, in persons with EH the defense pathway has become sensitized, with substantial reduction in stress threshold (figure 11.9). Such synaptic strengthening is important in learning and its associated memory circuits (Edelman, 1989; Edelman and Tononi, 2000). In these neurons, synaptic sensitization is readily induced, which depends partly on genetic factors and partly on the frequency of usage of the pathway.

In normotensives, the DA synapses linking cortex to the hypothalamopituitary (HP) axis do not become sensitized, but they do in persons susceptible to EH. One hypothesis to explain this is that in those susceptible to EH, a mutant gene regulating DA neuron activity gives them the attributes of thalamocortical and memory synapses. This results in sensitization during reinforcement by the appropriate environmental factors. Once sensitization of the defense pathway has been established, the stimuli that evoke the defense response are generally too mild to affect normal subjects.

Support for this hypothesis comes from comparisons of the effects of stress on borderline hypertensive rats (BHR), which behave like persons susceptible to EH (figure 3.14). In BHR, the high BP outlasts the stressful stimulus (figure 11.19). In SHR, with twice the number of high-BP genes, sensitization develops without environmental reinforcement. Furthermore, destruction of DA neurons in young SHR attenuates or prevents development of hypertension (figure 8.21).

Timing of Sensitization and the BP Rise

The mutant defense pathway synapses are already present in the fetus. However, EH first develops in adults during exposure to increased stress and unfavorable lifestyle changes. This resembles the conditions under which BHR develop hypertension.

In EH, as in *Aplysia* and hippocampal neurons, the environmental input rapidly lowers the stress threshold (figures 8.7, 8.8). The early functional synaptic changes are later complemented by the growth of new synaptic contacts, which makes sensitization difficult to reverse. What is remarkable is that in both *Aplysia* and mammalian hippocampal neurons, sensitization develops after only a few stimuli (figures 2.10, 8.8). For the hippocampus, this is a characteristic trait for memory neurons linked to the thalamocortical system.

However, in BHR stress-related elevation in resting BP is a slow process (figure 11.19). A similar slow time course has been observed in normotensive rats in response to direct hypothalamic stimulation through implanted electrodes (figure 11.6). It suggests that the delay is due to moderating baroreflex and cortical influences. In BHR, the BP remains high after the stress is over, indicating that sensitization has taken place. In contrast, in the normotensive rats BP declines rapidly at the end of stimulation.

Similar inhibitory influences are probably responsible for the slow development of EH. In Timio et al.'s (1997) 30-year case control study, it took 5–10 years for the average BPs of the laywomen to rise above that of the nuns, marking the development of frank EH in a proportion of the laywomen (figure 4.8). With the range of genotypes probably similar in both groups, the difference in BP responses is due to the greater stresses experienced by the laywomen (chapter 4).

In Down syndrome, genetic factors appear to make the patients completely resistant to the development of EH (figure 4.10). Their synapses at the corticohypothalamic interface could be like normal ANS synapses, which do not become sensitized. Alternatively, their impaired cognitive functions may make it difficult for them to recognize whether a situation is stressful.

The Two Syndromes

The SSR-EH syndrome accounts for about 60% of EH and hypertensive obesity for about 40%. In mild SSR-EH and hypertensive obesity, the initial rise in BP is neurally mediated through the ready-for-action variant of the defense response. The DA synapses linking the cortex with the hypothalamic defense area have become sensitized (figure 17.1), so that the defense response is maintained by stimuli of trivial magnitude.

Stress-and-Salt-related EH

Mental stress initiates this constrictor type of hypertension, with MAP increasing by 10–15 mmHg in mild EH. Average resting SNA is raised but plasma adrenaline is mostly normal, except during phasic rise in the level of stress. The stress-induced constrictor hypertension increases BP responsiveness to salt (1) by reducing the size of the extracellular fluid space, which raises its Na^+ concentration; and (2) by raising blood-brain barrier permeability to the ion through reduced production of NO. The latter is partly due to greater cortisol secretion, an indicator that the hyperresponsiveness extends to other parts of the HP axis.

Once sodium concentration increases in the brain, the activity of endogenous ouabain (EO) neurons rises, stimulating the defense area (figures 12.11, 17.1). This increases MAP by a further 5 mmHg. The increase in permeability is small, so that it takes several days for SNA to rise (figure 12.17). In very severe stress, blood-brain

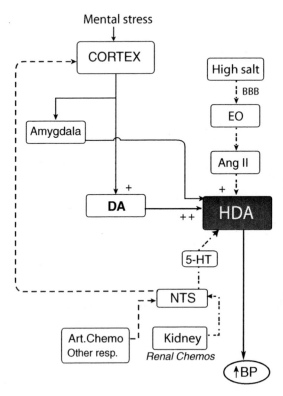

Figure 17.1. Diagram of pathways to hypothalamic defense area (HDA) including (1) from cortex via DA neurons, activated by mental stress, which is sensitized in EH; (2) from endogenous ouabain (EO) neurons, via neurons releasing angiotensin II (Ang II), after activation by high salt following entry of Na$^+$ into blood-brain barrier (BBB); (3) from arterial chemoreceptors (Art.Chemo) to nucleus tractus solitarius (NTS, dotted lines) via 5-HT neuron (dashed line) and via cortex; (4) from ischemic kidney (renal chemoreceptors) via NTS and 5-HT neuron. +, excitation.

barrier permeability may increase further (Uno et al., 1989; Hanin, 1996; Sapolsky, 1998).

Humans, like all mammals, have a hedonistic hunger for salt. Hence, it is fortunate that the sodium permeability of their blood-brain barrier is much smaller than in Dahl-S rats or SHR; otherwise, malignant hypertension would be common. However, even though the extra rise due to salt accounts for only a few millimeters of mercury, it has substantial effects on morbidity and mortality (figure 1.3).

The psychological profile of persons with EH is also established by the time mild EH has developed. It includes anxiety, depression, and repressed anger. These increase the subject's awareness of environmental challenges, accentuating the autonomic responses (figures 11.14, 11.24).

In moderate or more severe benign hypertension, SNA does not usually increase beyond the levels reached in mild EH (figure 5.14). However, MAP continues to increase by some further 20–40 mmHg, indicating that the additional rise is due to nonneural factors.

The factors raising R_1 vessel tone include raised SNA, lowered NO, and increased superoxide concentration. These narrow the vessels additively, with the net effect on TPR and BP further enhanced by the structural changes in R_1 vessel geometry, that is

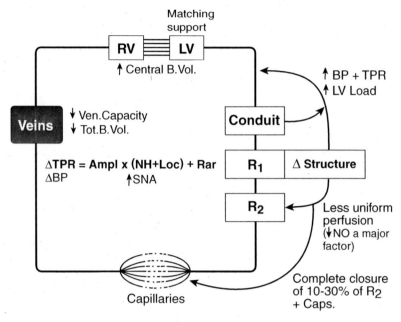

Figure 17.2. Diagram of peripheral effects of constrictor EH. Change in total peripheral resistance (ΔTPR) equals R_1 vessel structural amplification factor (Ampl) $\times$ sum of neurohumoral plus local constrictors (NH+Loc) plus rarefaction (Rar); not shown in diagram the decrease in conduit artery distensibility, which amplifies pulse pressure. Upstream of R_1 vessels there are rises in BP, TPR, and LV afterload and in central blood volume. Raised cardiac SNA and LVH support pumping by right and left ventricle (RV, LV). Downstream perfusion becomes less uniform, with more closed small R_2 arterioles and capillaries, a reduction in venous capacity and in total blood volume.

narrowing of the internal radius (r_i) and an increase in the ratio of wall thickness to r_i. The altered geometry provides each vessel with a mechanical advantage, whereby a given constrictor stimulus elicits greater rises in Vas R, TPR, and BP (figures 2.11, 6.16, 6.18, 17.2).

The above changes are accompanied by the development of concentric LVH, with myocyte enlargement and normal contractile activity (figure 7.9). The hypertrophy plus the high cardiac SNA allow the heart to match the increased vascular performance, allowing it to maintain CO against the raised BP better than the normal heart (figure 7.12).

As EH becomes more severe, VSM hypertrophy also develops in the conduit arteries together with reduction in arterial wall distensibility. The latter is responsible for the greater rise in pulse pressure and elevation of systolic BP (figures 4.3, 5.6). It places a substantial additional load on the left ventricle, causing further LVH. The high systolic BP increases the risk of stroke and cardiac failure.

The increasing R_1 vessel vasoconstriction has adverse effects on the downstream vasculature (figure 17.2). In addition, the lower endothelial NO production accentuates the normal heterogeneity of microcirculatory perfusion, with closure of a greater proportion of smaller arterioles, capillaries, and veins (chapter 6). Venous capacity declines and is associated with a 20% decrease in total blood volume, although the central blood volume is raised (chapter 5). This is characteristic of constrictor hypertension, in the absence of excessive renal impairment.

One downstream consequence of the enhanced vasoconstriction is rarefaction, in which the capillary area available for blood tissue exchanges is reduced. Initially rarefaction is transient, but in time the vascular closures become permanent. This causes focal damage in most body organs, including the brain, heart, and kidney. In the brain, cortical rarefaction is common and may be asymptomatic (chapter 6). In the kidney, the process leads to a gradual decline in nephron number (figure 15.1).

Steal syndromes are another mechanism by which focal organ damage is produced through faulty metabolic regulation. For example, in LVH myocardial metabolism in exercise increases much more in the inner compared to the outer layers of the LV myocardium. At high rates of work, the inner layer's requirements for oxygen can only be met if, in addition to maximum arteriolar vasodilation, there is also dilation of larger vessels right up to the conduit arteries. The ascending vasodilation depends on increased flow-related production of NO, which is attenuated in EH and SHR hypertension (figures 6.12, 6.14). Under these conditions, the active tissue diverts (steals) blood from a less active region nearby, which then becomes ischemic (figure 6.11). In brain, myocardium, and kidney, these ischemic attacks are usually transient.

As cardiopulmonary load increases in severe EH, the baroreflexes not only cause the vagal deficit but also tonically inhibit SNA. This may explain the return of SNA to normal values in older persons with systolic hypertension.

When renal functional deterioration becomes pronounced, SNA and BP may increase through the renal chemoreflex (figure 15.7). This may end in malignant hypertension, owing to ever-increasing renal impairment (cf. figure 15.6).

Other Factors

In SSR-EH (and SHR), genetically determined abnormalities in renal tubular transport have been described that increase reabsorption of sodium and water (chapter 3). Their effect on BP is barely measurable when compared to primary aldosteronism, in which reabsorption of sodium and water causes volume overload (figure 15.3). In EH and SHR, other tubular mechanisms may compensate for the above abnormalities, or their action may be masked by the large neurally mediated vasoconstriction.

Genetically determined neural and steroid hypertension coexist in some genetic rat models. In Dahl-S rats, the mineralocorticoid 18-OH-DOC accounts for about 15% of the otherwise neurally mediated rise in BP (figure 3.8; chapters 3, 12). Similarly, in young SHR there is a well-documented, albeit transient, rise in 19-noraldosterone. It suggests that such mixed neuroendocrine syndromes also occur in persons deemed to have predominantly neural EH. The past controversies have been about whether EH is an endocrine disorder, rather than whether it is a neuroendocrine syndrome. Williams et al. (2006) have provided persuasive evidence of such coexistence. This is supported by much evidence of the beneficial effects of spironolactone in some difficult-to-treat patients with EH.

Hypertensive Obesity

Hypertensive obesity accounts for about 40% of persons with EH. It arises through the superposition of obesity on SSR-EH. It is a volume overload hypertension that partially masks the constrictor effects of SSR-EH. Epidemiological findings suggest that a predisposition to EH also increases the chances of becoming obese. This has obviously been held in check by those with with SSR-EH, who are either lean or only slightly overweight.

In these lean hypertensives, the control system regulating energy balance functions effectively. If fat accumulates, plasma leptin concentration increases, inhibiting activity of hypothalamic neurons that release NPY (figure 13.3). This curbs appetite and reduces food intake. Restoration of body weight is helped further if accompanied by recreational and other forms of physical activity (figure 13.1).

In persons developing hypertensive obesity, these regulatory signals are ignored or suppressed by forebrain mechanisms. Persons with SSR-EH are often anxious and depressed and internalize their anger, and the excess eating is a response that transiently alleviates the stress-related anxieties. This may be through an increase in activity of the DA neurons that link cortex with hypothalamus, raising defense pathway activity as well as stimulating appetite. Food intake rises until a new body weight equilibrium is reached. Those with hypertensive obesity tend to eat as much as those with normotensive obesity, but they enjoy it less and often find social eating rather stressful (figure 13.4). Indeed, eating may become an addiction, rather than a joyful social occasion.

As fat accumulates in the adipocytes, glucose transport into the tissues becomes impaired. The rise in plasma glucose after a meal is a measure of the degree of impairment of glucose transport. The latter is partly due to signals from adipocytes to insulin receptors and to the transporters that carry glucose across cell membranes (figure 13.12). The latter are impermeable to glucose but are readily permeable to circulating free fatty acids and glycerol. All cells, except those of the brain, are therefore obliged to use them as sources of energy. In turn, this raises the breakdown of neutral lipids and increases the plasma concentration of atherogenic particles.

Owing to the high plasma glucose levels, the pancreas increases the secretion of insulin to overcome the apparent tissue resistance to the hormone's action (figure 13.2). Eventually the pancreas becomes exhausted, resulting in noninsulin dependent diabetes mellitus (NIDDM).

As normotensive obesity develops, SNA is raised. However, when body weight and fat have become stable, average SNA (NA spillover) returns close to normal (figure 13.19). In contrast, in hypertensive obesity, average SNA remains high (figure 13.20). The associated increase in muscle SNA is also raised, reducing the capillary area available for glucose transport into muscle. This accentuates insulin resistance and hastens development of NIDDM.

In hypertensive obesity, CO and blood volume are greater and TPR is lower than in SSR-EH. However, MAP is only 6 mmHg greater than in SSR-EH, but is 20–30 mmHg greater than in lean normotensives (figure 13.6). In normotensive obesity, the elevation of MAP is similar, that is, 6 mmHg greater than in lean normotensives. It indicates that obesity alone causes only a small increase in BP.

The elevated plasma insulin is the main determinant of the low TPR and high CO and blood volume. It is a powerful vasodilator (figures 13.9, 13.10) and raises blood volume through its direct action on renal tubular reabsorption of sodium and water, which is reinforced by the SNA-mediated renal vasoconstriction.

Constrictor and cardiac SNA are increased due to the sensitization of the defense pathway and they moderate the insulin-mediated vasodilation. The raised SNA and high CO account for the hypertension.

In hypertensive obesity, SNA, though raised, is lower than in lean hypertensives (figure 13.20). This is due to baroreflex-mediated sympathetic inhibition in response to the higher cardiopulmonary load in hypertensive obesity.

In the latter condition, salt sensitivity is smaller than in SSR-EH (Tuck, 1994). This may be due to a less permeable blood-brain barrier. One reason could be the smaller rise in plasma cortisol (figure 5.18), which causes less impairment of endothelial NO production than in SSR-EH.

Neural and Nonneural Phases

It is envisaged that after sensitization of the defense pathway, development of SSR-EH is slightly ahead of that of obesity. Hence the rise in BP is at first SNA mediated as in lean SSR-EH (figure 17.1). When body weight has become stable, the underlying vasoconstriction is partially masked by the dilator action of insulin (figure 13.6). The SNA pattern is an attenuated form of that in SSR-EH (figure 13.20).[1]

As the BP increases further, there is little additional rise in constrictor and cardiac SNA, except if renal ischemia becomes pronounced. Structural R_1 vessel changes develop as in SSR-EH. However, their lumen is wider, so that constrictor stimuli elicit smaller rises in TPR and BP. This is offset by the greater renal deterioration, which becomes further enhanced by the increases in renal renin production.

Accordingly, in hypertensive obesity (1) eccentric LVH and cardiac failure develop early; (2) nephropathy is severe and may lead to renal failure; and (3) atherosclerotic complications are widespread, affecting coronary, cerebral, and limb conduit arteries. All these factors shorten the time to the development of serious complications.

Conclusions and Comment

Each syndrome of EH develops when the dopaminergic synaptic link between cortex and the defense pathway has become sensitized (figure 17.1).

In SSR-EH, the constrictor hypertension is established by mild stress mainly in sedentary individuals, with further constriction due to high salt intake added soon afterward (figures 12.16, 12.17). Later, secondary structural and functional changes enhance the neurally mediated vasoconstriction, raising BP to two to three times the values in mild EH. The associated rarefaction is responsible for the gradual deterioration of vital organs such as the kidney, brain, and heart.

In hypertensive obesity, the superposition of obesity on SSR-EH represents a behavioral response to alleviate stress-related anxiety. The high BP is due to the effect of SNA-mediated vasoconstriction plus that of the insulin-dependent elevation of CO. The volume overload leads to early eccentric LVH, renal and atherosclerotic complications, and more rapid development of NIDDM.

The ready-for-action mental stress variant of the defense response allows normotensive individuals to respond to challenges as they arise. The ANS responses are related to the intensity of the stress (figure 11.14). This relationship is compromised in EH, where substantial responses are evoked by trivial stimuli. The hypertension-induced secondary structural and functional vascular changes have disastrous long-term effects on health.

The genetic determinants of EH remain unknown. In both syndromes, the sensitizable DA synapse may be due to genetic differences between hypertensives and normotensives. Probably some of the factors affecting blood-brain barrier permeability to Na^+ are genetically determined. For hypertensive obesity, the link between susceptibility to SSR-EH and obesity may also have a genetic basis. In both syndromes, there is much variation in the magnitude of the nonneural effects on BP and the development of complications (Perera, 1955; Pickering, 1968). This could reflect polymorphism in the many genes regulating vascular growth and repair, which probably account for some of the BP-related QTLs that have been described to date (chapter 3).

Last, the question now arises, when does EH stop being "essential," that is, of unknown cause? This seems the time to refer to each syndrome as a "lifestyle-related genetic hypertension."

Prevention and Treatment

Regular exercise, dietary salt reduction, and weight reduction programs have long been recommended as nonpharmacological forms of treating EH. This section examines their role in the possible prevention of EH and the desirability of using them more frequently in conjunction with antihypertensive drugs in established EH.

The Potential for Prevention

Nonpharmacological interventions that have been recommended for the treatment of EH include regular submaximal exercise (figure 4.12), reduction in dietary salt intake (figures 4.15, 12.13), weight reduction when appropriate (figure 4.16), qualitative dietary changes as in the DASH diet (table 12.10), avoidance of excessive intake of alcohol and smoking (Beilin, 1994, 1995), and owning a pet (figure 11.23).

Enthusiasm for these measures has been relatively muted. This is probably due to the lack of appreciation of (1) the importance of lifestyle factors in the pathogenesis of EH, and (2) that some of the interventions specifically antagonize the factors that initially elevate BP.

We now know that the rise in BP during exercise is mediated through hypothalamic defense neurons that inlude some that are activated by mental stress. Submaximal exercise training lowers BP partly by reducing SNA (figures 10.14, 10.15). It may also attenuate the responsiveness to stress. Its effects on synaptic transmission are induced relatively quickly, but it is not known to what extent a prolonged period of exercise training desensitizes defense pathway synapses.

By lowering salt intake, cerebrospinal fluid sodium is reduced and the EO neurons are stimulated less strongly (figure 17.1). If combined with exercise training, reduction in SNA is greater and salt sensitivity may also be reduced.

Excess alcohol and smoking may become addictive. A by-product of this is that stress-induced sensitization of the defense pathway becomes accentuated.

A combined program of weight reduction and exercise training addresses the initiating causes of hypertensive obesity. However, the reasons for the health benefits of the other components of the DASH diet are not well understood (Sacks et al., 2001).

Last, pet ownership reduces susceptibility to stress (figure 11.23). It is said to simulate the effect of social support, which has a small BP-lowering action (Pickering, 1994). More important, social support affects mood and emotions in both recipient and donor.

Together, the various nonpharmacological interventions lower MAP by some 30 mmHg (table 17.1). Their effects on BP are largely independent. With a selection of exercise training, salt reduction, and one of the other three interventions, reducing MAP by 15–20 mmHg seems a realistic goal.

The aim of the program is to prevent the development of EH by maintaining a healthy lifestyle from late adolescence through much of adult life. This will prevent the development of the high BP phenotype, as suggested in figure 3.14.

However, before making such recommendations, the feasibility and physiological and psychological effects of such a program need to be assessed. Current knowledge about long-term effects of the various interventions needs to be increased. This is probably best achieved through relatively small scale detailed investigations, of the type used in relation to exercise.

More Specific Treatment for Established EH?

The control of BP by antihypertensive drugs in EH has been one of the great achievements in medicine during the last century. It has improved the quality of life of the individual patient and reduced overall cardiovascular morbidity and mortality. Hence, it seems like gilding the lily to seek further improvements, particularly as many hypertensives who should be treated with antihypertensive drugs are not at present receiving adequate treatment (Swales, 1994d, 1994e; Persson et al., 2000, 2002; Persson, 2003). Yet the success of current treatment is almost entirely due to the

Table 17.1. Effects of Various Nonpharmacological Interventions on Mean Arterial Pressure (MAP), Based on Data from Earlier Chapters

Intervention	ΔMAP (mmHg)
Exercise training	−8
Reduction in salt intake	−5
Body weight reduction	−7
Other dietary factors	−4
Social support, pets	−4

reduction of BP, which is achieved in different ways by the various classes of antihypertensive drugs. In other words, a very significant benefit is achieved through nonspecific reduction in BP. Hence it seems logical to add an element of specificity to treatment by systematically combining nonpharmacological interventions with antihypertensive drugs. This would seem most appropriate in young and middle-aged hypertensives.

Chapter 4 gave an example of the lack of effect of drug therapy with β-blockers and diuretics on the underlying causes of EH. After 1 year's good control of BP in patients with moderate EH, TPR was now in the normal range, including its nonautonomic component (figure 4.17, table 6.1). The reduction in MAP reduces the myogenic component of R_1 vessel tone, the reduction being greater in hypertensives than in normotensives because the structural vascular amplifier also enhances dilator stimuli (figures 6.9, 6.20). This is a therapeutically desirable outcome. Reducing resting R_1 vessel tone substantially diminishes functional rarefaction and the likelihood of organ damage. Yet in these well-treated patients, BP recovered very rapidly after the drugs were withdrawn, returning to pretreatment levels within weeks (figure 17.3). In 85% of a group of 49 patients treated with a greater variety of drugs, BP returned to pretreatment values in less than 20 weeks (Jennings, Korner et al., 1991; Korner et al., 1991). However, there were 7 patients (15%) in whom BP remained low for over 1 year.

The above data suggest that drug treatment had little effect on the underlying sensitization or the structural changes that maintain high BP.[2] They are in accord with the universally accepted view that drug treatment must be maintained indefinitely. The question now arises whether greater knowledge of role of the environmental causes and the initiating and secondary mechanisms that raise BP in EH would make it possible to raise the proportion of patients whose BP remains normal and who remain in good health after a better targeted course of treatment.

Treatment should positively influence (1) the environmental causes of EH; (2) the mechanisms that raise SNA and negatively affect mood and emotions; (3) secondary mechanisms, including functional changes that increase constrictor tone in R_1 vessels and structural changes that amplify overall constrictor drive and decrease conduit artery distensibility; and (4) additional secondary factors mainly relevant to hypertensive obesity, that is, development of cardiac, renal, atherosclerotic, and diabetic complications.

Data obtained in the genetic rat models support the importance of reducing SNA, increasing availability of NO, and causing regression of structural changes. Some of these when applied to very young animals prevent the development of hypertension. Had they been applied to slightly older animals, a "cure" might still have been obtained. However, in much older animals, as in humans, treatment lowers BP without greatly affecting the underlying pathology (Weiss, 1974).

Support of Concept Studies

In young SHR, inactivation of the sympathoadrenal system prevents development of both hypertension and the associated structural changes (figures 16.15, 16.16). In view of the hyperresponsiveness of immature VSM cells and cardiac myocytes, the findings suggest that even these hyperresponsive R_1 vessels never become structural

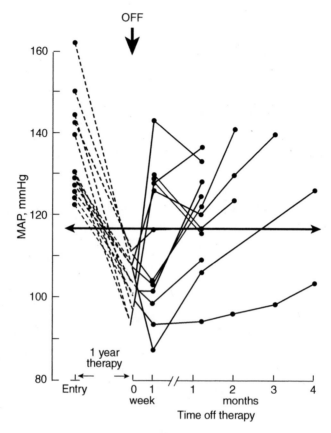

Figure 17.3. Data from 13 patients (1) before (black circles); (2) at the end of 1 year of excellent β-blocker + diuretic-induced control of BP (diuretic stopped 4 weeks and β-blocker 1 week before BP measurement at end of dashed line); and (3) changes after drug withdrawal. From Korner (1982), with permission of *Clinical Science*.

amplifiers in the absence of elevation of BP. The early vascular and cardiac responsiveness in SHR probably has no counterpart in EH, except possibly for septal hypertrophy that has been observed in young normotensives with a family history of EH (Radice et al., 1986; Safar, 1989).

A corollary of the results of sympathectomy in SHR is that hypertension would be prevented if one could reverse the synaptic fault that results in sensitization of the defense pathway. This is in accord with the attenuation of hypertension following destruction of DA neurons in young SHR (figure 8.21).

The lower production of endothelial NO is greatly exacerbated in Dahl-S rats on a high salt intake, particularly in the kidney. It contributes to the elevation of BP, and the hypertension is reduced by the provision of extra L-arginine (chapters 12, 15). This and scavengers of superoxide are potential therapeutic measures for reducing renal functional deterioration (figure 12.2).

As regards vascular development, which resembles later formation of structural changes, the administration of ACE inhibitors or AT_1 antagonists to young SHR greatly attenuates hypertension (figures 16.18, 16.19). The drugs cause spectacular long-term remodeling of R_1 and conduit vessels. Such long-term changes do not occur in WKY, pointing to a likely genetic difference. It underlines the importance of vascular widening in reducing the amount of rarefaction during chronic vasoconstriction.

Application to EH

Viewed against the earlier objectives of treatment, exercise training tends to reduce responsiveness to stress, as do social support activities. Reducing salt intake removes one environmental cause of SSR-EH. Exercise reliably lowers SNA, as does cessation of smoking. Body weight reduction decreases the hyperinsulinemia and its cardiovascular actions and if combined with regular exercise is often accompanied by "feel-good" emotions. From table 17.1, a BP reduction of about 20 mmHg should be a realistic target and tends to be accompanied by diminished perception of stress.

Of course, reduction in BP and SNA (or its effects) can be achieved with less effort on the part of the patient, through the administration of centrally and peripherally acting antiadrenergic drugs, including α-methyldopa (α-MD), clonidine, and prazosin. They generally do not give rise to the positive emotions associated with nonpharmacological interventions. In addition, their clinical usage has diminished because of side effects such as postural hypotension and somnolence. The centrally acting drugs, used in small doses, may accentuate the reduction in SNA, which may help desensitize the defense pathway.

Where antihypertensive drugs are of great potential importance is in causing regression of vascular and cardiac structural changes. Some of the large clinical trials have found little difference between the various classes of antihypertensive drugs, such as ALLHAT Collaborative Research Group (2002). However, others have found that ACE inhibitors and AT_1 antagonists provide more protection against stroke and produce more satisfactory reversal of LVH (Sheridan, 2000; PROGRESS Collaborative and Group, 2001; Dahlöf et al., 2002). All subjects in these studies were old hypertensives, to boost the number of "hard" end points.

Trying to reverse structural changes at this point is like closing the stable door after the horse has bolted. Treatments should be applied in young and middle-aged hypertensives with mild and moderate EH to prevent the development of structural changes or cause their early regression soon after VSM growth processes have begun. Such regression has been observed over a relatively short period of treatment (Schiffrin et al., 1994). This is in accord with findings in animals, in which the role of Ang II as an important growth promoter in VSM cells and cardiac myocytes is well established (e.g., figure 6.23). Once too much collagen has developed, reversing the structural changes becomes more difficult.

ACE inhibitors and AT_1 antagonists also moderate some of the intrarenal hemodynamic actions of Ang II, thereby reducing the rate of functional deterioration (chapter 15). This also occurs with other classes of drugs, including antiadrenergic drugs and nonpharmacological forms of treatment such as exercise, in which renal SNA is reduced.

In conclusion, it seems logical to apply some of the conclusions about causes and mechanisms of EH to the treatment of EH. Combining nonpharmacological treatments with drug therapy will, as stated earlier, require detailed clinical investigations. Not least among them is further work on how the various classes of drug lower BP. No reference has been made to antidiabetic drugs, which have a place in the management of diabetic obesity. One crucial question from the viewpoint of whether EH is curable is determining the extent to which reducing SNA by drugs or nonpharmacological measures desensitizes the defense pathway. Tests such as that illustrated in figure 11.9 seem ideal for assessing the effects of these maneuvers.

Concluding Remarks

EH begins as a variant autonomic response to mental stress in genetically susceptible individuals, particularly if they have a sedentary life style. It involves sensitization of synapses that link the thalamo-cortical system with the hypothalamus. As a result, and after repeated environmental reinforcement, the defense response is eventually elicited by levels of stress that are too low to affect normal individuals without the particular mutation. Once mild EH has become established, further elevation of BP results from a high salt intake, excessive consumption of calories, and several other factors. The sustained elevation of BP is a major contributor to "adaptive" vascular remodeling, which enhances the neural vasoconstriction and causes further elevation of BP. In addition, development of LV hypertrophy facilitates cardiac pump performance in hypertension. The vascular responses are further affected by changes in the profile of local autacoids such as NO, associated with the high BP.

Although the adverse life style changes initiate EH through predominantly neural autonomic mechanisms, after several years non-neural factors make an even greater contribution of the to the rise in BP. The overall consequence of the increasing vasoconstriction is gradual deterioration of vital organ structure and function, including the heart, brain and kidney. While the kidney does not initiate EH, it makes a major contribution to the elevation of BP throughout the natural history of the disorder.

The present account of EH suggests that the mammalian organism is not designed to withstand many years of chronic hypertension. By the same token, the encouraging therapeutic message is that simple lowering of BP with antihypertensive drugs greatly improves the prognosis. Furthermore, from what we now know about the pathogenesis of "lifestyle-related genetic hypertension" the adoption of a healthy lifestyle from an early age adds an element of specificity to treatment and offers hope that EH may be prevented.

The present work has provided an account of the macro-operation of the circulatory control system in hypertension. To paraphrase Winston Churchill, this type of analysis represents an end of the beginning of our understanding of EH.[3] I hope it has highlighted targets for detailed study by geneticists and cell biologists, which will illuminate the operation of critical components of the control system at the molecular level and lead to new specific therapeutic measures.

Notes

Chapter 1

1. The enzyme renin had been discovered some 30 years earlier by Tigerstedt and Bergman (1898), but the discovery was virtually ignored until the above work on renal hypertension.

Chapter 2

1. Rosen illustrates this by a physical example, where a harmonic oscillator of mass m oscillates in a viscous fluid, with displacement distance x from an equilibrium point. The viscous fluid offers a viscous resistance of magnitude β dx/dt and the restoring force acts toward the equilibrium point and is of magnitude kx, that is, is proportional to the displacement x. This is an open-loop system, and the differential equation of motion is the linear equation for simple harmonic motion: m $d^2x + \beta$. $dx/dt + kx$ where m, β, and k are constants. Now imagine an oscillator, where the resistance factor β is no longer constant, but increases as a monotonic function that is related to the displacement x. The greater the value of x, the more frictional resistance that will be encountered, owing to the rise in β. Intuitively, it is apparent that the resistance acts as a brake on the oscillations and that by suitable choice of the function of $\beta(x)$, the amplitude can be made to fall below any preassigned value in as short a time as is desired, regardless of the size of the initial displacement. What has been done is to introduce negative feedback into the operation of the system by making the degree of damping a function of the displacement. By doing this, the simple open-loop system has been converted into a closed-loop system, greatly increasing its effectiveness as a regulator. At the same time, the linear equation of motion has become nonlinear, because one of its parameters has been adjusted to a new value.

2. Long before biologists had thought about problems of regulation, they had speculated about the nature of living organisms. The physicalists thought animals and plants resembled machines. These views were opposed by the vitalists and teleologists, who postulated that special vital forces distinguished living beings from inanimate objects (Singer, 1928; Mayr, 1997).

3. The switch is prevented by prior intravenous or intracisternal administration of the opioid antagonist naloxone.

4. BHR are the F_1 hybrids of the mating between inbred SHR and normotensive WKY, and thus have half the complement of high BP genes of SHR (see chapter 3).

5. The following are additional references that give arguments for and against long-term autoregulation: Borst and Borst-de Geus (1963); Ledingham and Cohen (1964); Granger and Guyton (1969); Fletcher et al. (1976); Korner et al. (1980b); Hinojosa-Laborde et al. (1989); Cowley (1992).

Chapter 3

1. The hypertensive strain was originally bred by selecting rats with the highest BPs from an outbred founder stock and mating brothers with sisters (Okamoto and Aoki, 1963; Okamoto, 1969; Phelan, 1970; Ganten and De Jong, 1994; Yamori, 1994). Sometimes additional selection criteria were used, such as BP responsiveness to salt (Rapp, 1982). Low-BP strains have also been bred (Schlager, 1972).

2. These arise from inherited variation in the recognition sequences of restriction enzymes along DNA, which produce different sizes of genomic fragments on Southern blotting due to phenotypic differences at the molecular level. If a population has two or more phenotypes attributable to the alleles of one gene, this is called a polymorphism, and the term RFLP refers to two or more restriction fragment patterns, as revealed by hybridization to a particular probe. RFLPs provide landmarks along the chromosomal DNA to which other markers can be linked, including a disease locus (Griffiths et al., 1993; Roberts and Towbin, 1993).

3. Guanabenz is a centrally acting α_2-AR agonist, with actions similar to those of clonidine (Korner and Angus, 1981).

4. These are mostly small highly repetitive DNA sequences that occur throughout the genome and are known as satellite or microsatellite markers. Their exact localization is accomplished by using specific DNA sequences on each side of the marker locus, which are amplified by the polymerase chain reaction (PCR). For technical requirements for constructing linkage maps, see Vogel and Motulsky (1997); Rapp (2000).

Chapter 4

1. In each population, linear regression equations between BP and age were calculated between the ages of 20 and 60 years, and characterized by a slope and intercept. Many differentiate populations mainly on the basis of slope.

2. The patients are often elderly. The neuropathy has several causes and is common in severe diabetes. The postural hypotension may reduce patients to life "on all fours." Treatment aims to maintain cardiac filling pressures by reducing pooling of blood by wearing elastic stockings, constricting veins with dihydroergotamine, and giving steroids to cause fluid retention.

3. The difference was not due to different degrees of obesity.

4. The reduction in resting BP affects resting supine and upright SBP and DBP, and the BP reached during exercise (Jennings, Nelson et al., 1986; Georgiades et al., 2000).

5. That over 10% of subjects remained normotensive is interesting, but that EH redeveloped in 90% indicates that stopping treatment is unacceptably risky.

6. The slope of the age-BP relationship in the laywomen was the same as the average for Italian women, so that the proportion of those developing EH is also likely to be the same.

Chapter 5

1. Some early studies and reviews include Werkö and Lagerlöf (1949); Widimský et al. (1957); Rowe et al. (1961); Bello et al. (1965, 1967); Finkielman et al. (1965); Eich et al. (1966);

Sannerstedt (1966); Julius and Conway (1968); Kuramoto et al. (1968); Frohlich et al. (1969); Sannerstedt (1969); Molzahn et al. (1972); Safar et al. (1973, 1976); Julius et al. (1975, 1980); Sannerstedt and Sivertsson (1975); Korner and Fletcher (1977); Lund-Johansen (1980, 1995); Conway (1984).

2. It has been suggested that the rarefaction could have a congenital rather than a constrictor basis (Antonios et al., 1999a, 1999b).

3. Vasoconstriction is associated with a fall in conductance (C) and vasodilation with a rise in C in relation to control. From table 5.2, in mild EH renal C fell by 30% and gastrointestinal C by 16%, with the sum 46%, which is close to the rises in C of skeletal plus other beds of 44%.

4. The diastolic wave is an argument against a Windkessel function of the proximal aorta, which would result in an exponential decline in pressure (O'Rourke, 1982a, 1995).

5. The higher venous pressure is an indicator of an increase in central blood volume. In humans, Ulrych et al. (1971) observed a greater pressure rise during rapid IV infusions.

6. This agrees with estimates by the cardiac NA spillover method, as discussed later in this chapter. The advantage of the latter estimate is that they are obtained without altering BP, which avoids reflex heart rate changes.

7. Angiotensin III and angiotensin-(1–7) have distinctive cardiovascular actions. For example, the latter is a vasodilator and inhibitor of cell proliferation (Chappell et al., 2000).

8. An ecchymosis is a blotch in the skin due to extravasation of blood.

Chapter 6

1. Other NOS inhibitors include L-NMMA (N^G-monomethyl-L-arginine), L-NNA (N^w-nitro-L-arginine), and L-NAA (N^G-nitro-L-arginine).

2. The study was performed in Brattleboro rats, which lack AVP in their posterior pituitary and have diabetes insipidus and a high water intake. This makes it easy to give them drugs in desired quantities in their drinking water.

3. This included blocking the cardiac effectors with propranolol and atropine and the sympathoadrenal system with guanethidine and phentolamine. The regimen was used to avoid reflex changes in Vas R during administration of the vasoactive drugs (West et al., 1975).

4. Renal cellophane wrap hypertension is induced by wrapping both kidneys in cellophane, which results in renal capsular fibrosis, which compresses the renal parenchyma; MAP increases gradually by about 30–40 mmHg, which is associated with cardiovascular hypertrophy (for other types of renal hypertension, see chapter 15).

5. The drugs were given as brief infusions rather than boluses over several minutes, to allow steady-state concentrations to be reached and to allow the heart to adjust to the greater pressure load through the Frank-Starling mechanism.

6. The drugs used included the constrictor drugs NA and methoxamine Ang II and the dilator drugs ACh, adenosine, and serotonin (Wright et al., 1987).

7. Details of the blocking regimen are in chapter 9 in relation to the response to nonhypotensive hemorrhage (see Korner et al., 1990).

8. Myogenic tone has not been included because it is a consequence of BP rather than a cause of its increase. Some adjustment might be considered if there were significant differences in pulse pressure, as discussed in an earlier section.

9. When $E = 1.0$, distensibility is normal; at $E < 1.0$ distensibility, is reduced; at $E > 1.0$, distensibility is increased.

10. In the microcirculation, blood flow varies in different parts of a given bed. Borders and Granger (1986) estimated power dissipation (PoD, energy loss) in all parts of the microcirculatory network, from the formula PoD $= (P_1 - P_2) \times Q = 8 \times \pi \times v^2 \times \eta \times L$, where $(P_1 - P_2)$ is the pressure gradient; Q, blood flow; v, velocity; η, viscosity; L, vascular length. Power dissipation is a function of the product of (velocity)^2, viscosity, and vascular length.

From in vivo microscopy data, power dissipation is greatest in channels in which velocity is high, and these make the greatest contribution to a rise in Vas R.

11. In neonatal SHR, the R_1 vessel VSM cells are very immature and remain in the synthetic phenotype for the first 4–6 weeks of life, when they are more susceptible to mitogens than the corresponding cells in WKY (see chapter 16).

12. At that age, the MAP in the stenotic limb of SHR was the same as in the intact limb of WKY and medial structures were virtually identical, as emphasized by Bund et al. (1991).

Chapter 7

1. Creatine phosphate (PCr) in the cytosol is another energy-rich phosphorylated compound that gives rise to ATP, but it is present in amounts too small to contribute sufficient energy.

2. LV mass is linearly related to body surface area (BSA) and is expressed as LV mass index (LVMI), that is, LV mass per m^2 BSA. LV mass per body height has also been used, but this relationship is nonlinear (Devereux et al., 1994).

3. With echocardiography, numerical integration using Simpson's rule can be performed in theory, but this requires multiple measurements in parallel axis planes, each in a well-defined location, which is impractical (Marshall et al., 1992).

4. In some subjects, one cannot obtain quantifiable echocardiographic images, for example, in obese persons, those with chronic lung disease (Levy et al., 1990; Devereux and Roman, 1995).

5. The coronary blood flow (Q) reserve is $Q_{max\,dil}/Q_{rest}$, with the vasodilation produced by vasodilator drugs (Vas R_{dil}).

6. Hypertrophy in RV pressure overload is also maximal in regions where wall stress is greatest (Smith and Bishop, 1985).

7. The capacity for proliferation appears to be abolished permanently, except after severe myocardial damage when some hyperplasia has been reported (Linzbach, 1960; Anversa et al., 1990; Bugaisky et al., 1992; Kozlovskis et al., 1996).

8. A phenotype in spontaneous mutations in mice is similar to that of transgenic mice with β_2-AR overexpression. This is caused by a point mutation within the third intracellular domain of receptor protein, which allows more receptors to exist in the R* conformation (Koch et al., 1996).

Chapter 8

1. Reviews and monographs providing more detailed information about the properties of the cardiovascular pathways of the CNS include Guyenet (1990); Loewy and Spyer (1990); Chalmers and Pilowsky (1991); Kunos and Ciriello (1991/2); Chalmers et al. (1994); Dampney (1994a); Guyenet and Koshiya (1995); Pilowsky and Goodchild (2002).

2. RVLM neurons have axon collaterals that project to centers in hindbrain, pons, midbrain, hypothalamus, and many forebrain regions, from all of which they receive reciprocal innervation.

3. It was called pseudoaffective behaviour by Sherrington (1906/1947).

4. In other hippocampal neurons (e.g., the CA3 group), LTPs are induced by an opiate mechanism rather than through the NMDA receptor.

5. 6-OHDA has a high affinity for the NA and DA reuptake pumps at the noradrenergic and dopaminergic terminals (Jonsson, 1980; Korner and Angus, 1981). In the terminal, the neurotoxin is oxidized to H_2O_2, superoxide radicals, and quinones, which cause release of DA and NA from their vesicles, after which the terminals gradually degenerate over hours to weeks. The range of local tissue concentration for selective destruction of terminals is relatively narrow. In the optimum range, most CA terminals of cardiovascular significance are destroyed. After systemic administration of 6-OHDA, similar transmitter release followed by degeneration occurs in peripheral sympathetic nerve terminals (Haeusler, 1971).

6. In an earlier acute study, Chalmers and Reid (1972) gave i.c.v. 6-OHDA to pentobarbitone anesthetized rabbits, in which a sustained fall in MAP of about 15 mmHg was observed for the duration of the anesthesia.

7. This is in accord with findings by Neil and Loewy (1982) and Stanek et al. (1984) that both dilator and constrictor responses can be evoked from A5 neurons. Elam et al. (1984) showed that A6 neurons respond to baroreceptor stimuli, and their responses are closely linked to evoked sympathetic SNA.

8. See chapter 9 for details of characterizing baroreflexes.

9. Unfortunately, the same type of analysis was not performed on midbrain DA neurons to provide an additional control.

Chapter 9

1. Giving vasoconstrictor or vasodilator drugs sequentially alters plasma renin and angotensin II concentrations, which affect peripheral vagal function, as discussed later in this chapter.

2. The alternative explanation is that cardiopulmonary baroreceptors play a negligible role, which is known to be incorrect (Linden, 1973; Paintal, 1971, 1973; Thorén et al., 1979).

3. From the changes in G_{av}, it may be that in Group I rabbits the NA neuron also sends a collateral to CVLM and RVLM destined to the cardiac sympathetic motoneurons.

4. The shift in BP_{50} is largely due to rapid resetting of arterial baroreceptor P_{th}; changes in other reflex parameters are due to afferent interactions within the CNS or to the actions of Ang II.

5. The administration of a β-blocker tends to minimize elevation in PRA or PRC induced by diuretic therapy (Chalmers, Horvath et al., 1976).

6. Plasma Ang II is approximately $6.8 \times PRC$ (Korner, Oliver, and Casley, 1981 unpublished data).

7. The diets were administered according to a Latin square experimental design to eliminate bias (Korner, Oliver, and Casley, 1980).

8. Saralasin has partial agonist properties, but within-animal comparisons suggest that its effects on the reflex are closely similar to those of captopril.

9. On each day, the plateau of the reference calibration curves was set at 100 units (Dorward et al., 1985). This is unrelated to the true level of sympathetic activity in vivo. The effect of sinoaortic denervation on the latter has been controversial. In normal rabbits, SAD has little effect on cardiac NA turnover (Snell et al., 1986).

10. Neurohumoral blockade (NHB) antagonizes autonomic effector function. It involves infusing mecamylamine (ganglion blocker) and methscopolamine bromide (muscarinic antagonist). In addition, the systemic actions of Ang II and AVP are prevented by giving an ACE inhibitor and the vascular AVP antagonist penicillamine-o-methyl tyrosine (Korner et al., 1990). The marked hypotension due to mecamylamine is prevented by infusing NA at a constant rate to maintain prehemorrhage MAP at ± 10 mmHg of baseline and continuing at the same rate throughout the experiment. The response to bleeding is not affected; that is, the control system remains open-loop.

11. Similar changes in RSNA have been observed during this phase of hemorrhage in both dogs and rabbits (Morita and Vatner, 1985; Morita et al., 1988; Burke and Dorward, 1988).

12. The greater depression of the plateau during hemorrhage in the presence of procaine (figure 9.22, lower panel) emanates from pulmonary baroreceptors and high-threshold arterial baroreceptors (Coleridge and Coleridge, 1980; Kunze, 1986).

13. The rise in Ang II enhances the vagal deficit, providing a small amount of cardiac support; high plasma AVP levels tend to depress myocardial function, probably by affecting coronary blood flow (Pullan et al., 1980).

14. The relationships between EP and RAP (or VP) are the same whatever the effector status (figure 9.25), indicating that the rises in RAP (and VP) are mechanical consequences of ΔEP.

Chapter 10

1. This is a congenital condition in mice that resembles Duchenne muscular dystrophy.

2. My first research project was to reinvestigate Lewis's findings, using an antigravity suit that had been developed for the Allied air forces during World War II by my supervisor, Professor Frank Cotton of the University of Sydney. Occluding the limbs eliminated the BP trough, but to our surprise BP remained high during occlusion. We had rediscovered the muscle chemoreflex some 10 years after Alam and Smirk.

3. Typical rates of work are 1–2.5 W/kg body weight in various grades of bicycle exercise and 1.5–6.5 W/kg in mild to heavy 30-second sprint exercise. This contrasts with the work rates used by Alam and Smirk of about 0.2 W/kg.

4. The above explanation is not in accord with the results of Kozelka et al. (1987) (Rowell, 1993), who trained dogs to use only their hindlimbs during treadmill exercise at speeds increasing from 2 to 4 to 6 km/h. Only low rates of work were performed, raising MAP by less than 10 mmHg. This resulted in low levels of central command and elevation of muscle chemoreceptor activity only when exercise was performed in the presence of limb ischemia. The protocol has little relevance to the exercise performed by human subjects.

5. In normal rats and rabbits, the cardiac sympathetic component ranges from 30–40% of G_{av} when both effectors are intact (Head and McCarty, 1987; Weinstock et al., 1988).

6. The rabbits are habitual hoppers but were trained to exercise on a treadmill at 13 m/min for 60 seconds, which was an unusual and probably mildly stressful experience. This may be the reason for the increase in their plasma adrenaline during exercise, which does not occur in humans or dogs.

7. The data of Miki et al. (2003) were obtained under steady-state conditions, but central command is normally responsible for the large early changes. Hence the assumption that the initial reflex resetting is close to the steady-state changes, but that the early rise in resting RSNA is greater than under steady-state conditions. The decline would ensure depression of sympathetic baroreflexes already after the first bout of exercise by the effects on Purkinje neurons discussed later in this chapter.

8. These findings are similar to other studies at the Baker Institute and to those of Georgiades et al. (2000) in the United States. But one group of Japanese investigators found a fall in BP, associated with reduction in CI and blood volume and little change in TPRI (Urata et al., 1987; Arakawa, 1993), which differs from the findings described here. The reasons for this have not been determined.

9. Total and renal SNA were determined by the NA spillover, while muscle SNA was estimated by microneurography. The percentage changes refer to the corresponding sedentary controls.

10. The work was performed by Dr. Gillian Deakin, who was physician to the expedition. She had prepared herself for the project by spending 1 year at the Baker Institute in Dr. Garry Jenning's laboratory in Melbourne.

11. The effect on ΔMAP of the fall in TPR was offset by elevation in CO in all the tests.

12. Abolition of vagal tone probably involves interruption of the loop from barororeceptors → A1 and A2 NA neurons → hypothalamus → vagal medullary motoneurons (chapter 8).

13. Glutamate release from mossy and climbing fibers stimulates two glutamate receptors on Purkinje neurons—the AMPA and metabotropic receptors; the first is coupled to a gated ion channel. The second activates an enzymatic cascade characteristic of slow transmitter neurons, causing an increase in cytosolic Ca^{2+} and activation of phosphokinase C (PKC). PKC phosphorylates the AMPA receptor, which has become desensitized after binding to glutamate. NO diffuses into the Purkinje cell from an adjoining basket cell and inhibits the neuron's phosphatases; this

increases the duration of nonresponsiveness of the phosphorylated AMPA receptor. The role of the AMPA receptor in LTD differs from LTDs observed in *Aplysia* and mammalian hippocampal neurons that are mediated through the NMDA receptor, which is absent from Purkinje cells (Crepel and Audinate, 1991; Crepel et al., 1995).

Chapter 11

1. The sparse number of reactive sites with glutamate is in accord with the small number and discrete location of the cell bodies (Goodchild et al., 1982). Although glutamate may induce depolarization block of some neurons (Lipski et al., 1988), sufficient responsive neurons remained through which the defense response was evoked from the medial hypothalamus.

2. ΔMAP in the two groups may be similar because of offsetting by the modest increase in constrictor SNA by enhanced secretion of small amounts of adrenaline.

3. A similar cage had been used by Wexler and Greenberg (1978), who found that BPs were lower and cardiovascular pathology was less in male and female breeder rats when the animals were housed in small rather than large population cages.

4. This is in accord with findings in the South East Asian tree shrew, in which, during defense of the nest, the rises in sympathetic activity are greater in the losers than in the winners (Holst 1986, 1997).

5. When the animals were asleep, there were still significant differences between dominant and subordinate rats in SHR and SHR/y, but they were smaller than when the animals were active.

6. The firms were all in New York City and included a newspaper typography department, a federal health agency, a stock brokerage firm, a liquor marketer, a private hospital, a sanitation collection and repair facility, a department store warehouse, and the head office of an insurance company.

7. The subjects came from Birmingham, AL; Chicago, IL; Minneapolis, MN; and Oakland, CA.

8. The other variants are the autonomic responses to exercise, high salt intake, strong arterial chemoreceptor stimulation, obstructive sleep apnea, and the diving response.

9. At one time it was thought that baroreflexes were suppressed during the defense response (Hilton, 1963; Coote et al., 1979). This is not the case in EH (figure 9.19), in SHR hypertension, or during acute arterial hypoxic stress mediated through the defense area (Iriki et al., 1977a).

Chapter 12

1. Salt sensitivity and salt resistance in this chapter always refer to BP sensitivity to alterations in salt intake.

2. NO is normally the most important of the so-called antihypertensive factors produced by the kidney. Another mechanism is medullipin, described by Muirhead et al. (1991), the structure and function of which are still uncertain, as discussed briefly in chapter 15.

3. Secretion of aldosterone is greatly enhanced in primary aldosteronism, when sodium reabsorption is greatly increased as is blood volume and body sodium, causing pronounced hypertension (chapter 15).

4. At the time, we did not realize that the responses at these high ANP concentrations would be so different qualitatively.

5. During the body weight clamp, the dogs receive a constant amount of food each day by mouth and 1100 mL/day of water (IV). Weight was monitored by a special electronic balance. An increase in weight during salt loading + Ang II was prevented by reducing the dog's water intake (Cowley et al., 1984).

6. Reducing water intake in the clamped dogs in figure 12.8 was associated with a three- to fourfold increase in plasma AVP, thus increasing the constrictor factors compared to those in the uncontrolled animals (Krieger and Cowley, 1990). The reduction in blood volume will

thus accentuate the discrepancy between cardiac pump performance and peripheral vasoconstriction (chapter 7). Thus factors additional to blood volume are introduced by the maneuver.

7. NA neurons projecting to the hypothalamic defense area may also play a role in salt loading (Oparil et al., 1995; de Wardener, 2001).

8. In SHR, neonatal chemical sympathectomy plus inactivation of the effects of adrenal catecholamines completely prevents the hypertension, as discussed in chapter 16. The combination has not been tried in Dahl-S hypertension.

9. See chapter 15 for discussion of results of renal transplantation in Dahl rats.

10. Intrinsic impairment is the residual impairment remaining despite compensation through alternative transport mechanisms.

11. The order of diets varied in different animals according to a Latin square experimental design to eliminate bias.

12. The main interest in this section is to determine what distinguishes those who respond to salt loading with a pressure rise. Many of the present methods of defining salt sensitivity are not geared to answering this question; hence, the selection of the four groups seemed the best available compromise.

Chapter 13

1. In heavy drinkers, alcohol accounts for up to about 10% of energy consumption. At moderate ethanol intake the body can metabolize this through alcohol dehydrogenase, but at high intakes there is an increase in fat storage.

2. Body composition was measured with dual energy x-ray absorptiometry, and the various components of energy output were measured by indirect calorimetry using double-labeled water to measure daily CO_2 production.

3. The brain depends critically on glucose for its metabolism, but insulin does not regulate the transport of glucose from plasma to the neurons.

4. Lipoprotein lipase activity increases the greater the ratio of insulin to glucagon. As the triglycerides are progressively removed from chylomicrons, the latter become smaller and are termed chylomicron remnants. They contain cholesterol and $\sim 10\%$ of the original amount of triglyceride. They are finally taken up by the liver and degraded further.

5. The atherogenic particles involved in cholesterol transport are the very-low-, intermediate-, and low-density lipoproteins, which resemble the structure of chylomicrons. The high-density lipoprotein particle is probably antiatherogenic and helps move cholesterol out of tissues (Elliott and Elliott, 1997).

6. Sometimes the animals stop eating and drinking altogether after LHA lesions.

7. Disrupting the insulin receptor gene does not affect neuronal glucose uptake in the brain, which is independent of the action of insulin. In contrast, in peripheral tissues such as skeletal muscle, glucose uptake depends on insulin (Elliott and Elliott, 1997).

8. The effects on food and fluid intake were first examined on the day after administration of 6-OHDA or 5,6-DHT and have been assumed to be due to loss of function of CA or 5-HT neurons rather than acute transmitter release.

9. Glucose entry into the brain occurs independently of the action of insulin, but depends on an adequate plasma glucose concentration.

10. They consumed a high-energy liquid diet of about 3000 kCal, with a composition of 53% carbohydrate, 32% fat, and 15% protein.

11. The 6 subjects (5 M, 1 F) had an average BMI of 22.1 kg/m^2.

12. Grassi et al. (1995) observed a nearly 100% elevation in MSNA in grossly obese subjects, which is not in accord with the average NA spillover data in figure 13.19. The reason for the discrepancy is not known, but may have been due to the greater level of obesity in the Grassi study.

Chapter 14

1. Stimulation of the trigeminal nerve alone does not fully simulate the diving response or the smoke reflex, but elicits bradycardia and inhibits constrictor tone (Kumada et al., 1977).

2. For the apnea without smoke and smoke without apnea experiments, the rabbits were intubated under light anesthesia, and, after recovery from the anesthetic, were artificially ventilated after treatment with a muscle relaxant; they were subjected to 10–15 seconds apnea before ventilation was resumed (White et al., 1975).

3. Total autonomic blockade consisted of prior adrenalectomy performed 2 weeks before the study, followed by fixed steroid maintenance; guanethidine treatment started 4 days later (12.5 mg/kg/day IV), and the animals received atropine during the experiment (Korner and Uther, 1969).

4. In rabbits and rats, virtually all arterial chemoreceptor afferents are in the carotid sinus nerves, while 50% of arterial baroreceptor fibers are in the carotid sinus and 50% in the aortic nerves (Schmidt, 1932, 1968; Neil et al., 1949; D'Agostini, 1954; Douglas et al., 1956; Douglas and Schaumann, 1956; Chalmers et al., 1967b; Dawes, 1968). This makes it possible to assess the approximate role of the arterial chemoreceptors and baroreceptors by comparing the effects of graded hypoxia in intact animals, animals subjected to selective section of carotid sinus nerves or aortic nerves, and animals with combined sinoaortic denervation, as described by Korner and Uther (1970).

5. Each animal was exposed to only a single level of arterial hypoxia.

6. In TAB monkeys, respiration was less well maintained over the 20-minute period of arterial hypoxia (Brown, 1973; White, personal communication). It suggests that the sympathetic innervation of the carotid body may help to maintain receptor discharge as the receptors adapt (Neil and O'Regan, 1971a, 1971b; Carmody and Scott, 1974). In TAB rabbits, the respiratory response was largely the same as in intact rabbits (Korner and Uther, 1970).

7. Apnea was evoked by stimulation of either the superior laryngeal nerve or by perfusing the nasopharynx with a mixture of water and room air bubbles (Daly et al., 1978b).

Chapter 15

1. Recall from chapter 3 that BHR are the F_1 hybrids of SHR $\times$ WKY.

2. The very early postnatal structural changes in SHR are mostly unrelated to BP and are probably genetically determined, as discussed in chapter 16. However, from about 6–9 weeks of age onward the increase in structural remodeling is largely due to the rise in BP.

3. The donor kidney always replaces the native kidney of a uninephrectomized recipient.

4. Secondary hypertension was excluded, as were diabetes, alcoholism, and drug abuse. The subjects had no evidence of renal disease.

5. Renin secretion rate was calculated as RBF $\times$ arteriovenous renin difference.

6. To test whether stenosis resistance had declined because of cuff hysteresis, the artery was narrowed with a wire snare, but the results were the same as with the cuff (Anderson, Johnston, and Korner, 1979; Anderson, Korner, and Johnston, 1979).

7. The power dissipation formula $PoD = (P_1 - P_2) \times Q = 8 \times \pi \times v^2 \times \eta \times L$, where PoD is power dissipation; $P_1 - P_2$, lateral pressure gradient; v, blood flow velocity; η, viscosity; L, vascular length.

8. The reason for the large reduction in RBF was that Lupu et al. (1972) used surgical plication under anesthesia to narrow the artery; that is, the renal bed was constricted and the required reduction in RBF was greater than in conscious dogs.

9. There were 3–4 cuff adjustments over the first 90 minutes in awake dogs, in which RMAP$_{distal}$ was finally lowered to ~20 mmHg. Another adjustment was made on the following day, which resulted in stable mild hypertension for the 25 days of stenosis.

10. The individual kidney conductances were calculated from RBF/MAP, using the Doppler flowmeters on each renal artery.

11. This was done by continuous IV infusion of enalapril, using an implanted minipump.

12. Removal of the stenosis in animals (figures 15.12 and 15.16, left) leads to immediate falls in BP, as does surgical correction or angioplastic amelioration of clinical renal artery stenosis (Wilkinson, 1994; Pickering and Mann, 1995). In wrap hypertension, the technically demanding renal decompression by removal of the fibrous capsule was successfully performed 4 weeks after wrapping, resulting in normalization of BP (Fletcher, 1984).

13. The hypertension and the high resistance offered by the stenosis permit the maintenance of a reasonable level of RBF. Complete occlusion of the renal artery reduces RBF to zero, without raising MAP or TPR (Anderson and Korner, 1985).

14. Bex contained aspirin, phenacetin, and caffeine.

Chapter 16

1. There appears to be no increase in sympathetic innervation to the heart of SHR.

2. Earlier findings about POMC levels in the SHR pituitary have been conflicting (Haeusler et al., 1984; Gaida et al., 1985; Ardekani et al., 1989; Li et al., 1992). More recently, Braas and Hendley (1994) found that POMC levels and mRNA in the anterior pituitary of SHR were reduced to fewer POMC-producing cells, which may be the result of feedback from the high plasma corticosteroid levels.

3. Vincent et al. (1994) could not confirm Ely and Turner's original findings. Their SHR, which was another substrain of SHR in which there was no sexual BP dimorphism, came from a different commercial supplier (Turner and Ely, 1995).

4. A role for α_1-AR stimulation in myocardial and VSM hypertrophy agrees with in vitro studies (Simpson et al., 1982; Simpson, 1985; Bobik et al., 1990). However, in transgenic mice in which α_1-ARs are overexpressed in the heart, inotropic activity is enhanced without resulting in cardiac hypertrophy (Lin et al., 2001). The reason for the difference is unclear.

5. The results in SHR suggest that it might be worthwhile to perform more extensive sympathoadrenalectomies in the Dahl S, New Zealand GH, and Lyon hypertensive strains (Rapp, 1982; Simpson et al., 1994). In all of them, early administration of NGF antiserum produced attenuation of the hypertension (Clarke, 1971; Takeshita et al., 1979). In Dahl S rats, i.c.v. 6-OHDA also attenuated the hypertension (Haeusler et al., 1972; Haeusler, 1976).

6. Antisense RNA hybridises with the active mRNA in the cytoplasm, which prevents normal translation of mRNA to protein (Raizada et al., 2000).

7. Considering the number of publications on SHR hypertension, it is extraordinary how few observations there are on mortality data. These are largely due to the interest of the pharmaceutical industry.

Chapter 17

1. The elevation of BP is caused by factors resembling those operating during exercise: high CO (reflecting raised active muscle blood flow) plus neural vasoconstriction of the non-active beds.

2. Local endothelial NO production improves when BP is well controlled.

3. During World War II following the British victory in the Battle of Egypt in November 1942, Prime Minister Winston Churchill said in a speech at the Mansion House in London: "This is not the end. It is not even the beginning of the end. But it is, perhaps, the end of the beginning."

References

Aalkjaer, C., Eiskjaer, H., Mulvany, M. J., Jespersen, B., Kjaer, T., Sorensen, S. S., and Pedersen, E. B. (1989). Abnormal structure and function of isolated subcutaneous resistance vessels from essential hypertensive patients despite antihypertensive treatment. *J Hypertens* **7,** 305–310.

Aaronson, P. I., and Smirnov, S. V. (1996). Membrane ion channels in vascular smooth muscle excitation-contraction coupling. In *Pharmacology of Vascular Smooth Muscle*, Garland, C. J., and Angus, J. A., Eds., pp. 136–159. Oxford University Press, Oxford.

Abboud, F. M., and Thames, M. D. (1983). Interaction of cardiovascular reflexes in circulatory control. In *Handbook of Physiology: Section 2. The Cardiovascular System*, Abboud, F. M., and Shepherd, J. T., Eds., Vol. III, pp. 675–753. American Physiological Society, Washington, DC.

Abi-Samra, F., Fouad, F. M., and Tarazi, R. C. (1983). Determinants of left ventricular hypertrophy and function in hypertensive patients. *Am J Med* **75,** (supp 3A) 26–43.

Abrahams, V. C., Hilton, S. M., and Zbrožyna, A. (1960). Active muscle vasodilatation produced by stimulation of the brainstem: its significance in the defence reaction. *J Physiol (Lond)* **154,** 491–513.

Abrahams, V. C., Hilton, S. M., and Zbrožyna, A. W. (1964). The role of active muscle vasodilatation in the alerting stage of the defence reaction. *J Physiol (Lond)* **171,** 189–202.

Abramson, D. I., and Fierst, S. M. (1942). Resting blood flow and peripheral vascular response in hypertensive subjects. *Am Heart J* **23,** 84–98.

Adams, D. B., Baccelli, G., Mancia, G., and Zanchetti, A. (1968). Cardiovascular changes during preparation for fighting behavior in the cat. *Nature* **220,** 1239.

Adams, D., Bacelli, G., Mancia, G., and Zanchetti, A. (1969). Cardiovascular changes during naturally elicited fighting behavior in the cat. *Am J Physiol* **216,** 1226–1235.

Adams, N., and Blizard, D. A. (1987). Defeat and cardiovascular response. *Psychol Rec* **37,** 349–368.

Adams, M. A., Bobik, A., and Korner, P. I. (1989). Differential development of vascular and cardiac hypertrophy in genetic hypertension: relation to sympathetic function. *Hypertension* **14,** 191–202.

Adams, M. A., Bobik, A., and Korner, P. I. (1990). Enalapril can prevent vascular amplifier development in spontaneously hypertensive rat. *Hypertension* **16,** 252–260.

Agapitov, A. V., Correia, M. L. G., Sinkey, C. A., Dopp, J. M., and Haynes, W. G. (2002). Impaired skeletal muscle and skin microcirculatory function in human obesity. *J Hypertens* **20,** 1401–1405.

Aghajanian, G. K., and Vandermaelen, C. P. (1986). Specific systems of the reticular core: serotonin. In *Handbook of Physiology, Section 1: The Nervous System,* Bloom, F. E., Ed., Vol. IV, pp. 237–255. American Physiological Society, Bethesda, MD.

Akhter, S. A., Luttrell, L. M., Rockman, H. A., Iaccarino, G., Lefkowitz, R. J., and Koch, W. J. (1998). Targeting the receptor-Gq interface to inhibit in vivo pressure overload myocardial hypertrophy. *Science* **280,** 574–577.

Akinkugbe, O. O. (1985). World epidemiology of hypertension in blacks. In *Hypertension in Blacks: Epidemiology, Pathophysiology and Treatment,* Hall, W. D., Saunders, E., and Shulman, N. B., Eds., pp. 3–16. Year Book Medical Publishers, Chicago.

Alam, M., and Smirk, F. H. (1937a). Observations in man on a pulse accelerating reflex arising from the voluntary muscles of the leg. *J Physiol (Lond)* **92,** 167–177.

Alam, M., and Smirk, F. H. (1937b). Observations in man upon a blood pressure raising reflex arising from the voluntary muscles. *J Physiol (Lond)* **89,** 372–383.

Alam, M., and Smirk, F. H. (1938). Unilateral loss of a blood pressure raising, pulse accelerating reflex from voluntary muscle due to a lesion of the spinal cord. *Clin Sci* **3,** 247–252.

Albaladejo, P., Bouaziz, H., Duriez, M., Gohlke, P., Levy, B. I., Safar, M. E., and Benetos, A. (1994). Angiotensin converting enzyme inhibition prevents the increase in aortic collagen in rats. *Hypertension* **23,** 74–82.

Alberts, B., Bray, D., Lewis, J., Raff, M., Roberts, K., and Watson, J. D. (1989). *Molecular Biology of the Cell.* Garland Publishing, New York.

Albus, J. S. (1971). A theory of cerebellar function. *Math Biosci* **10,** 25–61.

Alexander, R. (1946). Tonic and reflex functions of medullary sympathetic cardiovascular centers. *J Neurophysiol* **9,** 205–217.

Allbutt, T. C. (1915). *Diseases of the Arteries Including Angina Pectoris.* Macmillan, London.

Allemann, Y., Hutter, D., Aeschbacher, B. C., Fuhrer, J., Delacretaz, E., and Weidmann, P. (2001). Increased central body fat deposition precedes a significant rise in resting blood pressure in male offspring of essential hypertensive parents: a 5 year follow-up study. *J Hypertens* **19,** 2143–2148.

Allen, F. M. (1925). *Treatment of Kidney Diseases and High Blood Pressure.* The Physiatric Institute, Morristown, NJ.

Allen, D. G., and Kentish, J. C. (1985). The cellular basis of the length-tension relation in cardiac muscle. *J Mol Cell Cardiol* **17,** 821–840.

Allen, A. M., Zhuo, J., Maric, C., Chai, S. Y., and Mendelsohn, F. A. O. (2000). Physiological insights derived from mapping the distributions of angiotensin receptors. In *Drugs, Enzymes and Receptors of the Renin-Angiotensin System: Celebrating a Century of Discovery,* Husain, A., and Graham, R., Eds., Vol. 1, pp. 93–108. Harwood, Amsterdam.

Allen, K., Shykoff, B., and Izzo, J. L., Jr. (2001). Pet ownership but not ACE inhibitor therapy blunts home blood pressure responses to mental stress. *Hypertension* **38,** 815–820.

Allen, A. M. (2002). Inhibition of the hypothalamic paraventricular nucleus in spontaneously hypertensive rats dramatically reduces sympathetic vasomotor tone. *Hypertension* **39**, 275–280.

ALLHAT Collaborative Research Group. (2002). Major outcomes in high-risk hypertensive patients randomized to angiotensin-converting enzyme inhibitor or calcium channel blocker versus diuretic: the antihypertensive and lipid lowering treatment to prevent heart attack. *JAMA* **288**, 2981–2997.

Allison, J., Sagawa, K., and Kumdada, M. (1969). An open-loop analysis of the aortic barostatic reflex. *Am J Physiol* **217**, 1576–1584.

Alpern, R. J., Emmett, M., and Seldin, D. W. (1992). Metabolic alkalosis. In *The Kidney: Physiology and Pathophysiology*, Seldin, D. W., and Giebisch, G., Eds., Vol. 2, pp. 2733–2836. Raven Press, New York.

Alvarez, W. C., and Stanley, L. L. (1930). Blood pressure in six thousand prisoners and four hundred guards. *Arch Int Med* **46**, 17–39.

Ambard, Z., and Beaujard, E. (1904). Causes de l'hypertension arterielle. *Arch Gen Med* **1**, 520–533.

Amery, A., Julius, S., Whitlock, L. S., and Conway, J. (1967). Influence of hypertension on the hemodynamic response to exercise. *Circulation* **36**, 231–237.

Amery, A., Bossaert, H., and Verstraete, M. (1969). Muscle blood flow in normal and hypertensive subjects. Influence of age, exercise and body position. *Am Heart J* **78**, 211–216.

Anand, B. K., and Brobeck, J. R. (1951). Localisation of a "feeding" centre in the hypothalamus of the rat. *Proc Soc Exp Biol Med* **77**, 323–324.

Andersen, P., and Henriksson, J. (1977). Capillary supply of the quadriceps femoris in man: adaptive response to exercise. *J Physiol (Lond)* **270**, 677–690.

Anderson, W. P., Johnston, C. I., and Korner, P. I. (1979). Acute renal haemodynamic and renin-angiotensin system responses to graded renal artery stenosis in the dog. *J Physiol (Lond)* **287**, 231–245.

Anderson, W. P., Korner, P. I., and Johnston, C. I. (1979). Acute angiotensin II-mediated restoration of distal renal artery pressure in renal artery stenosis and its relationship to the development of sustained one-kidney hypertension in conscious dogs. *Hypertension* **1**, 292–298.

Anderson, W., and Korner, P. (1980). The importance of renal vascular tone in determining the severity of renal artery stenosis in dogs. *J Physiol (Lond)* **303**, 31–41.

Anderson, W. P., Korner, P. I., Angus, J. A., and Johnston, C. I. (1981). Contribution of stenosis resistance to the rise in total peripheral resistance during experimental renal hypertension in conscious dogs. *Clin Sci* **61**, 663–670.

Anderson, W. P., Korner, P. I., and Selig, S. E. (1981). Mechanisms involved in the renal responses to intravenous and renal artery infusions of noradrenaline in conscious dogs. *J Physiol (Lond)* **321**, 21–30.

Anderson, D. E., Kearns, W. D., and Better, W. E. (1983). Progressive hypertension in dogs by avoidance conditioning and saline infusion. *Hypertension* **5**, 286–291.

Anderson, D. E. (1984). Interactions of stress, salt, and blood pressure. *Annu Rev Physiol* **46**, 143–153.

Anderson, W. P., Selig, S. E., and Korner, P. I. (1984). Role of angiotensin II in the hypertension induced by renal artery stenosis. *Clin Exper Hypertens (Part A)* **A6**, 299–314.

Anderson, B. D. O. (1985). Adaptive systems, lack of persistency of excitation and bursting phenomena. *Automatica* **21**, 247–258.

Anderson, W. P., and Korner, P. I. (1985). Haemodynamics of renal artery stenosis. Authors' reply. *Clin Sci* **68**, 480–482.

Anderson, W. P., and Woods, R. L. (1987). Intrarenal effects of angiotensin II in renal artery stenosis. *Kidney Internat* **31** (suppl 20), S157–S167.

Anderson, E. A., Sinkey, C. A., Lawton, W. J., and Mark, A. L. (1988). Elevated sympathetic activity in borderline hypertensive humans: evidence from direct intraneuronal recording. *Hypertension* **14**, 1277–1283.

Anderson, W. P., Denton, K. M., Woods, R. L., and Alcorn, D. (1990). Angiotensin II and the maintenance of GFR and renal blood flow during renal artery narrowing. *Kidney Internat* **30**, S109–S113.

Anderson, W. P., Ramsey, D. E., and Takata, M. (1990). Development of hypertension from unilateral renal artery stenosis in conscious dogs. *Hypertension* **16**, 441–451.

Anderson, E. A., Hoffman, R. P., Balon, T. W., Sinkey, C. A., and Mark, A. L. (1991). Hyperinsulinemia produces both sympathetic neural activation and vasodilatation in normal humans. *J Clin Invest* **87**, 2246–2252.

Anderson, B. D. O. (1992). Control engineering from the 17th to the 21st century (Flinders Lecture). In *Public Lectures 1991–2, Australian Academy of Science*. Australian Academy of Science, Canberra.

Anderson, E. A., and Mark, A. L. (1993). The vasodilator action of insulin: implications for the insulin hypothesis of hypertension. *Hypertension* **21**, 136–141.

Anderson, S., and Brenner, B. M. (1995). The role of nephron mass and of intraglomerular pressure in initiation and progression of experimental hypertensive-renal disorders. In *Hypertension: Pathophysiology, Diagnosis and Management*, Laragh, J. H., and Brenner, B. M., Eds., Vol. 1, pp. 1553–1568. Raven Press, New York.

Andrade, R., and Aghajanian, G. K. (1982). Single cell activity in the noradrenergic A5 region: responses to drugs and peripheral manipulations of blood pressure. *Brain Res* **242**, 125–135.

Andresen, M. C., and Yang, M. (1989). Arterial baroreceptor resetting: contributions of chronic and acute processes. *Clin Exp Pharmacol Physiol* (Suppl 15), 19–39.

Angell-James, J. E., and Daly, M. d. B. (1970). Comparison of the reflex vasomotor responses to separate and combined stimulation of the carotid sinus and aortic arch baroreceptors by pulsatile and non-pulsatile pressures in the dog. *J Physiol (Lond)* **209**, 257–293.

Angell-James, J. E. (1973). Characteristics of single aortic and right subclavian baroreceptor fiber actvity in rabbits with chronic renal hypertension. *Circ Res* **32**, 149–161.

Angell-James, J., and Lumley, J. (1974). The effects of carotid endarterectomy on the mechanical properties of the carotid sinus and carotid sinus nerve activity in atherosclerotic patients. *Br J Surg* **61**, 805–810.

Angus, J. A., West, M. J., and Korner, P. I. (1976). Assessment of autonomic and non-autonomic components of resting hindlimb vascular resistance and reactivity to pressor substances in renal hypertensive rabbits. *Clin Sci Mol Med* **51**, 57s–59s.

Angus, J. A., and Korner, P. I. (1980). Evidence against presynaptic alpha-adrenoceptor modulation of cardiac sympathetic transmission. *Nature* **286**, 288–291.

Angus, J. A., Bobik, A., Jackman, G. P., Kopin, I. J., and Korner, P. I. (1984). Role of auto-inhibitory feed-back in cardiac sympathetic transmission assessed by simultaneous measurements of changes in 3H-efflux and atrial rate in guinea-pig atrium. *Br J Pharmacol* **81**, 201–214.

Angus, J. A., and Cocks, T. M. (1987). The half-life of endothelium-derived relaxing factor released from bovine aortic endothelial cells in culture. *J Physiol (Lond)* **388**, 71–81.

Angus, J. A., Broughton, A., and Mulvany, M. J. (1988). Role of alpha-adrenoceptors in constrictor responses of rat, guinea-pig and rabbit small arteries to neural activation. *J Physiol (Lond)* **403**, 495–510.

Angus, J. A., and Cocks, T. M. (1989). Endothelium-derived relaxing factor. *Pharmacol Ther* **41**, 303–351.

Angus, J. A., Dyke, A. C., and Korner, P. I. (1990). Estimation of the role of presynaptic α_2- adrenoceptors in the circulation: influence of neuronal uptake. *Ann NY Acad Sci* **604**, 55–68.

Angus, J. A., Dyke, A. C., Jennings, G. L., Korner, P. I., Sudhir, K., Ward, J. E., and Wright, C. E. (1992). Release of endothelium-derived relaxing factor from resistance arteries in hypertension. *Kidney Internat* **41** (suppl 37), S73–S78.

Angus, J. A., and Lew, M. J. (1992). Interpretation of the acetylcholine test in hypertension. *J Hypertens* **10** (suppl 7), S179–S186.

Angus, J. A., Lew, M. J., Ward, J. E., and Murphy, R. (1995). Evidence for a functional role of neuropeptide Y in sympathetic vasoconstriction in rat small mesenteric arteries. *Clin Exp Pharmacol Physiol* **22**, 131.

Annest, J. L., Sing, C. F., Biron, P., and Mongeau, J. G. (1979a). Familial aggregation of blood pressure and weight in adoptive families. I. Comparisons of blood pressure and weight statistics among families with adopted, natural or both adopted and natural children. *Am J Epidemiol* **110**, 479–491.

Annest, J. L., Sing, C. F., Biron, P., and Mongeau, J. G. (1979b). Familial aggregation of blood pressure and weight in adoptive families. II. Estimation of the relative contributions of genetic and common environmental factors to blood pressure correlations between family members. *Am J Epidemiol* **110**, 492–503.

Anrep, G. (1912). On local vascular reactions and their interpretation. *J Physiol (Lond)* **45**, 318–327.

Antonaccio, M. J., and Kerwin, L. (1980). Evidence of prejunctional inhibition of norepinephrine release by captopril in spontaneously hypertensive rats. *Eur J Pharm* **68**, 209–212.

Antonaccio, M. J., and Kerwin, L. (1981). Pre- and postjunctional inhibition of vascular sympathetic function by captopril in SHR. Implication of vascular angiotensin II in hypertension and antihypertensive action of captopril. *Hypertension* **3** (suppl I), I-54–I-62.

Antonios, T. F. T., Singer, D. R. J., Markandu, N. D., Mortimer, P. S., and MacGregor, G. A. (1999a). Rarefaction of skin capillaries in borderline essential hypertension suggests an early structural abnormality. *Hypertension* **34**, 655–658.

Antonios, T. F. T., Singer, D. R. J., Markandu, N. D., Mortimer, P. S., and MacGregor, G. A. (1999b). Structural skin capillary rarefaction in essential hypertension. *Hypertension* **33**, 998–1001.

Anversa, P., Palckal, T., Sonnenblick, E. H., Olivetti, G., and Capasso, J. M. (1990). Hypertensive cardiomyopathy: myocyte nuclei hyperplasia in the mammalian rat heart. *J Clin Invest* **85**, 994–997.

Appel, L. J., Moore, T. J., Obarzanek, E. et al. (1997). A clinical trial of the effects of dietary patterns on blood pressure. *N Engl J Med* **336**, 1117–1124.

Arakawa, K. (1993). Antihypertensive mechanism of exercise. *J Hypertens* **11**, 223–231.

Arbib, M. A. (1995). Dynamics, self-organization and cooperativity: learning in artificial neural networks. In *The Handbook of Brain Theory and Neural Networks*, Arbib, M. A., Ed., pp. 34–41. MIT Press, Cambridge, MA.

Ardekani, A. M., Walker, S. J., Donohue, S. J., Stitzel, R. E., Connors, J. M., and Vrana, K. (1989). Adrenocorticotropin and corticosterone levels in pre-weanling spontaneously hypertensive rats. *Life Sci* **44**, 919–925.

Arendshorst, W., and Beierwaltes, W. (1979). Renal and nephron hemodynamics in spontaneously hypertensive rats. *Am J Physiol* **236**, F246–F251.

Arribas, S. M., Gonzalez, C., Graham, D., Dominiczak, A. F., and McGrath, J. C. (1997). Cellular changes induced by chronic nitric oxide inhibition in intact rat basilar arteries revealed by confocal microscopy. *J Hypertens* **15**, 1685–1693.

Aston-Jones, G., and Bloom, F. E. (1981). Norepinephrine-containing locus coeruleus neurons in behaving rats exhibit pronounced responses to non-noxious environmental stimuli. *J Neurosci* **1**, 887–900.

Astrand, P.-O., and Christensen, E. H. (1963). The hyperpnoea of exercise. In *The Regulation of Human Respiration*, Cunningham, D. J. C., and Lloyd, B. B., Eds., pp. 515–524. Blackwell, Oxford.

Astrand, P.-O., and Rodahl, K. (1986). *Textbook of Work Physiology: Physiological Bases of Exercise*. McGraw-Hill, New York.

Aström, A., and Crafoord, J. (1968). Afferent and efferent activity in the renal nerves of cats. *Acta Physiol Scand* **74**, 69–78.

Aström, K. J. (1995). Adaptive control systems: general methodology. In *The Handbook of Brain Theory and Neural Networks*, Arbib, M. A., Ed., pp. 66–69. MIT Press, Cambridge, MA.

Augustyniak, R. A., Tuncel, M., Zhang, W., Toto, R. D., and Victor, R. G. (2002). Sympathetic overactivity as a cause of hypertension in chronic renal failure. *J Hypertens* **20**, 3–9.

Aukland, K. (1989). Myogenic mechanisms in the kidney. *J Hypertens* **7** (suppl 4), S71–S78.

Australian National Health and Medical Research Council. (1989). Fall in blood pressure with modest reduction in dietary salt intake in mild hypertension. *Lancet* **i**, 399–402.

Aviv, A., Hollenberg, N. K., and Weder, A. (2004). Urinary potassium excretion and sodium sensitivity in blacks. *Hypertension* **43**, 707–713.

Avolio, A. (1995). Genetic and environmental factors in the function and structure of the arterial wall. *Hypertension* **26**, 34–37.

Ayers, C. R., Vaughan, E. D., Yancey, M. R., Bing, K. T., Johnson, C. C., and Morton, C. (1974). Effect of 1-sarcosine-8-alanine angiotensin II and converting enzyme inhibitor on renin release in dog acute renovascular hypertension. *Circ Res* **34 & 35** (suppl I), I-27–I-33.

Ayers, C. R., Katholi, R. E., Vaughan, E. D., Carey, R. M., Kimbrough, H. M., Yancey, M. R., and Morton, C. L. (1977). Intrarenal renin-angiotensin-sodium interdependent mechanism controlling postclamp renal artery pressure and renin release in the concious dog with chronic one-kidney Goldblatt hypertension. *Circ Res* **40**, 238–242.

Ayman, D., and Goldshine, A. D. (1940). Blood pressure determinations by patients with essential hypertension: the difference between clinic and home readings before treatment. *Am J Med Sci* **200**, 465–474.

Azar, S., Johnson, M. A., Hertel, B., and Tobian, L. (1977). Single-nephron pressures, flows and resistances in hypertensive kidneys with nephrosclerosis. *Kidney Internat* **12**, 28–40.

Azar, S., Johnson, M. A., Iwai, J., Bruno, L., and Tobian, L. (1978). Single-nephron dynamics in "post-salt" rats with chronic hypertension. *J Lab Clin Med* **91**, 156–166.

Azar, S., Ernsberger, P., Livingston, S., Azar, P., and Iwai, J. (1981). Paraventricular-suprachiasmatic lesions prevent salt-induced hypertension in Dahl rats. *Clin Sci* **61**, 49S.

Baba, S., Ozawa, H., Nakamoto, Y., Ueshima, H., and Omae, T. (1990). Enhanced blood pressure response to regular daily stress in urban hypertensive men. *J Hypertens* **8**, 647–655.

Bacakova, L., and Mares, V. (1995). Cell kinetics of aortic smooth muscle cells in long-term cultures prepared from rats raised under conventional and SPF conditions. *Physiol Res* **44**, 389–398.

Badoer, E., Head, G. A., and Korner, P. I. (1983). Effects of intracisternal and intravenous alpha-methyldopa and clonidine on haemodynamics and baroreceptor-heart rate reflex properties in conscious rabbits. *J Cardiovasc Pharmacol* **5**, 760–767.

Badoer, E., Head, G. A., Aberdeen, J. A., and Korner, P. I. (1987). Localization of the main noradrenergic neuron groups in the pons and medulla of the rabbit and the importance of cathodal lesions for prolonged survival. *J Neurosci Meth* **19**, 11–27.

Baker, K. M., Booz, G. W., and Dostal, D. E. (1992). Cardiac actions of angiotensin II: role of an intracardiac renin-angiotensin system. *Annu Rev Physiol* **54**, 227–241.

Ballermann, B. J., and Zeidel, M. L. (1992). Atrial natriuretic peptide. In *The Kidney: Physiology and Pathophysiology*, Seldin, D. W., and Giebisch, G., Eds., Vol. 2, pp. 1843–1884. Raven Press, New York.

Ballignand, J. L., Kelly, R. A., Marsden, P. A., Smith, T. W., and Michel, T. (1993). Control of cardiac muscle cell function by an endogenous nitric oxide signalling system. *Proc Natl Acad Sci, USA* **90**, 347–351.

Bandler, R., and Carrive, P. (1988). Integrated defence response elicited by excitatory amino acid microinjection in the midbrain periaqueductal gray region of the unrestrained cat. *Brain Res* **439**, 95–106.

Bannister, R., Sever, P., and Gross, M. (1977). Cardiovascular reflexes and biochemical responses in progressive autonomic failure. *Brain* **100**, 327–344.

Barcroft, H., and Samaan, A. (1935). Explanation of the increase in systemic flow caused by occluding the descending aorta. *J Physiol (Lond)* **85**, 47–61.

Bard, P. (1928). A diencephalic mechanism for the expression of rage with special reference to the sympathetic nervous system. *Am J Physiol* **84**, 490–515.

Bard, P., and Mountcastle, V. B. (1948). Some forebrain mechanisms involved in the expression of rage with special reference to suppression of angry behaviour. *Res Publ Assoc Res Nerv Ment Dis* **27**, 362–404.

Barenbrock, M., Spieker, C., Hoeks, A. P. G., Zidek, W., and Rahn, K.-H. (1994). Effect of lisinopril and metoprolol on arterial distensibility. *Hypertension* **23**, I-161–I-163.

Barger, A. C. (1979). Experimental renovascular hypertension (Goldblatt Lecture, Part I). *Hypertension* **1**, 447–455.

Barker, D. J. P., Bull, A. R., Osmond, C., and Simmonds, S. J. (1990). Fetal and placental size and risk of hypertension in adult life. *Br Med J* **301**, 259–262.

Barker, D. J. P., Godfrey, K. M., Osmond, C., and Bull, A. (1992). The relation of fetal length, ponderal index and head circumference to blood pressure and the risk of hypertension in adult life. *Paediatr Epidemiol* **6**, 35–44.

Barker, D. J. P. (1998). *Mothers and Babies and Health in Later Life*. Churchill Livingstone, London.

Baron, A. D., Brechtel-Hook, G., Johnson, A., and Hardin, D. (1993). Skeletal muscle blood flow: a possible link between insulin resistance and blood pressure. *Hypertension* **21**, 129–135.

Baron, A. D. (1996). The coupling of glucose metabolism and perfusion in human skeletal muscle. the potential role of endothelium-derived nitric oxide. *Diabetes* **45** (suppl 1), S105–S109.

Barraclough, M. A. (1966). Sodium and water depletion with acute malignant hypertension. *Am J Med* **40**, 265–272.

Bartha, G. T., and Thompson, R. F. (1995). Cerebellum and conditioning. In *The Handbook of Brain Theory and Neural Networks*, Arbib, M. A., Ed., pp. 169–172. MIT Press, Cambridge, MA.

Bar-Yam, Y. (1997). *Dynamics of Complex Systems*. Addison-Wesley, Reading, MA.

Baskin, D. G., Figlewicz, D. P., Woods, S. C., Porte, D., and Dorsa, D. M. (1987). Insulin in the brain. *Annu Rev Physiol* **39**, 335–347.

Batterham, R. L., Cowley, M. A., Small, C. J., Herzog, H., Cohen, M. A., Dakin, C. L., Wren, A. M., Brynes, A. E., Low, M. J., Ghatei, M. A., Cone, R. D., and Bloom, S. R. (2002). Gut hormone PYY$_{3-36}$ physiologically inhibits food intake. *Nature* **418**, 650–654.

Bauer, J. H., Brooks, C. S., and Burch, R. N. (1982). Renal function and haemodynamic studies in low- and normal-renin essential hypertension. *Arch Int Med* **142**, 1317–1323.

Baum, M. (1987). Insulin stimulates volume absorption in the rabbit proximal convoluted tubule. *J Clin Invest* **79**, 1104–1109.

Baumbach, G. L., and Heistad, D. D. (1988). Cerebral circulation in chronic arterial hypertension. *Hypertension* **12**, 89–95.

Baumbach, G. L., and Heistad, D. D. (1989). Remodeling of cerebral arterioles in chronic hypertension. *Hypertension* **13**, 968–972.

Baumbach, G. L., and Heistad, D. D. (1991). Adaptive changes in cerebral blood vessels during chronic hypertension [Editorial review]. *J Hypertens* **9**, 987–991.

Baumgarten, H. G., and Björklund, A. (1976). Neurotoxic indoleamines and monamine neurons. *Annu Rev Pharmacol Toxicol* **16**, 101–111.

Bayliss, W. M. (1902). On the local reactions of the arterial wall to changes in internal pressure. *J Physiol (Lond)* **28**, 230–241.

Beacham, W. S., and Kunze, D. L. (1969). Renal receptors evoking a spinal vasomotor reflex. *J Physiol (Lond)* **201**, 73–85.

Beaglehole, E. (1957). *Social Change in the South Pacific*. Allen and Unwin, London.

Beaglehole, R., Salmond, C. E., Hooper, A., Huntsman, J., Stanhope, J. M., Cassel, J. C., and Prior, I. A. M. (1977). Blood pressure and social interaction in Tokelau and migrants in New Zealand. *J Chronic Dis* **30**, 803–812.

Becker, H. F., Jerrentrup, A., Ploch, T., Grote, L., Penzel, T., Sullivan, C. E., and Peter, J. H. (2003). Effect of nasal continuous positive airway pressure treatment on blood pressure in patients with obstructive sleep apnea. *Circulation* **107**, 68–73.

Bedford, T. G., and Tipton, C. M. (1987). Exercise training and the arterial baroreflex. *J Appl Physiol* **63**, 1926–1932.

Beech, D. J. (2005). Emerging functions of 10 types of transient receptor potential (TRP) cationic channel in vascular smooth muscle. *Proc Aus Physiol Soc* **36**, 1–8.

Beilin, L. (1987). Diet and hypertension: critical concepts and controversies. State of the art lecture. *J Hypertens* **5**, S447–S457.

Beilin, L. J. (1994). Non-pharmacological management of hypertension: optimal strategies for reducing cardiovascular risk. *J Hypertens* **12** (suppl 10), S71–S81.

Beilin, L. J. (1995). Alcohol, hypertension and cardiovascular disease. *J Hypertens* **13**, 939–942.

Bell, E. T. (1950). *Renal Diseases*. Lea & Febiger, New York.

Bello, C. T., Sevy, R. W., and Harakal, C. (1965). Varying hemodynamic patterns in essential hypertension. *Am J Med Sci* **250**, 24–35.

Bello, C. T., Sevy, R. W., Harakal, C., and Hillyer, P. N. (1967). Relationship between clinical severity of disease and hemodynamic patterns in essential hypertension. *Am J Med Sci* **253**, 194–208.

Benetos, A., and Safar, M. E. (1993). Large arteries and sodium in hypertension. In *The Arterial System in Hypertension*, Safar, M. E., and O'Rourke, M. F., Eds., pp. 195–207. Kluwer Academic Publishers, Dordrecht.

Benetos, A., Topouchian, J., Ricard, S., Gautier, S., Bonnardeux, A., Asmar, A., Poirier, O., Soubrier, F., Safar, M., and Cambien, F. (1995). Influence of angiotensin II Type 1 receptor polymorphism on aortic stiffness in never-treated hypertensive patients. *Hypertension* **26**, 44–47.

Benison, S., Barger, A. C., and Wolfe, E. L. (1987). *Walter B. Cannon: The Life and Times of a Young Scientist*. Belknap Press, Cambridge, MA.

Bennett, T., Wilcox, R. G., and Macdonald, I. A. (1984). Post-exercise reduction of blood pressure in hypertensive men is not due to acute impairment of baroreflex function. *Clin Sci* **67**, 97–103.

Bennett, M. R. (2001). *History of the Synapse*. Harwood, Amsterdam.

Benzer, S. (1973). Genetic dissection of behavior. *Sci Am* **229**, 24–37.

Berecek, K. H. (1992). Role of vasopressin in central cardiovascular regulation. In *Central Neural Mechanisms in Cardiovascular Regulation*, Kunos, G., and Ciriello, J., Eds., Vol. 2, pp. 1–34. Birkhauser, Boston.

Beretta-Piccoli, C., Boddy, K., Brown, J. J., Davies, D. L., East, B. W., Lever, A. F., McAreavey, D., Robertson, I., Robertson, J. I. S., and Williams, E. D. (1983). Body sodium and potassium content in various hypertensive diseases. In *Clinical Aspects of Essential Hypertension*, Robertson, J. I. S., Ed., Vol. 1, pp. 267–277. Elsevier, Amsterdam.

Bergel, D. (1961a). The dynamic elastic properties of the arterial wall. *J Physiol (Lond)* **156**, 458–469.

Bergel, D. (1961b). The static elastic properties of the arterial wall. *J Physiol (Lond)* **156**, 445–457.

Berglund, A., Andersson, O., Berglund, G., and Fagerberg, B. (1989). Antihypertensive effect of diet compared with drug treatment in obese men with mild hypertension. *Brit Med J* **299**, 480–485.

Berguer, R., and Hwang, N. (1974). Critical arterial stenosis: a theoretical and experimental solution. *Ann Surg* **180**, 39–50.

Berk, B., and Alexander, R. (1989). Vasoactive effects of growth factors. *Biochem Pharmacol* **38**, 219–225.

Berk, B., Vallega, G., Muslin, A., Gordon, H., Canessa, M., and Alexander, R. W. (1989). Spontaneously hypertensive rat vascular smooth muscle in culture exhibit increased growth and Na+/H+ exchange. *J Clin Invest* **83**, 822–829.

Bernard, C. (1878). *Leçons sur les phenomenes de la vie, communs aux animaux et aux vegetaux.* Balliere, Paris.

Berne, R. (1964). Metabolic regulation of blood flow. *Circ Res* **14 & 15** (suppl I), I-261–I-268.

Berry, C. L., Sosa-Melgarejo, J. A., and Greenwald, S. E. (1993). The relationship between wall tension, lamellar thickness and intercellular junctions in the fetal and adult aorta: its relevance to the pathology of dissecting aneurysm. *J Pathol* **169**, 15–20.

Bevan, J. A., and Laher, I. (1991). Pressure and flow-dependent vascular tone. *FASEB J* **5**, 2267–2273.

Bianchi, G., Fox, U., Di Francesco, G., Giovanetti, A., and Pagetti, D. (1974). Blood pressure changes produced by kidney cross-transplantation between spontaneously hypertensive rats and normotensive rats. *Clin Sci Mol Med* **47**, 435–448.

Bickerton, R. K., and Buckley, J. P. (1961). Evidence for a central mechanism in angiotensin induced hypertension. *Proc Soc Exp Biol Med* **106**, 834–836.

Biglieri, E. G., Kater, C. E., and Mantero, F. (1995). Adrenocortical forms of hypertension. In *Hypertension: Pathophysiology, Diagnosis and Management, Second Edition*, Laragh, J. H., and Brenner, B. M., Eds., Vol. 2, pp. 2145–2162. Raven Press, New York.

Bill, A., and Linder, J. (1976). Sympathetic control of cerebral blood flow in acute arterial hypertension. *Acta Physiol Scand* **96**, 114–121.

Birkenhäger, W. H., and Schalekamp, M. A. D. H. (1976). *Control Mechanisms of Essential Hypertension*. Elsevier, Amsterdam.

Biron, P., Mongeau, J.-G., and Bertrand, D. (1976). Familial aggregation of blood pressure in 558 adopted children. *Can Med Assn J* **115**, 773–774.

Bishop, V. S., Hasser, E. M., and Nair, U. C. (1987). Baroreflex control of renal nerve activity in conscious animals. *Circ Res* **61**, I-76–I-81.

Bjoernberg, J., Graende, P., Maspers, M., and Mellander, S. (1988). Site of autoregulatory reactions in the vascular bed of cat skeletal muscle as determined with a new technique for segmental vascular resistance recordings. *Acta Physiol Scand* **133**, 199–210.

Björklund, A., and Lindvall, O. (1986). Catecholaminergic brain stem regulatory systems. In *Handbook of Physiology, Section 1: The Nervous System*, Bloom, F. E., Ed., Vol. IV, pp. 155–235. American Physiological Society, Bethesda, MD.

Björntorp, P. (1996). Behavior and metabolic diseases. *Int J Behav Med* **3**, 285–302.

Björntorp, P., Holm, G., Rosmond, R., and Folkow, B. (2000). Hypertension and the metabolic syndrome closely related central origin? *Blood Pressure* **9**, 71–82.

Black, M. J., Campbell, J. H., and Campbell, G. R. (1988). Does smooth muscle cell poly-ploidy occur in resistance vessels of spontaneously hypertensive rats? *Blood Vessels* **25**, 89–100.

Black, M., Adams, M., Bobik, A., Campbell, J., and Campbell, G. (1989). Effect of enalapril on aortic smooth muscle cell polyploidy in the spontaneously hypertensive rat. *J Hypertens* **7**, 997–1003.

Blair, D. A., Glover, W. E., and Roddie, I. C. (1961). Vasomotor responses in the human arm during led exercise. *Circ Res* **9**, 264–274.

Blake, D. W., and Korner, P. I. (1981). Role of baroreceptor reflexes in the hemodynamic and heart rate responses to Althesin, ketamine and thiopentone anesthesia. *J Auton Nerv Syst* **3**, 55–70.

Blake, D. W. (1983). Cardiovascular effects of intravenous anaesthesia. PhD thesis, Monash University (Baker Medical Research Institute), Melbourne.

Blaustein, M. P. (1977). Sodium ions, calcium ions, blood pressure regulation and hypertension: a reassessment and a hypothesis. *Am J Physiol* **232**, C165–C173.

Blaustein, M. P., and Lederer, W. J. (1999). Sodium/calcium exchange: its physiological implications. *Physiol Rev* **79**, 763–854.

Blessing, W. W., West, M. J., and Chalmers, J. (1981). Hypertension, bradycardia, and pul-monary edema in the conscious rabbit after brainstem lesions coinciding with the A1 group of catecholamine neurons. *Circ Res* **49**, 949–958.

Blessing, W. W. (1997). *The Lower Brainstem and Bodily Homeostasis*. Oxford University Press, New York.

Blix, A. S., Lundgren, O., and Folkow, B. (1975). The initial cardiovascular responses in the diving duck. *Acta Physiol Scand* **94**, 539–541.

Blombery, P. A. (1978). The circulatory response to a Valsalva-like manoeuvre: a method of assessing autonomic function in the unanaesthetized rabbit. PhD thesis, Monash University, Melbourne.

Blombery, P. A., and Korner, P. I. (1979). Relative contributions of aortic and carotid sinus baroreceptors to the baroreceptor-heart rate reflex of the conscious rabbit. *J Auton Nerv Syst* **1**, 161–171.

Blombery, P. A., and Korner, P. I. (1982). Role of aortic and carotid sinus baroreceptors on Valsalva-like vasoconstrictor and heart rate reflexes in the conscious rabbit. *J Auton Nerv Syst* **5**, 303–315.

Blombery, P. A., and Heinzow, B. G. J. (1983). Cardiac and pulmonary norepinephrine release and removal in the dog. *Circ Res* **53**, 688–694.

Bloom, F. E. (1996). Neurotransmission and the central nervous system. In *Goodman & Gilman's The Pharmacological Basis of Therapeutics, 9th ed.*, Hardman, J. G., Limbird, L. E., Molinoff, P. B., and Ruddon, R. W., Eds., pp. 267–293. Mc Graw-Hill, New York.

Blueher, M., Kahn, B. B., and Kahn, C. R. (2003). Extended longevity in mice lacking the insulin receptor in adipose tissue. *Science* **299**, 572–574.

Bobik, A., Oddie, C., Scott, P., Mill, G., and Korner, P. (1988). Relationship between the car-diovascular effects of L-methyldopa and its metabolism in pontomedullary adrenergic neurons of the rabbit. *J Cardiovasc Pharmacol* **11**, 529–537.

Bobik, A., Grinpukel, S., Little, P. J., Grooms, A., and Jackman, G. (1990). Angiotensin II and noradrenaline increase PDGF-BB stimulated DNA synthesis in vascular smooth muscle. *Biochem Biophys Res Com* **166**, 580–588.

Bobik, A., and Campbell, J. H. (1993). Vascular derived growth factors: cell biology, pathophysiology, and pharmacology. *Pharmacol Rev* **45**, 1–42.

Bobik, A., Neylon, C., and Little, P. (1994). Disturbances of vascular smooth muscle cation transport and the pathogenesis of hypertension. In *Textbook of Hypertension*, Swales, J., Ed., pp. 175–187. Blackwell, Oxford.

Bohlen, H. G. (1989). The microcirculation in hypertension. *J Hypertens* **7** (supp 4), S117–S124.

Bohlen, H. G., and Lash, J. M. (1994). Active and passive arteriolar regulation in spontaneously hypertensive rats. *Hypertension* **23**, 757–764.

Bolli, P., Amann, L., Hulthen, L., Kiowski, W., and Bühler, F. R. (1981). Elevated plasma adrenalin reflects sympathetic overactivity and enhanced alpha-mediated vasoconstriction in essential hypertension. *Clin Sci* **61**, 1615–1645.

Bolomey, A. A., Michie, A. J., Michie, C., Breed, E. S., Schreiner, G. E., and Lauson, H. D. (1949). Simultaneous measurement of effective renal blood flow and cardiac output in resting normal subjects and patients with essential hypertension. *J Clin Invest* **28**, 10–12.

Bonventre, J. V., and Leaf, A. (1982). Sodium homeostasis steady states without a set point. *Kidney Internat* **21**, 880–883.

Booz, G. W., and Baker, K. M. (1996). Role of type 1 and type 2 angiotensin receptors in angiotensin-induced cardiomyocyte hypertrophy. *Hypertension* **28**, 635–640.

Borders, J. L., and Granger, H. J. (1986). Power dissipation as a measure of peripheral resistance in vascular networks. *Hypertension* **8**, 184–191.

Borst, J. G. G., and Borst-de Geus, A. (1963). Hypertension explained by Starling's theory of circulatory homeostasis. *Lancet* **i**, 677–682.

Bouchard, C., and Perusse, L. (1988). Heredity and body fat. *Annu Rev Nutr* **8**, 259–277.

Bouchard, C. (1993). Genes and body fat. *Am J Hum Biol* **5**, 425–432.

Boulton, A. A., and Eisenhofer, G. (1998). Catecholamine metabolism: overview. In *Catecholamines: Bridging Basic Science With Clinical Medicine*, Goldstein, D. S., Eisenhofer, G., and McCarty, R., Eds., pp. 273–292. Academic Press, San Diego.

Bouriquet, N., Dupont, M., Herizi, A., Mimran, A., and Casellas, D. (1996). Preglomerular sudanophilia in L-NAME hypertensive rats. *Hypertension* **27** (part 1), 382–391.

Bowman, W. C., and Rand, M. J. (1980). *Textbook of Pharmacology*. Blackwell, Oxford.

Braas, K. M., and Hendley, E. D. (1994). Anterior pituitary proopiomelanocortin expression is decreased in hypertensive rat strains. *Endocrinology* **134**, 196–205.

Brace, R. A., Jackson, D. E., Ferguson, J. F., Norman, R. A. J., and Guyton, A. C. (1974). Pressure generated by scar tissue contractions: perinephritis hypertension. *Int Res Commun Syst Med Sci Cardiovasc Syst* **2**, 1683.

Bradley, D. J., Ghelarducci, B., Paton, J. F. R., and Spyer, K. M. (1987). The cardiovascular responses elicited from the posterior cerebellar cortex in the anaesthetised and decerebrate rabbit. *J Physiol (Lond)* **383**, 537–550.

Bradley, D. J., Pascoe, J. P., Paton, J. F. R., and Spyer, K. M. (1987). Cardiovascular and respiratory responses evoked from the posterior cerebellar cortex and fastigial nucleus in the cat. *J Physiol (Lond)* **393**, 107–121.

Bradley, D. J., Paton, J. F. R., and Spyer, K. M. (1987). Cardiovascular responses evoked from the fastigial region of the cerebellum in anesthetized and decerebrate rabbits. *J Physiol (Lond)* **392**, 475–491.

Brady, A. J. (1979). Mechanical properties of cardiac fibres. In *Handbook of Physiology, Section 2: The Cardiovascular System*, Berne, R. M., and Sperelakis, N., Eds., Vol. I, pp. 461–474. American Physiological Society, Bethesda, MD.

Brand, T., and Schneider, M. D. (1996). Transforming growth factor-β signal transduction [Mini review]. *Circ Res* **78**, 173–179.

Branson, R., Potoczna, N., Kral, J. G., Lentes, K.-U., Hoehe, M. R., and Horber, F. F. (2003). Binge eating as major phenotype of melanocortin 4 receptor gene mutations. *N Engl J Med* **348**, 1096–1104.

Braun-Menendez, E., Fasciolo, J., Leloir, L., and Munoz, J. (1939). La substancia hipertensora de la sangre del rinen isquemiado. *Revista de la Sociedad Argentina de Biologia* **15**, 420–425.

Braunwald, E. (1965). Control of ventricular function in man. *Brit Heart J* **27**, 1–16.

Braunwald, E., Ross, J. J., and Sonnenblick, E. H. (1967). *Mechanisms of Contraction of the Normal and Failing Heart*. Little, Brown and Company, Boston.

Braunwald, E., and Ross, J. J. (1979). Control of cardiac performance. In *Handbook of Physiology, Section 2: The Cardiovascular System*, Berne, R. M., and Sperelakis, N., Eds., Vol. 1, pp. 533–580. American Physiological Society, Bethesda, MD.

Bravo, E. L., Tarazi, R. C., and Dustan, H. P. (1977). Multifactorial analysis of chronic hypertension induced by electrolyte-active steroids in trained unanesthetized dogs. *Circ Res* **40**, I-140–I-145.

Bray, G. A., and York, D. A. (1979). Hypothalamic and genetic obesity in experimental animals: an autonomic and endocrine hypothesis. *Physiol Rev* **59**, 719.

Bray, G. A., York, D. A., and Fisler, J. S. (1989). Experimental obesity: a homeostatic failure due to defective nutrient stimulation of the sympathetic nervous system. *Vitam Horm* **45**, 1–125.

Brayden, J. E., and Nelson, M. T. (1992). Regulation of arterial tone by activation of calcium-dependent potassium channels. *Science* **256**, 532–535.

Brecher, G. A., and Galletti, P. M. (1963). Functional anatomy of cardiac pumping. In *Handbook of Physiology, Section 2: Circulation*, Hamilton, W. F., and Dow, P., Eds., Vol. 2, pp. 759–798. American Physiological Society, Washington, DC.

Brenner, B. M., Garcia, D. L., and Anderson, S. (1988). Glomeruli and blood pressure: less of one and more of the other? *Am J Hypertens* **1**, 335–347.

Brenner, B. M., Ballermann, B. J., Gunning, M. E., and Zeidel, M. L. (1990). Diverse biological actions of atrial natriuretic peptide. *Physiol Rev* **70**, 665–699.

Bright, R. (1836). Tabular view of the morbid appearances in one hundred cases connected with albuminous urine with observations. *Guy's Hosp Rep* **1**, 380–400.

Bristow, J. D., Honour, A. J., Pickering, G. W., Sleight, P., and Smyth, H. S. (1969). Diminished baroreflex sensitivity in high blood pressure. *Circulation* **39**, 48–54.

Brock, J. A., Van Helden, D. F., Dosen, P., and Rush, R. A. (1996). Prevention of high blood pressure by reducing sympathetic innervation in the spontaneously hypertensive rat. *J Auton Nerv Syst* **61**, 97–102.

Brod, J., Fencl, V., Hejl, Z., and Jirka, J. (1959). Circulatory changes underlying blood pressure elevation during acute emotional stress (mental arithmetic) in normotensive and hypertensive subjects. *Clin Sci* **18**, 269–279.

Brod, J. (1960). Essential hypertension: haemodynamic observations with a bearing on its pathogenesis. *Lancet* **ii**, 773–778.

Brod, J., Fencl, V., Hejl, Z., Jirka, J., and Ulrych, M. (1962). General and regional haemodynamic patterns underlying essential hypertension. *Clin Sci* **23**, 339–349.

Brod, J. (1963). Haemodynamic basis of acute pressor reactions and hypertension. *Br Heart J* **25**, 227–245.

Brodal, P., Ingjer, F., and Hermansen, L. (1977). Capillary supply of skeletal muscle in untrained and endurance trained men. *Am J Physiol* **232**, H705–H712.

Brodie, B. B., Costa, E., Dlabac, A., Neff, N. H., and Smookler, H. H. (1966). Application of steady-state kinetics to the estimation of synthesis rate and turnover time of tissue catecholamines. *J Pharmacol* **154**, 493–498.

Brodman, K., Erdman, A. J., Lorge, I., Wolff, H. G., and Broadbent, T. H. (1949). The Cornell Medical Index—an adjunct to medical interview. *JAMA* **140,** 530–534.

Brody, M. J., and Johnson, A. K. (1980). Role of the anteroventral third ventricle region in fluid and electrolyte balance, arterial pressure regulation and hypertension. In *Frontiers of Neuroendocrinology*, Martini, L., and Ganong, W. F., Eds., Vol. 6, pp. 249–291. Raven Press, New York.

Brody, M. J., Barron, K. W., Berecek, K. H., Faber, J. E., and Lappe, R. W. (1983). Nervous system and hypertension. In *Hypertension: Physiopathology and Treatment*, Genest, J., Ed., pp. 117–140. McGraw-Hill, New York.

Brody, M. J., Varner, K. J., Vasquez, E. C., and Lewis, S. J. (1991). Central nervous system and the pathogenesis of hypertension. *Hypertension* **18** (suppl III), III-7–III-12.

Brooks, D., Horner, R. L., Kozar, L. F., Render-Teixeira, C. L., and Phillipson, E. A. (1997). Obstructive sleep apnea as a cause of systemic hypertension evidence from a canine model. *J Clin Invest* **99,** 106–109.

Brooksby, G. A., and Donald, D. E. (1971). Dynamic changes in splanchnic blood flow and blood volume in dogs during activation of sympathetic nerves. *Circ Res* **31,** 105–118.

Broughton, A., and Korner, P. I. (1980). Steady-state effects of preload and afterload on isovolumic indices of contractility in autonomically blocked dogs. *Cardiovasc Res* **14,** 245–253.

Broughton, A. (1983). Left ventricular function in pressure overload hypertrophy: basal and maximal inotropic state and pumping capacity in the anaesthetised open chest dog, pp. 1–230. PhD thesis, Monash University and Baker Medical Research Institute, Melbourne.

Broughton, A., and Korner, P. I. (1983). Basal and maximal inotropic state in renal hypertensive dogs with cardiac hypertrophy. *Am J Physiol* **245,** H33–H41.

Broughton, A., and Korner, P. I. (1986). Left ventricular pump function in renal hypertensive dogs with cardiac hypertrophy. *Am J Physiol* **251,** H1260–H1266.

Brown, D. A. R. (1973). Arterial hypoxia in the unanaesthetised monkey: the relative roles of autonomic and circulatory mechanisms. BSc Hons thesis, Department of Medicine and Hallstrom Institute of Cardiology, University of Sydney, Sydney.

Brown, A. M., Saum, W. R., and Tuley, F. H. (1976). A comparison of aortic baroreceptor discharge in normotensive and spontaneously hypertensive rats. *Circ Res* **39,** 488–496.

Brown, A. M. (1980). Receptors under pressure. An update on baroreceptors. *Circ Res* **46,** 1–10.

Brownie, A. C. (1995). The adrenal cortex in hypertension: DOCA/salt hypertension and beyond. In *Hypertension: Pathophysiology, Diagnosis and Management, Second Edition*, Laragh, J. H., and Brenner, B. M., Eds., Vol. 2, pp. 2127–2144, Lippincott, Williams and Wilkins, New York.

Brunner, H. R., Kirshman, J. D., Sealey, J. E., and Laragh, J. H. (1971). Hypertension of renal origin: evidence for two different mechanisms. *Science* **174,** 1344–1346.

Brunner, H.-R., Laragh, J. H., Baer, L., Newton, M. A., Goodwin, F. T., Krakoff, L. R., Bard, R. H., and Bühler, F. R. (1972). Essential hypertension: renin and aldosterone, heart attack and stroke. *N Engl J Med* **286,** 441–449.

Bruno, L., Azar, S., and Weller, D. (1979). Absence of a prehypertensive stage in postnatal Kyoto hypertensive rats. *Jpn Heart J* **20** (suppl I), 90–92.

Brutsaert, D. L., and Sonnenblick, E. H. (1971). Nature of the force-velocity relation in cardiac muscle. *Cardiovasc Res* (suppl 1), 18–33.

Brutsaert, D., and Paulus, W. J. (1979). Contraction and relaxation of the heart as muscle and pump. In *Cardiovascular Physiology III: International Review of Physiology*, Guyton, A. C., and Young, D. B., Eds., Vol. 18, pp. 1–31. University Park Press, Baltimore, MD.

Brutsaert, D. L., and Andries, L. J. (1992). The endocardial endothelium. *Am J Physiol* **263,** H985–H1002.

Brutsaert, D. (1993). Endocardial and coronary endothelial control of cardiac performance. *NIPS* **8,** 82–86.

Budzikowski, A. S., and Leenen, F. H. H. (1997). Brain ouabain in the median preoptic nucleus mediates sodium sensitive hypertension in spontaneously hypertensive rats. *Hypertension* **29,** 599–605.

Bugaisky, L. B., Gupta, M., Gupta, M. P., and Zak, R. (1992). Cellular and molecular mechanisms of cardiac hypertrophy. In *The Heart and Cardiovascular System,* Fozzard, H. A., Haber, E. A., Jennings, R. B., Katz, A. M., and Morgan, H. E., Eds., Vol. 2. Raven Press, New York.

Bulpitt, C., Beevers, D., Butler, A., Coles, E., Hunt, D., Munro-Faure, A., Newson, R., O'Riordan, P., Petrie, J., Rajagopalan, B., Rylance, P., Twallin, G., Webster, J., and Dollery, C. (1986). The survival of treated hypertensive patients and their causes of death: a report from the DHSS Hypertensive Care Computing Project (DHCCP). *J Hypertens* **4,** 93–99.

Bulpitt, C., Beevers, D., Butler, A., Coles, E., Hunt, D., Munro-Faure, A., Newson, R., O'Riordan, P., Petrie, J., Rajagopalan, B., Rylance, P., Twallin, G., Webster, J., and Dollery, C. (1988). Treated blood pressure rather than pretreatment, predicts survival in hypertensive patients. A report from the DHSS Hypertension Care Computing Project (DHCCP). *J Hypertens,* **6,** 627–632

Bunag, R. D., and Barringer, D. L. (1988). Obese Zucker rats, though still normotensive, already have impaired chronotropic baroreflexes. *Clin Exper Hypertens (Part A)* **10** (suppl 1), 257–262.

Bunag, R. D., Eriksson, L., and Krizsan, D. (1990). Baroreceptor reflex impairment and mild hypertension in rats with dietary-induced obesity. *Hypertension* **15,** 397–406.

Bund, S., West, K., and Heagerty, A. (1991). Effects of protection from pressure on resistance artery morphology and reactivity in spontaneously hypertensive and Wistar-Kyoto rats. *Circ Res* **68,** 1230–1240.

Bund, S. J., and Lee, R. M. K. W. (2003). The vascular amplifier and persisting resisters. *J Hypertens* **21,** 643–645.

Burcher, E., and Garlick, D. (1973). Antagonism of vasoconstrictor responses by exercise in the gracilis muscle of the dog. *J Pharmacol* **187,** 78–85.

Burke, S. L., Dorward, P. K., and Korner, P. I. (1986). Rapid resetting of rabbit aortic baroreceptors and reflex heart rate responses by directional changes in blood pressure. *J Physiol (Lond)* **378,** 391–402.

Burke, S. L., and Dorward, P. K. (1988). Influence of endogenous opiates and cardiac afferents on renal nerve activity during haemorrhage in conscious rabbits. *J Physiol (Lond)* **402,** 9–27.

Burke, S. L., Malpas, S. C., and Head, G. A. (1998). Effect of rilmenidine on the cardiovascular responses to stress in the conscious rabbit. *J Auton Nerv Syst* **72,** 177–186.

Burke, V., Beilin, L. J., and Sciarrone, S. (1994). Vegetarian diets, proteins and fibre. In *Textbook of Hypertension,* Swales, J. D., Ed., pp. 619–632. Blackwell, Oxford.

Burke, V., Gracey, M. P., Beilin, L. J., and Milligan, R. A. K. (1998). Family history as a predictor of blood pressure in a longitudinal study of Australian children. *J Hypertens* **16,** 269–276.

Burnstock, G., and Holman, M. E. (1963). Smooth muscle: autonomic nerve transmission. *Annu Rev Physiol* **25,** 61–90.

Burnstock, G., Evans, B., Gannon, B. J., Heath, J. W., and James, V. (1971). A new method for destroying adrenergic nerves in adult animals using guanethidine. *Brit J Pharmacol* **43,** 295–301.

Burnstock, G., and Costa, M. (1975). *Adrenergic Neurons.* Chapman and Hall, London.

Burnstock, G. (1986). Vascular control by purines with emphasis on the coronary system. *Eur Heart J* **10** (Suppl F), 15–21.

Bursztyn, M. R., Bresnahan, M., Gavras, I., and Gavras, H. (1990). Pressor hormones in elderly hypertensive persons—racial differences. *Hypertension* **15** (suppl I), I-88–I-92.

Burton, A. C. (1962). Physical principles of circulatory phenomena: the physical equilibria of the heart and blood vessels. In *Handbook of Physiology, Section 2: Circulation*, Hamilton, W. F., and Dow, P., Eds., Vol. I, pp. 85–106. American Physiological Society, Washington, DC.

Byrom, F. B. (1954). The pathogenesis of hypertensive encephalopathy and its relation to the malignant phase of hypertension. Experimental evidence from the hypertensive rat. *Lancet* **ii**, 201–208.

Caldini, P., Permutt, S., Waddell, J. A., and Riley, R. L. (1972). Effect of epinephrine on pressure, flow and volume relationships in the systemic circulation of dogs. *Circ Res* **34**, 606–623.

Calhoun, D. A., Zhu, S., Wyss, J. M., and Oparil, S. (1994). Diurnal blood pressure variation and dietary salt in spontaneously hypertensive rats. *Hypertension* **24**, 1–7.

Cameron, J. D., and Dart, A. M. (1994). Exercise training increases total systemic arterial compliance in humans. *Am J Physiol* **266**, H693–H701.

Campbell, M. (1968). The incidence and later distribution of malformations of the heart. In *Paediatric Cardiology*, Watson, H., Ed., pp. 71–83. Lloyd-Luke (Medical Books), London.

Campbell, D. J., Skinner, S. L., and Day, A. J. (1973). Cellophane perinephritis hypertension and its reversal in rabbits. *Circ Res* **33**, 105–111.

Campbell, W. B., Gebremedhin, D., Pratt, P. F., and Harder, D. R. (1996). Identification of epoxycoseicosatrienoic acids as endothelium-derived hyperpolarizing factors. *Circ Res* **78**, 415–423.

Campese, V. M., Parise, M., Karubian, F., and Bigazzi, R. (1991). Abnormal renal haemodynamics in black salt-sensitive patients with hypertension. *Hypertension* **18**, 805–812.

Campese, V. M., and Kogosov, E. (1995). Renal afferent denervation prevents hypertension in rats with chronic renal failure. *Hypertension* **25**, 878–882.

Canessa, M., Adragna, N., Solomon, H. S., Connolly, T. M., and Tosteson, D. C. (1980). Increased sodium-lithium countertransport in red cells of patients with essential hypertension. *N Engl J Med* **302**, 772–776.

Canessa, M., Laski, C., and Falkner, B. (1990). Red blood cell Na$^+$ transport as a predictor of blood pressure response to Na$^+$ load in young blacks and whites. *Hypertension* **16**, 508–514.

Canessa, M., Romero, J. R., Ruiz-Opazo, N., and Herrera, V. L. M. (1993). The alpha 1 Na$^+$-K$^+$ pump of Dahl salt-sensitive rat exhibits altered Na$^+$ modulation of K$^+$ transport in red blood cells. *J Membr Biol* **134**, 107–122.

Cannon, W. B. (1915). *Bodily Changes in Pain, Hunger, Fear and Rage*. Appleton-Century-Crofts, New York.

Cannon, W. B., and Britton, S. W. (1925). Studies on the conditions of activity in endocrine glands. XV. Pseudoaffective medulliadrenal secretion. *Am J Physiol* **72**, 283–294.

Cannon, W. B. (1929a). Organization for physiological homeostasis. *Physiol Rev* **9**, 399–431.

Cannon, W. B. (1929b). *The Wisdom of the Body*. W.W. Norton, New York.

Capasso, J. M., Palackal, T., Olivetti, G., and Anversa, P. (1990). Left ventricular failure induced by long-term hypertension in rats. *Circ Res* **66**, 1400–1412.

Caples, S. M., Gami, A. S., and Somers, V. K. (2005). Obstructive sleep apnea. *Ann Int Med* **142**, 187–197.

Cappucio, F. P. (1994). Electrolyte intake and human hypertension—calcium and magnesium. In *Textbook of Hypertension*, Swales, J. D., Ed., pp. 551–566. Blackwell, Oxford.

Caravaggi, A. M., Bianchi, G., Brown, M. B., Lever, A. F., Morton, J. J., Powell-Jackson, J. D., Robertson, J. I. S., and Semple, P. F. (1976). Blood pressure and plasma angiotensin, II: concentration after renal artery constriction and angiotensin infusion in the dog. *Circ Res* **38**, 315–321.

Carlsson, A. (1988). The current status of the dopamine hypothesis of schizophrenia. *Neuropsychopharmacology* **1**, 179–186.

Carlsson, A., Hansson, L. O., Waters, N., and Carlsson, M. L. (1997). Neurotransmitter aberrations in schizophrenia: new perspectives and therapeutic implications. *Life Sci* **61**, 75–94.

Carlsson, A. (2001). A paradigm shift in brain research. *Science* **294**, 1021–1024.

Carlyle, M., Jones, O. B., Kuo, J. J., and Hall, J. E. (2002). Chronic cardiovascular and renal actions of leptin. *Hypertension* **39**, 496–501.

Carmody, J. J., and Scott, M. J. (1974). Respiratory and cardiovascular responses to prolonged stimulation of the carotid body chemoreceptors in the cat. *Aust J Exp Biol Med Sci* **52**, 271–283.

Carrive, P., Dampney, R. A. L., and Bandler, R. (1987). Excitation of neurons in a restricted portion of the periaqueductal grey elicits both behavioral and cardiovascular components of the defense reaction in the unanaesthetized decerebrate cat. *Neurosci Lett* **81**, 273–278.

Carroll, J. F., Huang, M., Hester, R. L., Cockrell, K., and Mizelle, H. L. (1995). Hemodynamic alterations in hypertensive obese rabbits. *Hypertension* **26**, 465–470.

Cattell, R. B., and Schreier, I. H. (1967). *Handbook for the IPAT Anxiety Scale Questionnaire*. Institute for Personality and Ability Testing, Chicago, IL.

Cechetto, D. F., and Saper, C. B. (1990). Role of the cerebral cortex in autonomic function. In *Central Regulation of Autonomic Functions*, Loewy, A. D., and Spyer, K. M., Eds., pp. 208–223. Oxford University Press, New York.

Chabanel, A., and Chien, S. (1995). Blood viscosity as a factor in human hypertension. In *Hypertension: Pathophysiology, Diagnosis and Management*, Laragh, J. H., and Brenner, B. M., Eds., Vol. 1, pp. 365–376. Raven Press, New York.

Chalmers, J. P., and Korner, P. I. (1966). Effects of arterial hypoxia on the cutaneous circulation of the rabbit. *J Physiol (Lond)* **184**, 685–697.

Chalmers, J. P., Korner, P. I., and White, S. W. (1966). The control of the circulation in skeletal muscle during arterial hypoxia in the rabbit. *J Physiol (Lond)* **184**, 698–716.

Chalmers, J. P., Korner, P. I., and White, S. W. (1967a). Distribution of peripheral blood flow in primary tissue hypoxia induced by inhalation of carbon monoxide. *J Physiol (Lond)* **192**, 549–559.

Chalmers, J. P., Korner, P. I., and White, S. W. (1967b). The relative roles of the aortic and carotid sinus nerves in the rabbit in the control of respiration and circulation during arterial hypoxia and hypercapnia. *J Physiol (Lond)* **188**, 435–450.

Chalmers, J., and Reid, J. L. (1972). Participation of central noradrenergic neurons in arterial baroreceptor reflexes in the rabbit: a study with intracisternally administered 6-hydroxydopamine. *Circ Res* **31**, 789–804.

Chalmers, J., Dollery, C., Lewis, P., and Reid, J. (1974). The importance of central adrenergic neurones in renal hypertension in rabbits. *J Physiol (Lond)* **238**, 403–411.

Chalmers, J. (1975). Brain amines and models of experimental hypertension. *Circ Res* **36**, 469–480.

Chalmers, J., Horvath, J., Tiller, D., and Bune, A. (1976). Effects of timolol and hydrocholorothiazole on blood pressure and plasma renin activity. *Lancet* **ii**, 328–331.

Chalmers, J., and Pilowsky, P. (1991). Brainstem and bulbospinal neurotransmitter systems in the control of blood pressure. *J Hypertens* **9**, 675–694.

Chalmers, J., Arnolda, L., Lelwellyn-Smith, I., Minson, J., and Pilowsky, P. (1994). Central nervous control of blood pressure. In *Textbook of Hypertension*, Swales, J. D., Ed., pp. 409–426. Blackwell, Oxford.

Chalmers, J., Arnolda, L., Llewellyn-Smith, I., Minson, J., and Pilowsky, P. (1997). Central neural control of the cardiovascular system. In *Handbook of Hypertension, Volume 17: Pathophysiology of Hypertension*, Zanchetti, A., and Mancia, G., Eds., p. 524. Elsevier, Amsterdam.

Chalmers, J. (1998). Volhard lecture: brain, blood pressure and stroke. *J Hypertens* **16,** 1849–1858.

Chalmers, J., for the Guidelines Committee. (1999). World Health Organization-International Society of Hypertension guidelines for the management of hypertension. *J Hypertens* **17,** 151–183.

Chamley-Campbell, J., Campbell, G. R., and Ross, R. (1979). The smooth muscle cell in culture. *Physiol Rev* **59,** 1–61.

Chan, R. K. W., Chan, Y. S., and Wong, T. M. (1991). Electrophysiological properties of neurons in the rostral ventrolateral medulla of normotensive and spontaneously hypertensive rats. *Brain Res* **549,** 118–126.

Chapleau, M. W., Hajduczok, G., and Abboud, F. M. (1989). Peripheral and central mechanisms of baroreflex resetting. *Clin Exp Pharmacol Physiol* **16** (suppl 15), 31–43.

Chapleau, M. W., Hajduczok, G., Sharma, R. V., Wachtel, R. E., Cunningham, J. T., Sullivan, M. J., and Abboud, F. M. (1995). Mechanisms of baroreceptor activation. *Clin Exper Hypertens* **17,** 1–14.

Chappell, M. C., Tallant, E. A., Diz, D. I., and Ferrario, C. M. (2000). The renin-angiotensin system and cardiovascular homeostasis. In *Drugs, Enzymes and Receptors in the Renin-Angiotensin System: Celebrating a Century of Discovery*, Husain, A., and Graham, R. M., Eds., pp. 3–22. Harwood, Amsterdam.

Charvat, J., Dell, P., and Folkow, B. (1964). Mental factors and cardiovascular disease. *Cardiologia* **44,** 124–141.

Chau, N., Safar, M., London, G., and Weiss, Y. (1979). Essential hypertension: an approach to clinical data by the use of models. *Hypertension* **1,** 86–97.

Chen, I. I. H., Prewitt, R. L., and Dowell, R. F. (1981). Microvascular rarefaction in spontaneously hypertensive rat cremaster muscle. *Am J Physiol* **241,** H306–H310.

Chiang, B. W., Perlman, L. V., and Epstein, F. H. (1969). Overweight and hypertension: a review. *Circulation* **39,** 403–421.

Chien, K. R., Zhu, H., Knowlton, K. U., Miller-Hance, W., Van Bilsen, M., O'Brien, T. X., and Evans, S. M. (1993). Transcriptional regulation during cardiac growth and development. *Annu Rev Physiol* **55,** 77–95.

Christenfeld, N., Gerin, W., Linden, W., Sanders, M., Mathur, J., Deich, J. D., and Pickering, T. G. (1997). Social support effects on cardiovascular reactivity: is a stranger as effective as a friend? *Psychosom Med* **59,** 388–398.

Christensen, K. L., Jespersen, L. T., and Mulvany, M. J. (1989). Development of blood pressure in spontaneously hypertensive rats after withdrawal of long-term treatment related to vascular structure. *J Hypertens* **7,** 83–90.

Christensen, K. L. (1991). Reducing pulse pressure in hypertension may normalize small artery structure. *Hypertension* **18,** 722–727.

Christy, I. J., Woods, R. L., Courneya, C. A., Denton, K. M., and Anderson, W. P. (1991). Evidence for a renomedullary vasodepressor system in rabbits and dogs. *Hypertension* **18,** 325–333.

Christy, I. J., Woods, R. L., and Anderson, W. P. (1993). Mediators of hypotensive response to increased renal perfusion in rabbits. *Hypertension* **21,** 149–154.

Chu, A., Lin, C.-C., Chambers, D. E., Kuehl, W. D., Palmer, R. M. J., Moncada, S., and Cobb, F. R. (1991). Effects of inhibition of nitric oxide formation on basal tone and endothelium-dependent responses of the coronary arteries in awake dogs. *J Clin Invest* **87,** 1964–1968.

Churchill, E. D., and Cope, O. (1929). Rapid shallow breathing resulting from pulmonary congestion and edema. *J Exp Med* **49,** 531–537.

Cicila, G., Rapp, J., Wang, J., St. Lezin, E., Ng, S., and Kurtz, T. (1993). Linkage of 11beta-hydroxylase mutations with altered steroid biosynthesis and blood pressure in the Dahl rat. *Nat Gen* **3,** 346–353.

Ciriello, J., Kline, R. L., Zhang, T. X., and Caverson, M. M. (1984). Lesions of the paraventricular nucleus alter the development of spontaneous hypertension in the rat. *Brain Res* **310,** 355–359.

Clark, J. H., Schrader, W. T., and O'Malley, B. W. (1992). Mechanism of action of steroid hormones. In *Williams Textbook of Endocrinology, 8th Edition,* Wilson, J. D., and Foster, D. W., Eds., pp. 35–90. W.B. Saunders, Philadelphia.

Clarke, N. P., Smith, O. A., and Shearn, D. W. (1968). Topographical representation of vascular smooth muscle of limbs in primate motor cortex. *Am J Physiol* **214,** 122–129.

Clarke, D. W. J. (1971). Effects of immunosympathectomy on the development of high blood pressure in genetically hypertensive rats. *Circ Res* **28,** 330–336.

Clarke, W. R., Schrott, H. G., Leaverton, P. E., Connor, W. E., and Lauer, R. M. (1978). Tracking of blood pressure of school age children. The Muscatine study. *Circulation* **58,** 626–634.

Clausen, J. P. (1977). Effect of physical training on cardiovascular adjustments to exercise in man. *Physiol Rev* **57,** 779–815.

Clement, D. L., De Buyzere, M. L., De Bacquer, D. A., de Leeuw, P. W., Duprez, D. A., Fagard, R. H., Gheeraert, P. J., Missault, L. H., Braun, J. J., Six, R. O., Van Der Niepen, P., and O'Brien, E. (2003). Prognostic values of ambulatory blood-pressure recordings in patients with treated hypertension. *N Engl J Med* **348,** 2407–2415.

Cleroux, J., Kouamè, N., Nadeau, A., Coulombe, D., and Larcourcière, Y. (1992). After-effects of exercise on regional and systemic haemodynamics in hypertension. *Hypertension* **19,** 183–191.

Cleutjens, J. P. M. (1996). The role of matrix metalloproteinases in heart disease. *Cardiovasc Res* **32,** 816–821.

Clynes, M. (1960). Computer dynamic analysis of the pupil light reflex. In *Proceedings of the 3rd International Conference on Medical Electronics,* pp. 356–358. International Federation of Medical Electronics & Biomedical Engineering and Institute of Electrical Engineers (London), London.

Coates, J. C., and de Bono, M. (2002). Antagonistic pathways in neurons exposed to body fluid regulate social feeding in *Caenorhabditis elegans. Nature* **419,** 925–928.

Coats, A. J. S., Conway, J., Isea, J. E., Pannarale, G., Sleight, P., and Somers, V. K. (1989). Systemic and forearm vascular resistance changes after upright bicycle exercise in man. *J Physiol (Lond)* **413,** 289–298.

Cochrane, K. L., and Nathan, M. A. (1989). Normotension in conscious rats after placement of bilateral electrolytic lesions in the rostral ventrolateral medulla. *J Auton Nerv Syst* **26,** 199–211.

Cocks, T. M. (1997). Endothelium-dependent vasodilator mechanisms. In *Pharmacology of Vascular Smooth Muscle,* Garland, C. J., and Angus, J. A., Eds., pp. 233–251. Oxford University Press, Oxford.

Cohen, J. (1974). Role of endocrine factors in the pathogenesis of cardiac hypertrophy. *Circ Res* **34 & 35** (suppl II), II-49–II-57.

Cohen, S., and Hoberman, H. M. (1983). Positive events and social support as buffers of life changes to stress. *J Appl Soc Psychol* **13,** 99–125.

Cohn, J. H., Liptak, T. E., and Freis, E. D. (1963). Hemodynamic effect of guanethidine in man. *Circ Res* **12**, 298–307.

Coleman, T. G., and Guyton, A. C. (1969). Hypertension caused by salt loading in the dog. III. Onset transients of cardiac output and other circulatory variables. *Circ Res* **25**, 153–169.

Coleman, T. G., Bower, J. D., Langford, H. G., and Guyton, A. C. (1970). Regulation of arterial pressure in the anephric state. *Circulation* **42**, 509–514.

Coleridge, H. M., Coleridge, J. C. G., and Kidd, C. (1964a). Cardiac receptors in the dog, with particular reference to two types of afferent ending in the ventricular wall. *J Physiol (Lond)* **174**, 323–339.

Coleridge, H. M., Coleridge, J. C. G., and Kidd, C. (1964b). Role of the pulmonary arterial baroreceptors in the effects produced by capsaicin in the dog. *J Physiol (Lond)* **170**, 272–285.

Coleridge, J. C. G., and Coleridge, H. M. (1979). Chemoreflex regulation of the heart. In *Handbook of Physiology, Section 2: The Cardiovascular System (Vol. I)*, Berne, R. M., Ed., pp. 653–676. American Physiological Society, Bethesda, MD.

Coleridge, H. M., and Coleridge, J. C. G. (1980). Cardiovascular afferents involved in regulation of peripheral vessels. *Annu Rev Physiol* **42**, 413–427.

Coleridge, H. M., Coleridge, J. C. G., Kaufman, M. P., and Dangel, A. (1981). Operational sensitivity and acute resetting of aortic baroreceptors in dogs. *Circ Res* **48**, 676–684.

Coleridge, H. M., Coleridge, J. C. G., Poore, E. R., Roberts, A. M., and Schultz, H. D. (1984). Aortic wall properties and baroreceptor behaviour at normal arterial pressure and in acute hypertensive resetting in dogs. *J Physiol (Lond)* **350**, 309–326.

Collins, R., Peto, R., MacMahon, S., Hebert, P., Fiebach, N. H., Eberlein, K. A., Godwin, J., Qizilbash, N., Taylor, J. O., and Hennekens, C. H. (1990). Blood pressure, stroke and coronary heart disease. Part 2, short term reductions in blood pressure: overview of randomised drug trials in their epidemiological context. *Lancet* **335**, 827–838.

Comroe, J. H., and Mortimer, L. (1964). The respiratory and cardiovascular responses of temporally separated aortic and carotid bodies to cyanide, nicotine, phenyldiguanide and serotonin. *J Pharmacol* **146**, 33–41.

Conn, J. W. (1964). Plasma renin activity in primary aldosteronism. Importance in differential diagnosis and in research of essential hypertension. *JAMA* **190**, 222–225.

Consentino, F., Sill, J. C., and Katusic, Z. S. (1994). Role of superoxide anions in the mediation of endothelium-dependent contractions. *Hypertension* **23**, 229–235.

Considine, P., Sinha, M. K., Heiman, M. L., Kriauciunas, A., Stephens, T. W., Nyce, M. R., Ohannesian, J. P., Marco, C. C., McKee, L. J., and Bauer, T. L. (1996). Serum immunoreactive-leptin concentrations in normal weight and obese humans. *N Engl J Med* **334**, 292–295.

Converse, R. L., Jacobsen, T. N., Toto, R. D., Jost, C. M., Consentino, F., Fouad-Tarazi, F., and Victor, R. G. (1992). Sympathetic overactivity in patients with chronic renal failure. *N Engl J Med* **327**, 1912–1918.

Conway, J. (1963). A vascular abnormality in hypertension. A study of blood flow in the forearm. *Circulation* **27**, 520–529.

Conway, J. (1968). Changes in sodium balance and hemodynamics during development of experimental renal hypertension in dogs. *Circ Res* **22**, 763–767.

Conway, J. (1984). Hemodynamic aspects of essential hypertension in humans. *Physiol Rev* **64**, 617–660.

Cooper, J. R., Bloom, F. E., and Roth, R. H. (1991). *The Biochemical Basis of Neuropharmacology*. Oxford University Press, New York.

Cooper, R., and Rotimi, C. (1994). Hypertension in populations of West African origin: is there a genetic predisposition [editorial review]. *J Hypertens* **12**, 215–227.

Cooper, G. M. (1997). *The Cell: A Molecular Approach*. ASM Press, Washington, DC.

Cooper, R. S., Rotimi, C. N., and Ward, R. (1999). The puzzle of hypertension in African-Americans. *Sci Am* **279**, 36–43.

Coote, J. H., Hilton, S. M., and Perez-Gonzalez, J. F. (1971). The reflex nature of the pressor response to muscular exercise. *J Physiol (Lond)* **215**, 789–804.

Coote, J., Hilton, S., and Perez-Gonzalez, J. (1979). Inhibition of the baroreceptor reflex on stimulation in the brain stem defence centre. *J Physiol (Lond)* **288**, 549–560.

Coote, J. H. (1988). The organisation of cardiovascular neurons in the spinal cord. *Rev Physiol Biochem Pharmacocol* **110**, 147–285.

Corcoran, A. C., Taylor, R. D., and Page, I. H. (1948). Functional patterns in renal disease. *Ann Int Med* **28**, 560–582.

Cornish, K. G., and Gilmore, J. P. (1985). Sino-aortic denervation in the monkey. *J Physiol (Lond)* **360**, 423–432.

Correia, M. L. G., Morgan, D. A., Sivitz, W. I., Mark, A. L., and Haynes, W. G. (2001). Leptin acts in the central nervous system to produce dose-dependent changes in arterial pressure. *Hypertension* **37**, 936–942.

Corvol, P., Persu, A., Gimenez-Roqueplo, A.-P., and Jeunemaitre, X. (1999). Seven lessons from two candidate genes in human essential hypertension: angiotensinogen and epithelial sodium channel. *Hypertension* **33**, 1324–1331.

Cottier, P. (1960). Renal hemodynamics, water and electrolyte excretion in essential hypertension. In *Essential Hypertension: An International Symposium*, Bock, K. D., and Cottier, P., Eds., p. 66. Springer, Berlin.

Cotton, T. S., Rapport, D. L., and Lewis, T. (1915–17). After effects of exercise on pulse rate and systolic blood pressure in case of normal subjects and patients with "irritable heart." *Heart* **6**, 269–281.

Courneya, C. A., and Korner, P. I. (1991). Neurohumoral mechanisms and the role of the arterial baroreceptors in the reno-vascular response to haemorrhage in rabbits. *J Physiol (Lond)* **437**, 393–407.

Courneya, C. A., Korner, P. I., Oliver, J. R., and Woods, R. L. (1991). Afferent vascular resistance control during hemorrhage in normal and autonomically blocked rabbits. *Am J Physiol* **261**, H380–H391.

Courtice, F. C., and Yoffey, J. M. (1970). *Lymphatics Lymph and the Lymphomyeloid Complex*. Academic Press, London.

Cowley, A. W., Liard, J. F., and Guyton, A. C. (1973). Role of the baroreceptor reflex in daily control of arterial blood pressure and other variables in dogs. *Circ Res* **32**, 564–576.

Cowley, A. W., Merill, D. C., Quillen, M. E. W., and Skelton, M. M. (1984). Long-term blood pressure and metabolic effects of vasopressin with servo-controlled fluid volume. *Am J Physiol* **247**, R537–R545.

Cowley, A. W., Jr. (1992). Long-term control of arterial blood pressure. *Physiol Rev* **72**, 231–300.

Cowley, A. W., Mattson, D. L., Lu, S., and Roman, R. J. (1995). The renal medulla and hypertension. *Hypertension* **25** (part 2), 663–673.

Cowley, A. W., Jr., and Roman, R. J. (1997). Renal mechanisms in hypertension. In *Handbook of Hypertension, Volume 17: Pathophysiology of Hypertension*, Zanchetti, A., and Mancia, G., Eds., pp. 740–784. Elsevier Science, Amsterdam.

Cox, R. H., and Bagshaw, R. J. (1988). Effects of hypertension and its reversal on canine arterial wall properties. *Hypertension* **12**, 301–309.

Cox, K. L., Puddey, I. B., Morton, A. R., Beilin, L. J., Vandongen, R., and Masarei, J. R. L. (1993). The combined effects of aerobic exercise and alcohol restriction on blood pressure and serum lipids: a two-way factorial study in sedentary men. *J Hypertens* **11**, 191–201.

Cox, K. (1994). Life style modification of cardiovascular risk factors: the relative roles of exercise, alcohol and calorie restriction. PhD thesis, University of Western Australia, Perth.

Cox, H. S., Kaye, D. M., Thompson, J. M., Turner, A. G., Jennings, G. L., Itsiopoulos, C., and Esler, M. D. (1995). Regional sympathetic nervous activation after a large meal in humans. *Clin Sci* **89**, 145–154.

Crepel, F., and Audinat, E. (1991). Excitatory amino acid receptors of cerebellar Purkinje cells: development and plasticity. *Prog Biophys Mol Biol* **55**, 31–46.

Crepel, F., Hemart, N., Jaillard, D., and Daniel, H. (1995). Long-term depression in the cerebellum. In *The Handbook of Brain Theory and Neural Networks*, Arbib, M. A., Ed., pp. 560–563. MIT Press, Cambridge, MA.

Crocker, E. F., Johnson, R. O., Korner, P. I., Uther, J. B., and White, S. W. (1968). Effects of hyperventilation on the circulatory response of the rabbit to arterial hypoxia. *J Physiol (Lond)* **199**, 267–282.

Crone, C. (1963). The permeability of capillaries in various organs as determined by use of the "indicator diffusion" method. *Acta Physiol Scand* **58**, 292–305.

Cross, C. E., Rieben, P. A., Barron, C. I., and Salisbury, P. F. (1963). Effects of arterial hypoxia on the heart and circulation: an integrative study. *Am J Physiol* **205**, 963–970.

Cruickshank, J. M., Thorp, J. M., and Zacharias, F. J. (1987). Benefits and potential harm of lowering high blood pressure. *Lancet* **i**, 581–584.

Cruickshank, J. M. (1988). Coronary flow reserve and the J-curve relation between diastolic blood pressure and myocardial infarction. *Br Med J* **297**, 1227–1230.

Cruz-Coke, R., Etcheverry, R., and Nagel, R. (1964). Influence of migration on the blood pressure of Easter Islanders. *Lancet* **i**, 697–699.

Cruz-Coke, R. (1983). Genetic aspects of essential hypertension. In *Handbook of Hypertension, Volume 1: Clinical Aspects of Essential Hypertension*, Robertson, J. I. S., Ed., pp. 21–29. Elsevier, Amsterdam.

Cryer, P. E., Haymond, M. W., Santiago, J. W., and Shah, S. D. (1976). Norepinephrine and epinephrine release and adrenergic mediation of smoking associated with hemodynamic and metabolic events. *N Engl J Med* **295**, 573–577.

Culbertson, J. W., Wilkins, R. W., Ingelfinger, F. J., and Bradley, S. E. (1951). The effect of the upright posture on hepatic blood flow in normotensive and hypertensive subjects. *J Clin Invest* **30**, 305–311.

Cullen-McEwen, L. A., Kett, M. M., Dowling, J., Anderson, W. P., and Bertram, J. F. (2003). Nephron number, renal function and arterial pressure in aged GDNF heterozygous mice. *Hypertension* **41**, 335–340.

Culpepper, W. S., Sodt, P. C., Messerli, F. H., Ruschhaupt, D. G., and Arcilla, R. (1983). Cardiac status of juvenile borderline hypertension. *Ann Int Med* **98**, 1–7.

Cunningham, D. J. C., Howson, M. G., Peterson, E. S., Pickering, T. G., and Sleight, P. (1972). Changes in the sensitivity of the baroreflex in muscular exercise [abstract]. *Acta Physiol Scand* **79**, 16A–17A.

Curtis, J. J., Luke, R. G., Dustan, H. P., Kashgarian, M., Whelchel, J. D., Jones, P., and Diethelm, A. G. (1983). Remission of essential hypertension after renal transplantation. *N Engl J Med* **309**, 1009–1015.

Cutiletta, A. F., Erinoff, L., Heller, A., Low, J., and Oparil, S. (1977). Development of left ventricular hypertrophy in young spontaneously hypertensive rats after peripheral sympathectomy. *Circ Res* **40**, 428–434.

D'Agostini, N. (1954). Osservazioni istologiche sul paranganglio succlavio del coniglio. *Bolletino Societa Italiana Biologica Sperementale* **30**, 922–934.

Dahl, L. K. (1961). Possible role of chronic excess salt consumption in the pathogenesis of essential hypertension. *Am J Cardiol* **8**, 571–581.

Dahl, L. K., Heine, M., and Tassinari, L. (1962). Role of genetic factors in suceptibility to experimental hypertension due to chronic excess salt ingestion. *Nature* **194**, 480–482.

Dahl, L. K., Heine, M., and Thompson, K. (1974). Genetic influence of the kidneys on blood pressure. *Circ Res* **34**, 94–101.

Dahl, L. K., and Heine, M. (1975). Primary role of renal homografts in setting blood pressure level in rats. *Circ Res* **36**, 692–696.

Dahlöf, B., and Hansson, L. (1992). Regression of left ventricular hypertrophy in previously untreated essential hypertension: different effects of enalapril and hydrochlorothiazide. *J Hypertens* **10**, 1513–1524.

Dahlöf, B., Pennert, K., and Hansson, L. (1992). Reversal of left ventricular hypertrophy in hypertensive patients. A meta-analysis of 109 treatment studies. *Am J Hypertens* **5**, 95–110.

Dahlöf, B., Devereux, R. B., Kjeldsen, S. E., Julius, S., Beevers, G., de Faire, U., Fyhrquist, F., Ibsen, H., Kristiansson, K., Lederballe-Pedersen, O., Lindholm, L. H., Nieminen, M. S., Omvik, P., Oparil, S., and Wedel, H. (2002). Cardiovascular morbidity and mortality in the Losartan Intervention for Endpoint reduction in hypertension study (LIFE): a randomised trial against atenolol. *Lancet* **359**, 995–1003.

Dahlström, A., and Fuxe, K. (1964). Evidence for the existence of monoamine-containing neurons in the central nervous system. I. Demonstration of monoamines in the cell bodies of brain stem neurons. *Acta Physiol Scand* **62** (suppl 232), 1–55.

Dahlström, A., and Fuxe, K. (1965). Evidence for the existence of monoamine-containing neurons in the central nervous system. II. Experimentally induced changes in the intraneuronal amine levels of bulbospinal neuron systems. *Acta Physiol Scand* **64** (suppl 247), 1–36.

Daly, M. d. B., and Hazzledine, J. L. (1963). The effects of artificially induced hyperventilation on the primary cardiac reflex responses to stimulation of the carotid bodies in the dog. *J Physiol (Lond)* **168**, 872–889.

Daly, M. d. B., and Scott, M. J. (1963). The cardiovascular responses to stimulation of the carotid body chemoreceptors in the dog. *J Physiol (Lond)* **165**, 179–197.

Daly, M. d. B., Hazzledine, J. L., and Ungar, A. (1967). The reflex effects of alterations in lung volume on systemic vascular resistance in the dog. *J Physiol (Lond)* **188**, 331–351.

Daly, M. d. B., and Robinson, B. H. (1968). An analysis of the reflex systemic vasodilator response elicited by lung inflation in the dog. *J Physiol (Lond)* **195**, 387–406.

Daly, M. d. B., Korner, P. I., Angell-James, J. E., and Oliver, J. R. (1978a). Cardiovascular and respiratory effects of carotid body stimulation in the monkey. *Clin Exp Pharmacol Physiol* **5**, 511–524.

Daly, M. d. B., Korner, P. I., Angell-James, J. E., and Oliver, J. R. (1978b). Cardiovascular-respiratory reflex interactions between carotid bodies and upper airways receptors in the monkey. *Am J Physiol* **234**, H293–H299.

Daly, M. d. B. (1986). Interaction between respiration and circulation. In *Handbook of Physiology, Section 3: The Respiratory System. Vol. II: Control of Breathing*, pp. 529–594. American Physiological Society, Bethesda, MD.

Damasio, A. R. (1994). *Descartes' Error*. G.P. Putnam's Sons, New York.

Damasio, A. R. (1997). Towards a neuropathology of emotion and mood. *Nature* **386**, 769–770.

Dampney, R. A. L., Stella, A., Gorlin, R., and Zanchetti, A. (1979). Vagal and sinoaortic reflexes in postural control of circulation and renin release. *Am J Physiol* **237**, H146–H152.

Dampney, R. A. L., and Moon, E. A. (1980). Role of ventrolateral medulla in vasomotor response to cerebral ischemia. *Am J Physiol* **239**, H349–H358.

Dampney, R. A. L. (1981). Brain stem mechanisms in the control of arterial pressure. *Clin Exper Hypertens* **A3**, 379–391.

Dampney, R. A. L., Goodchild, A. K., and Tan, E. (1985). Vasopressor neurons in the rostral ventrolateral medulla of the rabbit. *J Auton Nerv Syst* **14**, 239–254.

Dampney, R. A. L. (1994a). Functional organization of central pathways regulating the cardiovascular system. *Physiol Rev* **74**, 323–364.

Dampney, R. A. L. (1994b). The subretrofacial vasomotor nucleus: anatomical, chemical and pharmacological properties and role in cardiovascular regulation. *Progr Neurobiol* **42**, 197–227.

Dampney, R. A. L., Coleman, M. J., Fontes, M. A. P., Hirooka, Y., Horiuchi, J., Li, Y.-W., Polson, J. W., Potts, P. D., and Tagawa, T. (2002). Central mechanisms underlying short- and long-term regulation of the cardiovascular system. *Clin Exp Pharmacol Physiol* **29**, 261–268.

Dampney, R. A. L., and Horiuchi, J. (2003). Functional organisation of central cardiovascular pathways: studies using c-*fos* gene expression. *Progr Neurobiol* **71**, 359–384.

Darian-Smith, I. (1982). Touch in primates. *Annu Rev Psychol* **33**, 155–194.

Darian-Smith, I., Galea, M. P., Darian-Smith, C., Sugitani, M., Tan, A., and Burman, K. (1996). The anatomy of manual dexterity. *Adv Anat Embryol Cell Biol* **133**, 1–142.

Darnell, J., Lodish, H., and Baltimore, D. (1990). *Molecular Cell Biology.* W.H. Freeman, New York.

Darwin, C. (1872). *The Expression of the Emotions in Man and Animals.* HarperCollins, London.

D'Atri, D. A., and Ostfeld, A. M. (1975). Crowding in prison—its effects on blood pressure in prison setting. *Behav Med* **4**, 550–556.

D'Atri, D. A., Fitzgerald, E. F., Kasl, S. K., and Ostfeld, A. M. (1981). Crowding in prison: the relationship between changes in housing mode and blood pressure. *Psychosom Med* **43**, 95–105.

Davidson, A. O., Schork, N., Jaques, B. C., Kelman, A. W., Sutcliffe, R. G., Reid, J. L., and Dominiczak, A. F. (1995). Blood pressure in genetically hypertensive rats: influence of the Y chromosome. *Hypertension* **26**, 452–459.

Davies, P. F., and Barbee, K. A. (1994). Endothelial cell surface imaging: insights into hemodynamic force transduction. *NIPS* **9**, 153–157.

Davies, P. F. (1995). Flow-mediated endothelial mechanotransduction. *Physiol Rev* **75**, 519–560.

Davis, J. O., and Freeman, R. H. (1976). Mechanisms regulating renin release. *Physiol Rev* **56**, 1.

Davis, M. J., and Hill, M. A. (1999). Signalling mechanisms underlying the vascular myogenic response. *Physiol Rev* **79**, 387–423.

Dawes, G. S. (1968). *Foetal and Neonatal Physiology.* Year Book Medical Publishers, Chicago.

Day, M. D., Roach, A. G., and Whiting, R. L. (1973). The mechanism of the antihypertensive action of α-methyldopa in hypertensive rats. *Eur J Pharm* **21**, 271–280.

Dean, C., and Coote, J. H. (1986). A ventromedullary relay involved in the hypothalamic and chemoreceptor activation of sympathetic postganglionic neurons to skeletal muscle kidney and splanchnic area. *Brain Res* **377**, 279–285.

de Bold, A. J. (1982). Atrial natriuretic factor of the rat heart: studies on isolation and properties. *Proc Soc Exp Biol Med* **170**, 133–138.

de Bono, M., Tobin, D. M., Davis, M. W., Avery, L., and Bargmann, C. I. (2002). Social feeding in *Caenorhabtitis elegans* is induced by neurons that detect aversive stimuli. *Nature* **419**, 899–903.

De Champlain, J., Cousineau, D., and Lapointe, L. (1979). The significance of circulating catecholamines in the evolution and treatment of hypertension. In *Nervous System and Hypertension*, Meyer, P., and Schmitt, H., Eds., pp. 277–286. Wiley-Flammarion, Paris.

Dejours, P. (1963). The regulation of breathing during muscular exercise in man. In *The Regulation of Human Respiration*, Cunningham, D. J. C., and Lloyd, B. B., Eds., pp. 535–547. Blackwell, Oxford.

de Leeuw, P. W., Kho, T. L., Falke, H. E., Birkenharger, W. H., and Wester, A. (1978). Haemodynamic and endocrinological profile of essential hypertension. *Acta Med Scand* **622** (suppl), 5–86.

de Leeuw, P. W., Schalekamp, M. A. D. H., and Birkenhaeger, W. H. (1983). The renal circulation in hypertension. In *Handbook of Hypertension, Volume I: Clinical Aspects of Essential Hypertension*, Robertson, J. I. S., Ed., pp. 202–215. Elsevier, Amsterdam.

de Leeuw, P. W., De Bos, R., Van Es, P. N., and Birkenhäger, W. H. (1985). Effect of sympathetic stimulation and intrarenal alpha-blockade on the secretion of renin by the human kidney. *Eur J Clin Invest* **15**, 166–170.

Delius, W., Hagbarth, K. E., Hongell, A., and Wallin, B. G. (1972a). Manoeuvres affecting sympathetic outflow in human muscle nerves. *Acta Physiol Scand* **84**, 82–94.

Delius, W., Hagbarth, K. E., Hongell, A., and Wallin, B. G. (1972b). Manoeuvres affecting sympathetic outflow in human skin nerves. *Acta Physiol Scand* **84**, 177–186.

Dell'Italia, L. J., and Husain, A. (2000). Chymase: a critical evaluation of its role in angiotensin II formation and cardiovascular disease. In *Enzymes and Receptors of the Renin-Angiotensin System: Celebrating a Century of Discovery*, Husain, A., and Graham, R. M., Eds., pp. 347–364. Harwood Academic Publishers, Amsterdam.

De Mey, J. G. R., and Schiffers, P. M. (1993). Effects of endothelium on growth responses in arteries. *J Cardiovasc Pharmacol* **21** (suppl 1), S22–S25.

Denton, D. (1982). *The Hunger for Salt*. Springer-Verlag, Berlin.

Denton, K. M., Anderson, W. P., and Korner, P. I. (1983). Renal blood flow and glomerular filtration rate in renal wrap hypertension in rabbits. *J Hypertens* **1**, 351–355.

Denton, K. M., and Anderson, W. P. (1985). Role of angiotensin II in renal wrap hypertension. *Hypertension* **7**, 893–898.

Denton, K. M. (1989). Renal venous wedge pressure in renal wrap hypertension in rabbits. *Clin Exp Pharmacol Physiol* **16**, 681–684.

Denton, D., Weisinger, R., Mundy, N. I., Wickings, E. J., Dixson, A., Ardaillou, R., Paillard, F., Chapman, J., Thillet, J., and Michel, J. B. (1995). The effect of increased salt intake on blood pressure of chimpanzees. *Nat Med* **1**, 1009–1016.

Denton, K. M., Anderson, W. P., and Sinniah, R. (2000). Effects of angiotensin II on regional afferent and efferent arteriole dimensions and the glomerular pole. *Am J Physiol* **279**, R629–R638.

Denton, K. M., Flower, R. L., Stevenson, K. M., and Anderson, W. P. (2003). Adult rabbit offspring of mothers with secondary hypertension have increased blood pressure. *Hypertension* **41**(2), 634–639.

Denton, K. M., Luff, S. E., Shweta, A., and Anderson, W. P. (2004). Differential neural control of glomerular ultrafiltration. *Clin Exp Pharmacol Physiol* **31**, 380–386.

de Pomerai, D. (1986). *From Gene to Animal*. Cambridge University Press, Cambridge.

Derkx, F., and Schalekamp, M. (1994). Renal artery stenosis and hypertension. *Lancet* **344**, 237–239.

Deter, H. C., Buchholz, K., Schorr, U., Schachinger, H., Turan, S., and Sharma, A. M. (1997). Psychophysiological reactivity of salt sensitive normotensive subjects. *J Hypertens* **15**, 839–844.

Devereux, R. B., and Reichek, N. (1977). Echocardiographic determination of left ventricular mass. Anatomic validation of the method. *Circulation* **55**, 613–615.

Devereux, R. B., Pickering, T. G., Harshfield, G. A., Kleinert, H. D., Denby, L., Clark, L., Pregibon, D., Jason, M., Kleiner, B., Borer, J. S., and Laragh, J. H. (1983). Left ventricular hypertrophy in patients with hypertension: importance of BP in response to regularly occurring stress. *Circulation* **68**, 470–476.

Devereux, R. B., Pickering, T. G., Alderman, M. H., Chien, S., Borer, J. A., and Laragh, J. (1987). Left ventricular hypertrophy in hypertension. Prevalence and relationship to pathophysiologic variables. *Hypertension* **9**(II), II-53–II-60.

Devereux, R., de Simone, G., Ganau, A., and Roman, M. (1994). Left ventricular hypertrophy and geometric remodeling in hypertension: stimuli, functional consequences and prognostic implications. *J Hypertens* **12** (suppl 10), S117–S127.

Devereux, R. B., and Roman, M. J. (1995). Hypertensive cardiac hypertrophy: pathophysiologic and clinical characteristics. In *Hypertension: Pathophysiology, Diagnosis and Management*, Laragh, J. H., and Brenner, B. M., Eds., Vol. 1, pp. 409–432. Raven Press, New York.

Devereux, R. B., Pini, R., Aurigemma, G. P., and Roman, M. J. (1997). Measurement of left ventricular mass: methodology and expertise. *J Hypertens* **15**, 801–809.

de Wardener, H. E., and MacGregor, G. A. (1980). Dahl's hypothesis that a saluretic substance may be responsible for a sustained rise in arterial pressure: its possible role in essential hypertension. *Kidney Internat* **18**, 1–9.

de Wardener, H. E. (1990). The primary role of the kidney and salt intake in the aetiology of essential hypertension: parts I and II. *Clin Sci* **79**, 193–200, 289–297.

de Wardener, H. E. (1996). Franz Volhard Lecture: sodium transport inhibitors and hypertension. *J Hypertens* **14** (suppl 5), S9–S18.

de Wardener, H. E. (2001). The hypothalamus and hypertension. *Physiol Rev* **81**, 1599–1658.

De Wit, C., Jahrbeck, B., Schafer, C., Bolz, S.-S., and Pohl, U. (1998). Nitric oxide opposes myogenic pressure responses predominantly in large arterioles in vivo. *Hypertension* **31**, 784–794.

Dhital, K. K., Gerli, R., Lincoln, J., Milner, P., Tanganelli, P., Weber, G., Fruschelli, C., and Burnstock, G. (1988). Increased density of perivascular nerves to the major cerebral vessels of the spontaneously hypertensive rat. *Brain Res* **444**, 33–45.

DiBona, G. F. (1989). Neural control of renal function: cardiovascular implications. *Hypertension* **13**, 539–548.

DiBona, G. F. (1991). Stress and sodium intake in neural control of renal function in hypertension. *Hypertension* **17** (suppl III), III-2–III-6.

DiBona, G. F., Jones, S. Y., and Sawin, L. L. (1996). Renal sympathetic neural mechanisms as intermediate phenotype in spontaneously hypertensive rats. *Hypertension* **27** (part 2), 626–630.

DiBona, G. F., and Kopp, U. C. (1997). Neural control of renal function. *Physiol Rev* **77**, 75–197.

DiCarlo, S. E., and Bishop, V. S. (1988). Exercise training attenuates baroreflex regulation of nerve activity in rabbits. *Am J Physiol* **255**, H974–H979.

Dickinson, C. J. (1995). Cerebral oxidative metabolism in essential hypertension: a meta-analysis. *J Hypertens* **13**, 653–658.

Dilley, R. J., and Schwartz, S. M. (1989). Vascular remodelling in the growth hormone transgenic mouse. *Circ Res* **65**, 1233–1240.

Dilley, R., Kanellakis, P., Oddie, C., and Bobik, A. (1994). Vascular hypertrophy in renal hypertensive spontaneously hypertensive rats. *Hypertension* **24**, 8–15.

DiMicco, J. A., Soltis, R. P., Anderson, J. J., and Wible, J. H. (1992). Hypothalamic mechanisms and the cardiovascular response to stress. In *Central Neural Mechanisms in Cardiovascular Regulation*, Kunos, G., and Ciriello, J., Eds., Vol. 2, pp. 52–79. Birkhauser, Boston.

Dimsdale, J. E., Mills, P., Ziegler, M., Leitz, K., and Nelesen, R. (1992). Converting enzyme inhibition and blood pressure reactivity to psychological stressors. *Hypertension* **20**, 210–213.

Dimsdale, J. E., Loredo, J. S., and Profant, J. (2000). Effect of continuous positive airway pressure on blood pressure: a placebo trial. *Hypertension* **35**, 144–147.

Ding, B., Price, R. L., Borg, T. H., Weinberg, E. O., Halloran, P. F., and Lorell, B. H. (1999). Presssure overload induces severe hypertrophy in mice treated with cyclosporine, an inhibitor of calcineurin. *Circ Res* **84**, 729–734.

Dobrian, A. D., Davies, M. J., Prewitt, R. L., and Lauterio, T. J. (2000). Development of hypertension in a rat model of diet induced obesity. *Hypertension* **35**, 1009–1015.

Dobrin, P. B., Littooy, F. N., and Endean, E. D. (1989). Mechanical factors predisposing to intimal hyperplasia and medial thickening in autogenous vein grafts. *Surgery* **105**, 393–400.

Dobrin, P. B. (1995). Mechanical factors associated with the development of intimal and medial thickening in vein grafts subjected to arterial pressure: a model of arteries exposed to hypertension. *Hypertension* **26**, 38–43.

Dodge, H. T., Frimer, M., and Stewart, D. K. (1974). Functional evaluation of hypertrophied heart in man. *Circ Res* **34, 35** (suppl II), II-122–II-127.

Dodic, M., May, C. N., Wintour, E. M., and Coghlan, J. P. (1998). An early prenatal exposure to excess glucocorticoid leads to hypertensive offspring in sheep. *Clin Sci* **94**, 149–155.

Dodt, C., Breckling, U., Derad, I., Fehm, H. L., and Born, J. (1997). Plasma epinephrine and norepinephrine concentrations of healthy humans associated with nighttime sleep and morning arousal. *Hypertension* **30** (part 1), 71–76.

Dodt, C., Keyser, B., Molle, M., Fehm, H. L., and Elam, M. (2000). Acute suppression of muscle sympathetic nerve activity by hydrocortisone in humans. *Hypertension* **35**, 758–763.

Dominiczak, A. F., Devlin, A. M., Lee, W. K., Anderson, N. H., Bohr, D. F., and Reid, J. L. (1996). Vascular smooth muscle polyploidy and cardiac hypertrophy in genetic hypertension. *Hypertension* **27** (part 2), 752–759.

Dominiczak, A. F., Clark, J. S., Jeffs, B., Anderson, N. H., Negrin, C. D., Lee, W. K., and Brosnan, M. J. (1998). Genetics of experimental hypertension. *J Hypertens* **16**, 1859–1869.

Dominiczak, A. F., Negrin, D. C., Clark, J. S., Brosnan, M. J., McBride, M. W., and Alexander, M. Y. (2000). Genes and hypertension: from gene mapping in experimental models to vascular gene transfer strategies. *Hypertension* **35** (part 2), 164–172.

Dominiczak, A. F., Graham, D., McBride, M. W., Brain, N. J. R., Lee, W. K., Charchar, F. J., Tomaszewski, M., Delles, C., and Hamilton, C. A. (2005). Cardiovascular genomics and oxidative stress. *Hypertension* **45** (part 2), 636–642.

Donald, D., and Shepherd, J. (1963). Response to exercise in dogs with cardiac denervation. *Am J Physiol* **205**, 393–400.

Donald, D. E. (1981). Splanchnic circulation. In *Handbook of Physiology, Section 2, The Cardiovascular System: Peripheral Circulation and Organ Blood Flow*, Shepherd, J. T., and Abboud, F. M., Eds., Vol. III, pp. 219–240. American Physiological Society, Bethesda, MD.

Dorward, P. K., Andresen, M. C., Burke, S. L., Oliver, J. R., and Korner, P. I. (1982). Rapid resetting of the aortic baroreceptors in the rabbit and its implications for short-term and longer term reflex control. *Circ Res* **50**, 428–439.

Dorward, P. K., Riedel, W., Burke, S. L., Gipps, J., and Korner, P. I. (1985). The renal sympathetic baroreflex in the rabbit. Arterial and cardiac baroreceptor influences, resetting and effect of anesthesia. *Circ Res* **57**, 618–633.

Dorward, P. K., and Korner, P. I. (1987). Does the brain "remember" the absolute blood pressure? *NIPS* **2**, 10–13.

Dorward, P. K., Bell, L. B., and Rudd, C. D. (1990). Cardiac afferents attenuate renal sympathetic baroreceptor reflexes during acute hypertension. *Hypertension* **16**, 131–139.

Douglas, W. W., Ritchie, J. M., and Schaumann, W. (1956). Depressor reflexes from medullated and non-medullated fibres in the rabbit's aortic nerve. *J Physiol (Lond)* **132,** 187–198.

Douglas, W. W., and Schaumann, W. (1956). A study of the depressor and pressor components of the cat's carotid sinus and aortic nerves using electrical stimuli of different intensities and frequencies. *J Physiol (Lond)* **132,** 176–186.

Downer, J. L. d. (1961). Changes in visual gnostic functions and emotional behaviour following unilateral temporal pole damage in the "split-brain" monkey. *Nature* **191,** 50–51.

Doyle, A. E., Fraser, J. R. E., and Marshall, R. J. (1959). Reactivity of forearm vessels to vasoconstrictor substances in hypertensive and normotensive subjects. *Clin Sci* **18,** 441–454.

Dragunow, M., and Faull, R. (1989). The use of *c-fos* as a metabolic marker in neuronal pathway tracing. *J Neurosci Meth* **29,** 261–265.

Dressler, W. W. (1990). Life style, stress and blood pressure in a southern black community. *Psychosom Med* **52,** 182–198.

Drevets, W. C., and Raichle, M. E. (1994). Positron emission tomographic imaging studies of human emotional disorders. In *The Cognitive Neurosciences*, Gazzaniga, M. S., Ed., pp. 1153–1164. MIT Press, Cambridge, MA.

Drevets, W. C., Price, J. L., Simpson, J. R., Todd, R. D., Reich, T., Vannier, M., and Raichle, M. E. (1997). Subgenual prefrontal cortex abnormalities in mood disorders. *Nature* **386,** 824–827.

Drummond, H. A., and Seagard, J. L. (1996). Acute baroreflex resetting: differential control of pressure and nerve activity. *Hypertension* **27,** 442–448.

Dudai, Y., Jan, Y. N., Byers, D., Quinn, W. G., and Benzer, S. (1976). Dunce, a mutant of *Drosophila* deficient in learning. *Proc Natl Acad Sci, USA* **73,** 1684–1688.

Dudai, Y. (1988). Neurogenic dissection of learning and short term memory in *Drosophila*. *Annu Rev Neurosci* **11,** 537–563.

Duff, F., and Shepherd, J. T. (1953). The circulation in the chronically denervated forearm. *Clin Sci* **12,** 407–416.

Duling, B. R., and Berne, R. M. (1970). Longitudinal gradients in periarteriolar oxygen tension. *Circ Res* **27,** 669–678.

Dunn, W. R., and Gardiner, S. M. (1995). No evidence for vascular remodelling during hypertension induced by chronic inhibition of nitric oxide synthase in Brattleboro rats. *J Hypertens* **13,** 849–857.

Dustan, H. P., Tarazi, R. C., Bravo, E. L., and Dart, R. A. (1973). Plasma and extracellular fluid volumes in hypertension. *Circ Res* **32–33,** 73–83.

Dustan, H. P. (1990). Legacies of Irvine H. Page (Irvine Page Lecture). *J Hypertens* **8,** S29–S34.

Dusting, G. J. (1995). Nitric oxide in cardiovascular disorders. *J Vascular Res* **32,** 143–161.

Dworkin, L. D., and Brenner, B. M. (1992). Biophysical basis of glomerular filtration. In *The Kidney: Physiology and Pathophysiology*, Seldin, D. W., and Giebisch, G., Eds., Vol. 1, pp. 979–1016. Raven Press, New York.

Dyke, A. C. (1989). Function of the cardiovascular sympathetic nerve varicosities during maturation in the SHR and WKY rat. Department of Pharmacology, Monash University, Melbourne, Australia.

Dyke, A. C., Angus, J. A., and Korner, P. I. (1989). A functional study of the development of the cardiac sympathetic neuroeffector junction in the SHR. *J Hypertens* **7,** 345–353.

Dzau, V. J., Siwek, L. G., Rosen, S., Fahri, E. R., Mizoguchi, H., and Barger, A. C. (1981). Sequential renal hemodynamics in experimental benign and malignant hypertension. *Hypertension* **3,** I-63–I-68.

Dzau, V., and Gibbons, G. (1987). Autocrine-paracrine mechanisms of vascular myocytes in systemic hypertension. *Am J Cardiol* **60,** 99–103I.

Dzau, V. J., Gibbons, G. H., Morishita, R., and Pratt, R. E. (1994). New perspectives in hypertension research: potentials of vascular biology. *Hypertension* **23** (part 2), 1132–1140.

East, E. M. (1915). Studies on size inheritance in *Nicotiana*. *Genetics* **1**, 164–176.

Ebihara, A., and Grollman, A. (1968). Pressor activity of renal venous effluent following constriction of renal artery in dogs. *Am J Physiol* **214**, 1–5.

Eccles, J. C., Ito, M., and Szenthágotai, J. (1967). *The Cerebellum as a Neuronal Machine*. Springer-Verlag, New York.

Eckberg, D. L., and Sleight, P. (1992). *Human Baroreflexes in Health and Disease*. Clarendon Press, Oxford.

Edelman, G. M. (1989). *Neural Darwinism: The Theory of Neuronal Group Selection*. Oxford University Press, Oxford.

Edelman, G. M., and Tononi, G. (2000). *Consciousness: How Matter Becomes Imagination*. Penguin Books, London.

Edmunds, M. E., Russell, G. I., Burton, P. R., and Swales, J. D. (1990). Baroreceptor-heart rate reflex function before and after surgical reversal of two-kidney, one-clip hypertension in the rat. *Circ Res* **66**, 1673–1680.

Edwards, A. W. T., Korner, P. I., and Thorburn, G. D. (1959). The cardiac output of the unanaesthetized rabbit, and the effects of preliminary anaesthesia, environmental temperature and carotid occlusion. *Q J Exp Physiol* **44**, 309–321.

Edwards, G., Dora, K. A., Gardener, M. J., Garland, C. J., and Weston, A. H. (1998). K^+ is an endothelium derived hyperpolarizing factor in rat arteries. *Nature* **396**, 269–272.

Egan, B., Schork, N., Panis, R., and Hinderliter, A. (1988). Vascular structure enhances regional resistance responses in mild essential hypertension. *J Hypertens* **6**, 41–48.

Eghbali, M., Tomek, R., Sukhatme, V., Woods, C., and Bhambi, B. (1991). Differential effects of transforming growth factor-beta1 and phorbol myristate acetate on cardiac fibroblasts. Regulation of fibrillar collagen mRNAs and expression of early transcription factors. *Circ Res* **69**, 483–490.

Eich, R. H., Cuddy, R. P., Smulyan, H., and Lyons, R. H. (1966). Hemodynamics in labile hypertension. A follow up study. *Circulation* **34**, 299–307.

Eilam, R., Malach, R., Bergmann, F., and Segal, M. (1991). Hypertension induced by hypothalamic transplantation from genetically hypertensive to normotensive rats. *J Neurosci* **11**, 401–411.

Eisenberg, B. R., Edwards, J. A., and Zak, R. (1985). Transmural distribution of isomyosin in rabbit ventricle during maturation examined by immunofluorescence and staining for calcium-activated adenosine triphosphatase. *Circ Res* **56**, 548–555.

Ekblom, P. (1992). Renal development. In *The Kidney: Physiology and Pathophysiology*, Seldin, D. W., and Giebisch, G., Eds., Vol. 1, pp. 475–501. Raven Press, New York.

Ekelund, U., Bjoernberg, J., Graende, P. O., and Albert, U. (1992). Myogenic vascular regulation in skeletal muscle in vivo is not dependent of endothelium-derived nitric oxide. *Acta Physiol Scand* **144**, 199–207.

Ekman, P. (1998). Introduction to the third edition. In *Darwin's The Expression of the Emotions in Man and Animals*, Ekman, P., Ed., pp. xxi–xxxvi. HarperCollins, New York.

Elam, M., Yao, T., Thorén, P., and Svensson, T. H. (1981). Hypercapnia and hypoxia: chemoreceptor mediated control of locus coeruleus neurons and splanchnic sympathetic nerves by cardiovascular afferents. *Brain Res* **222**, 373–381.

Elam, M., Yao, T., Svensson, T. H., and Thorén, P. (1984). Regulation of locus coeruleus neurons and splanchnic, sympathetic nerves by cardiovascular afferents. *Brain Res* **290**, 281–287.

Elam, M., Svensson, T. H., and Thorén, P. (1985). Differentiated cardiovascular afferent regulation of locus coeruleus neurons and sympathetic nerves. *Brain Res* **358**, 77–84.

Elam, M., Thorén, P., and Svensson, T. H. (1986). Locus coeruleus neurons and sympathetic nerves: activation by visceral afferents. *Brain Res* **375**, 117–125.

Elbert, T., Ray, W. J., Kowalik, Z. J., Skinner, J. E., Graf, K. E., and Birbaumer, N. (1994). Chaos and physiology: deterministic chaos in excitable cell assemblies. *Physiol Rev* **74**, 1–47.

Elghozi, J.-L., Head, G. A., Wolf, W. A., Anderson, C. R., and Korner, P. I. (1989). Importance of spinal noradrenergic pathways in cardiovascular reflexes and central actions of clonidine and L-methyldopa in the rabbit. *Brain Res* **499**, 39–52.

Elias, C. F., Kelly, J. F., Lee, C. E., Ahima, R. S., Drucker, D. J., and Saper, C. B. (2000). Chemical characterisation of leptin activated neurons in the rat brain. *J Comp Neurol* **423**, 261–281.

Eliasson, S., Folkow, B., Lindgren, P., and Uvnas, B. (1951). Activation of sympathetic vasodilator nerves to the skeletal muscle in the cat by hypothalamic stimulation. *Acta Physiol Scand* **23**, 333–351.

Elliott, W. H., and Elliott, D. C. (1997). *Biochemistry and Molecular Biology*. Oxford University Press, Oxford.

Elmquist, J. K. (2001). Hypothalamic pathways underlying the endocrine, autonomic and behavioral effects of leptin. *Physiol Behav* **74**, 703–708.

Elsner, R. W., Franklin, D. L., and Van Citters, R. L. (1964). Cardiac output during diving in an unrestrained sea lion. *Nature* **202**, 809–810.

Elsner, R., and Scholander, P. F. (1965). Circulatory adaptations to diving in animals and man. In *Physiology of Breath-Hold Diving and the Ama of Japan*, Rahn, H., and Yokoyama, T., Eds. National Academy of Sciences and National Research Council (Publication 1341), Washington, DC.

Elsner, R., and Gooden, B. (1983). *Diving and Asphyxia*. Cambridge University Press, Cambridge.

Ely, D. L., and Turner, M. E. (1990). Hypertension in the spontaneously hypertensive rat is linked to the Y chromosome. *Hypertension* **16**, 277–281.

Ely, D. L., Falvo, J., Dunphy, G., Caplea, A., Salisbury, R., and Turner, M. E. (1994). The spontaneously hypertensive rat Y chromosome produces an early testosterone rise in normotensive rats. *J Hypertens* **12**, 769–774.

Ely, D., Caplea, A., Dunphy, G., and Smith, D. (1997a). Physiological and neuroendocrine correlates of social position in normotensive and hypertensive rat colonies. *Acta Physiol Scand* **161** (suppl 640), 92–95.

Ely, D. L., Caplea, A., Dunphy, G., Daneshvar, H., Turner, M., Milsted, A., and Taiyyuddin, M. (1997b). Spontaneous hypertensive rat Y chromosome increases indexes of sympathetic nervous system activity. *Hypertension* **29**, 613–618.

Elzinga, G., and Westerhof, N. (1976). The pumping ability of the left heart and the effect of coronary occlusion. *Circ Res* **38**, 297–302.

Elzinga, G., Noble, M. I. M., and Stubbs, J. (1977). The effect of an increase in aortic pressure upon the inotropic state of cat and dog left ventricles. *J Physiol (Lond)* **273**, 597–615.

Engelmann, G. L., Vitullo, J. C., and Gerrity, R. G. (1987). Morphometric analysis of cardiac hypertrophy during development, maturation and senescence in spontaneously hypertensive rats. *Circ Res* **60**, 487–494.

Engelmann, G. L., Boehm, K. D., Haskell, J. F., Khairallah, P. A., and Ilan, J. (1989). Insulin-like growth factors and neonatal cardiomyocyte development: ventricular gene expression and membrane receptor variations in normotensive and hypertensive rats. *Mol Cell Endocrinology* **63**, 1–14.

Engelmann, G. L., Dionne, C. A., and Jaye, M. C. (1993). Acidic fibroblast growth factor and heart development: role in myocyte proliferation and capillary angiogenesis. *Circ Res* **72**, 7–19.

Eppel, G. A., Malpas, S. C., Denton, K. M., and Evans, R. G. (2004). Neural control of renal medullary perfusion. *Clin Exp Pharmacol Physiol* **31**, 387–396.

Epstein, F. H., and Eckoff, R. D. (1967). *The Epidemiology of High Blood Pressure—Geographical Distributions and Etiological Factors*. Grune & Stratton, New York.

Erickson, J. C., Clegg, K. E., and Palmiter, R. D. (1996). Sensitivity to leptin and susceptibility to seizures of mice lacking neuropeptide Y. *Nature* **381**, 415–418.

Ernsberger, P., Koletsky, R. J., Collins, L. A., and Douglas, J. G. (1993). Renal angiotensin receptor mapping in obese spontaneously hypertensive rats. *Hypertension* **21**, 1039–1045.

Esler, M. D., Julius, S., Randall, O. S., Ellis, C. N., and Kashima, T. (1975). Relation of renin status to neurogenic vascular resistance in borderline hypertension. *Am J Cardiol* **36**, 708–715.

Esler, M., Julius, S., and Randall, O. (1976). Relationship of volume factors, renin and neurogenic vascular resistance in borderline hypertension. In *The Arterial Hypertensive Diseases*, Rorive, G., and Van Cauwenberge, H., Eds., pp. 231–249. Masson, Paris.

Esler, M., Jackman, G., Bobik, A., Kelleher, D., Jennings, G., Leonard, P., Skews, H., and Korner, P. (1979). Determination of norepinephrine apparent release rate and clearance in humans. *Life Sci* **25**, 1461–1470.

Esler, M., Jackman, G., Kelleher, D., Skews, H., Jennings, G., Bobik, A., and Korner, P. (1980). Norepinephrine kinetics in patients with idiopathic autonomic insufficiency. *Circ Res* **46**, I-47–I-48.

Esler, M., Jackman, G., Leonard, P., Bobik, A., Skews, H., Jennings, G., Kelleher, D., and Korner, P. (1980). Determination of noradrenaline uptake, spillover to plasma and plasma concentration in patients with essential hypertension. *Clin Sci* **59** (suppl 6), 311s–313s.

Esler, M., Jackman, G., Leonard, P., Skews, H., Bobik, A., and Korner, P. (1981). Effect of norepinephrine uptake blockers on norepinephrine kinetics. *Clin Pharmacol Ther* **29**, 12–20.

Esler, M. (1982). Assessment of sympathetic nervous function in humans from noradrenaline plasma kinetics. *Clin Sci* **62**, 247–254.

Esler, M., Jennings, G., Korner, P., Blombery, P., Burke, F., Willett, I., and Leonard, P. (1984). Total, and organ-specific, noradrenaline plasma kinetics in essential hypertension. *Clin Exp Hypertens* **A6**, 507–521.

Esler, M., Jennings, G., Korner, P., Blombery, P., Sacharias, N., and Leonard, P. (1984). Measurement of total and organ-specific norepinephrine kinetics in humans. *Am J Physiol* **247**, E21–E28.

Esler, M., Jennings, G., Lambert, G., and Korner, P. (1987). Local autonomic activity in primary hypertension. In *Early Pathogenesis of Primary Hypertension*, Hofman, A., Grobbee, D. E., and Schalekamp, M. A. D. H., Eds. Elsevier Science Publishers, Amsterdam.

Esler, M., Lambert, G., and Jennings, G. (1989). Regional norepinephrine turnover in human hypertension. *Clin Exp Hypertens (Part A)* **11** (suppl 1), 75–89.

Esler, M., Jennings, G., Lambert, G., Meredith, I., Horne, M., and Eisenhofer, G. (1990). Overflow of catecholamine neurotransmitters to the circulation: source, fate and functions. *Physiol Rev* **70**, 963–986.

Esler, M. (1995). The sympathetic nervous system and catecholamine release and plasma clearance in normal blood pressure control, in aging, and in hypertension. In *Hypertension: Pathophysiology, Diagnosis and Management*, Laragh, J. H., and Brenner, B. M., Eds., Vol. 1, pp. 755–773. Raven Press, New York.

Espiner, E. E., and Nicholls, M. G. (1993). Renin and the control of aldosterone. In *The Renin-Angiotensin System*, Robertson, J. I. S., and Nicholls, M. G., Eds., Vol. 1, pp. 33.1–33.24. Gower Medical Publishing, London.

Evans, R., Ludbrook, J., and Potocnik, S. (1989). Intracisternal naloxone and cardiac nerve blockade prevent vasodilatation during simulated hemorrhage in awake rabbits. *J Physiol (Lond)* **409**, 1–14.

Evans, R., Szenasi, G., and Anderson, W. (1995). Effects of N^G-nitro-L-arginine on pressure natriuresis in anaesthetized rabbits. *Clin Exp Pharmacol Physiol* **22**, 94–101.

Evans, R. G., Majid, D. S. A., and Eppel, G. (2005). Mechanisms mediating pressure natriuresis: what we know and what we need to find out. *Clin Exp Pharmacol Physiol* **32**, 400–409.

Evenwel, R. T., Kasbergen, C. M., and Struyker-Boudier, H. A. J. (1983). Central and regional hemodynamics and plasma volume distribution during the development of spontaneous hypertension in rats. *Clin Exp Hypertens (Part A)* **A5**(9), 1511–1536.

Everett, A., Tufro-McReddie, A., Fisher, A., and Gomez, R. A. (1994). Angiotensin receptor regulates cardiac hypertrophy and transforming growth factor-β1 expression. *Hypertension* **23**, 587–592.

Everson, S. A., Kaplan, G. A., Goldberg, D. E., and Salonen, J. T. (2000). Hypertension incidence is predicted by high levels of hopelessness in Finnish men. *Hypertension* **35**, 561–567.

Faber, J. E., and Brody, M. J. (1985). Afferent renal nerve-dependent hypertension following acute renal artery stenosis in the conscious rat. *Circ Res* **57**, 676–688.

Fabiato, A. (1983). Calcium-induced release of calcium from the cardiac sarcoplasmic reticulum. *Am J Physiol* **245**, C1–C14.

Fagard, R., and Amery, A. (1995). Physical exercise in hypertension. In *Hypertension: Pathophysiology, Diagnosis and Management*, Laragh, J. H., and Brenner, B. M., Eds., Vol. 2, pp. 2669–2681. Raven Press, New York.

Falck, B., and Hillarp, N.-A. (1959). On the cellular localisation of catecholamines in the brain. *Acta Anatomica* **38**, 277–279.

Falconer, D. S. (1960). *Introduction to Quantitative Genetics*. Ronald Press, New York.

Falkner, B. (1987). Reactivity to mental stress in hypertension and prehypertension. In *Handbook of Hypertension, Volume 9: Behavioral Factors in Hypertension*, Julius, J., and Bassett, D., Eds., pp. 94–103. Elsevier, Amsterdam.

Falkner, B., Hulman, S., and Kushner, H. (1998). Birth weight versus childhood growth as determinants of adult blood pressure. *Hypertension* **31** (part 1), 145–150.

Falsetti, H. L., Mates, R. E., Greene, D. G., and Bunnell, I. L. (1971). V_{max} as an index of contractile state in man. *Circulation* **43**, 467–479.

Fan, X.-M., Hendley, E. D., and Forehand, C. J. (1995). Enhanced vascular neuropeptide Y-immunoreactive innervation in two hypertensive rat strains. *Hypertension* **26**, 758–763.

Faraci, F. M., and Heistad, D. D. (1998). Regulation of the cerebral circulation: role of endothelium and potassium channels. *Physiol Rev* **78**, 53–97.

Fareh, J., Touyz, R. M., Schiffrin, E. L., and Thibault, G. (1996). Endothelin-1 and angiotensin II receptors in cells from rat hypertrophied heart. *Circ Res* **78**, 302–311.

Faris, I. B., Iannos, J., Jamieson, G. G., and Ludbrook, J. (1980). Comparison of methods for eliciting the baroreceptor-heart rate reflex in conscious rabbits. *Clin Exp Pharmacol Physiol* **7**, 281–291.

Farooqi, I. S., Keogh, J. M., Yeo, G. S. H., Lank, E. J., Cheetham, T., and O'Rahilly, S. (2003). Clinical spectrum of obesity and mutations in the melanocortin 4 receptor gene. *N Engl J Med* **348**, 1085–1095.

Fedorova, O. V., Lakatta, E. G., and Bagrov, A. Y. (2000). Endogenous Na,K pump ligands are differentially regulated during acute NaCl loading of Dahl rats. *Circulation* **102**, 3009–3014.

Fedorova, O. V., Kolodkin, N. I., Agalakova, N. I., Lakatta, E. G., and Bagrov, A. Y. (2001). Marinobufagenin, an endogenous alpha-1 sodium pump ligand, in hypertensive salt-sensitive rats. *Hypertension* **37**, 462–466.

Fedorova, O. V., Agalakova, N. I., Talan, M. I., Lakatta, E. G., and Bagrov, A. Y. (2005). Brain ouabain stimulates peripheral marinobufagenin via angiotensin II signalling in NaCl loaded Dahl-S rats. *J Hypertens* **23**, 1515–1523.

Feigl, E., Johansson, B., and Lofving, B. (1964). Renal vasoconstriction and the "defense reaction." *Acta Physiol Scand* **62**, 429–435.

Feigl, E. O. (1983). Coronary physiology. *Physiol Rev* **63**, 1–205.

Feldberg, W., and Guertzenstein, P. G. (1976). Vasodepressor effects obtained by drugs acting on the ventral surface of the brain stem. *J Physiol (Lond)* **258**, 337–355.

Fenoy, F. J., Ferrer, P., Carbonell, L., and Garcia-Salom, M. (1995). Role of nitric oxide on papillary blood flow and pressure natriuresis. *Hypertension* **25**, 408–414.

Ferrannini, E. (1992). The haemodynamics of obesity: a theoretical analysis. *J Hypertens* **10**, 1417–1424.

Ferrannini, E. (1995). The phenomenon of insulin resistance: its possible relevance to hypertensive disease. In *Hypertension: Pathophysiology, Diagnosis and Management*, Laragh, J. H., and Brenner, B. M., Eds., Vol. 2, pp. 2281–2300. Raven Press, New York.

Ferrans, V. J., and Rodriguez, E. R. (1987). Morphology of the heart in left ventricular hypertrophy. In *The Heart and Hypertension*, Messerli, F. H., Ed., pp. 75–86. Yorke Medical Books, New York.

Ferrario, C., Page, I., and McCubbin, J. (1970). Increased cardiac output as a contributory factor in experimental renal hypertension in dogs. *Circ Res* **27**, 799–810.

Ferrario, C., and McCubbin, J. (1973). Hemodynamics of experimental renal hypertension. In *Hypertension: Mechanisms and Management, 26th Hahnemann Symposium*, Onesti, G., Kim, K., and Moyer, J., Eds., pp. 591–600. Grune & Stratton, New York.

Ferrario, C. M., Barnes, K. L., Diz, D. I., Block, C. H., and Averill, D. B. (1987). Role of area postrema mechanisms in the regulation of arterial pressure. *Can J Physiol Pharmacol* **65**, 1591–1597.

Ferrier, C., Jennings, G. L., Eisenhofer, G., Lambert, G., Cox, H. S., Kalff, V., Kelly, M., and Esler, M. D. (1993). Evidence for increased noradrenaline release from subcortical brain regions in essential hypertension. *J Hypertens* **11**, 1217–1227.

Filipovsky, J., Ducimetiere, P., Eschwege, E., Richard, J. L., Rosselin, G., and Claude, J. R. (1996). The relationship of blood pressure with glucose, insulin, heart rate, free fatty acid and plasma cortisol levels according to the degree of obesity in middle-aged men. *J Hypertens* **14**, 229–235.

Finch, L., and Haeusler, G. (1973). Further evidence for a central hypotensive action of alpha-methyldopa in both the rat and cat. *Brit J Pharmacol* **47**, 217–228.

Finer, J. F., Simmons, R. M., and Spudich, J. A. (1994). Single myosin molecule mechanics: piconewton forces and nanometre steps. *Nature* **368**, 113–119.

Fink, G. D., and Brody, M. J. (1979). Renal vascular resistance and reactivity in the spontaneously hypertensive rat. *Am J Physiol* **237**, F128–F132.

Finkielman, S., Worcel, M., and Agrest, A. (1965). Hemodynamic patterns in essential hypertension. *Circulation* **31**, 356–368.

Fiorillo, C. D., Tobler, P. N., and Schultz, W. (2003). Discrete coding of reward probability and uncertainty by dopamine neurons. *Science* **299**, 1898–1902.

Fisher, R. A. (1918). The correlation between relatives on the supposition of Mendelian inheritance. *Trans R Soc Edinb* **52**, 399–433.

Fisher, R. A. (1930). *The Genetical Theory of Natural Selection*. Oxford University Press, Oxford.

Fisher, R. A. (1946). *Statistical Methods for Research Workers*. Oliver and Boyd, Edinburgh.

Fisher, R. A. (1947). *The Design of Experiments*. Oliver and Boyd, Edinburgh.

Fisher, L. A., and Brown, M. R. (1983). Corticotropin-releasing factor: central nervous system effects on the sympathetic nervous system and cardiovascular regulation. In *Current*

Topics in Neuro-endocrinology: Central Cardiovascular Control, Ganten, D., and Pfaff, D., Eds., pp. 87–101. Springer-Verlag, Berlin.

Fisher, L. A. (1989). Central autonomic modulation of cardiac baroreflex by corticotropin-releasing factor. *Am J Physiol* **256**, H949–H955.

Fisher, D. A. (1992). Endocrinology of fetal development. In *Williams Textbook of Endocrinology*, Wilson, J. D., and Foster, D. W., Eds., pp. 1049–1078. W.B. Saunders, Philadelphia.

Fitzsimons, J. (1994). Physiology and pathophysiology of thirst and sodium appetite. In *The Kidney*, Seldin, D., and Giebisch, G., Eds., Vol. 2, pp. 1615–1648. Raven Press, New York.

Fleckenstein, A., Fleckenstein-Grün, G., Frey, M., and Zorn, J. (1987). Future direction in the use of calcium antagonists. *Am J Cardiol* **59**, 177B–187B.

Fletcher, P. J., Korner, P. I., Angus, J. A., and Oliver, J. R. (1976). Changes in cardiac output and total peripheral resistance during development of renal hypertension in the rabbit: lack of conformity with the autoregulation theory. *Circ Res* **39**, 633–639.

Fletcher, P. J. (1984). Baroreceptor heart rate reflex in rabbits after reversal of renal hypertension. *Am J Physiol* **246**, H261–H266.

Fletcher, E. C., Lesske, J., Qian, W., Miller, C. C., and Unger, T. (1992). Repetitive episodic hypoxia cause diurnal elevation of blood pressure in rats. *Hypertension* **19**, 555–561.

Floras, J. S., Hassan, M. O., Vann Jones, J., Osikowska, B. A., Sever, P. S., and Sleight, P. (1988). Consequences of impaired arterial baroreflexes in essential hypertension: effects on pressor responses, plasma noradrenaline and blood pressure variability. *J Hypertens* **6**, 525–535.

Floras, J. S., Sinkey, C. A., Aylward, P. E., Seals, D. R., Thorén, P. N., and Mark, A. L. (1989). Postexercise hypotension and sympathoinhibition in borderline hypertensive men. *Hypertension* **14**, 28–35.

Floras, J. S., and Hara, K. (1993). Sympathoneural and haemodynamic characteristics of young subjects with mild essential hypertension. *J Hypertens* **11**, 647–655.

Fokkema, D. S. (1985). Social behavior and blood pressure: a study of rats. Thesis for Doctorate in Natural Sciences, University of Groningen, Groningen, Netherlands.

Fokkema, D. S., and Koolhaas, J. M. (1985). Psychosocial behaviour and blood pressure in individual rats. *Physiol Behav* **34**, 33–38.

Folkow, B. (1949). Intravascular pressure as a factor regulating the tone of the small vessels. *Acta Physiol Scand* **17**, 289–310.

Folkow, B. (1956). Structural, myogenic, humoral and nervous factors controlling peripheral resistance. In *Hypotensive Drugs*, Harrington, M., Ed., pp. 163–174. Pergamon Press, London.

Folkow, B., and Löfving, B. (1956). The distensibility of the systemic resistance blood vessels. *Acta Physiol Scand* **38**, 37–52.

Folkow, B., Grimby, G., and Thulesius, O. (1958). Adaptive structural changes of the vascular walls in hypertension and their relation to the control of the peripheral resistance. *Acta Physiol Scand* **44**, 255–272.

Folkow, B. (1964). Description of the myogenic hypothesis. *Circ Res* **14 & 15** (suppl I), I-279–I-287.

Folkow, B., and Rubinstein, E. H. (1966). Cardiovascular effects of acute and chronic stimulation of the hypothalamic defence area in the rat. *Acta Physiol Scand* **68**, 48–57.

Folkow, B., Hallbäck, M., Lundgren, Y., and Weiss, L. (1970). Background of increased flow resistance and vascular reactivity in spontaneously hypertensive rats. *Acta Physiol Scand* **80**, 93–106.

Folkow, B., and Neil, E. (1971). *Circulation*. Oxford University Press, New York.

Folkow, B., Hallbäck, M., Lundgren, Y., and Weiss, L. (1972). The effects of "immunosympathectomy" on blood pressure and "vascular reactivity" in normal and spontaneously hypertensive rats. *Acta Physiol Scand* **84**, 512–523.

Folkow, B., Gothberg, G., Lundin, S., and Ricksten, S. E. (1977). Structural renal vascular changes in renal hypertensive rats (RHR). *Acta Physiol Scand* **101**, 254–256.

Folkow, B. (1978). Cardiovascular structural adaptation: its role in the initiation and maintenance of primary hypertension (Fourth Volhard Lecture). *Clin Sci Mol Med* **55**, 3s–22s.

Folkow, B. (1982). Physiological aspects of primary hypertension. *Physiol Rev* **62**, 347–504.

Folkow, B., and Karlström, G. (1984). Age- and pressure-dependent changes of systemic resistance vessels concerning the relationships between geometric design, wall distensibility, vascular reactivity and smooth muscle sensitivity. *Acta Physiol Scand* **122**, 17–33.

Folkow, B. (1987). Physiology of behaviour and blood pressure regulation in animals. In *Handbook of Hypertension, Volume 9: Behavioural Factors in Hypertension*, Julius, S., and Bassett, D. R., Eds., pp. 1–18. Elsevier, Amsterdam.

Folkow, B., and Ely, D. L. (1987). Dietary sodium effects on cardiovascular and sympathetic neuroeffector functions as studied in various rat models. *J Hypertens* **5**, 383–395.

Folkow, B., and Karlström, G. (1987). Vascular reactivity in hypertension: importance of structural changes. *J Cardiovasc Pharmacol* **10** (suppl 4), S25–S30.

Folkow, B., Hansson, L., and Johansson, B. E. (1989). Myogenic mechanisms in the control of systemic resistance. *J Hypertens* **7** (suppl 4), S1–S173.

Folkow, B. (1993). Physiological organization of neurohormonal responses to psychosocial stimuli: implications for health and disease. *Ann Behav Med* **15**, 236–244.

Folkow, B., and Svanborg, A. (1993). Physiology of cardiovascular aging. *Physiol Rev* **73**, 725–764.

Folkow, B. (1995a). Hypertensive structural changes in systemic precapillary resistance vessels: how important are they for *in vivo* haemodynamics. *J Hypertens* **13**, 1546–1559.

Folkow, B. (1995b). The structural factor in hypertension with special emphasis on the altered geometric design of the systemic resistance arteries. In *Hypertension: Pathophysiology, Diagnosis and Management*, Laragh, J. H., and Brenner, B. M., Eds., Vol. 1, pp. 481–502. Raven Press, New York.

Folkow, B. (2000). The debate on the amplifier hypothesis: some comments. *J Hypertens* **18**, 375–378.

Fontana, A. M., Diegnan, T., Villeneuve, A., and Lepore, S. (1999). Nonevaluative social support reduces cardiovascular reactivity in young women during acutely stressful performance situations. *J Behav Med* **22**, 75–91.

Foote, S. L., Bloom, F. E., and Aston-Jones, G. (1983). Nucleus locus ceruleus: new evidence of anatomical and physiological specificity. *Physiol Rev* **63**, 844–914.

Force, T., Pombo, C. M., Avruch, J. A., Bonventre, J. V., and Kyriakis, J. M. (1996). Stress-activated protein kinases in cardiovascular disease. *Circ Res* **78**, 947–953.

Forsyth, R. P. (1968). Blood pressure and avoidance conditioning. *Psychosom Med* **30**, 125–135.

Frame, M. D. S., and Sarelius, I. H. (1993). Regulation of capillary perfusion by small arterioles is spatially organized. *Circ Res* **73**, 155–163.

Frame, M. D. S., and Sarelius, I. H. (1995). L-arginine induced conducted signals alter upstream arteriolar responsivity to l-arginine. *Circ Res* **77**, 695–701.

Franco-Morselli, R., De Mendonca, M., Baudouin-Legros, M., Guicheney, P., and Meyer, P. (1979). Plasma catecholamines in essential human hypertension and in DOCA-salt hypertension of the rat. In *Nervous System and Hypertension*, Meyer, P., and Schmitt, H., Eds., pp. 287–296. Wiley-Flammarion, Paris.

Frank, O. (1905). Der Pulse in den Arterien. *Ztschr f Biol* **46**, 441–553.

Frank, E. (1911). Bestehen Beziehungen zwischen chromafinem System und der chronischen hypertonie des Menschen? Ein kritischer Beitrag zu der Lehre von der physiopathologischen Bedeutund des Adrenalins. *Deutsch Arch Klin Med* **103**, 397.

Frankenhaeuser, M. (1978). Psychoneuroendocrine approaches to the study of emotion as related to stress and coping. *Nebr Symp Motivation* **26,** 123–162.

Frankenhaeuser, M. (1983). The sympathetic-adrenal and pituitary-adrenal response to challenge: comparison between the sexes. In *Biobehavioral Bases of Coronary Heart Disease,* Denbuoski, T. M., Schmidt, T. H., and Blomchen, G., Eds., pp. 91–105. Karger, Basel.

Frankenhaeuser, M. (1987). Stress. In *The Oxford Companion to the Mind,* Gregory, R. L., Ed., pp. 748–750. Oxford University Press, Oxford.

Fraticelli, A., Josephson, R., Danziger, R., Lakatta, E., and Spurgeon, H. (1989). Morphological and contractile characteristics of rat cardiac myocytes from maturation to senescence. *Am J Physiol* **257,** H259–H265.

Fredrikson, M., and Matthews, K. A. (1990). Cardiovascular responses to behavioral stress and hypertension: a meta-analytic review. *Ann Behav Med* **12,** 30–39.

Freeman, R., Davis, J., and Watkins, B. (1977). Development of chronic perinephritic hypertension in dogs without volume expansion. *Am J Physiol* **233,** F278–F281.

Freis, E. D. (1976). Salt, volume and the prevention of hypertension. *Circulation* **53,** 589–595.

Freund, P. R., Rowell, L. B., Murphy, T. M., Hobbs, S. F., and Butler, S. H. (1979). Blockade of the pressor response to muscle ischemia by sensory nerve block in man. *Am J Physiol* **237,** H433–H439.

Freyschuss, U., Hjemdahl, P., Juhlin-Dannfelt, A., and Linde, B. (1988). Cardiovascular and sympathoadrenal responses to mental stress: influence of beta-blockade. *Am J Physiol* **255,** H1443–H1451.

Friberg, P., Folkow, B., and Nordlander, M. (1985). Structural adaptation of the rat left ventricle in response to changes in pressure and volume loads. *Acta Physiol Scand* **125,** 67–80.

Friberg, P., Rupp, H., and Nordlander, M. (1989). Functional and biochemical analyses of isolated rat hearts in renal and reversed renal hypertension. *Acta Physiol Scand* **135,** 123–132.

Friberg, P., Meredith, I., Jennings, G., Lambert, G., Fazio, V., and Esler, M. (1990). Evidence for increased renal norepinephrine overflow during sodium restriction in humans. *Hypertension* **16,** 121–130.

Friberg, P., and Nordlander, M. (1990). Influence of left ventricular and coronary vascular hypertrophy on cardiac performance [Editorial review]. *J Hypertens* **8,** 879–889.

Friberg, P., Sundelin, B., Bohman, S.-O., Bobik, A., Nilsson, H., Wickman, A., Gustafsson, H., Petersen, J., and Adams, M. A. (1994). Renin-angiotensin system in neonatal rats: induction of a renal abnormality in response to ACE inhibition or angiotensin II antagonism. *Kidney Internat* **45,** 485–492.

Friedman, R., and Dahl, L. (1975). The effect of chronic conflict on the blood pressure of rats with a genetic susceptibility to experimental hypertension. *Psychosom Med* **37,** 402–416.

Friedman, R., Tassinari, L. M., Heine, M., and Iwai, J. (1979). Differential development of salt-induced and renal hypertension in Dahl hypertension sensitive rats after neonatal sympathectomy. *Clin Exp Hypertens* **1,** 779–786.

Friedman, J. M., and Halas, J. L. (1998). Leptin and the regulation of body weight in mammals. *Nature* **395,** 763–770.

Friedmann, E., and Thomas, S. A. (1995). Pet ownership, social support and one-year survival after acute myocardial infarction in the Cardiac Arrhythmia Suppression Trial (CAST). *Am J Cardiol* **76,** 1213–1217.

Frohlich, E. D., Tarazi, R. C., and Dustan, H. P. (1969). Reexamination of the hemodynamics of hypertension. *Am J Med Sci* **257,** 9–23.

Frohlich, E. D., and Pfeffer, M. A. (1989). Heart and hypertension: the magnitude of the problem. In *The Heart in Hypertension,* Safar, M. E., and Fouad-Tarazi, F. M., Eds., pp. 169–178. Kluwer Academic Publishers, Dordrecht.

Frühbeck, G. (2004). The adipose tissue as a source of vasoactive factors. *Curr Med Chem Cardiovasc Haematol Agents* **2,** 197–208.

Fujii, K., Sadoshima, S., Okada, Y., Yao, H., Kuwabara, Y., and Ichiya, Y. (1990). Cerebral blood flow and metabolism in normotensive and hypertensive patients with transient neurological deficits. *Stroke* **21,** 283–290.

Fujita, T., Henry, W. L., Bartter, F. C., Lake, C. R., and Delea, C. S. (1980). Factors influencing blood pressure in salt-sensitive patients with hypertension. *Am J Med* **69,** 335–344.

Fujita, T., Ando, K., and Ogata, E. (1990). Systemic and regional hemodynamics in patients with salt sensitive hypertension. *Hypertension* **16,** 235–244.

Fukuda, T., and Kobayashi, T. (1961). On the relation of chemoreceptor stimulation to epinepherine secretion in anoxemia. *Jpn J Physiol* **11,** 467–475.

Fukuda, Y., Sato, A., and Trzebski, A. (1986). Carotid chemoreceptor discharge responses to hypoxia and hypercapnia in normotensive and spontaneously hypertensive rats. *J Auton Nerv Syst* **19,** 1–11.

Fuller, P. J., and Young, M. J. (2005). Mechanisms of mineralocorticoid action. *Hypertension* **46,** 1227–1235.

Funder, J. W., Pearce, P. T., Smith, R., and Smith, A. I. (1988). Mineralocorticoid action: target tissue specificity is enzyme, not receptor, mediated. *Science* **242,** 583–585.

Funder, J. W. (1994). Adrenal steroids. In *Textbook of Hypertension*, Swales, J., Ed., pp. 388–396. Blackwell, Oxford.

Fung, Y. (1984). *Biodynamics: Circulation*. Springer-Verlag, New York.

Fung, Y. (1990). Biomechanics: Motion, Flow, Stress, and Growth. Springer-Verlag, New York.

Fung, Y. (1993). Biomechanics: Mechanical Properties of Living Tissues. Springer-Verlag, New York.

Furchgott, R. F., and Zawadski, J. V. (1980). The obligatory role of endothelial cells in the relaxation of arterial smooth muscle by acetylcholine. *Nature* **288,** 373–376.

Furuyama, M. (1962). Histometrical investigations of arteries in reference to arterial hypertension. *Tohoku J Exp Med* **76,** 388–414.

Gabbai, F. B., Gushwa, L. C., Peterson, O. W., Wilson, C. B., and Blantz, R. C. (1987). Analysis of renal function in the two kidney Goldblatt model. *Am J Physiol* **252,** F131–F137.

Gaida, W., Lang, R. E., Kraft, K., Unger, T., and Ganten, D. (1985). Altered neuropeptide concentrations in spontaneously hypertensive rats: cause or consequence. *Clin Sci* **68,** 35–43.

Gajjar, D., Egan, B., Curé, J., Rust, P., VanTassel, P., and Patel, S. J. (2000). Vascular compression of the rostral ventrolateral medulla in sympathetic mediated essential hypertension. *Hypertension* **36,** 78–82.

Gally, J. A., Montague, P. R., Reeke, G. N., and Edelman, G. M. (1990). The NO hypothesis: possible effects of a short-lived, rapidly diffusible signal in the development and function of the nervous system. *Proc Natl Acad Sci, USA* **87,** 3547–3551.

Galton, F. (1865). Hereditary talent and character. *Macmillan's Magazine* **12,** 157.

Gandevia, S. C., Killian, K., McKenzie, D. K., Crawford, M., Allen, G. M., Gorman, R. B., and Hales, J. P. (1993). Respiratory sensations, cardiovascular control, kinaesthesia and transcranial stimulation during paralysis in humans. *J Physiol (Lond)* **470,** 85–107.

Ganguli, M., Tobian, L., and Iwai, J. (1979). Cardiac output and peripheral resistance in strain of rats sensitive and resistant to chronic excess salt ingestion. *Hypertension* **1,** 3–7.

Ganote, C., and Armstrong, S. (1993). Ischaemia and the myocyte cytoskeleton: review and speculation. *Cardiovasc Res* **27,** 1387–1403.

Ganten, D., Hutchinson, S., and Schelling, P. (1975). The intrinsic brain iso-renin angiotensin system its possible role in central mechanisms of blood pressure. *Clin Sci Mol Med* **48** (suppl), 265S–268S.

Ganten, U., Schroeder, G., Witt, M., Zimmermann, F., Ganten, D., and Stock, G. (1989). Sexual dimorphism of blood pressure in spontaneously hypertensive rats: effects of anti-androgen treatment. *J Hypertens* **7**, 721–726.

Ganten, D., Lindpaintner, K., Ganten, U., Peters, J., Zimmermann, F., Bader, M., and Mullins, J. (1991). Transgenic rats: new animal models in hypertension research. *Hypertension* **17**, 843–855.

Ganten, D., and De Jong, W. (1994). Experimental and genetic models of hypertension. In *Handbook of Hypertension*, Birkenhäger, W. H., and Reid, J. T., Eds., Vol. 16, p. 642. Elsevier, Amsterdam.

Gardiner, S. M., Kemp, P. A., Bennett, T. R., Palmer, R. M. J., and Moncada, S. (1992). Nitric oxide synthase inhibitors cause sustained but reversible hypertension and hindquarter vasoconstriction in Brattleboro rats. *Eur J Pharm* **213**, 449–451.

Gardiner, S. M., Kemp, P. A., and Bennett, T. (1993). Regional haemodynamics in Brattleboro rats during chronic ingestion of N^G-nitro-l-arginine methyl ester. *Blood Pressure* **2**, 228–232.

Gardner-Medwin, D. (1996). Developmental abnormalities of the nervous system. In *Oxford Textbook of Medicine*, Weatherall, D. J., Ledingham, J. G. G., and Warrell, D. A., Eds., Vol. 3, pp. 4105–4122. Oxford University Press, Oxford.

Garrod, A. E. (1902). The incidence of alcaptonuria: a study in chemical individuality. *Lancet* **ii**, 1616–1620.

Garrod, A. E. (1923). *Inborn Errors of Metabolism*. Frowde, London (reprinted 1963 by Oxford University Press, London).

Garthwaite, J. (1991). Glutamate, nitric oxide and cell-cell signalling in the nervous system. *Trends Neurosci* **14**, 60–67.

Gaskell, W. H. (1880). On the tonicity of the heart and blood vessels. *J Physiol (Lond)* **3**, 48–74.

Gattone, V. H., Evan, A. P., Willis, L. R., and Luft, F. C. (1983). Renal afferent arteriole in the spontaneously hypertensive rat. *Hypertension* **5**, 8–16.

Gauer, O. H., and Henry, J. P. (1963). Circulatory basis of fluid volume control. *Physiol Rev* **43**, 423–481.

Gauthier, P., Reis, D. J., and Nathan, M. A. (1981). Arterial hypertension elicited either by lesions or by electrical stimulations of the rostral hypothalamus in the rat. *Brain Res* **211**, 91–105.

Gavras, H., Brunner, H. R., Thurston, H., and Laragh, J. H. (1979). Reciprocation of renin dependency with sodium volume dependency in renal hypertension. *Science* **188**, 1316–1317.

Gavras, I., and Gavras, H. (1995). Role of vasopressin in hypertensive disorders. In *Hypertension: Pathophysiology, Diagnosis and Treatment*, Laragh, J. H., and Brenner, B. M., Eds., Vol. 1, pp. 789–800. Raven Press, New York.

Gazzaniga, M. S. (1997). *The Cognitive Neurosciences*. Bradford MIT Press, Cambridge, MA.

Gebber, G. (1990). Central determinants of sympathetic nerve discharge. In *Central Regulation of Autonomic Function*, Loewy, A., and Spyer, K., Eds., pp. 126–144. Oxford University Press, New York.

Gebber, G. L. (2001). A defence-like reaction an emergent property of a system of coupled non-linear oscillators. *Clin Exp Pharmacol Physiol* **28**, 125–129.

Geer, P. A., Wang, B. C., and Goetz, K. L. (1986). Blood pressure of sino-aortic dogs is not increased by cranial denervation. *Proc Soc Exp Biol Med* **181**, 33–40.

Gehring, W. J., and Hiromi, Y. (1986). Homeotic genes and the homeobox. *Ann Rev Gen* **20**, 147–173.

Georgiades, A., Sherwood, A., Gullette, E. C. D., Babyak, M. A., Hinderliter, A., Waugh, R., Tweedy, D., Craighead, L., Bloomer, R., and Blumenthal, J. A. (2000). Effects of exercise and weight loss on mental stress-induced cardiovascular responses in individuals with high blood pressure. *Hypertension* **36,** 171–176.

Gerdes, A. M., Onodera, T., Wang, X., and McCune, S. A. (1996). Myocyte remodeling during the progression to failure in rats with hypertension. *Hypertension* **28,** 609–614.

Gerin, W., Chaplin, W., Schwartz, J. E., Holland, J., Alter, R., Wheeler, R., Duong, D., and Pickering, T. G. (2005). Sustained blood pressure increase after an acute stressor: the effects of the 11 September 2001 attack on the New York City World Trade Center. *J Hypertens* **23,** 279–284.

Ghez, C. (1991). The cerebellum. In *Principles of Neural Science, 3rd Edition,* Kandel, E. R., Schwartz, J. H., and Jessell, T. M., Eds., pp. 626–646. Prentice-Hall International, London.

Gibbins, I. L., Furness, J. B., Costa, M., MacIntyre, I., Hillyard, C., and Girgis, S. (1985). Co-localization of calcitonin-gene related peptide-like immunoreactivity with substance P in cutaneous, vascular and visceral sensory neurons of guinea pigs. *Neurosci Lett* **1,** 131–136.

Girerd, X., London, G., Boutouyrie, P., Mourad, J.-J., Safar, M., and Laurent, S. (1996). Remodeling of the radial artery in response to a chronic increase in shear stress. *Hypertension* **27** (part 2), 799–803.

Girgis, M., and Shih-Chang, W. (1981). *A New Stereotaxic Atlas of the Rabbit Brain.* Warren H Green, St. Louis.

Girouard, H., Chulak, C., LeJossec, M., Lamontage, D., and De Champlain, J. (2003). Chronic antioxidant treatment improves sympathetic function and β-adrenergic pathway in the spontaneously hypertensive rat. *J Hypertens* **21,** 179–188.

Gleibermann, L. (1973). Blood pressure and dietary salt in human hypertension. *Ecol Food Nutr* **2,** 143–156.

Glick, G., and Braunwald, E. (1965). Relative roles of the sympathetic and parasympathetic nervous system in the reflex control of heart rate. *Circ Res* **16,** 363–375.

Gluckman, P., and Hanson, M. (2005). *The Fetal Matrix: Evolution, Development and Disease.* Cambridge University Press, Cambridge.

Glynn, I. (1999). An Anatomy of Thought: The Origin and Machinery of the Mind. Weidenfeld & Nicolson, London.

Gödecke, A., Decking, U. K., Ding, Z., Hirchenhain, J., Bidmain, H.-J., Gödecke, S., and Schrader, J. (1997). Coronary haemodynamics in endothelial NO synthase knockout mice. *Circ Res* **82,** 186–194.

Goldblatt, H., Lynch, J., Hanzal, R. F., and Summerville, W. W. (1934). Studies on experimental hypertension: I. Production of persistent elevation of systolic blood pressure by means of renal ischemia. *J Exp Med* **59,** 374–379.

Goldblatt, H. (1937). Studies on experimental hypertension: III. Production of persistent hypertension in monkeys (Macaque) by renal ischemia. *J Exp Med* **65,** 671–675.

Goldblatt, H. (1964). Hypertension of renal origin: historical and experimental background. *American Journal of Surgery* **107,** 21–25.

Goldman-Rakic, P. S. (1987). Circuitry of primate prefrontal cortex and regulation of behavior by representational memory. In *Handbook of Physiology, Section 1: The Nervous System, Vol. 5, Higher Functions of the Brain,* Mountcastle, V. B., Ed., pp. 373–417. American Physiological Society, Bethesda, MD.

Goldring, W., Chasis, H., Ranges, H. A., and Smith, H. W. (1941). Effective renal blood flow in subjects with essential hypertension. *J Clin Invest* **20,** 637–653.

Goldring, W., and Chasis, H. (1944). *Hypertension and Hypertensive Disease,* pp. 39–95. Commonwealth Fund, New York.

Goldstein, D. S. (1983). Plasma catecholamines and essential hypertension: an analytical review. *Hypertension* **5,** 86–99.

Goldstein, D. S. (1992). Central catecholamines and the control of sympathetic tone. In *Central Neural Mechanisms in Cardiovascular Regulation*, Kunos, G., and Ciriello, J., Eds., Vol. 2, pp. 113–208. Birkhauser, Boston.

Gomez, A. M., Valdivia, H. H., Cheng, H., Lederer, M. R., Santana, L. F., Cannell, M. B., McCune, S. A., Altschuld, R. A., and Lederer, W. J. (1997). Defective excitation-contraction coupling in experimental cardiac hypertrophy and heart failure. *Science* **276**, 800–806.

Goodchild, A. K., Dampney, R. A. L., and Bandler, R. (1982). A method for evoking physiological responses by stimulation of cell bodies but not axons of pasage within localized regions of the central nervous system. *J Neurosci Meth* **6**, 351–363.

Goodwin, G. M., McCloskey, D. I., and Mitchell, J. H. (1972). Cardiovascular and respiratory responses to changes in central command during isometric exercise at constant muscle tension. *J Physiol (Lond)* **226**, 173–190.

Gordon, R. D., Stowasser, M., Klemm, S. A., and Tunny, T. J. (1994). Primary aldosteronism and other forms of mineralocorticoid hypertension. In *Textbook of Hypertension*, Swales, J. D., Ed., pp. 865–892. Blackwell, Oxford.

Gorzelniak, K., Engeli, S., Janke, J., Luft, F. C., and Sharma, A. M. (2002). Hormonal regulation of the human adipose tissue renin angiotensin system relationship to obesity and hypertension. *J Hypertens* **20**, 965–973.

Göthberg, G. (1982). Structural adaptation of the renal vascular bed in rats. Effects of hypertension, hypotension, kidney hypertrophy and ageing on renal flow resistance and glomerular filtration. Department of Physiology, University of Göteborg.

Göthberg, G., Hallbäck, M., Lundin, S., Ricksten, S., and Folkow, B. (1976). A comparison of renal flow resistance in normotensive control rats and spontaneously hypertensive rats. *Clin Exp Pharmacol Physiol* (suppl 3), 79–82.

Goto, A., Ikeda, T., Tobian, L., Iwai, J., and Johnson, M. A. (1981). Brain lesions in the paraventricular nuclei and catecholaminergic neurons minimize salt hypertension in Dahl salt-sensitive rats. *Clin Sci* **61**, 53S.

Gotoh, E. (1982). Cerebrospinal fluid sodium concentrations and blood pressure in essential hypertension: a comparison between salt sensitive and salt resistant groups. *Nippon Naika Gakkai Zasshi* **71**, 1528–1533.

Gould, K. L., and Lipscomb, K. (1974). Effects of coronary stenoses on coronary flow reserve and resistance. *Am J Cardiol* **34**, 48–55.

Gould, K. L. (1980). Dynamic coronary stenosis. *Am J Cardiol* **45**, 286–292.

Grady, C. L., McIntosh, A. R., Horwitz, B., Maisog, J. M., Ungerleider, L. G., Mentis, M. J., Pietrini, P., Schapiro, M. B., and Haxby, J. V. (1995). Age-related reductions in human recognition memory due to impaired encoding. *Science* **269**, 218–221.

Graef, I., and Page, I. (1940). The pathological anatomy of cellophane perinephritis. *Am J Path* **16**, 211–221.

Graham, J. D. P. (1945). High blood pressure after battle. *Lancet* ii, 239–240.

Graham, R. M., Perez, D. M., Hwa, J., and Piascik, M. T. (1996). Alpha 1–adrenergic receptor subtypes: molecular structure, function and signaling. *Circ Res* **78**, 737–749.

Granata, A. R., Kumada, M., and Reis, D. J. (1985). Sympathoinhibition by A1 noradrenergic neurons is mediated by neurons in the C1 area of the rostral medulla. *J Auton Nerv Syst* **14**, 387–395.

Granger, H. J., and Guyton, A. C. (1969). Autoregulation of the total systemic circulation following destruction of the central nervous system in the dog. *Circ Res* **25**, 379–388.

Grant, L. D., and Stumpf, W. E. (1975). Hormone uptake sites in relation to CNS biogenic amine systems. In *Anatomical Neuroendocrinology*, Grant, L. D., and Stumpf, W. E., Eds., pp. 445–463. Karger, Basel.

Grassi, G., Giannatasio, C., Cleroux, J., Cuspidi, C., Sampieri, Bolla, G. B., and Mancia, G. (1988). Cardiopulmonary reflex before and after regression of left ventricular hypertrophy in essential hypertension. *Hypertension* **12,** 227–237.

Grassi, G., Seravalle, G., Calhoun, D. A., and Mancia, G. (1994). Physical training and baroreceptor control of sympathetic nerve activity in humans. *Hypertension* **23,** 294–301.

Grassi, G., Seravalle, G., Cattaneo, B. M., Bolla, G. B., Lamfranchi, A., Colombo, M., Giannatasio, C., Brunani, A., Cavagnini, F., and Mancia, G. (1995). Sympathetic activation in obese normotensive subjects. *Hypertension* **25,** 560–563.

Grassi, G. (1998). Role of the sympathetic nervous system in human hypertension. *J Hypertens* **16,** 1979–1987.

Grassi, G., Cattaneo, B. M., Seravalle, G., Lanchfranchi, A., and Mancia, G. (1998). Baroreflex control of sympathetic nerve activity in essential and secondary hypertension. *Hypertension* **31** (part 1), 68–72.

Grassi, G., Seravalle, G., Colombo, M., Bolla, G. B., Cattaneo, B. M., Cavagnini, F. et al. (1998). Body weight reduction, sympathetic nerve traffic and arterial baroreflex in obese normotensive humans. *Circulation* **97,** 2037–2042.

Grassi, G. (1999). Debating sympathetic overactivity as a hallmark of human obesity: a pro's position. *J Hypertens* **17,** 1059–1060.

Gray, S. D. (1982). Anatomical and physiological aspects of cardiovascular function in Wistar-Kyoto and spontaneously hypertensive rats at birth. *Clin Sci* **63,** 383s–385s.

Gray, S. (1984). Spontaneous hypertension in the neonatal rat: a review. *Clin Exp Hypertens Theory Pract* **A6,** 755–781.

Gray, J. A. (1994). A model of the limbic system and basal ganglia: applications to anxiety and schizophrenia. In *The Cognitive Neurosciences*, Gazzaniga, M. S., Ed., pp. 1165–1176. MIT Press, Cambridge, MA.

Greene, A. S., Tonellato, P. J., Lui, J., Lombard, J. H., and Cowley, A. J., Jr. (1989). Microvascular rarefaction and tissue vascular resistance in hypertension. *Am J Physiol* **256,** H126–H131.

Greengard, P. (2001). The neurobiology of slow synaptic transmission. *Science* **294,** 1024–1030.

Greenland, P. (2001). Beating high blood pressure with low-sodium DASH [Editorial]. *N Engl J Med* **201,** 53–55.

Gregg, D. (1950). *Coronary Circulation in Health and Disease.* Lea & Febiger, Philadelphia.

Gribbin, B., Pickering, T. G., Sleight, P., and Peto, R. (1971). Effect of age and high blood pressure on baroreflex sensitivity in man. *Circ Res* **29,** 424–431.

Griffith, T. M., Edwards, D. H., Davies, R. L., Harrison, T. J., and Evans, K. T. (1987). EDRF coordinates the behaviour of vascular resistance vessels. *Nature* **329,** 442–445.

Griffith, T. M., Edwards, D. H., and Davies, R. L. (1990). EDRF in intact vascular networks. *Blood Vessels* **27,** 230–237.

Griffiths, A. J. F., Miller, J. H., Suzuki, D. T., Lewontin, R. C., and Gelbart, W. M. (1993). *An Introduction to Genetic Analysis.* W.H. Freeman, New York.

Grim, C. E., Luft, F. C., Miller, J. Z., Brown, P. L., Gannon, M. A., and Weinberger, M. H. (1979). Effects of sodium loading and depletion in normotensive first degree relatives of essential hypertensives. *J Lab Clin Med* **94,** 764–771.

Grim, C. E., Miller, J. Z., Luft, F., Christian, J. C., and Weinberger, M. H. (1979). Genetic influences on renin, aldosterone, and the renal excretion of sodium and potassium following volume expansion and contraction in man. *Hypertension* **1,** 583–590.

Grim, C. E., Henry, J. P., and Myers, H. (1995). High blood pressure in blacks: salt, slavery, survival, stress and racism. In *Hypertension: Pathophysiology, Diagnosis and Management*, Laragh, J. H., and Brenner, B. M., Eds., Vol. 1, pp. 171–208. Raven Press, New York.

Grobbee, D. E. (1991). Methodology of sodium sensitivity assessment: the example of age and sex. *Hypertension* **17** (suppl I), I-109–I-114.

Grobbee, D. E. (1994). Electrolyte intake and human hypertension: sodium and potassium. In *Textbook of Hypertension*, Swales, J. D., Ed., pp. 539–551. Blackwell, Oxford.

Grodins, F. S., and Buoncristiani, J. F. (1967). General formulation of the cardiovascular control problem: mathematical models of the mechanical system. In *Physical Bases of Circulatory Transport*, Reeve, E. B., and Guyton, A. C., Eds., pp. 61–75. W.B. Saunders, Philadelphia.

Grollman, A., Muirhead, E. E., and Vanatta, J. (1949). Role of the kidney in the pathogenesis of hypertension as determined by a study of the effects of bilateral nephrectomy and other experimental procedures on the blood pressure of the dog. *Am J Physiol* **157**, 21–30.

Grollman, A. (1951). Experimental studies on hypertension. In *Hypertension: A Symposium*, Bell, E. T., Clawson, B. J., and Fahr, G. E., Eds. University of Minnesota Press, Minneapolis.

Groppelli, A., Giorgi, D. M. A., Omboni, S., Parati, G., and Mancia, G. (1992). Persistent blood pressure increase induced by heavy smoking. *J Hypertens* **10**, 495–499.

Grossman, W., Jones, D., and McLaurin, L. P. (1975). Wall stress and patterns of hypertrophy. *J Clin Invest* **56**, 56–64.

Grunfeld, S., Hamilton, C. A., Mesaros, S., McClain, S. W., Dominiczak, A. F., Bohr, D. F., and Malinski, T. (1995). Role of superoxide in the depressed nitric oxide production by the endothelium of genetically hypertensive rats. *Hypertension* **26** (part 1), 854–857.

Guidi, E., Bianchi, G., Rivolta, E., Ponticelli, C., Quarto di Palo, F., Minetti, L., and Polli, E. (1985). Hypertension in man with a kidney transplant: role of familial versus other factors. *Nephron* **41**, 14–21.

Guidi, E., Menghetti, D., Milani, S., Montagnino, G., Palazzi, P., and Bianchi, G. (1996). Hypertension may be transplanted with the kidney in humans: a long-term historical perspective. *J Am Soc Nephrol* **7**, 1131–1138.

Guidicelli, J. F., Freslon, J. L., Glasson, S., and Richer, C. (1980). Captopril and hypertension: development in SHR. *Clin Exp Hypertens* **A:2**, 1083–1096.

Guilleminault, C., Motta, J., Mihm, F., and Melvin, K. (1986). Obstructive sleep apnea and cardiac index. *Chest* **89**, 331–334.

Guron, G., and Friberg, P. (2000). An intact renin angiotensin system is a prerequisite for normal renal development. *J Hypertens* **18**, 123–137.

Gutkowska, J., Antunes-Rodrigues, J., and McCann, S. M. (1997). Atrial natriuretic peptide in brain and pituitary gland. *Physiol Rev* **77**, 465–515.

Guyenet, P. G. (1990). Role of the ventral medulla oblongata in blood pressure regulation. In *Central Regulation of Autonomic Functions*, Loewy, A. D., and Spyer, K. M., Eds., pp. 145–167. Oxford University Press, New York.

Guyenet, P. G., and Koshiya, N. (1995). Working model of the sympathetic chemoreflex in rats. *Clin Exp Hypertens (Part A)* **17**, 167–179.

Guyton, A. (1955). Determination of cardiac output by equating venous return curves with cardiac response curves. *Physiol Rev* **35**, 123–129.

Guyton, A. C., and Coleman, T. G. (1967). Long-term regulation of the circulation: interrelationships with body fluid volumes. In *Physical Bases of Circulatory Transport: Regulation and Exchange*, Reeve, E. B., and Guyton, A. C., Eds., pp. 179–201. W.B. Saunders, Philadelphia.

Guyton, A. C., Coleman, T. G., Cowley, A. W. J., Liard, J.-F., Norman, R. A. J., and Manning, R. D. J. (1972). Systems analysis of arterial pressure regulation and hypertension. *Ann Biomed Eng* **1**, 254–281.

Guyton, A. C., Coleman, T. G., and Granger, H. J. (1972). Circulation: overall regulation. *Annu Rev Physiol* **34**, 13–46.

Guyton, A. C., Coleman, T. G., Cowley, A. W., Jr, Manning, R. D., Norman, R. A., and Ferguson, J. D. (1974). A systems analysis approach to understanding long range arterial blood pressure control and hypertension. *Circ Res* **35,** 159–176.

Guyton, A. C. (1980). *Arterial Pressure and Hypertension.* W.B. Saunders, Philadelphia.

Guyton, A. C. (1990). The surprising kidney-fluid mechanism for pressure control—its infinite gain! *Hypertension* **16,** 725–730.

Guyton, A. C., Hall, J. E., Coleman, T. G., Manning, R. D., Jr., and Norman, R. A., Jr. (1995). The dominant role of the kidneys in long-term arterial pressure regulation in normal and hypertensive states. In *Hypertension: Pathophysiology, Diagnosis and Management,* Laragh, J. H., and Brenner, B. M., Eds., Vol. 1, pp. 1311–1326. Raven Press, New York.

Haddy, F. J., and Overbeck, H. W. (1976). The role of humoral agents in volume expanded hypertension. *Life Sci* **19,** 935–948.

Hadrava, V., Tremblay, J., Sekaly, R. P., and Hamet, P. (1992). Accelerated entry of aortic smooth muscle cells from spontaneously hypertensive rats in the S phase of the cell cycle. *Biochem Cell Biol* **70,** 599–604.

Haeusler, G. (1971). Early pre- and postjunctional effects of 6–hydroxydopamine. *J Pharmacol* **178,** 49–62.

Haeusler, G., Finch, L., and Thoenen, H. (1972). Central adrenergic neurons and the initiation and development of experimental hypertension. *Experientia* **28,** 1200–1203.

Haeusler, G. (1976). Central adrenergic neurons in experimental hypertension. In *Regulation of Blood Pressure by the Central Nervous System,* Onesti, G., Fernandes, M., and Kim, K. E., Eds., pp. 53–64. Grune & Stratton, New York.

Haggendal, E., and Johansson, B. B. (1971). Pathophysiological aspects of the blood barrier change in acute arterial hypertension. *Eur Neurol* **6,** 24–28.

Haldane, J. S., and Priestley, J. G. (1935). *Respiration.* Clarendon Press, Oxford.

Hales, S. (1733). *Statical Essays: Containing Haemastaticks.* (No. 22, History of Medicine Series) Hafner Publishing, New York.

Hall, W. D. (1985). Secondary causes of hypertension in blacks. *In Hypertension in Blacks: Epidemiology, Pathophysiology and Treatment* (W. D. Hall, E. Saunders, and N. B. Shulman, Eds.), pp. 144–155. Year Book Publishers, Inc, Chicago.

Hall, J. E., Brands, M. W., Hildebrandt, D. A., and Mizelle, H. L. (1992). Obesity-associated hypertension: hyperinsulinaemia and renal mechanisms. *Hypertension* **19** (suppl I), I-45–I-55.

Hall, J. E., Brands, M. W., Dixon, W. N., and Smith, M. J. (1993). Obesity-induced hypertension: renal function and systemic hemodynamics. *Hypertension* **22,** 292–299.

Hall, J. E., and Granger, J. P. (1994). Role of sodium and fluid excretion in hypertension. In *Textbook of Hypertension,* Swales, J. D., Ed., pp. 360–387. Blackwell, Oxford.

Hall, J. E. (2003a). Arthur C. Guyton, MD (1919–2003): in memoriam. *Hypertension* **41,** 1175–1177.

Hall, J. E. (2003b). The kidney, hypertension and obesity. *Hypertension* **41** (2), 625–633.

Hallbäck, M. (1975). Consequence of social isolation on blood pressure, cardiovascular reactivity and design in spontaneously hypertensive rats. *Acta Physiol Scand* **93,** 455–465.

Hallbäck-Nordlander, M. (1980). Left/right ventricular weight ratio: an estimate of "cardiac adaptation to hypertension." *Clin Sci* **59,** 415s–417s.

Hambling, J. (1951). Emotions and symptoms in essential hypertension. *B J Med Psychol* **24,** 242.

Hamet, P., Hadrava, V., Kruppa, U., and Tremblay, J. (1988). Vascular smooth muscle cell hyper-responsiveness to growth factors in hypertension. *J Hypertens* **6** (suppl 4), S36–S39.

Hamet, P., Richard, L., Dam, T.-V., Teiger, E., Orlov, S. N., Gaboury, L., Gossard, F., and Tremblay, J. (1995). Apoptosis in target organs of hypertension. *Hypertension* **26,** 642–648.

Hamet, P., Pausova, Z., Adarichev, V., Adaricheva, K., and Tremblay, J. (1998). Hypertension: genes and environment. *J Hypertens* **16,** 397–418.

Hamilton, W. F., Woodbury, R. A., and Harper, H. T. (1936). Physiologic relationships between intrathoracic, intraspinal and arterial pressures. *J Am Med Assoc* **107,** 853–856.

Hamilton, W. F., and Dow, P. (1939). An experimental study of the standing waves in the pulse propagated through the aorta. *Am J Physiol* **125,** 48–59.

Hamilton, W. F. (1944). Arterial pulse. In *Medical Physics*, Glasser, O., Ed., Vol. 1, pp. 7–9. Year Book Publishers, Chicago.

Hamilton, M., Pickering, G., Fraser Roberts, J., and Sowry, G. (1954a). The aetiology of essential hypertension. 1. The arterial pressure in the general population. *Clin Sci* **13,** 11–35.

Hamilton, M., Pickering, G., Fraser Roberts, J., and Sowry, G. (1954b). The aetiology of essential hypertension. 2. Scores for arterial blood pressures adjusted for differences in age and sex. *Clin Sci* **13,** 37–49.

Hamilton, M., Pickering, G. W., Fraser Roberts, J. A., and Sowry, G. S. C. (1954c). The aetiology of essential hypertension. 4. The role of inheritance. *Clin Sci* **14,** 273–304.

Hamilton, C. A., and Reid, J. L. (1983). Alpha adrenoceptors and autonomic mechanisms in perinephritic hypertension in the rabbit. *Hypertension* **5,** 958–967.

Hamilton, C. A., Brosnan, M. J., McIntyre, M., Graham, D., and Dominiczak, A. F. (2001). Superoxide excess in hypertension and aging: a common cause of endothelial dysfunction. *Hypertension* **37** (part 2), 529–534.

Hamlyn, J. M., Hamilton, B. P., and Manunta, P. (1996). Endogenous ouabain sodium balance and blood pressure: a review and a hypothesis. *J Hypertens* **14,** 151–167.

Hanin, I. (1996). The Gulf War, stress and a leaky blood brain barrier. *Nat Med* **2,** 1307–1308.

Hanis, C. L., Sing, C. F., Clarke, W. R., and Schrott, H. G. (1983). Multivariate models for human genetic analysis: aggregation, co-aggregation and tracking of systolic blood pressure and weight. *Am J Hum Genet* **35,** 1196–1205.

Hannan, R. D., Luyken, J., and Rothblum, L. I. (1995). Regulation of rDNA transcription factors during cardiomyocyte hypertrophy induced by adrenergic agents. *J Biol Chem* **270,** 8290–8297.

Hansen, M. J., Jovanovska, V., and Morris, M. J. (2005). Adaptive responses in hypothalamic neuropeptide Y in the face of prolonged high fat feeding in the rat. *J Neurochem* **88,** 909–916.

Hansson, J. H., Nelson-Williams, C., Susuki, H., Schild, L., Shimkets, R. A., Lu, Y., Canessa, C., Iwasaki, T., Rossier, B. C., and Lifton, R. P. (1995). Hypertension caused by a truncated epithelial sodium channel γ-subunit: genetic heterogeneity of Liddle syndrome. *Nat Gen* **11,** 76–82.

Hansson, L., Hedner, T., and Jern, S. (1997). Psychosocial factors and blood pressure. Why are nuns better off? [Editorial]. *Blood Pressure* **6,** 68.

Harada, K., Komuro, I., Zou, Y., Kudoh, S., Kiijima, K., Matsubara, H., Sugaya, T., Murakami, K., and Yazaki, Y. (1998). Acute pressure overload could induce hypertrophic responses in the heart of angiotensin II type 1a knockout mice. *Circ Res* **82,** 779–785.

Harburg, E., Erfurt, J. C., Chape, C., Hauenstein, L. S., Schull, W. J., and Schork, M. A. (1973). Socioecological stressor areas and black-white blood pressure: Detroit. *J Chronic Dis* **26,** 595–611.

Harburg, E., Erfurt, J. C., Hauenstein, L. S., Schull, W. J., and Schork, M. A. (1973). Socioecological stress, suppressed hostility, skin color and black-white blood pressure (in Detroit). *Psychosom Med* **35,** 276–296.

Harper, R. N., Moore, M. A., Marr, M. C., Watts, L. E., and Hutchins, P. M. (1978). Arteriolar rarefaction in the conjunctiva of human essential hypertensives. *Microvasc Res* **16,** 369–372.

Harper, S. L., and Bohlen, H. G. (1984). Microvascular adaptation in the cerebral cortex of adult spontaneously hypertensive rats. *Hypertension* **6,** 408–419.

Harrap, S. B., Louis, W. J., and Doyle, A. E. (1984). Failure of psychosocial stress to induce chronic hypertension in the rat. *J Hypertens* **2,** 653–662.

Harrap, S. B. (1986). Genetic analysis of blood pressure and sodium balance in spontaneously hypertensive rats. *Hypertension* **8,** 572–582.

Harrap, S. B., Nicolaci, J. A., and Doyle, A. E. (1986). Persistent effects on blood pressure and renal haemodynamics following chronic angiotensin converting enzyme inhibition with perindopril. *Clin Exp Pharmacol Physiol* **13,** 753–765.

Harrap, S. B. (1988). Causes and effects of high blood pressure: a longitudinal approach to cosegregational analysis. *J Cardiovasc Pharmacol* **12,** S99–S109.

Harrap, S. B., Macpherson, F., Wilson, W. G., Davies, D. L., Isaksson, O. P. G., Folkow, B., and Lever, A. F. (1988). Failure of chronic administration of growth hormone to affect blood pressure, vascular reactivity and sodium metabolism in normal rats. *J Hypertens* **6** (suppl 4), S170–S172.

Harrap, S. B., Van der Merwe, W. M., Griffin, S. A., Macpherson, F., and Lever, A. F. (1990). Brief angiotensin converting enzyme inhibitor treatment in young spontaneously hypertensive rats reduces blood pressure long-term. *Hypertension* **16,** 603–614.

Harrap, S. B., Wang, B.-Z., and MacLellan, D. G. (1992). Renal transplantation between male and female spontaneously hypertensive rats. *Hypertension* **19,** 431–434.

Harrap, S. (1994). Genetic approaches to hypertension. In *Textbook of Hypertension*, Swales, J., Ed., pp. 504–518. Blackwell, Oxford.

Harrap, S., Datodi, S., Crapper, E., and Bach, L. (1994). Hypertension and cardiac hypertrophy in growth hormone deficient rats. *Clin Sci* **87,** 239–243.

Harrap, S. B., Cumming, A. D., Davies, D. L., Foy, C. J. W., Fraser, R., Kamitani, A., Connor, J. M., Lever, A. F., and Watt, G. C. M. (2000). Glomerular hyperfiltration high renin and low extracellular volume in high blood pressure. *Hypertension* **35,** 952–957.

Harrington, M., Kincaid-Smith, P., and McMichael, J. (1959). Results of treatment in malignant hypertension. A seven year experience in 94 cases. *Brit Med J* **ii,** 969–980.

Harris, A. K., Stopak, D., and Wild, P. (1981). Fibroblast traction as a mechanism for collagen morphogenesis. *Nature* **290,** 249–251.

Harshfield, G. A., Pickering, T. G., James, G. D., and Blank, S. G. (1990). Blood pressure variability and reactivity in the natural environment. In *Blood Pressure Measurements: New Techniques in Autonomic and 24-Hour Indirect Blood Pressure Monitoring*, Meyer-Sabellek, W., Anlauf, M., Cotzen, R., and Steinfeld, L., Eds., pp. 241–252. Steinkopff, Darmstadt.

Harshfield, G. A., and Grim, C. E. (1997). Stress hypertension: the "wrong" genes in the "wrong" environment. *Acta Physiol Scand* **161** (suppl. 640), 129–132.

Haselton, J. R., and Guyenet, P. G. (1989). Electrophysiological characterisation of putative C1 adrenergic neurons in the rat. *Neuroscience* **30,** 199–214.

Hasenfuss, G., Reinecke, H., Studer, R., Meyer, M., Pieske, B., Holtz, J. et al. (1994). Relation between myocardial function and expression of sarcoplasmic reticulum Ca^{2+}-ATPase in failing and nonfailing human myocardium. *Circ Res* **75,** 434–442.

Hashimoto, K., Makino, S., Hirasawa, R., Takao, T., Sugawara, M., Murakami, K., Ono, K., and Ota, Z. (1989). Abnormalities in the hypothalamo-pituitary-adrenal axis in spontaneously hypertensive rats during development of hypertension. *Endocrinology* **125,** 1161–1167.

Hasking, G. J., Esler, M. D., Jennings, G. L., Burton, D., Johns, J. A., and Korner, P. I. (1986). Norepinephrine spillover to plasma in patients with congestive heart failure: evidence of increased overall and cardiorenal sympathetic nervous activity. *Circulation* **73,** 615–621.

Hattori, T., Hashimoto, K., and Ota, Z. (1986). Adrenocorticotropin responses to corticotropin releasing factor and vasopressin in spontaneously hypertensive rats. *Hypertension* **8**, 386–390.

Hausberg, M., Morgan, D. A., Chapleau, M. A., Sivitz, W. I., Mark, A. L., and Haynes, W. G. (2002). Differential modulation of leptin-induced sympathoexcitation by baroreflex activation. *J Hypertens* **20**, 1633–1641.

Hausler, A., Girard, J., Baumann, J. B., Ruch, W., and Otten, U. H. (1983). Stress-induced secretion of ACTH and corticosterone during development of spontaneous hypertension in rats. *Clin Exp Hypertens*, **A5**, 11–19.

Hausler, A., Oberholzer, M., Baumann, J. B., Girard, J., and Heitz, P. (1984). Quantitative analysis of ACTH-immunoreactive cells in the anterior pituitary of young spontaneously hypertensive and normotensive rats. *Cell Tiss Res* **236**, 229–235.

Haynes, W. G., Morgan, D. A., Djalali, A., Sivitz, W. I., and Mark, A. L. (1999). Interactions between the melanocortin system and leptin in the control of sympathetic nerve traffic. *Hypertension* **33** (part II), 542–547.

He, F. J., Markandu, N. D., and MacGregor, G. A. (1998). Importance of the renin system for determining blood pressure fall with acute salt restriction in hypertensive and normotensive whites. *Hypertension* **38**, 321–325.

He, F. J., and MacGregor, G. A. (2003). How far should salt intake be reduced? *Hypertension* **42**, 1093–1099.

Head, G. A., and Korner, P. I. (1980). Mechanisms of acute hypertension and bradycardia following intracisternal 6–hydroxydopamine in conscious rabbits. *Eur J Pharm* **66**, 111–115.

Head, G. A. (1981). The role of central monoaminergic pathways in cardiovascular control. PhD thesis, Baker Medical Research Institute and Monash University, Melbourne.

Head, G. A., and Korner, P. (1982). Cardiovascular functions of brain serotonergic neurons in the rabbit as analysed from the acute and chronic effects of 5,6–dihydroxytryptamine. *J Cardiovasc Pharmacol* **4**, 398–408.

Head, G. A., Korner, P. I., Lewis, S. L., and Badoer, E. (1983). Contributions of noradrenergic and serotonergic neurons to the circulatory effects of centrally acting clonidine and alpha-methyldopa in rabbits. *J Cardiovasc Pharmacol* **5**, 945–953.

Head, G., and de Jong, W. (1986). Differential blood pressure responses to intracisternal clonidine, alpha-methyldopa, and 6–hydroxydopamine in conscious normotensive and spontaneously hypertensive rats. *J Cardiovasc Pharmacol* **8**, 735–742.

Head, G. A., Badoer, E., and Korner, P. I. (1987). Cardiovascular role of A1 catecholaminergic neurons in the rabbit. Effect of chronic lesions on responses to methyldopa, clonidine and 6–OHDA induced transmitter release. *Brain Res* **412**, 18–28.

Head, G. A., and McCarty, R. (1987). Vagal and sympathetic components of the baroreceptor-heart rate reflex in conscious rats. *J Auton Nerv Syst* **21**, 203–213.

Head, G. A., and Adams, M. A. (1988). Time course of changes in baroreceptor reflex control of heart rate in conscious SHR and WKY: contribution of the cardiac vagus and sympathetic nerves. *Clin Exp Pharmacol Physiol* **15**, 289–292.

Head, R. J. (1989). Hypernoradrenergic innervation: its relationship to functional and hyperplastic changes in the vasculature of the spontaneously hypertensive rat. *Blood Vessels* **26**, 1–20.

Head, R. J. (1991). Hypernoradrenergic innervation and vascular smooth muscle hyperplastic changes. *Blood Vessels* **28**, 173–178.

Head, G. A., and Adams, M. A. (1992). Characterisation of the baroreceptor-heart rate reflex during development in spontaneously hypertensive rats. *Clin Exp Pharmacol Physiol* **19**, 587–597.

Head, G. A. (1995). Baroreflexes and cardiovascular regulation in hypertension. *J Cardiovasc Pharmacol* **26,** S7–S16.

Head, G. A., and Burke, S. L. (2000). Comparison of renal sympathetic baroreflex effects of rilmenidine and alpha-methylnoradrenaline in the ventrolateral medulla of the rabbit. *J Hypertens* **18,** 1263–1276.

Head, G. A. (2002). Spontaneous baroreflex sensitivity towards an ideal index of cardiovascular risk. *J Hypertens* **20,** 829–831.

Heagerty, A., Bund, S., and Aalkjaer, C. (1988). Effects of drug treatment on human resistance arteriole morphology in essential hypertension: direct evidence for structural remodelling of resistance vessels. *Lancet* **ii,** 1209–1210.

Heagerty, A., Aalkjaer, C., Bund, S., Korsgaard, N., and Mulvany, M. (1993). Small artery structure in hypertension: dual processes of remodelling and growth. *Hypertension* **21,** 391–397.

Hebb, D. O. (1949). *The Organisation of Behaviour.* Wiley, New York.

Heesch, C. M., Thames, M. D., and Abboud, F. M. (1984). Acute resetting of carotid sinus baroreceptors. I. Dissociation between discharge and wall changes. *Am J Physiol* **247,** H824–H832.

Heesen, W. E., Beltman, F. W., May, J. F., Smit, A. J., de Graeff, P. A., Havinga, T. K., Schuurman, F. H., van der Veur, E., Hamer, J. P. M., Meyboom-de Jong, B., and Lie, K. I. (1997). High prevalence of concentric remodeling in elderly individuals with isolated systolic hypertension from a population survey. *Hypertension* **29,** 539–543.

Hein, L., Stevens, M. E., Barsh, G. S., Pratt, R. E., Kobilka, B. K., and Dzau, V. J. (1997). Overexpression of angiotensin AT1 receptor transgene in the mouse myocardium produces a lethal phenotype associated with myocyte hyperplasia and heart block. *Proc Natl Acad Sci, USA* **94,** 6391–6396.

Helber, A., Wambach, G., Hummerich, W., Bonner, G., Muerer, K. A., and Kaufmann, W. (1980). Evidence for a subgroup of essential hypertensives with non-suppressible excretion of aldosterone during sodium loading. *Klin Wochenschr* **58,** 439–447.

Hendley, E. D., Cierpial, M. A., and McCarty, R. (1988). Sympathetic-adrenal medullary response to stress in hypertensive and hyperactive rats. *Physiol Behav* **44,** 47–51.

Hendley, E. D., and Ohlsson, W. G. (1991). Two new inbred rat strains derived from SHR: WKHA hyperactive, and WKHT hypertensive rats. *Am J Physiol* **261,** H583–H589.

Henrich, W. L. (1992). Functional and organic ischemic renal disease. In *The Kidney: Physiology and Pathophysiology*, Seldin, D. W., and Giebisch, G., Eds., Vol. 3, pp. 3289–3304. Raven Press, New York.

Henry, J. P., Meehan, J. P., and Stephens, P. M. (1967). The use of psychological stimuli to induce prolonged systolic hypertension in mice. *Psychosom Med* **29,** 408–432.

Henry, J. P., and Cassel, J. C. (1969). Psychosocial factors in essential hypertension: recent epidemiological and animal experimental evidence. *Am J Epidemiol* **90,** 171–200.

Henry, J. P., Stephens, P. M., Axelrod, J., and Mueller, R. A. (1971). Effect of psychosocial stimulation on the enzymes involved in the biosynthesis and metabolism of noradrenaline and adrenaline. *Psychosom Med* **33,** 227–237.

Henry, J., Ely, D., and Stephens, P. (1972). Blood pressure, catecholamines and social role in relation to the development of cardiovascular disease in mice. In *Neural and Psychological Mechanisms in Cardiovascular Disease*, Zanchetti, A., Ed., pp. 211–223. Casa Editrice Il Ponte, Milan.

Henry, J. P., and Grim, C. E. (1990). Psychosocial mechanisms of primary hypertension. *J Hypertens* **8,** 783–794.

Henry, J. P. (1993a). Biological basis of the stress response. *NIPS* **8,** 69–73.

Henry, J. P. (1993b). Psychological and physiological responses to stress: the right hemisphere and the hypothalamo-pituitary-adrenal axis, an inquiry into problems of human bonding. *Int Physiol Behav Sci* **28,** 368–386.

Henry, J. P., Liu, Y.-Y., Nadra, W. E., Qian, C., Mormède, P., Lemaire, V., Ely, D., and Hendley, E. D. (1993). Psychosocial stress can induce chronic hypertension in normotensive strains of rats. *Hypertension* **21**, 714–723.

Henry, J. P., Liu, J., and Meehan, W. P. (1995). Psychosocial stress and experimental hypertension. In *Hypertension: Pathophysiology, Diagnosis and Management*, Laragh, J. H., and Brenner, B. M., Eds., Vol. 1, pp. 905–921. Raven Press, New York.

Henry, J. P. (1997a). *Cultural Change and High Blood Pressure*. LIT Verlag, Münster.

Henry, J. P. (1997b). Psychological and physiological responses to stress: the right hemisphere and the hypothalamo-pituitary adrenal axis, an inquiry into problems of human bonding. *Acta Physiol Scand* **161** (suppl 640), 10–25.

Herd, J. A., Morse, W. H., Kelleher, R. T., and Jones, L. G. (1969). Arterial hypertension in the squirrel monkey during behavioral experiments. *Am J Physiol* **217**, 24–29.

Herd, J. A. (1991). Cardiovascular response to stress. *Physiol Rev* **71**, 305–330.

Hermansen, L., and Wachtlová, M. (1971). Capillary density of skeletal muscle in well trained and untrained men. *J Appl Physiol* **30**, 860–863.

Herrera, V. L. M., and Ruiz-Opazo, N. (1990). Alteration of $\tilde{\alpha}1Na^+,K^+$-ATPase ^{86}Rb influx by a single amino acid substitution. *Science* **249**, 1023–1026.

Herzig, T. C., Buchholz, R. A., and Haywood, J. R. (1991). Effects of paraventricular nucleus lesions on chronic renal hypertension. *Am J Physiol* **261**, H860–H867.

Hess, W. R., and Brugger, M. (1943). Das subkortikale Zentrum der affektiven-Abwehrreaktion. *Helv Physiol Acta* **1**, 33–52.

Hess, W. R. (1957). *The Functional Organization of the Diencephalon*. Grune & Stratton, New York.

Hetherington, A. W., and Ranson, S. W. (1940). Hypothalamic lesions and adiposity in rats. *Anat Rec* **78**, 149–172.

Heusser, K., Tank, J., Luft, F. C., and Jordan, J. (2005). Baroreflex failure. *Hypertension* **45**, 834–839.

Heymans, C., and Neil, E. (1958). *Reflexogenic Areas of the Cardiovascular System*. J. & A. Churchill, London.

Higashi, Y., Oshima, T., Watanabe, M., Matsuura, H., and Kajiyama, G. (1996). Renal response to L-arginine in salt sensitive patients with essential hypertension. *Hypertension* **27** (part 2), 643–648.

Hilden, T. (1948). Diodrast clearance in essential hypertension. *Acta Med Scand* **206**, 242–245.

Hill, A. V. (1970). *First and Last Experiments in Muscle Mechanics*. Cambridge University Press, London.

Hill, J. O., Wyatt, H. R., Reed, G. W., and Peters, J. C. (2003). Obesity and the environment: where do we go from here? *Science* **299**, 853–858.

Hille, B. (1992). *Ionic Channels of Excitable Membranes*. Sinauer, Sunderland, MA.

Hilsted, J., Parving, H.-H., Christensen, N. J., Benn, J., and Galbo, H. (1981). Hemodynamics in diabetic orthostatic hypotension. *J Clin Invest* **68**, 1427–1434.

Hilton, S. M. (1959). A peripheral arterial conducting mechanism, underlying dilatation of the femoral artery and concerned in functional dilatation of skeletal muscle. *J Physiol (Lond)* **149**, 93–111.

Hilton, S. M. (1963). Inhibition of baroreceptor reflexes on hypothalamic stimulation [Abstract]. *J Physiol (Lond)* **165**, P56–P57.

Hilton, S. M. (1982). The defence-arousal system and its relevance for circulatory and respiratory control. *J Exp Biol* **100**, 159–174.

Hilton, S. M., and Marshall, J. M. (1982). The pattern of cardiovascular response to carotid chemoreceptor stimulation in the cat. *J Physiol (Lond)* **326**, 495–513.

Hinman, A. T., Engel, B. T., and Bickford, A. F. (1962). Portable blood pressure recorder. Accuracy and preliminary use in evaluating intra-daily variations in pressure. *Am Heart J* **63,** 663–668.

Hinojosa-Laborde, C., Greene, A., and Cowley, A., Jr. (1989). Whole body autoregulation in conscious areflexic rats during hypoxia and hyperoxia. *Am J Physiol* **256,** H1023–H1029.

Hirst, G. D. S., and Neild, T. O. (1980). Evidence for two populations of excitatory receptors for noradrenaline on arteriolar smooth muscle. *Nature* **283,** 767–768.

Hirst, G. D., and Edwards, F. R. (1989). Sympathetic neuro-effector transmission in arteries and arterioles. *Physiol Rev* **69,** 546–604.

Hittinger, L., Mirsky, I., Shen, Y.-T., Patrick, T. A., Bishop, S. P., and Vatner, S. F. (1995). Hemodynamic mechanisms responsible for reduced subendocardial coronary reserve in dogs with left ventricular hypertrophy. *Circulation* **92,** 978–986.

Hjemdahl, P., Freyschuss, U., Juhlin-Dannfelt, A., and Linde, B. (1984). Differentiated sympathetic activation during mental stress evoked by the Stroop test. *Acta Physiol Scand* (suppl 527), 25–29.

Hjemdahl, P., and Friberg, P. (1996). Biochemical assessment of sympathetic activity and prejunctional modulation of noradrenaline release in humans. *J Hypertens* **14,** 147–150.

Hobbs, S. F., and Gandevia, S. C. (1985). Cardiovascular responses and the sense of effort during attempts to contract paralysed muscles: role of the spinal cord. *Neurosci Lett* **57,** 85–90.

Hobson, J. A. (2005). Sleep is of the brain, by the brain and for the brain. *Nature* **437,** 1254–1256.

Hoff, E. C., Kell, J. F., and Carroll, M. N. (1963). Effects of cortical stimulation and lesions on cardiovascular function. *Physiol Rev* **43,** 68–114.

Hoffer, B. J., Siggins, G. R., Oliver, A. P., and Bloom, F. E. (1973). Activation of the pathways from locus coeruleus to rat cerebellar Purkinje neurons: pharmacological evidence of noradrenergic central inhibition. *J Pharmacol* **184,** 553–569.

Hoffman, J. I. E., and Spaan, J. A. E. (1990). Pressure-flow relations in coronary circulation. *Physiol Rev* **70,** 331–390.

Hoffmann, P., and Thorén, P. (1986). Long-lasting cardiovascular depression induced by acupuncture-like stimulation of the sciatic nerve in unanaesthetized rats. Effects of arousal and type of hypertension. *Acta Physiol Scand* **127,** 119–126.

Hohenbleicher, H., Schmitz, S. A., Koennecke, H.-C., Offermann, R., Offermann, J., Zeytountchian, H., Wolf, K.-J., Distler, A., and Sharma, A. M. (2001). Neurovascular contact of cranial nerve IX and X root entry zone in hypertensive patients. *Hypertension* **37,** 176–181.

Hohimer, A., and Smith, O. (1979). Decreased renal blood flow in the baboon during mild dynamic leg exercise. *Am J Physiol* **236,** H141–H150.

Hollenberg, N. K., Epstein, M., Basch, R. I., Couch, N. P., Hickler, R. B., and Merrill, J. P. (1969a). "No man's land" of the renal vasculature: an arteriographic and haemodynamic assessment of the interlobar and arcuate arteries in essential and accelerated hypertension. *Am J Med* **47,** 845–854.

Hollenberg, N. K., Epstein, M., Basch, R. I., Couch, N. P., Hickler, R. B., and Merrill, J. P. (1969b). Renin secretion in essential and accelerated hypertension. *Am J Med* **47,** 855–859.

Hollenberg, N. K., Borucki, L. J., and Adams, D. F. (1978). The renal vasculature in early essential hypertension: evidence for a pathogenic role. *Med Baltimore* **57,** 167–178.

Hollenberg, N. K. (1980). Set point for sodium homeostasis: surfeit, deficit and their implications. *Kidney Internat* **17,** 423–429.

Hollenberg, N. K., Williams, G. H., and Adams, D. F. (1981). Essential hypertension abnormal renal vascular and endocrine responses to a mild psychological stimulus. *Hypertension* **3,** 11–17.

Hollenberg, N. K., and Williams, G. H. (1995). Abnormal renal function, sodium-volume homeostasis and renin system behavior in normal-renin essential hypertension: the evolution of the nonmodulator concept. In *Hypertension: Pathophysiology, Diagnosis and Management*, Laragh, J. H., and Brenner, B. M., Eds., Vol. 2, pp. 1837–1856. Raven Press, New York.

Holst, D. v. (1986). Vegetative and somatic components of tree shrews' behaviour. *J Auton Nerv Syst* (suppl), 657–670.

Holst, D. v. (1997). Social relations and their health impact in tree shrews. *Acta Physiol Scand* **161** (suppl 640), 77–82.

Honig, C. R., and Bourdeau-Martini, J. (1974). Extravascular component of oxygen transport in normal and hypertrophied hearts with special reference to oxygen therapy. *Circ Res* **34 & 35** (suppl II), II-97–II-103.

Hope, B. T., Michael, G. J., Knigge, K. M., and Vincent, S. R. (1991). Neuronal NADPH diaphorase is a nitric oxide synthetase. *Proc Natl Acad Sci, USA* **88**, 2811–2814.

Hopkins, P. N., Lifton, R. P., Hollenberg, N. K., Jeunemaitre, X., Hallouin, M.-C., Skuppin, J., Williams, C. S., Dluhy, R. G., Lalouel, J.-M., Williams, R. R., and Williams, G. H. (1996). Blunted renal vascular response to angiotensin II is associated with a common variant of the angiotensinogen gene and obesity. *J Hypertens* **14**, 199–207.

Horiuchi, J., Wakabayashi, S., and Dampney, R. A. L. (2005). Activation of 5–hydroxytryptamine 1A receptors suppress the cardiovascular response evoked from the dorsomedial hypothalamic nucleus. *Hypertension* **46**, 173–179.

Hornbein, T. F., Griffo, Z. J., and Ross, A. (1961). Quantitation of chemoreceptor activity: interrelation of hypoxia and hypercapnia. *J Neurophysiol* **24**, 561–568.

Hostetter, T. H., Olson, J. L., Rennke, H. G., Venkatachalam, M. A., and Brenner, B. M. (1981). Hyperfiltration in remnant nephrons a potentially adverse response to renal ablation. *Am J Physiol* **241**, F85–F93.

Hotamisligil, G. S., Budavari, A., Murray, D., and Spiegelman, B. M. (1994). Internet search. *J Clin Invest* **94**, 1543–1549.

Hotamisligil, G. S., Johnson, R. S., Distel, R. J., Ellis, R., Papaioannou, V. E., and Spiegelman, B. M. (1996). Uncoupling of obesity from insulin resistance through a targeted mutation in aP2, the adipocyte fatty acid binding protein. *Science* **274**, 1377–1379.

Houk, J. C. (1988). Control strategies in physiological systems. *FASEB J* **2**, 97–107.

Howard, J. (1994). Clamping down on myosin. *Nature* **368**, 98–99.

Hoy, W. E., Douglas-Denton, R. N., Hughson, M. D. et al. (2003). A stereological study of glomerular number and volume: preliminary findings in a multiracial study of kidneys at autopsy. *Kidney Internat* **63** (suppl 83).

Hu, L., Manning, R. D., Jr., and Brands, M. W. (1994). Long-term cardiovascular role of nitric oxide in conscious rats. *Hypertension* **23**, 185–194.

Hu, E., Kim, J. B., Sarraf, P., and Spiegelman, B. M. (1996). Inhibition of adipogenesis through MAP-kinase mediated phosphorylation of PPARγ. *Science* **274**, 2100–2103.

Huang, B. S., Harmsen, E., Yu, H., and Leenen, F. H. H. (1992). Brain ouabain-like activity and the sympathoexcitatory and pressor effects of central sodium in rats. *Circ Res* **71**, 1059–1066.

Huang, B. S., and Leenen, F. H. H. (1992). Dietary sodium, age and baroreflex control of heart rate and renal sympathetic activity in rats. *Am J Physiol* **262**, H1441–H1448.

Huang, B. S., Huang, X., Harmsen, E., and Leenen, F. H. H. (1994). Chronic central versus peripheral ouabain blood pressure and sympathetic activity in rats. *Hypertension* **23** (part 2), 1087–1090.

Huang, B. S., and Leenen, F. H. H. (1994). Dietary Na and baroreflex modulation of blood pressure and RSNA in normotensive vs. spontaneously hypertensive rats. *Am J Physiol* **266**, H496–H502.

Huang, P. L., Huang, Z., Mashimo, H., Bloch, K. D., Moskowitz, M. A., Bevan, J. A., and Fishman, M. C. (1995). Hypertension in mice lacking the gene for endothelial nitric oxide synthase. *Nature* **377,** 239–242.

Huang, B. S., and Leenen, F. H. H. (1996). Brain "ouabain" and angiotensin II in salt-sensitive hypertension in spontaneously hypertensive rats. *Hypertension* **28,** 1005–1012.

Huang, B. S., and Leenen, F. H. H. (1998). Both brain angiotensin II and "ouabain" contribute to sympathoexcitation and hypertension in Dahl S rats on high salt intake. *Hypertension* **32,** 1028–1033.

Huang, B. S., and Leenen, F. H. H. (2002). Brain amiloride sensitive Phe-Met-Arg-Phe-NH_2 gated Na^+ channels and Na^+ induced sympathoexcitation and hypertension. *Hypertension* **39,** 557–561.

Hudlicka, O. (1991). What makes blood vessels grow. *J Physiol (Lond)* **444,** 1–24.

Hudlicka, O., Brown, M., and Eggington, S. (1992). Angiogenesis in skeletal and cardiac muscle. *Physiol Rev* **72,** 369–417.

Hughson, M. D., Faris, A. B., and Douglas-Denton, R. N. (2003). Glomerular number and size in autopsy kidney: the relationship to birth weight. *Kidney Internat* **63,** 2113–2122.

Huisman, R. M., and De Zeeuw, D. (1985). Haemodynamics of renal artery stenosis (a comment based on Ohm's law). *Clin Sci* **68,** 479–480.

Hulthén, U. L., Bolli, P., Amann, F. W., Kiowski, W., and Bühler, F. R. (1982). Enhanced vasodilation in essential hypertension by calcium channel blockade with verapamil. *Hypertension* **4,** II-26–II-31.

Hunt, J. C., Sheps, S. G., Harrison, E. G., Strong, C. G., and Bernatz, P. E. (1978). Renal and renovascular hypertension. A reasoned approach to diagnosis and management. *Arch Int Med* **133,** 988–999.

Hunt, S. C., Stephenson, S. H., Hopkins, P. N., and Williams, R. R. (1991). Predictors of increased risk of future hypertension in Utah. *Hypertension* **17,** 969–976.

Husain, A., and Graham, R. M. (2000). *Drugs, Enzymes and Receptors of the Renin-Angiotensin System: Celebrating a Century of Discovery.* Victor Chang Molecular Cardiology Series, Vol. 1. Harwood, Sydney.

Hutchins, P. M., and Darnell, A. E. (1974). Observation of a decreased number of small arterioles in spontaneously hypertensive rats. *Circ Res* **34–35** (suppl 1), I-161–I-165.

Hutchins, P. M., Lynch, C. D., Cooney, P. T., and Curseen, K. A. (1996). The microcirculation in experimental hypertension and aging. *Cardiovasc Res* **32,** 772–780.

Huxley, A. F. (1957). Muscle structure and theories of contraction. *Prog Biophys Biophys Chem* **7,** 255–318.

Iams, S. G., and Wexler, B. C. (1979). Inhibition of the development of spontaneous hypertension in SH rats by gonadectomy or estradiol. *J Lab Clin Med* **10,** 608–616.

Ichikawa, M., Suzuki, H., Kumagai, K., Kumagai, H., Ryuzaki, M., Nishizawa, M., and Saruta, T. (1995). Differential modulation of baroreceptor sensitivity by long-term antihypertensive treatment. *Hypertension* **26,** 425–431.

Ignarro, L. J., and Kadowitz, P. J. (1985). The pharmacological and physiological role of cyclic GMP in vascular smooth muscle relaxation. *Annu Rev Pharmacol Toxicol* **25,** 171–191.

Imai, Y., Abe, K., Munakata, M., Sakuma, H., Hashimoto, J., Imai, K., Sekino, H., and Yoshinaga, K. (1990). Circadian blood pressure variations under different pathophysiological conditions. *J Hypertens* **8** (suppl 7), S125–S132.

Intersalt Research Group. (1988). Intersalt: an international study of electrolyte excretion and blood pressure. Results for 24 hour urinary sodium and potassium excretion. *Br Med J* **297,** 319–328.

Iriki, M., Dorward, P., and Korner, P. I. (1977a). Baroreflex "resetting" by arterial hypoxia in the renal and cardiac sympathetic nerves of the rabbit. *Eur J Physiol (Pflügers Archiv)* **370,** 1–7.

Iriki, M., Dorward, P., and Korner, P. I. (1977b). Baroreflex "resetting" in various regional sympathetic nerves during arterial hypoxia in rabbits [Abstract]. *Proc 27th Int Congr Physiol Sci* **13**, 345.

Iriki, M., and Korner, P. I. (1979). Central nervous interactions between chemoreceptor and baroreceptor control mechanisms. In *Integrative Functions of the Autonomic Nervous System*, Brooks, C. M., Koizumi, K., and Sato, A., Eds., pp. 415–426. Elsevier, Amsterdam.

Iriki, M., Kozawa, E., Korner, P. I., and Dorward, P. K. (1979). Arterial and cardiopulmonary baroreceptor and chemoreceptor influences and interactions on ear sympathetic nerve discharge in the rabbit. *Jpn J Physiol* **29**, 551–558.

Iriki, M., and Kozawa, E. (1983). Renal sympathetic baroreflex during normoxia and during hypoxia in conscious and in anesthetized animals. *Eur J Physiol (Pflügers Archiv)* **398**, 23–26.

Irving, L. (1963). Bradycardia in human divers. *J Appl Physiol* **18**, 489–491.

Ishibashi, Y., Duncker, D. J., Zhang, J., and Bache, R. J. (1998). ATP-sensitive K^+ channels, adenosine and nitric oxide-mediated mechanisms account for coronary vasodilatation during exercise. *Circ Res* **82**, 346–359.

Ishikawa, Y., and Homcy, C. J. (1997). The adenyl cyclases as integrators of transmembrane signal transduction. *Circ Res* **80**, 297–304.

Ito, C. S., and Scher, A. M. (1981). Hypertension following arterial baroreceptor denervation in the unanesthetised dog. *Circ Res* **48**, 576–586.

Ito, M., Sakurai, M., and Tongroach, P. (1982). Climbing fibre induced depression of both mossy fibre responsiveness and glutamate sensitivity of cerebellar Purkinje cells. *J Physiol (Lond)* **324**, 113–134.

Ito, M. (1984). *The Cerebellum and Neural Control*. Raven Press, New York.

Ito, M. (1989). Long-term depression. *Ann. Rev. Neurosci.* **12**, 85–102.

Iwamoto, T., Kita, S., Zhang, J., Blaustein, M. P., Arai, Y., Yoshida, S., Wakimoto, K., Komuro, I., and Katsuragi, T. (2004). Salt-sensitive hypertension is triggered by Ca^{2+} entry via Na^+/Ca^{2+} exchanger type-1 in vascular smooth muscle. *Nat Med* **10**, 1193–1199.

Iwase, M., Bishop, S. P., Uechi, M., Vatner, D. E., Shannon, R. P., Kudej, R. K., Wight, D. C., Wagner, T. E., Ishikawa, Y., Homcy, C. J., and Vatner, S. F. (1996). Adverse effects of chronic endogenous sympathetic drive induced by cardiac $G_{s\alpha}$ overexpression. *Circ Res* **78**, 517–524.

Izzard, A. S., Heagerty, A. M., and Leenen, F. H. H. (1999). The amplifier hypothesis: permission to dissent? *J Hypertens* **17**, 1667–1669.

Izzard, A. S., Heagerty, A. M., and Leenen, F. H. H. (2002). Amplifiers and resisters: reply. *J Hypertens* **20**, 2522–2524.

Jablonskis, L. T., and Howe, P. R. C. (1994). Elevated plasma adrenaline in spontaneously hypertensive rats. *Blood Pressure* **3**, 106–111.

Jackson, E. K., and Garrison, J. C. (1996). Renin and angiotensin. In *Goodman and Gilman's Pharmacological Basis of Therapeutics*, Hardman, J. G., Limbird, L. E., Molinoff, P. B., and Ruddon, R. W., Eds., pp. 733–758. McGraw-Hill, New York.

Jacob, H. J. (1999). Physiological genetics application to hypertension research. *Clin Exp Pharmacol Physiol* **26**, 530–535.

Jacobs, B. L. (1987). Brain monoaminergic activity in behaving animals. *Prog Psychobiol Physiol Psychol* **12**, 171–206.

Jacobs, B. L., and Azmitia, E. C. (1992). Structure and function of the brain serotonin systems. *Physiol Rev* **72**, 165–229.

Jacobson, M. (1991). *Developmental Neurobiology*. Plenum Press, New York.

Jahn, R., and Sudhof, T. C. (1994). Synaptic vesicles and exocytosis. *Annu Rev Neurosci* **17**, 219–246.

Jamerson, K. A., Julius, S., Gudbrandsson, T., Andersson, O., and Brant, D. O. (1993). Reflex sympathetic activation induces acute insulin resistance in the human forearm. *Hypertension* **21,** 618–623.

James, T. N., James, M. D., and Isobe, J. H. (1975). Analysis of components in a cardiogenic hypertensive chemoreflex. *Circulation* **52,** 179–192.

James, S. A., Hartnett, S. A., and Kalsbeck, W. (1983). John Henryism and blood pressure differences among black men. *J Behav Med* **6,** 259–278.

James, G. D., and Baker, P. T. (1995). Human population biology and blood pressure: evolutionary and ecological considerations and interpretations of population studies. In *Hypertension: Pathophysiology, Diagnosis and Management*, Laragh, J. H., and Brenner, B. M., Eds., Vol. 1, pp. 115–126. Raven Press, New York.

Janetta, P. J. (1980). Neurovascular compression in cranial nerve and systemic disease. *Ann Surg* **192,** 518–525.

Janetta, P., Segal, R., and Wolfson, S. K. (1985). Neurogenic hypertension: etiology and surgical treatment—observations in 53 patients. *Ann Surg* **201,** 391–398.

Janeway, T. C. (1904). *The Clinical Study of Blood-Pressure*. Appleton, New York.

Jänig, W. (1985). Organization of the lumbar sympathetic outflow to skeletal muscle and skin of the cat hindlimb and tail. *Rev Physiol Biochem Pharmacol* **102,** 119–213.

Janke, J., Engeli, S., Gorzelniak, K., Luft, F. C., and Sharma, A. M. (2002). Mature adipocytes inhibit in vitro differentiation of human preadipocytes via angiotensin-type 1 receptors. *Diabetes* **51,** 1699–1707.

Jarrell, T. W., Gentile, C. G., Romanski, L. M., McCabe, P. M., and Schneiderman, N. (1987). Involvement of cortical and thalamic auditory regions in retention of differential bradycardia conditioning to acoustic conditioned stimuli in rabbits. *Brain Res* **412,** 285–294.

Jennings, G., Esler, M., Holmes, R., and Korner, P. (1979). Treatment of postural hypotension accompanying autonomic insufficiency, with dihydroergotamine, a relatively selective venoconstrictor. *Aust NZ J Med* **9,** 765–766.

Jennings, G. L., Esler, M. D., and Korner, P. I. (1980). Effect of prolonged treatment on haemodynamics of essential hypertension before and after autonomic block. *Lancet* **ii,** 166–169.

Jennings, G., Bobik, A., and Korner, P. (1981). Influence of intrinsic sympathomimetic activity of beta-adrenoceptor blockers on the heart rate and blood pressure responses to graded exercise. *Br J Clin Pharmacol* **12,** 355–362.

Jennings, G., Korner, P., Esler, M., and Restall, R. (1984). Redevelopment of essential hypertension after cessation of long-term therapy: preliminary findings. *Clin Exp Hypertens* **A6,** 493–505.

Jennings, G., Nelson, L., Dewar, E., Korner, P., Esler, M., and Laufer, E. (1986). Antihypertensive and haemodynamic effects of one year's regular exercise. *J Hypertens* **4** (suppl 6), S659–S661.

Jennings, G., Nelson, L., Nestel, P., Esler, M., Korner, P., Burton, D., and Bazelmans, J. (1986). The effects of changes in physical activity on major cardiovascular risk factors, hemodynamics, sympathetic function, and glucose utilization in man: a controlled study of four levels of activity. *Circulation* **73,** 30–40.

Jennings, G. L., Deakin, G., Dewar, E., Laufer, E., and Nelson, L. (1989). Exercise, cardiovascular disease and blood pressure. *Clin Exp Hypertens,* **A11,** 1035–1052.

Jennings, G., Dart, A., Meredith, I., Korner, P., Laufer, E., and Dewar, E. (1991). Effects of exercise and other nonpharmacological measures of blood pressure and cardiac hypertrophy. *J Cardiovasc Pharmacol* **17** (suppl 2), S70–S74.

Jennings, G. L., Deakin, G., Korner, P., Meredith, I., Kingwell, B., and Nelson, L. (1991). What is the dose-response relationship between exercise training and blood pressure? *Ann Med* **23,** 313–318.

Jennings, G., Korner, P. I., Sudhir, K., Esler, M., Angus, J. A., and Laufer, E. (1991). Evidence for a role for the cardiovascular amplifiers in human primary hypertension. *Clin Exp Pharmacol Physiol* **18**, 37–41.

Jennings, G. L., and Kingwell, B. A. (1994). Exercise. In *Textbook of Hypertension*, Swales, J. D., Ed., pp. 593–604. Blackwell, Oxford.

Jennings, G. L., and Wong, J. (1997). Reversibility of left ventricular hypertrophy and malfunction by antihypertensive treatment. Assessment of hypertensive organ damage. In *Handbook of Hypertension*, Hansson, L., and Birkenhäger, W., Eds., Vol. 18, pp. 184–223. Elsevier, Oxford.

Jequier, E. (1993). Body weight regulation in humans: the importance of nutrient balance. *NIPS* **8**, 273–276.

Jequier, E., and Tappy, L. (1999). Regulation of body weight in humans. *Physiol Rev* **79**, 451–480.

Jeunemaitre, X., Lifton, R., Hunt, S., Williams, R. R., and Lalouel, J. M. (1992). Absence of linkage between the angiotensin converting enzyme locus and human essential hypertension. *Nat Gen* **1**, 72–75.

Jeunemaitre, X., Rigat, B., Charru, A., Houot, A. M., Soubrier, F., and Corvol, P. (1992). Sib pair analysis of renin gene haplotypes in human essential hypertension. *Hum Genet* **88**, 301–306.

Jeunemaitre, X., Soubrier, F., Kotelvtsev, Y. V., Lifton, R. P., Williams, C. S., Charru, A., Hunt, S. C., Hopkins, P. N., Williams, R. R., Lalouel, J.-M., and Corvol, P. (1992). Molecular basis of human hypertension. Role of angiotensinogen. *Cell* **71**, 169–180.

Jia, L., Bonaventura, C., Bonaventura, J., and Stamler, J. S. (1996). S-nitrosohaemoglobin: a dynamic activity of blood involved in vascular control. *Nature* **380**, 221–226.

Johannsen, W. (1909). *Elemente der exakten Erblichkeitslehre*. Fischer, Jena.

Johansson, J. E. (1895). Über die Einwirkung der Muskeltätigkeit auf die Atmung und die Herztätigkeit. *Skand Arch Physiol* **5**, 20–66.

Johansson, B., and Somlyo, A. P. (1980). Electrophysiology and excitation-contraction coupling. In *Handbook of Physiology, Section 2: The Cardiovascular System, Vol. II: Vascular Smooth Muscle*, Bohr, D. F., Somlyo, A. P., and Sparks, H. V., Jr., Eds., pp. 301–324. American Physiological Society, Bethesda, MD.

Johansson, B. (1984). Cerebral vascular bed in hypertension and consequences for the brain. *Hypertension* **6** (suppl III), III-81–III-86.

Johansson, B. (1989). Myogenic tone and reactivity: definitions based on muscle physiology. *J Hypertens* **7** (suppl 4), S5–S8.

Johansson, B. B. (1992). Vascular mechanisms in hypertensive cerebrovascular disease. *J Cardiovasc Pharmacol* **19** (suppl 3), S11–S15.

Johansson, M., Elam, M., Rundqvist, B., Eisenhofer, G., Herlitz, H., Lambert, G., and Friberg, P. (1999). Increased sympathetic nerve activity in renovascular hypertension. *Circulation*, **99**, 2537–2542.

Johnson, P. C. E. (1964a). Autoregulation of blood flow. *Circ Res* **14 & 15** (suppl I), I-1–I-291.

Johnson, P. (1964b). Review of previous studies and current theories of autoregulation. *Circ Res* **14 & 15** (suppl I), I-2–I-9.

Johnson, P. (1980). The myogenic response. In *Handbook of Physiology, Section 2: The Cardiovascular System, Vol. II: Vascular Smooth Muscle*, Bohr, D., Somlyo, A., and Sparks, H., Jr., Eds., pp. 409–442. American Physiological Society, Bethesda, MD.

Johnson, A. K., and Loewy, A. D. (1990). Circumventricular organs and their role in visceral functions. In *Central Regulation of Autonomic Functions*, Loewy, A. D., and Spyer, K. M., Eds., pp. 247–267. Oxford University Press, New York.

Jones, J. V., and Floras, J. S. (1982). Baroreflex sensitivity changes during development of Goldblatt two-kidney one-clip hypertension in rats. *Clin Sci* **59**, 347–352.

Jonsson, G. (1980). Chemical neurotoxins as denervation tools in neurobiology. *Annu Rev Neurosci* **3**, 169–187.

Jordan, D. (1990). Autonomic changes in affective behavior. In *Central Regulation of Autonomic Functions*, Loewy, A. D., and Spyer, K. M., Eds., pp. 349–366. Oxford University Press, New York.

Jose, A. D., and Taylor, R. R. (1969). Autonomic blockade by propranolol and atropine to study intrinsic myocardial function in man. *J Clin Invest* **48**, 2019–2031.

Ju, H., Gros, R., You, X., Tsang, S., Husain, M., and Rabinovitch, M. (2001). Conditional and targeted overexpression of vascular chymase causes hypertension in transgenic mice. *Proc Natl Acad Sci, USA* **98**, 7469–7474.

Judy, W. V., Watanabe, A. M., Murphy, W. R., Aprison, B. S., and Yu, P.-L. (1979). Sympathetic nerve activity and blood pressure in normotensive backcross rats genetically related to the spontaneously hypertensive rat. *Hypertension* **1**, 598–604.

Julius, S., and Conway, J. (1968). Hemodynamic studies in patients with borderline blood pressure elevation. *Circulation* **38**, 282–288.

Julius, S., Pascual, A. V., and London, R. (1971). Role of parasympathetic inhibition in the hyperkinetic type of borderline hypertension. *Circulation* **44**, 413–418.

Julius, S., Pascual, A. V., Abbrecht, P. H., and London, R. (1972). Effect of beta-adrenergic blockade on plasma volume in human subjects. *Proc Soc Exp Biol Med* **140**, 982–985.

Julius, S., and Esler, M. (1975). Autonomic nervous cardiovascular regulation in borderline hypertension. *Am J Cardiol* **36**, 685–696.

Julius, S., Randall, O. S., Esler, M. D., Kashima, T., Ellis, C., and Bennet, J. (1975). Altered cardiac responsiveness and regulation in the normal cardiac output type of borderline hypertension. *Circ Res* **36 & 37** (suppl I), I-199–I-207.

Julius, S., and Esler, M. (1976). Increased central blood volume: a possible pathological factor in mild low renin essential hypertension. *Clin Sci* **51** (suppl 3), 207–210.

Julius, S., Hansson, L., Andren, L., Gudbrandsson, T., Sivertsson, R., and Svensson, A. (1980). Borderline hypertension. *Acta Med Scand* **208**, 481–489.

Julius, S., Jamerson, K., Mejia, A., Krause, L., Schork, N., and Jones, K. (1990). The association of borderline hypertension with target organ changes and higher coronary risk: Tecumseh Blood Pressure Study. *JAMA* **264**, 354–358.

Julius, S., Mejia, A., Krause, L., Schork, N., van de Ven, C., Johnston, E., Petrin, J., Sekkarie, A. M., Kjeldsen, S. E., Schmoudt, F., Gupta, R., Ferraro, J., Nazzaro, P., and Weissfeld, J. (1990). "White coat" versus "sustained" borderline hypertension in Tecumseh, Michigan. *Hypertension* **16**, 617–623.

Julius, S., Jones, K., Schork, N., Johnson, E., Krause, L., Nazzaro, P., and Zemva, A. (1991). Independence of pressure reactivity from pressure levels in Tecumseh, Michigan. *Hypertension* **17**, III-12–III-21.

Julius, S., Valentini, M., and Palatini, P. (2000). Overweight and hypertension: a two way street? *Hypertension* **35**, 807–813.

Julius, S., Nesbitt, S., Egan, B., Kaciroti, N., Schork, M. A., Grozinski, M., and Michelson, E. (2004). Trial of preventing hypertension: design and 2–year progress report. *Hypertension* **44**, 146–151.

Kahn, C. R., Smith, R. J., and Chin, W. W. (1992). Mechanism of action of hormones that act at the cell surface. In *Williams Textbook of Endocrinology, 8th Edition*, Wilson, J. D., and Foster, D. W., Eds., pp. 91–134. W.B. Saunders, Philadelphia.

Kahn, C. R. (1995). Causes of insulin resistance. *Nature* **373**, 384–385.

Kalis, B. L., Harris, R. E., Bennett, C. F., and Sokolow, M. (1961). Personality and life history factors in persons who are potentially hypertensive. *J Nerv Ment Dis* **132**, 457.

Kandel, E. R., and Schwartz, J. H. (1991). Directly gated transmission at central synapses. In *Principles of Neural Science, 3rd Edition*, Kandel, E. R., Schwartz, J. H., and Jessel, T. M., Eds., pp. 153–172. Prentice-Hall International, New York.

Kandel, E. R. (2001). The molecular biology of memory storage: a dialogue between genes and synapses. *Science* **294**, 1030–1038.

Kannel, W. B., Brand, N., Skinner, J. J., Dawber, T. R., and McNamara, P. M. (1967). The relation of adiposity to blood pressure and development of hypertension. *Ann Int Med* **67**, 48–59.

Kannel, W. B., Wolf, P. A., McGee, D. L., Dawber, T. R., McNamara, P., and Castelli, W. P. (1981). Systolic blood pressure, arterial rigidity and risk of stroke. The Framingham Study. *JAMA* **245**, 1225–1229.

Kannel, W. B. (1983). Prevalence and natural history of electrocardiographic left ventricular hypertrophy. *Am J Med* **75** (suppl 3A), 4–11.

Kannel, W. B. (1990). Hypertension and the risk of cardiovascular disease. In *Hypertension: Pathophysiology, Diagnosis and Management*, Laragh, J. H., and Brenner, B. M., Eds., Vol. 1, pp. 101–117. Raven Press, New York.

Kannel, W. B. (1991). Effect of current treatment of hypertension on metabolism and risk of cardiovascular disease. In *Hypertension as an Insulin-Resistant Disorder*, Smith, U., Bruun, N. E., Hedner, T., and Hokfelt, B., Eds., pp. 359–380. Elsevier, Amsterdam.

Kaplan, N. M., Kem, D. C., Holland, O. B., Kramer, N. J., Higgins, J., and Gomez-Sanchez, C. (1976). The intravenous furosemide test: a simple way to evaluate renin responsiveness. *Ann Int Med* **84**, 639–645.

Kaplan, N. M. (2002). *Kaplan's Clinical Hypertension*. Lippincott, Williams and Wilkins, Philadelphia.

Kapuscinski, M., Charchar, F., Innes, B., Mitchell, G. A., Norman, T. L., and Harrap, S. B. (1996). Nerve growth factor gene and hypertension in spontaneously hypertensive rats. *J Hypertens* **14**, 191–197.

Karasek, R. A., Baker, D., Marxer, F., Ahlbohm, A., and Theorell, T. (1981). Job decision latitude, job demands, and cardiovascular disease: a prospective study in Swedish men. *Am J Public Health* **75**, 694–705.

Karasek, R. A., Theorell, T., Schwartz, J. E., Schnall, P. L., Pieper, C. F., and Michela, J. L. (1988). Job characteristics in relation to the prevalence of myocardial infarction in the US: Health Examination Survey (HES) and Health and Nutrition Examination Survey (HANES). *Am J Public Health* **78**, 910–919.

Kardos, A., Watterich, G., de Menezes, R., Csanady, M., Casadei, B., and Rdas, L. (2001). Determinants of spontaneous baroreflex sensitivity in a healthy working population. *Hypertension* **37**, 911–916.

Karlström, G., Arnman, V., Folkow, B., and Göthberg, G. (1988). Activation of the humoral anti-hypertensive system of the kidney increases diuresis. *Hypertension* **11**, 597–601.

Katholi, R. E., and Woods, W. T. (1987). Afferent renal nerves and hypertension. *Clin Exp Hypertens* **A.9** (suppl 1), 211–226.

Kato, N., Sugiyama, T., Morita, H., Nabika, T., Kurihara, H., Yamori, Y., and Yazaki, Y. (1999). Lack of evidence for association between the endothelial nitric oxide synthase gene and hypertension. *Hypertension* **33**, 933–936.

Kato, M., Phillips, B. G., Sigurdsson, G., Narkiewicz, K., Pesek, C. A., and Somers, V. K. (2000). Effects of sleep deprivation on neural circulatory control. *Hypertension* **35**, 1173.

Kato, M., Roberts-Thompson, P., Phillips, B. G., Haynes, W. G., Winnicki, M., Accurso, V., and Somers, V. K. (2000). Impairment of endothelium-dependent vasodilatation of resistance vessels in patients with obstructive sleep apnea. *Circulation* **102**, 2607–2610.

Kato, N., Sugiyama, T., Morita, H., Kurihara, H., Furukawa, T., Isshiki, T., Sato, T., Yamori, Y., and Yazaki, Y. (2000). Comprehensive analysis of the renin-angiotensin gene polymorphisms with relation to hypertension in the Japanese. *J Hypertens* **18**, 1025–1032.

Katz, A. M. (1993). Cardiac ion channels. *N Engl J Med* **328**, 1244–1251.

Katzman, P. L., Henningsen, N. C., Fagher, B., Thulin, T., and Hulthen, U. L. (1990). Renal and endocrine effects of long-term converting enzyme inhibition as compared with calcium antagonism in essential hypertension. *J Cardiovasc Pharmacol* **15**, 360–364.

Kawabe, K., Watanabe, T. X., Shione, K., and Sokabe, H. (1979). Influence on blood pressure of renal isografts between spontaneously hypertensive and normotensive rats, utilising F1 hybrids. *Jpn Heart J* **20**, 886–894.

Kawasaki, T., Delea, C. S., Bartter, F. C., and Smith, H. (1978). The effect of high sodium and low sodium intakes on blood pressure and other related variables in human subjects with idiopathic hypertension. *Am J Med* **64**, 193–198.

Kawato, M. (1995). Cerebellum and motor control. In *The Handbook of Brain Theory and Neural Networks*, Arbib, M. A., Ed., pp. 172–178. MIT Press, Cambridge, MA.

Keeley, F. W., Elmoselhi, A., and Leenen, F. H. H. (1991). Effects of antihypertensive drug classes on regression of connective tissue components of hypertension. *J Cardiovasc Pharmacol* **17** (suppl 2), S64–S69.

Keith, N. M., Wagener, H. P., and Barker, N. W. (1939). Some different types of essential hypertension: their course and prognosis. *Am J Med Sci* **197**, 332–342.

Keller, G., Zimmer, G., Mall, G., Ritz, E., and Amann, K. (2003). Nephron numbers in patients with primary hypertension. *N Engl J Med* **348**, 101–108.

Kelly, R. P., and O'Rourke, M. F. (1995). Evaluation of arterial wave forms in hypertension and normotension. In *Hypertension: Pathophysiology, Diagnosis and Management*, Laragh, J. H., and Brenner, B. M., Eds., Vol. 1, pp. 343–364. Raven Press, New York.

Kelly, P. A. T., and Garland, C. J. (1996). Pharmacology of the cerebral circulation. In *Pharmacology of Vascular Smooth Muscle*, Garland, C. J., and Angus, J. A., Eds., pp. 252–275. Oxford University Press, Oxford.

Kelly, J. J., Tam, S. H., Williamson, P. M., Lawson, J., and Whitworth, J. A. (1998). The nitric oxide system and cortisol-induced hypertension in humans. *Clin Exp Pharmacol Physiol* **25**, 945–946.

Kelly, J. J., Williamson, P., Martin, A., and Whitworth, J. A. (2001). Effects of oral l-arginine on plasma nitrate and blood pressure in cortisol-treated humans. *J Hypertens* **19**, 263–268.

Kelm, M., Feelisch, M., Krebber, T., DeuBen, A., Motz, W., and Strauer, B. E. (1995). Role of nitric oxide in the regulation of coronary vascular tone in hearts from hypertensive rats: maintenance of nitric oxide-forming capacity and increased basal production of nitric oxide. *Hypertension* **25**, 186–193.

Kelm, M., Preik, M., Hafner, D. J., and Strauer, B. E. (1996). Evidence for a multifactorial process involved in the impaired flow response to nitric oxide in hypertensive patients, with endothelial dysfunction. *Hypertension* **27** (part 1), 346–353.

Kempner, W. (1948). Treatment of hypertensive vascular disease with rice diet. *Arch Int Med* **133**, 758–785.

Kennard, M. A. (1945). Focal autonomic representation in the cortex and its relation to sham rage. *J Neuropath Exp Neurol* **4**, 295–304.

Kennedy, G. C. (1953). The role of depot fat in the hypothalamic control of food intake in the rat. *Proc R Soc B* **140**, 578–592.

Kenney, M. J., Morgan, D. A., and Mark, A. L. (1991). Sympathetic nerve responses to sustained stimulation of somatic afferents in Dahl rats. *J Hypertens* **9**, 963–968.

Kett, M. M., Alcorn, D., Bertram, J. F., and Anderson, W. P. (1995). Enalapril does not prevent renal arterial hypertrophy in spontaneously hypertensive rats. *Hypertension* **25**, 335–342.

Kett, M. M., Alcorn, D., Bertram, J. F., and Anderson, W. P. (1996). Glomerular dimensions in spontaneously hypertensive rats: effects of AT_1 antagonism. *J Hypertens* **14**, 107–114.

Kett, M. M., and Bertram, J. F. (2004). Nephron endowment and blood pressure: what do we really know? *Current Hypertension Reports* **6**, 133–139.

Kezdi, P. (1962). Mechanism of the carotid sinus in experimental hypertension. *Circ Res* **11**, 145–152.

Khalil, R. A., and Breemen, C. v. (1995). Mechanisms of calcium mobilization and homeostasis in vascular smooth muscle and their relevance to hypertension. In *Hypertension: Pathophysiology, Diagnosis and Management*, Laragh, J. H., and Brenner, B. M., Eds., Vol. 1, pp. 523–539. Raven Press, New York.

Khayutin, V. M., Lukoshkova, E. V., Rogoza, A. N., and Nikolsky, V. P. (1995). Negative feedbacks in the pathogenesis of primary arterial hypertension: mechanosensitivity of the endothelium. *Blood Pressure* **4**, 70–76.

Kimura, G., Frem, G. J., and Brenner, B. M. (1994). Renal mechanisms of salt sensitivity in hypertension. *Curr Opin Nephrol Hypertens* **3**, 1–12.

Kincaid-Smith, P., McMichael, J., and Murphy, E. A. (1958). The clinical course and pathology of hypertension with papilloedema (malignant hypertension). *Q J Med* **27**, 117–153.

Kincaid-Smith, P. (1969). Analgesic nephropathy: a common form of renal disease in Australia. *Med J Aus* **ii**, 1131–1135.

Kincaid-Smith, P. (1980). Malignant hypertension: mechanisms and management. *Pharmacol Ther* **9**, 245–269.

Kincaid-Smith, P. (1985). What has happened to malignant hypertension? In *Handbook of Hypertension, Volume 6: Epidemiology of Hypertension*, Bulpitt, C. J., Birkenhäger, W. H., and Reid, J. L., Eds. Elsevier, Amsterdam.

Kingwell, B. A., McPherson, G. A., and Korner, P. I. (1991). Assessment of gain of tachycardia and bradycardia responses of cardiac baroreflex. *Am J Physiol* **260**, H1254–H1263.

Kingwell, B. A., Dart, A. M., Jennings, G. L., and Korner, P. I. (1992). Exercise training reduces the sympathetic component of the blood pressure-heart rate baroreflex in man. *CS* **82**, 357–362.

Kingwell, B. A., and Jennings, G. L. (1993). A comparison of the effects of walking and other exercise programs upon blood pressure in normal subjects. *Med J Aus* **158**, 234–238.

Kingwell, B. A., Tran, B., Cameron, J. D., Jennings, G. L., and Dart, A. M. (1996). Enhanced vasodilatation to acetylcholine in athletes is associated with lower plasma cholesterol. *Am J Physiol* **270**, H2008–H2013.

Kingwell, B. A., Berry, K. L., Cameron, J. D., Jennings, G. L., and Dart, A. M. (1997). Arterial compliance increases after moderate intensity cycling. *Am J Physiol* **273**, H2186–H2191.

Kingwell, B. A., Sherrard, B., Jennings, G. L., and Dart, A. M. (1997). Four weeks of cycle training increases basal production of nitric oxide from the forearm. *Am J Physiol* **272**, H1070–H1077.

Kingwell, B. A., Arnold, P. J., Jennings, G. L., and Dart, A. M. (1998). The effects of voluntary running on cardiac mss and aortic compliance in Wistar-Kyoto and spontaneously hypertensive rats. *J Hypertens* **16**, 181–185.

Kingwell, B. A., and Jennings, G. L. (1998). The role of aerobic training in the regulation of vascular tone. *Nutr Metab Cardiovasc Dis* **8**, 173–183.

Kinter, W. B., and Pappenheimer, J. R. (1956). Renal extraction of PAH and Diodrast-I[131] as a function of arterial red cell concentration. *Am J Physiol* **183**, 391–398.

Kiowski, W., Bühler, F. R., vanBrummelen, P., and Amann, F. W. (1981). Plasma noradrenalin concentration and alpha-adrenoceptor mediated vasoconstriction in normotensive and hypertensive man. *Clin Sci* **60**, 483–489.

Kirchheim, H. R. (1976). Systemic arterial baroreceptor reflexes. *Physiol Rev* **56**, 100–176.

Kishi, T., Hirooka, Y., Ito, K., Sakai, K., Shimokawa, H., and Takeshita, A. (2002). Cardiovascular effects of overexpression of endothelial nitric oxide synthase in the rostral ventrolateral medulla in stroke-prone spontaneously hypertensive rats. *Hypertension* **39**, 264–268.

Kissebah, A. H., Vydelingum, N., Murray, R., Evans, D., Hartz, A., Kalkhoff, R. K., and Adams, P. W. (1982). Relation of body fat distribution to metabolic complications of obesity. *J Clin Endocrinol Metab* **54**, 254–260.

Kissebah, A. H., and Krakower, G. R. (1994). Regional adiposity and morbidity. *Physiol Rev* **74**, 761–811.

Knardahl, S., and Hendley, E. D. (1990). Association between cardiovascular reactivity to stress and hypertension and behavior. *Am J Physiol* **259**, H248–H257.

Knorr, A., Garthof, B., Kazda, S., and Stasch, J.-P. (1991). Effects of different antihypertensive drug classes on survival in animal models. *J Cardiovasc Pharmacol* **17**, S94–S100.

Kobinger, W. (1984). Central anti-hypertensives. In *Discoveries in Pharmacology, Volume 2: Haemodynamics, Hormones and Inflammation*, Parnham, M. J., and Bruivels, J., Eds., pp. 107–123. Elsevier, Amsterdam.

Koch, E., and Mies, A. (1929). Chronischer arterieller Hochdruck durch experimentelle Dauerausschaltung der Blutdruckzuegler. *Krankheitsforschung* **7**, 241–256.

Koch, E. (1931). Die Reflektorische Selbsteuerung des Kreislaufes. Steinkopf, Leipzig.

Koch, E., and Mattonet, K. (1934). Versuche zur Frage der arteriellen Hypertonie nach Dauerasschaltung von pressorezeptorischen Kreislaufnerven. *Zeitschr f Biol* **94**, 105–113.

Koch, W. J., Milano, C. A., and Lefkowitz, R. J. (1996). Transgenic manipulation of myocardial G protein-coupled receptors and receptor kinases. *Circ Res* **78**, 511–516.

Koepke, J., Jones, S., and DiBona, G. (1987). α_2-adrenoceptors in amygdala control of renal symphathetic nerve activity and renal function in conscious spontaneously hypertensive rats. *Brain Res* **404**, 80–88.

Koh, G. Y., Klug, M. G., and Field, L. J. (1993). Atrial natriuretic factor and transgenic mice. *Hypertension* **22**, 634–639.

Koizumi, K., and Brooks, C. M. (1972). The integration of autonomic system reactions: a discussion of autonomic reflexes, their control and their association with somatic reactions. *Rev Physiol Biochem Exp Pharmacol* **67**, 1–68.

Koletsky, S. (1975). Pathologic findings and laboratory data in a new strain of obese hypertensive rats. *Am J Path* **80**, 129–142.

Koletsky, R. J., and Ernsberger, P. (1992). Obese SHR (Koletsky rat): a model for the interactions between hypertension and obesity. In *Genetic Hypertension*, Sassard, J., Ed., pp. 373–375. John Libbey, London.

Kolin, A. (1936). An electromagnetic flowmeter. Principle of the method and its application to blood flow measurements. *Proc Soc Exp Biol Med* **35**, 53–56.

Koller, A., Sun, D., and Kaley, G. (1993). Role of shear stress and endothelial prostaglandins in flow- and viscosity-induced dilatation of arterioles in vitro. *Circ Res* **72**, 1276–1284.

Koller, A., and Huang, A. (1994). Impaired nitric oxide-mediated flow-induced dilatation in arterioles of spontaneoulsy hypertensive rats. *Circ Res* **74**, 416–421.

Komuro, I., and Yazaki, Y. (1993). Control of cardiac gene expression by mechanical stress. *Annu Rev Physiol* **55**, 55–75.

Koolen, M. I., and Van Brummelen, P. (1984). Adrenergic activity and peripheral haemodynamics in relation to sodium sensitivity in patients with essential hypertension. *Hypertension* **6**, 820–825.

Kopelman, P. G. (2000). Obesity as a medical problem. *Nature* **404**, 635–643.

Kopp, U. C., Smith, L. A., and Di Bona, G. F. (1987). Impaired renal reflexes in spontaneously hypertensive rats. *Hypertension* **9**, 69–75.

Kopp, U. C., and Buckley-Bleier, R. L. (1989). Impaired renorenal reflexes in two-kidney, 1 clip hypertensive rats. *Hypertension* **14**, 445–452.

Kopp, U. C., and DiBona, G. F. (1992). The neural control of renal function. In *The Kidney: Physiology and Pathophysiology*, Seldin, D. W., and Giebisch, G., Eds., Vol. 1, pp. 1157–1204. Raven Press, New York.

Korner, P. I. (1947). Studies on human vasomotor responses to exercise. MSc thesis, Department of Physiology, University of Sydney, Sydney.

Korner, P. I. (1952a). The normal human blood pressure during and after exercise, with some related observations on changes in the heart rate and the blood flow in the limbs. *Aust J Exp Biol Med Sci* **30**, 375–384.

Korner, P. I. (1952b). Reflex regulation of post-exercise blood pressure. *Aust J Exp Biol Med Sci* **30**, 385–394.

Korner, P. I., and Courtice, F. C. (1954). The effects of acute anoxia and noradrenaline vaso-constriction on lymph flow and protein dynamics following transfusions of ringer locke solution. *Aust J Exp Biol Med Sci* **32**, 321–332.

Korner, P. I., Morris, B., and Courtice, F. C. (1954). An analysis of factors affecting lymph flow and protein compostion during gastric absorption of food and fluids and during intravenous infusion. *Aust J Exp Biol Med Sci* **32**, 301–320.

Korner, P. I. (1959). Circulatory adaptations in hypoxia. *Physiol Rev* **39**, 687–730.

Korner, P. I. (1963). Effects of low oxygen and of carbon monoxide on the renal circulation in the unanaesthetized rabbits. *Circ Res* **12**, 361–374.

Korner, P. I. (1964). Effects of hypoxia on the renal circulation. *Bull PostGrad Comm Univ Sydney* **20**, 67–77.

Korner, P. I. (1965a). The effect of section of the carotid sinus and aortic nerves on the cardiac output of the rabbit. *J Physiol (Lond)* **180**, 266–278.

Korner, P. I. (1965b). The role of the arterial chemoreceptors and baroreceptors in the circulatory response to hypoxia of the rabbit. *J Physiol (Lond)* **180**, 279–303.

Korner, P. I., Chalmers, J. P., and White, S. W. (1967). Some mechanisms of reflex control of the circulation by the sympatho-adrenal system. *Circ Res* **20 & 21** (suppl III), III-157–III-172.

Korner, P. I., Langsford, G., Starr, D., Uther, J. B., Ward, W., and White, S. W. (1968). The effects of chloralose-urethane and sodium pentobarbitone anaesthesia on the local and autonomic components of the circulatory response to arterial hypoxia. *J Physiol (Lond)* **199**, 283–302.

Korner, P., and Uther, J. (1969). Dynamic characteristics of the cardiovascular autonomic effects during severe arterial hypoxia in the unanesthetized rabbit. *Circ Res* **24**, 671–687.

Korner, P. I., Uther, J. B., and White, S. W. (1969). Central nervous integration of the circulatory and respiratory responses to arterial hypoxemia in the rabbit. *Circ Res* **24**, 757–776.

Korner, P. I. (1970). Central nervous control of autonomic function—possible implications in the pathogenesis of hypertension. *Circ Res* **26 & 27**, II-159–II-168.

Korner, P. I., and Uther, J. B. (1970). Stimulus-cardiorespiratory effector response profile during arterial hypoxia in the unanaesthetized rabbit. *Aust J Exp Biol Med Sci* **48**, 663–685.

Korner, P. (1971a). The central nervous system and physiological mechanisms of "optimal" cardiovascular control. *Aust J Exp Biol Med Sci* **49**, 319–343.

Korner, P. I. (1971b). Integrative neural cardiovascular control. *Physiol Rev* **51**, 312–367.

Korner, P. I., Shaw, J., West, M. J., and Oliver, J. R. (1972). Central nervous system control of baroreceptor reflexes in the rabbit. *Circ Res* **31**, 637–652.

Korner, P. I., Shaw, J., Uther, J. B., West, M. J., McRitchie, R. J., and Richards, J. G. (1973). Autonomic and non-autonomic circulatory components in essential hypertension in man. *Circulation* **48**, 107–117.

Korner, P. I., Shaw, J., West, M. J., Oliver, J. R., and Hilder, R. G. (1973). Integrative reflex control of heart rate in the rabbit during hypoxia and hyperventilation. *Circ Res* **33**, 63–73.

Korner, P. I., West, M. J., and Shaw, J. (1973). Central nervous resetting of baroreceptor reflexes. *Aust J Exp Biol Med Sci* **51**, 53–64.

Korner, P. I. (1974). Control of blood flow to special vascular areas: brain, kidney, muscle, skin, liver and intestine. In *Cardiovascular Physiology*, Guyton, A. C., and Jones, C. E., Eds., Vol. 1, pp. 123–162. University Park Press, Baltimore, MD.

Korner, P. I., Oliver, J. R., Sleight, P., Chalmers, J. P., and Robinson, J. S. (1974). Effect of clonidine on the baroreceptor-heart rate reflex and on single aortic baroreceptor fibre discharge. *Eur J Pharm* **28**, 189–198.

Korner, P. I., West, M. J., Shaw, J., and Uther, J. B. (1974). "Steady-state" properties of the baroreceptor-heart rate reflex in essential hypertension in man. *Clin Exp Pharmacol Physiol* **1**, 65–76.

Korner, P. I., Oliver, J. R., Sleight, P., Robinson, J. S., and Chalmers, J. P. (1975). Assessment of cardiac autonomic excitability in renal hypertensive rabbits using clonidine-induced resetting of the baroreceptor-heart rate reflex. *Eur J Pharm* **33**, 353–362.

Korner, P. I., and Uther, J. B. (1975). Reflex autonomic control of heart rate and peripheral blood flow. *Brain Res* **87**, 293–303.

Korner, P. I., Blombery, P. A., Bobik, A., Tonkin, A. M., and Uther, J. B. (1976). Valsalva vasoconstrictor reflex in human hypertension and after beta-adrenoceptor blockade in conscious rabbits. *Clin Sci Mol Med* **51**, 365s–368s.

Korner, P. I., Tonkin, A. M., and Uther, J. B. (1976). Reflex and mechanical circulatory effects of graded Valsalva maneuvers in normal man. *J Appl Physiol* **40**, 434–440.

Korner, P. I., and Fletcher, P. J. (1977). Role of the heart in causing and maintaining hypertension. *Cardiovasc Med* **2**, 139–155.

Korner, P. I., Anderson, W. P., Johnston, C. I., Angus, J. A., and Fletcher, P. J. (1978). The role of cardiac output in the pathogenesis of hypertension. In *Proceedings of the VIIth International Congress on Nephrology*. Presses de l'Université de Montréal, Montréal.

Korner, P. I., Oliver, J. R., Reynoldson, J. A., Head, G. A., Carson, V. J., and Walker, M. M. (1978). Cardiovascular and behavioural effects of intracisternal 6–hydroxydopamine in the rabbit. *Eur J Pharm* **53**, 83–93.

Korner, P. I. (1979a). Central nervous control of autonomic cardiovascular function. In *Handbook of Physiology. The Cardiovascular System: The Heart*, Berne, R. M., and Sperelakis, N., Eds., Vol. I, Section 2, pp. 691–739. American Physiological Society, Bethesda, MD.

Korner, P. I. (1979b). Role of cardiac output, volume and resistance factors in the pathogenesis of hypertension. *Clin Sci* **57**, 77s–82s.

Korner, P. I., and Dorward, P. K. (1979). Central nervous effects of propranolol on renal sympathetic baroreflex in the rabbit—relation to haemodynamic response in man. *Jpn Heart J* **20**, 195–197.

Korner, P. I., Oliver, J. R., Reynoldson, J. A., and Head, G. A. (1979). Circulatory, reflex and behavioural effects after intracisternal 6–hydroxydopamine. In *Perspectives in Nephrology and Hypertension Series: Nervous System and Hypertension*, Schmitt, H., and Meyer, P., Eds., pp. 115–122. Wiley, New York.

Korner, P. I., Reynoldson, J. A., Head, G. A., Oliver, J. R., and Carson, V. (1979). Effect of 6–hydroxydopamine on baroreceptor-heart rate and nasopharyngeal reflexes. *J Cardiovasc Pharmacol* **1**, 311–328.

Korner, P. I., Tonkin, A. M., and Uther, J. B. (1979). Valsalva constrictor and heart rate reflexes in subjects with essential hypertension and with normal blood pressure. *Clin Exp Pharmacol Physiol* **6**, 97–110.

Korner, P. I. (1980a). Operation of the central nervous system in reflex circulatory control. *Fed Proc* **39**, 2504–2512.

Korner, P. I. (1980b). The present status of the autoregulation theory of the pathogenesis of hypertension. *Clin Exp Pharmacol Physiol* **7**, 521–526.

Korner, P. I., Dorward, P. K., Blombery, P. A., and Frean, G. J. (1980). Central nervous beta-adrenoceptors and their role in the cardiovascular action of propranolol in rabbits. *Circ Res* **46**, I-26–I-32.

Korner, P. I., Oliver, J. R., and Casley, D. J. (1980). Effect of dietary salt on hemodynamics of established renal hypertension in the rabbit. Implications for the autoregulation theory of hypertension. *Hypertension* **2**, 794–801.

Korner, P. I., and Angus, J. A. (1981). Central nervous control of blood pressure in relation to antihypertensive drug treatment. *Pharmacol Ther* **13**, 321–356.

Korner, P. I., and Head, G. A. (1981). Effects of noradrenergic and serotonergic neurons on blood pressure, heart rate and baroreceptor-heart rate reflex of the conscious rabbit. *J Auton Nerv Syst* **3**, 511–523.

Korner, P. I. (1982). Volhard Lecture: Causal and homeostatic factors in hypertension. *Clin Sci* **63**, 5s–26s.

Korner, P. I. (1983). The role of the heart in hypertension. In *Handbook of Hypertension, Volume I: Clinical Aspects of Essential Hypertension*, Robertson, J., Ed., Vol. I, pp. 97–132. Elsevier, Amsterdam.

Korner, P. I., Oliver, J. R., Aberdeen, J., and Evans, B. K. (1983). Circulatory patterns evoked from the rabbit hypothalamus. In *29th International Congress of Physiological Sciences*, Vol. 15, pp. Abstract 123.25. Elsevier International Congress Series.

Korner, P. (1984). The pathogenesis of hypertension: the Baker Concerto. *Clin Exp Hypertens* **A6**, 565–586.

Korner, P. I., Head, G. A., and Badoer, E. (1984). Effects of sino-aortic denervation on the circulatory responses to centrally administered 6–hydroxydopamine and of clonidine in conscious rabbits. *J Cardiovasc Pharmacol* **6**, 909–913.

Korner, P. I., Head, G. A., Bobik, A., Badoer, E., and Aberdeen, J. A. (1984). Central and peripheral autonomic mechanisms involved in the circulatory actions of methyldopa. *Hypertension* **6** (suppl II), II-63–II-70.

Korner, P. I., Badoer, E., and Head, G. A. (1987). Cardiovascular role of the major noradrenergic cell groups in the rabbit: analysis based on 6–hydroxydopamine-induced transmitter release. *Brain Res* **435**, 258–272.

Korner, P. I., Jennings, G. L., Esler, M. D., Anderson, W. P., Bobik, A., Adams, M. A., and Angus, J. A. (1987). The cardiovascular amplifiers in human primary hypertension and their role in a strategy for detecting the underlying cause. *Can J Physiol Pharmacol* **65**, 1730–1738.

Korner, P. I., Jennings, G. L., Esler, M. D., and Broughton, A. (1987). A new approach to the identification of pathogenetic factors and to therapy in human primary hypertension. *J Clin Hypertens* **3**, 187–196.

Korner, P. I., Jennings, G. L., Nelson, L., and Esler, M. D. (1987). Long-term antihypertensive action of regular exercise: its role in a new treatment strategy. In *Prevention of Cardiovascular Diseases: An Approach to Active Long Life*, Yamori, Y., and Lenfant, C., Eds., pp. 213–223. Excerpta Medica, Amsterdam.

Korner, P. I. (1988). Neurohumoral circulatory regulation in hypertension. *Acta Physiol Scand* **133** (suppl 571), 83–96.

Korner, P. I. (1989). Baroreceptor resetting and other determinants of baroreflex properties in hypertension. *Clin Exp Pharmacol Physiol* **16** (suppl 15), 45–64.

Korner, P. I., Bobik, A., Angus, J. A., Adams, M. A., and Friberg, P. (1989). Resistance control in hypertension. *J Hypertens* **7** (suppl 4), S125–S134.

Korner, P. I., Oliver, J. R., Zhu, J. L., Gipps, J., and Hanneman, F. (1990). Autonomic, hormonal and local circulatory effects of hemorrhage in conscious rabbits. *Am J Physiol* **258**, H229–H239.

Korner, P., Bobik, A., Jennings, G., Angus, J., and Anderson, W. (1991). Significance of cardiovascular hypertrophy in the development and maintenance of hypertension. *J Cardiovasc Pharmacol* **17**, S25–S32.

Korner, P. I., and Angus, J. A. (1992). Structural determinants of vascular resistance properties in hypertension. *J Vascular Res* **29**, 293–312.

Korner, P. I., Bobik, A., and Angus, J. A. (1992). Are cardiac and vascular "amplifiers" both necessary for the development of hypertension? *Kidney Internat* **41**, S38–S44.

Korner, P. I., Bobik, A., Oddie, C., and Friberg, P. (1992). Sympathoadrenal system is critical for structural changes in resistance vessels. In *Genetic Hypertension: Proceedings of 7th International Symposium on SHR and Related Studies*, Sassard, J., Ed., Vol. 218, pp. 237–239. John Libbey Eurotex/EditionsINSERM, Montrouge, France.

Korner, P. I., and Head, G. A. (1992). Baroreflexes in hypertension. In *Central Neural Mechanisms in Cardiovascular Regulation*, Kunos, G., and Ciriello, J., Eds., Vol. 2, pp. 356–374. Birkhauser, Boston.

Korner, P., Bobik, A., Oddie, C., and Friberg, P. (1993). Sympathoadrenal system is critical for structural changes in genetic hypertension. *Hypertension* **22**, 243–252.

Korner, P. I. (1995a). Cardiac baroreflex in hypertension: role of the heart and angiotensin II. *Clin Exper Hypertens,* **A 17**, 425–439.

Korner, P. I. (1995b). Circulatory control and the supercontrollers (Bjorn Folkow Award Lecture). *J Hypertens* **13**, 1508–1521.

Korner, P. I., and Angus, J. A. (1995). Correction of error in article: Structural determinants of vascular resistance properties in hypertension. *J Vascular Res* **29**, 293–312. *J Vasc Res* **32**, 119.

Korner, P. I., and Bobik, A. (1995). Cardiovascular development after enalapril in spontaneously hypertensive and Wistar Kyoto rats. *Hypertension* **25**, 610–619.

Korner, P. I., and Angus, J. A. (1997). Vascular Remodeling [Letter to the Editor]. *Hypertension* **29**, 1065–1066.

Korner, P. I., and Jennings, G. L. (1998). Assessment of prevalence of left ventricular hypertrophy in hypertension. *J Hypertens* **16**, 715–723.

Korner, P. I., Angus, J. A., and Wright, C. E. (2000). Structure and the resistance amplifier in hypertension: reply to the dissenters. *J Hypertens* **18**, 235–239.

Korotkoff, N. S. (1905). K voprosu o metodoach eezldovania krovyonovo davlenia. *Izv Imperator Vorenno Med Akad* **11**, 365–367.

Korsgaard, N., and Mulvany, M. J. (1992). Effects of antihypertensive treatment on the characteristics of resistance arteries. *Acta Physiol Scand* **146** (suppl 608), 20.

Kostromina, E. Y., Rodionov, I. M., and Shinkarenko, V. S. (1991). Tone, autoregulatory properties, and wall thickness-to-radius ratio in skeletal muscle arterioles. *Am J Physiol* **261**, H1095–H1101.

Koushanpour, E. (1991). Baroreceptor discharge behaviour and resetting. In *Baroreceptor Refelexes*, Persson, P. B., and Kirchheim, H. R., Eds., pp. 9–44. Springer-Verlag, Berlin.

Kozelka, J. W., Christy, G. W., and Wurster, R. D. (1987). Ascending pathways mediating somatoautonomic reflexes in exercising dogs. *J Appl Physiol* **62**, 1186–1191.

Kozlovskis, P. L., Smets, M. J. D., Strauss, W. L., and Myerburg, R. J. (1996). DNA synthesis in adult feline ventricular myocytes: comparison of hypoxic and normoxic states. *Circ Res* **78**, 289–301.

Kremer, M., Wright, S., and Scarff, R. W. (1933). Experimental hypertension and the arterial lesions in the rabbit. *Br J Exp Pathol* **14**, 281–290.

Kreutz, R., Stock, P., Struk, B., and Lindpaintner, K. (1996). The Y chromosome: epistatic and ecogenetic interactions in genetic hypertension. *Hypertension* **28**, 895–897.

Krieger, E. M., Salgado, H. C., and Michelini, L. C. (1982). Resetting of the baroreceptors. In *Cardiovascular Physiology IV*, Guyton, A., and Hall, J. E., Eds., Vol. 26, pp. 119–146. University Park Press, Baltimore, MD.

Krieger, E. M. (1989). Arterial baroreceptor resetting in hypertension. J.W. McCubbin Memorial Lecture. *Clin Exp Pharmacol Physiol* **16** (suppl 15), 3–17.

Krieger, J., and Cowley, A., Jr. (1990). Prevention of salt angiotensin II hypertension by servo-control of body water. *Am J Physiol* **258**, H994–H1003.

Krieger, J. E., Liard, J. F., and Cowley, A. W., Jr. (1990). Hemodynamics, fluid volume, and hormonal responses to chronic high-salt intake in dogs. *Am J Physiol* **259**, H1629–H1636.

Krieger, D. R., and Landsberg, L. (1995). Obesity and hypertension. In *Hypertension: Pathophysiology, Diagnosis and Management*, Laragh, J., and Brenner, B., Eds., Vol. 2, pp. 2367–2390. Raven Press, New York.

Krogh, A. (1912). Regulation of the supply of blood to the right heart (with a description of a new circulation model. *Skand Arch Physiol* **27**, 227–248.

Krogh, A., and Lindhard, J. (1913). The regulation of respiration and circulation during the initial stages of muscular work. *J Physiol (Lond)* **47**, 112–136.

Krogh, A., and Lindhard, J. (1917). A comparison between voluntary and electrically induced work in man. *J Physiol (Lond)* **51**, 182–201.

Kuczmarski, R. J., Carroll, M. D., Flegal, K. M., and Troiano, R. P. (1997). Varying body mass index cut off points to describe overweight prevalence among U.S. adults: NHANES III (1988–1994). *Obesity Res* **5**, 542.

Kuhn, T. (1962). *The Structure of Scientific Revolutions*. University of Chicago Press, Chicago.

Kumada, M., Schramm, L. P., Altmansberger, R. A., and Sagawa, K. (1975). Modulation of carotid sinus baroreceptor reflex by hypothalamic defence response. *Am J Physiol* **228**, 34–45.

Kumada, M., Dampney, R., and Reis, D. (1977). The trigeminal depressor response: a novel vasodepressor response originating from the trigeminal system. *Brain Res* **119**, 305–326.

Küng, C. F., and Lüscher, T. F. (1995). Different mechanisms of endothelial dysfunction with aging and hypertension in rat aorta. *Hypertension* **25**, 194–200.

Küng, C. F., Moreau, P., Takase, H., and Lüscher, T. F. (1995). L-NAME hypertension alters endothelial and smooth muscle function in rat aorta: prevention by trandolapril and vera-pamil. *Hypertension* **26**, 744–751.

Kunos, G., and Ciriello, J. E. (1991/2). *Central Neural Mechanisms in Cardiovascular Regulation, Vols. 1 and 2*. Birkhauser, Boston.

Kunze, D. (1986). Acute resetting of baroreceptor reflex in rabbits: a central component. *Am J Physiol* **250**, H866–H870.

Kuo, L., Davis, M. J., and Chilian, W. M. (1988). Myogenic activity in isolated subepicardial and subendocardial coronary arterioles. *Am J Physiol* **255**, H1558–H1562.

Kupferman, I. (1991). Hypothalamus and limbic system: peptidergic neurons, homeostasis and emotional behaviour. In *Principles of Neural Science, 3rd Edition*, Kandel, E. R., Schwartz, J. H., and Jessell, T. M., Eds., pp. 735–749. Prentice-Hall International, London.

Kuramoto, K., Murata, K., Yazaki, Y., Ikeda, M., and Nakao, K. (1968). Hemodynamics in juvenile hypertension with special reference to the response to propranolol. *Jpn Circ J* **32**, 981–987.

Kurokawa, K., Fukagawa, M., Hayashi, M., and Saruta, T. (1992). Renal receptors and cellular mechanisms of hormone action in the kidney. In *The Kidney: Physiology and*

Pathophysiology, Seldin, D. W., and Giebisch, G., Eds., Vol. 1, pp. 1339–1372. Raven Press, New York.

Kuro-o, M., Hanaoka, K., Hiroi, Y., Noguchi, T., Fujimori, Y., Takewaki, S., Hayasaka, M., Katoh, H., Miyagishi, A., Nagai, R., Yazaki, Y., and Nabeshima, Y. (1995). Salt sensitive hypertension in transgenic mice overexpressing Na^+-proton exchanger. *Circ Res* **76**, 148–153.

Kurose, I., Kubes, P., Wolf, R., Anderson, D. C., Paulson, J., Miyasaka, M., and Granger, D. N. (1993). Inhibition of nitric oxide production: mechanisms of vascular albumin leakage. *Circ Res* **73**, 164–171.

Kurtz, T. W., and Morris, R. C., Jr. (1987). Biological variability in Wistar-Kyoto rats: implications for research with the spontaneously hypertensive rat. *Hypertension* **10**, 127–131.

Kurtz, T. W., Montano, M., Chan, L., and Kabra, P. (1989). Molecular evidence of genetic heterogeneity in Wistar-Kyoto rats: implications for research with the spontaneously hypertensive rat. *Hypertension* **13**, 188–192.

Kurtz, T. W., Casto, R., Simonet, L., and Printz, M. P. (1990). Biometric genetic analysis of blood pressure in the spontaneously hypertensive rat. *Hypertension* **16**, 718–724.

Kurtz, T. W., St. Lezin, E. M., and Pravenec, M. (1994). Development of hypertension strains. In *Textbook of Hypertension*, Swales, J. D., Ed., pp. 441–447. Blackwell, Oxford.

Kurtz, T. W. (1995). Possible genetic lesions in experimental and clinical forms of essential hypertension. In *Hypertension: Pathophysiology, Diagnosis and Management*, Laragh, J. H., and Brenner, B. M., Eds., Vol. 1, pp. 1281–1287. Raven Press, New York.

Labeit, S., Kolmerer, B., and Linke, W. A. (1997). The giant protein titin: emerging roles in physiology and pathophysiology. *Circ Res* **80**, 290–294.

Lack, A. (1949). Biomicroscopy of conjunctival vessels in hypertension. *Am Heart J* **38**, 654–664.

Lais, L., and Brody, M. (1978). Vasoconstrictor hyperresponsiveness: an early pathogenic mechanism in the spontaneously hypertensive rat. *Eur J Pharm* **47**, 177–189.

Lakatta, E. G. (1987). Is normotensive aging of the cardiovascular system a muted form of hypertensive cardiovascular disease? In *The Heart and Hypertension*, Messerli, F. H., Ed., pp. 261–272. Yorke Medical Books, New York.

Lakatta, E. (1993). Cardiovascular regulatory mechanisms in advanced age. *Physiol Rev* **73**, 413–467.

Lambert, G. W., Ferrier, C., Kaye, D. M., Kalff, V., Kelly, M. J., Cox, H. S., Turner, A. G., Jennings, G. L., and Esler, M. D. (1994). Monoaminergic neuronal activity in subcortical brain regions in essential hypertension. *Blood Pressure* **3**, 55–66.

Lambert, G. W., Ferrier, C., Jennings, G. L., Kalff, V., Kelly, M. J., and Cox, H. S. (1995). Central nervous system norepinephrine turnover in essential hypertension. *Ann NY Acad Sci* **763**, 679–694.

Lambert, G. W., Vaz, M., Rajkumar, C., Cox, H. S., Turner, A. G., Jennings, G. L., and Esler, M. D. (1996). Cerebral metabolism and its relationship with sympathetic nervous activity in essential hypertension: evaluation of the Dickinson hypothesis. *J Hypertens* **14**, 951–959.

Landas, S., Fischer, J., Wilkin, L. D., Mitchell, L., Johnson, A. K., Turner, J. W., Theriac, M., and Moore, K. C. (1985). Demonstration of regional blood brain barrier permeability in human brain. *Neurosci Lett* **57**, 251–256.

Lander, E. S., and Botstein, D. (1989). Mapping Mendelian factors underlying quantitative traits using RFLP linkage maps. *Genetics* **121**, 185–199.

Landis, E. M., and Pappenheimer, J. R. (1963). Exchange of substances through the capillary walls. In *Handbook of Physiology, Section 2: Circulation* Hamilton, W. F., and Dow, P., Eds., Vol. II, pp. 961–1034. American Physiological Society, Washington, DC.

Landsberg, L., and Young, J. B. (1978). Fasting, feeding and regulation of the sympathetic nervous system. *N Engl J Med* **298**, 1295–1301.

Landsberg, L., and Young, J. B. (1985). Insulin-mediated glucose metabolism in the relationship between dietary intake and sympathetic nervous system activity. *Int J Obes* **9** (suppl 2), 63–68.

Landsberg, L. (2001). Volhard Lecture: Insulin-mediated sympathetic stimulation: role in the pathogenesis of obesity-related hypertension, or how insulin affects blood pressure, and why. *J Hypertens* **19**, 523–528.

Langer, S. Z., Adler-Graschinsky, E., and Giorgi, O. (1977). Physiological significance of alpha-adrenoceptor-mediated negative feedback mechanism regulating noradrenaline release during nerve stimulation. *Nature* **265**, 648–650.

Langer, S. Z. (1981). Presynaptic regulation of the release of catecholamines. *Pharmacol Rev* **32**, 337–362.

Langer, S. Z., and Arbilla, S. (1990). Presynaptic receptors on peripheral noradrenergic neurons. *Ann NY Acad Sci* **604**, 7–16.

Langer, G. (1992). Calcium and the heart: exchange at the tissue, cell and organelle levels. *FASEB J* **6**, 894–902.

Langille, B. L., and O'Donnell, F. (1986). Reductions in arterial diameter produced by chronic decreases in blood flow are endothelium-dependent. *Science* **231**, 405–407.

Langille, B. L., Bendeck, M. P., and Keeley, F. W. (1989). Adaptations of carotid arteries of young and mature rabbits to reduced carotid blood flow. *Am J Physiol* **256**, H931–H939.

Langille, B. L. (1996). Arterial remodeling: relationship to haemodynamics. *Can J Physiol Pharmacol* **74**, 834–841.

Langston, J. B., Guyton, A. C., Douglas, B. H., and Dorsett, P. E. (1963). Effect of changes in salt intake on arterial pressure and renal function in nephrectomized dog. *Circ Res* **12**, 508–513.

Lantelme, P., Khettab, F., Custaud, M.-A., Rial, M.-O., Joanny, C., Gharib, C., and Milon, H. (2002). Spontaneous baroreflex sensitivity toward an ideal index of cardiovascular risk in hypertension? *J Hypertens* **20**, 935–944.

Laragh, J. H., Ulick, S., Januszewicz, W., Deming, Q. B., Kelly, W. G., and Lieberman, S. (1960). Aldosterone secretion and primary and malignant hypertension. *J Clin Invest* **139**, 1091–1106.

Laragh, J. H., and Brenner, B. M. (1995). *Hypertension: Pathophysiology, Diagnosis and Management*. Raven Press, New York.

Laragh, J. H., and Sealey, J. E. (1995). Renin system understanding for analysis and treatment of hypertensive patients: a means to quantify the vasoconstrictor elements, diagnose curable renal and adrenal causes, assess risk of cardiovascular morbidity and find the best-fit drug regimen. In *Hypertension: Pathophysiology, Diagnosis and Management*, Laragh, J. H., and Brenner, B. M., Eds., Vol. 2, pp. 1813–1836. Raven Press, New York.

Lariviere, R., Thibault, G., and Schiffrin, E. L. (1993). Increased endothelin-1 content in blood vessels of deoxycorticosterone acetate-salt hypertension but not in spontaneously hypertensive rats. *Hypertension* **21**, 294–300.

Larkin, S. W., and Williams, T. J. (1993). Evidence for sensory nerve involvement in cutaneous reactive hyperemia in humans. *Circ Res* **73**, 147–154.

La Rovere, M. T., Bigger, J. T., Marcus, F. I., Mortara, A., and Schwartz, P. J. (1998). Baroreflex sensitivity and heart rate variability in prediction of total cardiovascular mortality after myocardial infarction. ATRAMI (Autonomic Tone and Reflexes after Myocardial Infarction) investigators. *Lancet* **351**, 478–484.

Larsen, P. R., and Ingbar, S. H. (1992). The thyroid gland. In *Williams Textbook of Endocrinology*, Wilson, J. D., and Foster, D. W., Eds., pp. 357–487. W. B. Saunders, Philadelphia.

Larson, D. E., Xie, W. Q., Glibetic, M., O'Mahony, D., Sells, B. H., and Rothblum, L. I. (1993). Coordinated decreases in rRNA gene transcription factors and rRNA synthesis during muscle cell differentiation. *Proc Natl Acad Sci, USA* **90,** 7933–7936.

Latham, R. D., Rubal, B. J., Westerhof, N., Sipkema, P., and Walsh, R. A. (1987). Nonhuman primate model for regional wave travel and reflection along aortas. *Am J Physiol* **253,** H299–H306.

Laude, D., Elghozi, J.-L., Girard, A., Bellard, E., Bouhaddi, M., Castiglioni, P., Cerutti, C., Cividjian, A., DiRienzo, M., Fortrat, J.-O., Janssen, B., Karemaker, J. M., Leftheriotis, G., Parati, G., Persson, P. B., Porta, A., Quintin, L., Regnard, J., Rüdiger, H., and Stauss, H. M. (2004). Comparison of various techniques to estimate spontaneous baroreflex sensitivity (the EuroBaVar study). *Am J Physiol* **286,** R226–R231.

Laufer, E., Jennings, G. L., Korner, P. I., and Dewar, E. (1989). Prevalence of cardiac structural and functional abnormalities in untreated primary hypertension. *Hypertension* **13,** 151–162.

Lawler, J. E., Barker, G. F., Hubbard, J. W., and Schaub, R. G. (1981). Effects of stress on blood pressure and cardiac pathology in rats with borderline hypertension. *Hypertension* **3,** 496–505.

Law, C. M., de Swiet, M., Osmond, C., Fayers, P. M., Barker, D. J. P., Cruddas, A. M., and Fall, C. H. D. (1993). Initiation of hypertension in utero and its amplification throughout life. *Brit Med J* **306,** 24–27.

Law, C., and Barker, D. (1994). Fetal influences on blood pressure. *J Hypertens* **12,** 1329–1332.

Lawler, J. E., Barker, G. F., Hubbard, J. W., Cox, R. H., and Randall, G. W. (1984). Blood pressure and plasma renin activity responses to chronic stress in the borderline hypertensive rat. *Physiol Behav* **32,** 101–105.

Ledingham, J. M., and Cohen, R. D. (1964). Changes in the extracellular fluid volume and cardiac output during the development of experimental renal hypertension. *Can Med Assn J* **90,** 292–294.

Ledingham, J. M. (1989). Autoregulation in hypertension: a review. *J Hypertens* **7** (suppl 4), S97–S104.

Le Douarin, N. M. (1986). Ontogeny of the peripheral nervous system from the neural crest and the placodes. A developmental model studied on the basis of the quail-chicken chimera system. *Harvey Lect* **80,** 137–186.

LeDoux, J. E. (1994). In search of an emotional system in the brain: leaping from fear to emotion and consciousness. In *The Cognitive Neurosciences*, Gazzaniga, M. S., Ed., pp. 1049–1061. MIT Press, Cambridge, MA.

Lee, T. H., and Alderman, M. H. (1978). Malignant hypertension: declining mortality rate in New York City, 1958 to 1974. *N Y State J Med* **79,** 1389–1391.

Lee, R. M. K. W. (1985). Vascular changes at the prehypertensive phase in the mesenteric arteries from spontaneously hypertensive rats. *Blood Vessels* **22,** 105–126.

Lee, R. M. K. W., Triggle, C. R., Cheung, D. W. T., and Coughlin, M. D. (1987). Structural and functional consequence of neonatal sympathectomy on the blood vessels of spontaneously hypertensive rats. *Hypertension* **10,** 328–338.

Lee, R. M. K. W., Berecek, K. H., Tsoporis, J., McKenzie, R., and Triggle, C. R. (1991). Prevention of hypertension and vascular changes by captopril treatment. *Hypertension* **17,** 141–150.

Lee, R. M. K., Borkowski, K. R., Leenen, F. H. H., Tsoporis, J., and Coughlin, M. (1991). Interaction between sympathetic nervous system and adrenal medulla in the control of cardiovascular changes in hypertension. *J Cardiovasc Pharmacol* **17** (suppl 2), S114–S116.

Lee, C. K., Klopp, R. G., Weindruch, R., and Prolla, T. A. (1999). Gene expression profile of aging and its retardation by caloric restriction. *Science* **285**, 1390–1393.

Lee, R. M. K. W., and Bund, S. J. (2002). Amplifier and resisters. *J Hypertens* **20**, 2519–2522.

Leenen, F. H. H., Holliwell, D. L., and Cardella, C. J. (1991). Blood pressure and left ventricular anatomy and function after heart transplantation. *Am Heart J* **122**, 1087–1094.

Leenen, F. H. H., Yuan, B., Tsoporis, J., and Lee, R. M. K. W. (1994). Arterial hypertrophy and pressor responsiveness during development of hypertension in spontaneously hypertensive rats. *J Hypertens* **12**, 23–32.

Leenen, F. H. H., Ruzicka, M., and Huang, B. S. (2002). The brain and salt-sensitive hypertension. *Current Hypertension Reports* **4**, 129–135.

Leibowitz, S., Roossin, P., and Rosenn, M. (1984). Chronic norepinephrine injection into the hypothalamic paraventricular nucleus produces hyperphagia and increased body weight in the rat. *Pharmacol Biochem Behav* **21**, 801–808.

Leibowitz, S., and Alexander, J. (1998). Hypothalamic serotonin in control of eating behaviour, meal size and body weight. *Biol Psychiatry* **44**, 851–864.

Le Magnen, J. (1983). Body energy balance and food intake: a neuroendocrine regulatory mechanism. *Physiol Rev* **63**, 314–386.

Le Moal, M., and Simon, H. (1991). Mesocorticolimbic dopaminergic network: functional and regulatory roles. *Physiol Rev* **71**, 155–234.

Lesske, J., Fletcher, E. C., Bao, G., and Unger, T. (1997). Hypertension caused by chronic intermittent hypoxia—influence of chemoreceptors and sympathetic nervous system. *J Hypertens* **15**, 1593–1603.

Letcher, R. L., Chien, S., Pickering, T. G., Sealey, J. E., and Laragh, J. H. (1981). Direct relationship between blood pressure and blood viscosity in normal and hypertensive subjects role of fibrinogen and concentration. *Am J Med* **70**, 1195–1202.

Lever, A. F., Beretta-Piccoli, C., Brown, J. J., Davies, D. L., Fraser, R., and Robertson, J. I. S. (1981). Sodium and potassium in essential hypertension. *Br Med J* **283**, 463–468.

Lever, A. F., and Harrap, S. B. (1992). Essential hypertension: a disorder of growth with origins in childhood. *J Hypertens* **10**, 101–120.

Lever, A. F., and Swales, J. D. (1994). Investigating the hypertensive patient: an overview. In *Textbook of Hypertension,* J. D. Swales, Ed., pp. 1026–1032. Blackwell, Oxford.

Levi-Montcalcini, R. (1987). The nerve growth factor 35 years later. *Science* **237**, 1154–1162.

Levine, J. A., Eberhardt, N. L., and Jensen, M. D. (1999). Role of non-exercise activity thermogenesis in resistance to fat gain in humans. *Science* **283**, 212–214.

Levy, A. M., Tabakin, B. S., and Hanson, J. S. (1967). Hemodynamic responses to graded treadmill exercise in young untreated labile hypertensive patients. *Circulation* **35**, 1063–1072.

Levy, D., Garrison, R. J., Savage, D. D., Kannel, W. B., and Castelli, W. P. (1990). Prognostic implications of echocardiographically determined left ventricular mass in the Framingham Heart Study. *N Engl J Med* **322**, 1561–1566.

Levy, D. (1991). Clinical significance of left ventricular hypertrophy: insights from the Framingham study. *J Cardiovasc Pharmacol* **17** (suppl 2), S1–S6.

Lew, M., and Angus, J. (1992). Wall thickness to lumen diameter ratios of arteries from SHR and WKY: comparison of pressurised and wire-mounted preparations. *J Vascular Res* **29**, 435–442.

Lewis, P. J., and Haeusler, G. (1975). Reduction in sympathetic nervous activity as a mechanism for hypotensive effect of propranolol. *Nature* **256**, 440.

Lewis, E. B. (1978). A gene complex controlling segmentation in *Drosophila. Nature* **276**, 565–570.

Li, S.-J., Wong, S.-C., Hong, J.-S., and Ingenito, A. J. (1992). Age-related changes in opioid peptide concentrations in brain and pituitary of spontaneously hypertensive rats. *Pharmacology* **44,** 245–256.

Li, J.-M., and Brooks, G. (1997). Differential protein expression and subcellular distribution of TGF-β_1, β_2, and β_3 in cardiomyocytes during pressure overload induced hypertrophy. *J Mol Cell Cardiol* **29,** 2213–2224.

Li, S.-G., Lawler, J. E., Randall, D. C., and Brown, D. R. (1997). Sympathetic nervous activity and arterial pressure responses during rest and acute behavioral stress in SHR and WKY. *J Auton Nerv Syst* **62,** 147–154.

Liao, Y., and Husain, A. (1995). The chymase-angiotensin systems in humans: biochemistry, molecular biology and potential role in cardiovascular diseases. *Can J Cardiol* **11** (suppl F), 13F–19F.

Liard, J. F. (1981). Regional blood flows in salt loading hypertension in the dog. *Am J Physiol* **240,** H361–H367.

Lie, M., Sejersted, O. M., and Kiil, F. (1970). Local regulation of vascular cross section during changes in femoral arterial blood flow in dogs. *Circ Res* **27,** 727–737.

Lienhard, G. E. (1994). Life without IRS (insulin receptor substrate). *Nature* **372,** 128–129.

Lifton, R. P., Dluhy, R. G., Powers, M., Rich, G. M., Cook, S., Ulick, S., and Lalouel, J. M. (1992a). A chimaeric 11beta-hydroxylase/aldosterone synthase gene causes glucocorticoid-remedial aldosteronism and human hypertension. *Nature* **355,** 262–265.

Lifton, R. P., Dluhy, R. G., Powers, M., Rich, G. M., Gutkin, M., and Fallo, F. (1992b). Hereditary hypertension caused by chimaeric gene duplications and ectopic expression of aldosterone synthase. *Nat Gen* **2,** 66–74.

Lifton, R. P., and Jeunemaitre, X. (1993). Finding genes that cause human hypertension. *J Hypertens* **11,** 231–236.

Lifton, R. P. (1996). Molecular genetics of human blood pressure variation. *Science* **272,** 676–680.

Lim, P. O., Young, W. F., and MacDonald, T. M. (2001). A review of the medical treatment of primary aldosteronism. *J Hypertens* **19,** 353–361.

Lin, F., Owens, A., Chen, S., Stevens, M. E., Kesteven, S., Arthur, J. F., Woodcock, E. A., Feneley, M. P., and Graham, R. M. (2001). Targeted α_1 adrenergic receptor overexpression induces enhanced cardiac contractility but not hypertrophy. *Circ Res* **89,** 343–350.

Linden, R. J. (1973). Function of cardiac receptors. *Circulation* **68,** 463–480.

Linden, D. J., and Connor, J. A. (1991). Participation of postsynaptic PKC in cerebellar longterm depression in culture. *Science* **254,** 1656–1659.

Lindpaintner, K., Kreutz, R., and Ganten, D. (1992). Genetic variation in hypertensive and "control" strains. What are we controlling for anyway? *Hypertension* **19,** 428–430.

Linzbach, A. J. (1960). Heart failure from the point of view of quantitative anatomy. *Am J Cardiol* **5,** 370–382.

Lipski, J., Bellingham, M. C., West, M. J., and Pilowsky, P. (1988). Limitations of the technique of pressure microinjection of excitatory amino acids for evoking responses from localised regions of the CNS. *J Neurosci Meth* **26,** 169–179.

Lisander, B. (1970). Factors influencing the autonomic component of the defense reaction. *Acta Physiol Scand* (suppl 351), 1–42.

Lisander, B., and Martner, J. (1971). Cerebellar suppression of the autonomic components of the defence reaction. *Acta Physiol Scand* **81,** 84–95.

Liu, B. H. (1998). *Statistical Genomics: Linkage Mapping and QTL Analysis*. CRC, New York.

Ljungman, S., Aurell, M., Hartford, M., Wikstrand, J., Wilhelmsen, L., and Berglund, G. (1980). Blood pressure and renal function. *Acta Physiol Scand* **208,** 17–25.

Ljungman, S., and Granerus, G. (1995). The evaluation of kidney function in hypertensive patients. In *Hypertension: Pathophysiology, Diagnosis and Management*, Laragh, J. H., and Brenner, B. M., Eds., Vol. 2, pp. 1987–2004. Raven Press, New York.

Llewellyn-Smith, I., Phend, K. D., Minson, J., Pilowsky, P., and Chalmers, J. (1992). Glutamate immunoreactive synapses on retrogradely labeled sympathetic preganglionic neurons in rat thoracic spinal cord. *Brain Res* **581**, 67–80.

Loewy, A. D. (1990). Central autonomic pathways. In *Central Regulation of Autonomic Function*, Loewy, A. D., and Spyer, K. M., Eds., pp. 88–103. Oxford University Press, New York.

Loewy, A. D., and Spyer, K. M., Eds. (1990). *Central Regulation of Autonomic Function*. Oxford University Press, New York.

Löfving, B. (1961). Cardiovascular adjustments induced from the rostral cingulate gyrus. *Acta Physiol Scand* **53** (suppl 184), 2–82.

Lohmeier, T. E., Irwin, E. D., Rossing, M. A., Serdar, D. J., and Kieval, R. S. (2004). Prolonged activation of baroreflex produces sustained hypotension. *Hypertension* **43** (part 2), 306–311.

Loke, K. E., Sobey, C. G., Dusting, G. J., and Woodman, O. L. (1994a). Cholinergic neurogenic vasodilatation is mediated by nitric oxide in the dog hindlimb. *Cardiovasc Res* **28**, 542–547.

Loke, K. E., Sobey, C. G., Dusting, G. J., and Woodman, O. L. (1994b). Requirement for endothelium-derived nitric oxide in vasodilatation produced by stimulation of cholinergic nerves in rat hindquarters. *Br J Pharmacol* **112**, 630–634.

Lombard, J. H., Eskinder, H., Kauser, K., Osborn, J. L., and Harder, D. R. (1990). Enhanced norepinephrine sensitivity in renal arteries at elevated transmural pressure. *Am J Physiol* **259**, H29–H33.

London, G. M., Safar, M. E., Sassard, J. E., Levinson, J. A., and Simon, A. C. (1984). Renal and systemic hemodynamics in sustained essential hypertension. *Hypertension* **6**, 743–754.

London, G. M., and Levy, B. I. (1993). Large arteries and calcium in hypertension: pathophysiological and therapeutic aspects. In *The Arterial System in Hypertension*, Safar, M. E., and O'Rourke, M. F., Eds., pp. 209–219. Kluwer Academic Publishers, Dordrecht.

Long, C. S., Kariya, K., Karns, L., and Simpson, P. C. (1991). Sympathetic activity: modulator of myocardial hypertrophy. *J Cardiovasc Pharmacol* **17** (suppl 2), S20–S24.

Longhurst, P. A., Stitzel, R. E., and Head, R. J. (1986). Perfusion of the intact and partially isolated rat mesenteric vascular bed: application to vessels from hypertensive and normotensive rats. *Blood Vessels* **23**, 288–296.

Lopez, M. J., Wong, S. K.-F., Kishimoto, I., Dubois, S., Mach, V., Friesen, J., Garbers, D. L., and Beuve, A. (1995). Salt-resistant hypertension in mice lacking the guanylyl cyclase-A receptor for atrial natriuretic peptide. *Nature* **378**, 65–68.

Lou, Y., Wen, C., Li, M., Adams, D. J., Wang, M., Yang, F., Morris, B. J., and Whitworth, J. A. (2001). Decreased renal expression of nitric oxide synthase isoforms in adrenocorticotropin-induced and corticosterone-induced hypertension. *Hypertension* **37**, 1164–1170.

Loutzenhiser, R. D., and Parker, M. J. (1994). Hypoxia inhibits myogenic reactivity of renal afferent arterioles by activating ATP-sensitive K^+ channels. *Circ Res* **74**, 861–869.

Lovallo, W. R., Pincomb, G. A., Brackett, D. J., and Wilson, M. F. (1990). Heart rate reactivity as a predictor of neuroendocrine responses to aversive and appetitive challenges. *Psychosom Med* **52**, 17–26.

Lowell, B. B., and Spiegelman, B. M. (2000). Towards a molecular understanding of adaptive thermogenesis. *Nature* **404**, 652–660.

Lowenstein, J., Steinmetz, P. R., Effros, R. M., Demeester, M., Chasis, H., Baldwin, D. S., and Gomez, D. M. (1967). The distribution of intrarenal blood flow in normal and hypertensive man. *Circulation* **35**, 250–254.

Lowenstein, J., Beranbaum, E. R., Chasis, H., and Baldwin, D. S. (1970). Intrarenal pressure and exaggerated natriuresis in essential hypertension. *Clin Sci* **38**, 359–374.

Ludbrook, J. (1984). Comparison of the reflex effects of arterial baroreceptors and cardiac receptors on the heart rate of conscious rabbits. *Clin Exp Pharmacol Physiol* **11**, 245–260.

Ludbrook, J., and Graham, W. F. (1984). The role of cardiac receptor and arterial baroreceptor reflexes in control of the circulation during acute changes of blood volume in the conscious rabbit. *Circ Res* **54**, 424–435.

Ludbrook, J., and Rutter, P. C. (1988). Effect of naloxone on haemodynamic responses to acute blood loss in unanaesthetized rabbits. *J Physiol (Lond)* **400**, 1–14.

Luff, S. E., McLachlan, E. M., and Hirst, G. D. S. (1987). An ultrastructural analysis of the sympathetic neuromuscular junctions on arterioles of the submucosa of the guines pig ileum. *J Comp Neurol* **257**, 578–594.

Luff, S. E., and McLachlan, E. M. (1988). The form of sympathetic postganglionic axons at clustered neuromuscular junctions near branch points of arterioles in the submucosa of the guinea pig ileum. *J Neurocytol* **17**, 451–463.

Luff, S. E., and McLachlan, E. M. (1989). Frequency of neuromuscular junctions on arteries of different dimensions in the rabbit, guinea pig and rat. *Blood Vessels* **26**, 95–106.

Luff, S. E., Hengstberger, S. G., McLachlan, E. M., and Anderson, W. P. (1991). Two types of sympathetic axons innervating the juxtaglomerular arterioles of the rabbit and rat kidney differ structurally from those supplying other arteries. *J Neurocytol* **20**, 781–795.

Luff, S. E., Hengstberger, S. G., McLachlan, E. M., and Anderson, W. P. (1992). Distribution of sympathetic neuroeffector junctions in the juxtaglomerular region of the rabbit kidney. *J Auton Nerv Syst* **40**, 239–254.

Luft, F. C., Grim, C. E., Willis, L. R., Higgins, J. T., Jr., and Weinberger, M. H. (1977). Natriuretic responses to saline infusions in normotensive and hypertensive man. The role of renin suppression in exaggerated natriuresis. *Circulation* **55**, 779–784.

Luft, F. C., Grim, C. E., Fineberg, N., and Weinberger, M. C. (1979). Effects of volume expansion and contraction in normotensive whites, blacks, and subjects of different ages. *Circulation* **59**, 643–650.

Luft, F. C., Rankin, L. I., Bloch, R., Weyman, A. E., Willis, L. R., Murray, R. H., Grim, C. E., and Weinberger, M. H. (1979). Cardiovascular and humoral responses to extremes of sodium intake in normal black and white men. *Circulation* **60**, 697–706.

Luft, F. C., Grim, C. E., and Weinberger, M. H. (1985). Electrolyte and volume homeostasis in blacks. In *Hypertension in Blacks*, Hall, W., Saunders, E., and Shulman, N., Eds., pp. 115–131. Year Book, Chicago.

Luft, F. C., Miller, J. Z., Grim, C. E., Fineberg, N. S., Christian, J. C., Daugherty, S. A., and Weinberger, M. H. (1991). Salt sensitivity and resistance of blood pressure: age and race as factors in physiological responses. *Hypertension* **17** (suppl I), I-102–I-108.

Luft, F. C., and Dietz, R. (1993). Franz Volhard in historical perspective. *Hypertension* **22**, 253–256.

Luft, F. C. (1998). Molecular genetics of human hypertension. *J Hypertens* **16**, 1871–1878.

Luft, F. C. (2001). Twins in cardiovascular genetic research. *Hypertension* **37** (part II), 350–356.

Luft, F. C. (2004). Geneticism of essential hypertension. *Hypertension* **43**, 1155–1159.

Lundberg, U., and Frankenhaeuser, M. (1980). Pituitary-adrenal and sympathetic-adrenal correlates of distress and effort. *J Psychosom Res* **24**, 125–130.

Lundgren, Y. (1974). Regression of structural changes after reversal of experimental renal hypertension in rats. *Acta Physiol Scand* **91**, 275–285.

Lundgren, O. (1986). Microcirculation of the gastrointestinal tract and pancreas. In *Handbook of Physiology, Section 2: The Cardiovascular System: Volume IV, Microcirculation,*

Part 2, Renkin, E. M., and Michel, C. C., Eds., pp. 799–863. American Physiological Society, Washington, DC.

Lundin, S., and Thorén, P. (1982). Renal function and sympathetic activity during mental stress in normotensive and spontaneously hypertensive rats. *Acta Physiol Scand* **115**, 115–124.

Lundin, S., Friberg, P., and Ricksten, S.-E. (1983). Diastolic properties of the hypertrophied left ventricle in spontaneously hypertensive rats. *Acta Physiol Scand* **118**, 1–9.

Lund-Johansen, P. (1977). Haemodynamic alterations in hypertension—spontaneous changes and effects of drug therapy. A review. *Acta Med Scand* **201** (Suppl.603), 1–14.

Lund-Johansen, P. (1980). Haemodynamics in essential hypertension. *Clin Sci* **59**, 343s–354s.

Lund-Johansen, P. (1994). Haemodynamics of essential hypertension. In *Textbook of Hypertension*, Swales, J. D., Ed., pp. 61–76. Blackwell, Oxford.

Luo, W., Grupp, I. L., Harrer, J., Ponnia, S., Grupp, G., Duffy, J. J., Doetschman, T., and Kranias, E. G. (1994). Targeted ablation of the phospholamban gene is associated with markedly enhanced myocardial contractility and loss of β-agonist stimulation. *Circ Res* **75**, 401–409.

Lupu, A. N., Maxwell, M. H., Kaufman, J. J., and White, F. N. (1972). Experimental unilateral renal artery constriction in the dog. *Circ Res* **42**, 152–162.

Lüscher, T., Seo, B.-G., and Buehler, F. (1993). Potential role of endothelin in hypertension: controversy on endothelin in hypertension. *Hypertension* **21**, 752–757.

Lüscher, T. F. (1994). The endothelium in hypertension: bystander, target or mediator? *J Hypertens* **12** (suppl 10), S105–S116.

Luyken, J., Hannan, E. D., Cheung, J. Y., and Rothblum, L. I. (1996). Regulation of rDNA induced transcription during endothelin-1–induced hypertrophy of neonatal cardiomyocytes: hyperphosphorylation of upstream binding factor, an rDNA transcription factor. *Circ Res* **78**, 354–361.

MacGregor, G. A., Markandu, N. D., Best, F. E., Elder, D., Cam, J., and Squires, M. (1982). Double-blind randomised crossover trial of moderate sodium restriction in essential hypertension. *Lancet* **i**, 351–354.

MacGregor, G. A., Markandu, N. D., Sagnella, G. A., Singer, D. R., and Cappucio, F. P. (1989). Double-blind study of three sodium intakes and long-term effects of sodium restriction in essential hypertension. *Lancet* **ii**, 1244–1247.

Mackenzie, H. S., Garcia, D. L., Anderson, S., and Brenner, B. M. (1995). The renal abnormality in hypertension: a proposed defect in glomerular filtration surface area. In *Hypertension Pathophysiology Diagnosis and Management*, Laragh, J. H., and Brenner, B. M., Eds., Vol. 1, pp. 1539–1552. Raven Press, New York.

MacLean, P. D. (1970). The triune brain, emotion and scientific bias. In *The Neurosciences*, Schmitt, F. O., Ed., pp. 336–348. Rockefeller University, New York.

MacMahon, S. W., Blacket, R. B., Macdonald, G. J., and Hall, W. (1984). Obesity, alcohol consumption and blood pressure in Australian men and women. The National Heart Foundation of Australia Risk Factor Prevalence Study. *J Hypertens* **2**, 85–91.

MacMahon, S. W., Macdonald, G. J., Bernstein, L., Andrews, G., and Blacket, R. B. (1985). Comparison of weight reduction with metoprolol in treatment of hypertension in young overweight patients. *Lancet* **i**, 1233–1236.

MacMahon, S. (1987). Alcohol consumption and hypertension. *Hypertension* **9**, 111–121.

MacMahon, S. (1994). Blood pressure and the risks of cardiovascular disease. In *Textbook of Hypertension*, Swales, J. D., Ed., pp. 46–57. Blackwell, Oxford.

Maguire, E. A., Burgess, N., Donnett, J. G., Frackowiak, R. S. J., Frith, C. D., and O'Keefe, J. (1998). *Science* **280**, 921–924.

Majewski, H., and Rand, M. J. (1981a). Adrenaline-mediated hypertension: a clue to the antihypertensive effect of beta-adrenoceptor blocking drugs? *Trends Pharmacolog Sci* **2**, 24–26.

Majewski, H., and Rand, M. J. (1981b). An interaction between prejunctional alpha-adrenoceptors and prejunctional beta-adrenoceptors. *Eur J Pharm* **69,** 493–498.

Majewski, H., Rand, M. J., and Tung, L.-H. (1981). Activation of prejunctional α-adrenoceptors in rat atria by adrenaline applied exogenously or released as a co-transmitter. *Br J Pharmacol* **73,** 669–679.

Majewski, H., Tung, L. H., and Rand, M. J. (1981). Adrenaline-induced hypertension in rats. *J Cardiovasc Pharmacol* **3,** 179–185.

Majid, D. S. A., and Nishiyama, A. (2002). Nitric oxide blockade enhances renal responses to superoxide dismutase inhibition in dogs. *Hypertension* **39,** 293–297.

Malliani, A. (1982). Cardiovascular sympathetic afferent fibres. *Rev Physiol Biochem Pharmacocol* **94,** 11–74.

Mancia, G., Baccelli, G., and Zanchetti, A. (1972). Hemodynamic responses to different emotional stimuli in the cat: patterns and mechanisms. *Am J Physiol* **223,** 925.

Mancia, G., Shepherd, J. T., and Donald, D. E. (1975). Role of cardiac, pulmonary and carotid mechanoreceptors in the control of hind-limb and renal circulation in dogs. *Circ Res* **37,** 200–208.

Mancia, G., Lorenz, R. R., and Shepherd, J. T. (1976). Reflex control of circulation by heart and lungs. In *International Review of Physiology,Cardiovascular Physiology II*, Guyton, A. C., and Cowley, A. W., Eds., Vol. 9, pp. 111–144. University Park Press, Baltimore, MD.

Mancia, G., Ferrari, A., Gregorini, L., Parati, G., Pomidossi, G., Bertinieri, G., Grassi, G., Di Rienzo, M., Pedotti, A., and Zanchetti, A. (1983). Blood pressure and heart rate variabilities in normotensive and hypertensive human beings. *Circ Res* **53,** 96–104.

Mancia, G., and Mark, A. L. (1983). Arterial baroreflexes in humans. In *Handbook of Physiology, Section 2: The Cardiovascular System, Volume 3: Peripheral Circulation and Organ Blood Flow*, Shepherd, J. T., and Abboud, F. M., Eds., pp. 755–794. American Physiological Society, Bethesda, MD.

Mancia, G., and Parati, G. (1987). Reactivity to physical and behavioral stress and blood pressure variability in hypertension. In *Handbook of Hypertension*, Julius, S., and Bassett, D. R., Eds., Vol. 9, pp. 104–122. Elsevier, Amsterdam.

Mancia, G. (1990). Ambulatory blood pressure monitoring: research and clinical application (Presidential Lecture). *J Hypertens* **8** (suppl 7), S1–S13.

Mancia, G. (1997). Björn Folkow Award Lecture: The sympathetic nervous system in hypertension. *J Hypertens* **15,** 1553–1565.

Mandler, G. (1987). Emotion. In *The Oxford Companion to Mind*, Gregory, R. L., Ed., pp. 219–220. Oxford University Press, Oxford.

Mangos, G. J., Walker, B. R., Kelly, J. J., Lawson, J., Webb, D. J., and Whitworth, J. A. (2000). Cortisol inhibits vasodilatation in the human forearm. *Am J Hypertens* **36,** 912–916.

Manning, R. D., Hu, L., Mizelle, H. L., Montani, J.-P., and Norton, M. W. (1993). Cardiovascular responses to long-term blockade of nitric oxide synthesis. *Hypertension* **22,** 40–48.

Marcus, M. L. (1983). *The Coronary Circulation in Health and Disease*. McGraw-Hill, New York.

Margetts, B. M., Beilin, L. J., Vandongen, R., and Armstrong, B. K. (1986). Vegetarian diet in mild hypertension: a randomised controlled trial. *Br Med J* **293,** 1468–1471.

Margossian, S. S., White, H. D., Caulfield, J. B., Norton, P., Taylor, S., and Slayter, H. S. (1992). Light chain 2 profile and activity of human ventricular cardiomyopathy: identification of a causal agent for impaired myocardial junction. *Circulation* **85,** 1720–1733.

Mark, A. L., Gordon, F. J., and Takeshita, A. (1981). Sodium, vascular resistance, and genetic hypertension. In *Hypertension: Commentary Issues in Nephrology*, Brenner, B. M., and Stein, J. H., Eds., pp. 21–38. Churchill-Livingstone, New York.

Mark, A. L. (1984). Structural changes in resistance and capacitance vessels in borderline hypertension. *Hypertension* **6**, III-69–III-73.

Mark, A., Victor, R., Nerhed, C., and Wallin, B. (1985). Microneurographic studies of the mechanisms of sympathetic nerve response to static exercise in humans. *Circ Res* **57**, 461–469.

Mark, A. L., Shaffer, R. A., Correia, M. L. G., Morgan, D. A., Sigmund, C. D., and Haynes, W. G. (1999). Contrasting blood pressure effects of obesity in leptin deficient ob/ob mice and agouti yellow obese mice. *J Hypertens* **17**, 1949–1953.

Mark, A. L., Correia, M. L. G., Rahmouni, K., and Haynes, W. G. (2002). Selective leptin resistance: a new concept in leptin physiology with cardiovascular implications. *J Hypertens* **20**, 1245–1250.

Markovitz, J. H., Matthews, K. A., Wing, R. R., Kuller, L. H., and Meilahn, E. N. (1991). Psychological, biological and health behavior predictors of blood pressure changes in middle-aged women. *J Hypertens* **9**, 399–406.

Marr, D. (1969). A theory of cerebellar cortex. *J Physiol (Lond)* **202**, 437–470.

Marsh, A. J., Fontes, M. A. P., Killinger, S., Pawlak, D. B., Polson, J. W., and Dampney, R. A. L. (2003). Cardiovascular responses evoked by leptin acting on neurons in the ventromedial and dorsomedial hypothalamus. *Hypertension* **42**, 488–493.

Marshall, S. A., Levine, R. A., and Weyman, A. E. (1992). Echocardiography in cardiac research. In *The Heart and Cardiovascular System*, Fozzard, H. A., Haber, E., Jennings, R. B., and Katz, A. M., Eds., Vol. 1, pp. 745–838. Raven Press, New York.

Martinez-Maldonado, M., Benabe, J. E., and Cordova, H. R. (1992). Chronic clinical intrinsic renal failure. In *The Kidney: Physiology and Pathophysiology*, Seldin, D. W., and Giebisch, G., Eds., Vol. 3, pp. 3227–3288. Raven Press, New York.

Mather, K., and Jinks, J. L. (1982). *Biometrical Genetics*. Chapman and Hall, London.

Matsubara, H., Mori, Y., Takashima, H., and Inada, M. (1989). Simultaneous measurement of α-human atrial natriuretic factor (hANF) and NH_2 terminal fragments of pro-hANF in essential hypertension. *Am Heart J* **118**, 494–499.

Matthews, K. A., Kiefe, C. I., Lewis, C. E., Liu, K., Sidney, S., and Yunis, C. (2002). Socioeconomic trajectories and incident hypertension in a biracial cohort of young adults. *Hypertension* **39**, 772–776.

Mattson, D. L., Roman, R. J., and Cowley, A. W., Jr. (1992). Role of nitric oxide in renal papillary blood flow and sodium excretion. *Hypertension* **19**, 766–769.

Mattson, D. L., Lu, S., Nakanishi, K., Papanek, P. E., and Cowley, A. W. (1994). Effect of chronic renal medullary nitric oxide inhibition on blood pressure. *Am J Physiol* **266**, H1918–H1926.

Maxwell, M., Lupu, A., Viskoper, R., Aravena, L., and Waks, U. (1977). Mechanisms of hypertension during the acute and intermediate phases of the one-clip, two-kidney model in the dog. *Circ Res* **40** (suppl I), I-24–I-28.

May, A., Van de Berg, L., DeWeese, J., and Rob, C. (1963). Critical arterial stenosis. *Surgery* **54**, 250–259.

Mayet, J., Shahi, M., McGrath, K., Poulter, N. R., Sever, P. S., Foale, R. A., and Thom, S. A. M. (1996). Left ventricular hypertrophy and QT dispersion in hypertension. *Hypertension* **28**, 791–796.

Mayr, E. (1961). Cause and effect in biology: kinds of causes, predictability, and teleology as viewed by a practising biologist. *Science* **134**, 1501–1506.

Mayr, E. (1997). *This Is Biology: The Science of the Living World*. Belknap Press, Cambridge, MA.

McAllen, R. M. (1986). Action and specificity of ventral medullary vasopressor neurones in the cat. *Neuroscience* **18**, 51–59.

McAllen, R. M., and Dampney, R. (1989). The selectivity of descending vasomotor control by subretrofacial neurons. *Prog Brain Res* **81,** 233–242.

McCance, R. A., and Widdowson, E. M. (1974). The determinants of growth and form. *Proc R Soc B* **185,** 1–17.

McCarron, D. A., Henry, H. J., and Morris, C. D. (1992). Human nutrition and blood pressure regulation: an integrated approach. *Hypertension* **19** (suppl III), 2–13.

McCarty, R., and Lee, J. H. (1996). Preweanling administration of terazosin decreases blood pressure of hypertensive rats in adulthood. *Hypertension* **27,** 1115–1120.

McCloskey, D., and Mitchell, J. (1972). Reflex cardiovascular and respiratory responses originating in exercising muscle. *J Physiol (Lond)* **224,** 173–186.

McCubbin, J. W., Green, J. H., and Page, I. H. (1956). Baroreceptor function in chronic renal hypertension. *Circ Res* **4,** 205–210.

McDonald, D. A., and Taylor, M. G. (1959). The hydrodynamics of the arterial circulation. *Prog Biophysics* **9,** 105–173.

McDonald, D. A. (1960). *Blood Flow in Arteries.* Edward Arnold, London.

McEwan, J. R., Benjamin, N., Larkin, S., Fuller, R. W., Dollery, C. T., and MacIntyre, I. (1988). Vasodilatation by calcitonin-gene-related peptide and by substance P: a comparison of their effects on resistance and capacitance vessels of human forearms. *Circulation* **77,** 1072–1080.

McEwen, B. S. (1994). Stressful experience brain and emotions: developmental genetic and hormonal influences. In *The Cognitive Neurosciences,* Gazzaniga, M. S., Ed., pp. 1117–1135. MIT Press, Cambridge, MA.

McEwen, B. S. (1998). Protective and damaging effects of stress mediators. *N Engl J Med* **338,** 171–179.

McGarry, J. D., and Dobbins, R. L. (1999). Fatty acids, lipotoxicity and insulin secretion. *Diabetologia* **42,** 128–138.

McGrath, B. P., Tiller, D. J., Bune, A., Chalmers, J. P., Korner, P. I., and Uther, J. B. (1977). Autonomic blockade and the Valsalva maneuver in patients on maintenance hemodialysis: a hemodynamic study. *Kidney Internat* **12,** 294–302.

McNally, J. G., Muller, W. G., Walker, D., Wolford, R., and Hager, G. L. (2000). The glucocorticoid receptor rapid exchange with regulatory sites in living cells. *Science* **287,** 1262–1265.

McRitchie, R. J. (1973). Nasopharyngeal reflexes in the unanaesthetised rabbit: an integrative analysis of respiratory and cardiovascular effects. PhD thesis, Department of Medicine, University of Sydney, Sydney.

McRitchie, R. J., and White, S. W. (1974). Role of trigeminal, olfactory, carotid sinus and aortic nerves in the respiratory and circulatory response to nasal inhalation of cigarette smoke and other irritants in the rabbit. *Aust J Exp Biol Med Sci* **52,** 127–140.

Medgett, I. C., McCulloch, M. W., and Rand, M. J. (1978). Partial agonist action of clonidine on prejunctional and postjunctional α-adrenoceptors. *Naunyn-Schmiedeberg's Arch Pharmacol* **304,** 215–221.

Meerson, F. Z., Zaletayeva, T. A., Lagutchev, S. S., and Pshennikova, M. G. (1964). Structure and mass of mitochondria in the process of compensatory hyperfunction and hypertrophy of the heart. *Exp Cell Res* **36,** 568–573.

Meerson, F. Z. (1974). Development of modern (components) concepts of the mechanism of cardiac hypertrophy. *Circ Res* **34 & 35** (suppl II), II-58–II-63.

Meininger, G. A., Lubrano, V. M., and Granger, H. J. (1984). Hemodynamics and microvascular responses in the hindquarters during the development of renal hypertension in rats: evidence for the involvement of an autoregulatory component. *Circ Res* **55,** 609–622.

Meininger, G. A., Routh, L. K., and Granger, H. J. (1985). Autoregulation and vasoconstriction in the intestine during acute renal hypertension. *Hypertension* **7,** 364–373.

Meininger, G. A., Fehr, K. L., Yates, M. B., Borders, J. L., and Granger, H. J. (1986). Hemodynamic characteristics of the intestinal microcirculation in renal hypertension. *Hypertension* **8**, 66–75.

Meininger, G. A., and Trzeciakowski, J. P. (1988). Vasoconstriction is amplified by autoregulation during vasoconstrictor-induced hypertension. *Am J Physiol* **254**, H709–H718.

Meininger, G. A., and Faber, J. E. (1991). Adrenergic facilitation of myogenic response in skeletal muscle arterioles. *Am J Physiol* **263**, H1424–H1432.

Melby, J. C., Dale, S. L., Grekin, R. J., Gaunt, R., and Wilson, T. E. (1972). Hydroxy-11–deoxycorticosterone (18–OH-DOC) secretion in experimental and human hypertension. *Recent Prog Horm Res* **28**, 287–351.

Melkumyants, A. M., Balashov, S. A., and Khayutin, V. M. (1989). Endothelium-dependent control of arterial diameter by blood viscosity. *Cardiovasc Res* **23**, 741–747.

Mellander, S., and Johansson, B. (1968). Control of resistance, exchange and capacitance functions in the peripheral circulation. *Pharmacol Rev* **20**, 117–196.

Mellander, S., and Bjoernberg, J. (1992). Regulation of vascular smooth muscle tone and capillary pressure. *NIPS* **7**, 113–119.

Mendel, G. J. (1865). *Versuche über Pflanzenhybriden*. Verhandlungen des Naturforschenden Vereins, Brünn.

Meneton, P., Jeunemaitre, X., de Wardener, H. E., and MacGregor, G. A. (2005). Links between dietary salt intake, renal salt handling, blood pressure and cardiovascular diseases. *Physiol Rev* **85**, 679–715.

Meredith, I. T., Jennings, G. L., Esler, M. D., Dewar, E. M., Bruce, A. M., Fazio, V. A., and Korner, P. I. (1990). Time-course of the antihypertensive and autonomic effects of regular endurance exercise in human subjects. *J Hypertens* **8**, 859–866.

Meredith, I. T., Friberg, P., Jennings, G. L., Dewar, E. M., Fazio, V. A., Lambert, G. W., and Esler, M. D. (1991). Exercise training lowers resting renal but not cardiac sympathetic activity. *Hypertension* **18**, 575–582.

Messerli, F. H., Genest, J., Nowaczynski, W., Kuchel, O., Honda, M., Latour, Y., and Dumont, G. (1975). Splanchnic blood flow in essential hypertension and in hypertensive patients with renal artery stenosis. *Circulation* **51**, 1114–1119.

Messerli, F. H., De Carvalho, J. G. R., Christie, B., and Frohlich, E. D. (1978). Systemic and regional hemodynamics in low, normal and high cardiac output borderline hypertension. *Circ Res* **58**, 441–448.

Messerli, F. H., Christie, B., De Carvalho, J. G. R., Aristimuno, G. G., Suarez, D. H., Dreslinski, G. R., and Frohlich, E. D. (1981). Obesity and essential hypertension: hemodynamics, intravascular volume, sodium excretion and plasma renin activity. *Arch Int Med* **141**, 81–85.

Messerli, F. H. (1982). Cardiovascular effects of obesity and hypertension. *Lancet* **i**, 1165–1168.

Messerli, F. H., Sundgaard-Riise, K., Reisin, E., Dreslinski, G., Dunn, F. G., and Frohlich, E. (1983). Disparate cardiovascular effects of obesity and hypertension. *Am J Med* **74**, 808–812.

Messerli, F. H., Sundgaard-Riise, K., Ventura, H. O., Dunn, F. G., Glade, L. B., and Frolich, E. D. (1983). Essential hypertension in the elderly: Haemodynamics intravascular volume plasma renin activity and circulating catecholamine levels. *Lancet* **ii**, 983–986.

Messerli, F. H., Sundgaard-Riise, K., Ventura, H. O., Dunn, F. G., Oigman, W., and Frohlich, E. D. (1984). Clinical and haemodynamic determinants of left ventricular dimensions. *Arch Intern Med* **144**, 477–481.

Miall, W. E., and Oldham, P. D. (1958). Factors influencing arterial pressure in the general population. *Clin Sci* **17**, 409–444.

Miall, W. E., and Lovell, H. G. (1967). Relation between change of blood pressure and age. *Brit Med J* **2,** 660–662.

Miall, W. E., and Chinn, S. (1973). Blood pressure and ageing: results of a 15–17 year follow-up study in South Wales. *Clin Sci Mol Med* **45** (suppl I), 23s–33s.

Miall, W. E., and Brennan, P. J. (1981). Hypertension in the elderly: the South Wales study. In *Hypertension in the Young and the Old,* Onesti, G., and Kim, K. E., Eds., pp. 277–283. Grune & Stratton, New York.

Miall, W. E. (1982). Systolic or diastolic hypertension—which matters most? *Clin and Exper Hypertens* **A7,** 1121–1131.

Miano, J. M., Cserjesi, P., Ligon, K. L., Periasamy, M., and Olson, E. N. (1994). Smooth muscle myosin heavy chain exclusively marks the smooth muscle lineage during mouse embryogenesis. *Circ Res* **75,** 803–812.

Michel, C. C. (1984). The barrier to fluid and macromolecules at the capillary wall. In *Frontiers in Physiological Research (29th International Congress of Physiological Sciences, 1983),* Garlick, D. G., and Korner, P. I., Eds., pp. 134–146. Australian Academy of Science, Sydney.

Miki, K., Yoshimoto, M., and Tanimizu, M. (2003). Acute shifts of baroreflex control of renal sympathetic nerve activity induced by treadmill exercise in rats. *J Physiol (Lond)* **548,** 313–322.

Miksche, L. W., Miksche, U., and Gross, F. (1970). Effect of sodium restriction on renal hypertension and on renin activity in the rat. *Circ Res* **17,** 973–984.

Miller, E. D., Jr., Samuels, A. I., Haber, E., and Barger, A. C. (1975). Inhibition of angiotensin conversion and prevention of renal hypertension. *Am J Physiol* **228,** 448–453.

Mills, C. J., Gabe, I. T., Gault, J. H., Mason, D. T., Ross, J., Braunwald, E., and Shillingford, J. P. (1970). Pressure-flow relationships and vascular impedance in man. *Cardiovasc Res* **4,** 405–407.

Mills, E., Minson, J., Drolet, G., and Chalmers, J. P. (1989). Effect of intrathecal amino acid receptor antagonists on basal blood pressure and pressor responses to brainstem stimulation in normotensive and hypertensive rats. *J Cardiovasc Pharmacol* **15,** 877–883.

Milhorn, H., Jr. (1966). *The Application of Control Theory to Physiological Systems.* W.B. Saunders Company, Philadelphia.

Milnor, W. R. (1982). *Hemodynamics.* Williams & Wilkins, Baltimore, MD.

Milsum, J. H. (1966). *Biological Control Systems Analysis.* McGraw-Hill, New York.

Minamisawa, K., Tochikubo, O., and Ishii, M. (1994). Systemic hemodynamics during sleep in young or middle-aged and elderly patients with essential hypertension. *Hypertension* **23,** 167–173.

Minson, J. B., Llewellyn-Smith, I. J., Pilowsky, P. M., Oliver, J. O., and Chalmers, J. P. (1994). Disinhibition of the rostral ventrolateral medulla increases blood pressure and Fos expression in bulbospinal neurons. *Brain Res* **646,** 44–52.

Minson, J. B., Suzuki, S., Llewellyn-Smith, I. J., Pilowsky, P. M., Oliver, J. O., and Chalmers, J. P. (1995). *c-fos* expression in central cardiovascular pathways. *Clin Exp Hypertens* **A17,** 67–79.

Minson, J., Arnolda, L., Llewellyn-Smith, I., Pilowsky, P., and Chalmers, J. (1996). Altered *c-fos* in rostral medulla and spinal cord of spontaneously hypertensive rats. *Hypertension* **27** (part I), 433–441.

Mirsky, I. (1979). Elastic properties of the myocardium: a quantitative approach with physiological and clinical applications. In *Handbook of Physiology, Section 2: The Cardiovascular System, Volume I: The Heart,* Berne, R. M., and Sperelakis, N., Eds., pp. 497–532. American Physiological Society, Bethesda, MD.

Missouris, C. G., Forbat, S. M., Singer, D. R. J., Markandu, N. D., Underwood, R., and MacGregor, G. A. (1996). Echocardiography overestimates left ventricular mass: a comparative study with magnetic resonance imaging in patients with hypertension. *J Hypertens* **14**, 1005–1010.

Mitchell, P. (1961). Coupling of phosphorylation to electron and hydrogen transfer by a chemiosmotic type of mechanism. *Nature* **191**, 144–148.

Miura, M., and Takayama, K. (1988). The site of origin of the so-called fastigial pressor response. *Brain Res* **473**, 352–358.

Miyajima, E., Yamada, Y., Yoshida, Y., Matsukawa, T., Shionoiri, H., Tochikubo, O., and Ishii, M. (1991). Muscle sympathetic nerve activity in renovascular hypertension and primary aldosteronism. *Hypertension* **17**, 1057–1062.

Miyata, N., and Cowley, A. W. J. (1999). Renal intramedullary infusion of L-arginine prevents reduction of medullary blood flow and hypertension in Dahl salt-sensitive rats. *Hypertension* **33**, 446–450.

Mo, R., Omvik, P., and Lund-Johansen, P. (1995). The Bergen Blood Pressure Study: offspring of two hypertensive parents have significantly higher blood pressures than offspring of one hypertensive and one normotensive parent. *J Hypertens* **13**, 1614–1617.

Möhring, J., Petri, M., Szokol, M., Haack, D., and Möhring, B. (1976). Effects of saline drinking on malignant course of renal hypertension in rats. *Am J Physiol* **230**, 849–857.

Molkentin, J. D., and Olson, E. N. (1997). GATA4: a novel transcription regulator of cardiac hypertrophy. *Circulation* **96**, 3833–3835.

Molkentin, J. D., Lu, J.-R., Antos, C. L., Markham, B., Grant, S. R., and Olson, E. N. (1998). A calcineurin-dependent transcriptional pathway for cardiac hypertrophy. *Cell* **93**, 215–228.

Molkentin, J. D. (2000). Calcineurin and beyond cardiac hypertrophic signaling. *Circ Res* **87**, 731–738.

Molzahn, M., Dissmann, T. H., Halim, S., Lonman, F. W., and Oelkers, W. (1972). Orthostatic changes of haemodynamics renal function plasma catecholamines and plasma renin concentration in normal and hypertensive man. *Clin Sci* **42**, 209–222.

Moncada, S., Palmer, R. M. J., and Higgs, E. A. (1991). Nitric oxide: physiology, pathophysiology, and pharmacology. *Pharmacol Rev* **43**, 109–142.

Monos, E., Berczi, V., and Nadasy, G. (1995). Local control of veins: biomechanical, metabolic and humoral aspects. *Physiol Rev* **75**, 611–666.

Monroe, R. G., Gamble, W. J., Lafarge, C. G., Kumar, A. E., Stark, J., Sanders, G. L., Phornphutkul, C., and Davis, M. (1972). The Anrep effect reconsidered. *J Clin Invest* **51**, 2573–2583.

Moore, R. A. (1931). The total number of glomeruli in the normal human kidney. *Anat Rec* **48**, 153–168.

Moore, R. Y. (1999). A clock for the ages. *Science* **284**, 2102–2104.

Moore, V. M., Cockington, R. A., Ryan, P., and Robinson, J. S. (1999). The relationship between birth weight and blood pressure amplifies from childhood to adulthood. *J Hypertens* **17**, 883–888.

Moore-Ede, M. C. (1986). Physiology of circadian timing system: predictive versus reactive homeostasis (Bowditch Lecture). *Am J Physiol* **250**, R735–R752.

Morgan, D. A., DiBona, G. F., and Mark, A. L. (1990). Effects of interstrain renal transplantation on NaCl-induced hypertension in Dahl rats. *Hypertension* **15**, 436–442.

Morgan, J. I., and Curran, T. (1991). Stimulus-transcription coupling in the nervous system: involvement of the inducible proto-oncogenes *fos* and *jun*. *Ann Rev Neurosci* **14**, 421–451.

Morgan, H. E., Chua, B. H. L., and Russo, L. (1992). Protein synthesis and degradation. In *The Heart and Cardiovascular System: Scientific Foundations*, Fozzard, H. A., Haber, E.,

Jennings, R. B., Katz, A. M., and Morgan, H. E., Eds., Vol. 2, pp. 1505–1524. Raven Press, New York.

Morimoto, S., Sasaki, S., Itoh, H., Nakata, T., Takeda, K., Nakagawa, M., Furuya, S., Naruse, S., Fukuyama, R., and Fushiki, S. (1999). Sympathetic activation and contribution of genetic factors in hypertension with neurovascular compression of the rostral ventrolateral medulla. *J Hypertens* **17**, 1577–1582.

Morita, H., and Vatner, S. F. (1985). Effects of hemorrhage on renal nerve activity in conscious dogs. *Circ Res* **57**, 788–793.

Morita, H., Nishida, Y., Motochigawa, H., Uemura, N., Hosomi, H., and Vatner, S. F. (1988). Opiate receptor-mediated decrease in renal nerve activity during hypotensive hemorrhage in conscious rabbits. *Circ Res* **63**, 165–172.

Mormède, P., Lemaire, V., Castanon, N., Dulluc, J., Laval, M., and Le Moal, M. (1990). Multiple neuroendocrine responses to chronic social stress interaction between individual characteristics and situational factors. *Physiol Behav* **47**, 1099–1105.

Mormède, P. (1997). Genetic influences on the responses to psychosocial challenges in rats. *Acta Physiol Scand* **161** (suppl 649), 65–68.

Morris, J. L. (1995). Peptides as neurotransmitters in vascular autonomic neurons. *Clin Exp Pharmacol Physiol* **22**, 792–802.

Morris, B. J. (2005). A forkhead in the road to longevity: the molecular basis of lifespan becomes clearer. *J Hypertens* **23**, 1285–1309.

Morrison, R. A., McGrath, A., Davidson, G., Brown, J. J., Murray, G. D., and Lever, A. F. (1996). Low blood pressure in Down's syndrome: a link with Alzheimer's disease. *Hypertension* **28**, 569–575.

Morton, J. J., Beattie, E. C., Speirs, A., and Gulliver, F. (1993). Persistent hypertension following inhibition of nitric oxide formation in the young Wistar rat: role of renin and vascular hypertrophy. *J Hypertens* **11**, 1083–1088.

Moruzzi, G. (1940). Paleocerebellar inhibition of vasomotor and respiratory carotid sinus reflexes. *J Neurophysiol* **3**, 20–32.

Moruzzi, G., and Magoun, H. W. (1949). Brain stem reticular formation and activation of the EEG. *Electroencephalogr Clin Neurophysiol* **1**, 455–473.

Motz, W., and Strauer, B. (1989). Left ventricular function and collagen content after regression of hypertensive hypertrophy. *Hypertension* **13**, 43–50.

Mountcastle, V. B. (1984). Central nervous mechanisms in mechanoreceptive sensibility. In *Handbook of Physiology, Section 1: The Nervous System, Volume III: Sensory Processes, Part 2*, Darian-Smith, I., Ed., pp. 789–878. American Physiological Society, Bethesda, MD.

Mubagwa, K., Mullane, K., and Flameng, W. (1996). Role of adenosine in the heart and circulation. *Cardiovasc Res* **32**, 797–813.

Mueller, S. M. (1983). Longitudinal study of hindquarter vasculature during development in spontaneously hypertensive and Dahl salt-sensitive rats. *Hypertension* **5**, 489–497.

Muirhead, E. E., Rightsel, W. A., Leach, B. E., Byers, L. W., Pitcock, J. A., and Brooks, B. (1977). Reversal of hypertension by transplants and lipid extracts of cultured renomedullary interstitial cells. *Lab Invest* **35**, 162–172.

Muirhead, E. (1991). Renomedullary system of blood pressure control. *Am J Hypertens* **4**, 556s–568s.

Muirhead, E. E., Brooks, B., Byers, L. W., Brown, P., and Pitcock, J. A. (1991). Secretion of medullipin I by isolated kidneys perfused under elevated pressure. *Clin Exp Pharmacol Physiol* **18**, 409–417.

Muirhead, E. E. (1994). Renomedullary vasodepressor lipid: medullipin. In *Textbook of Hypertension,* Swales, J. D., Ed., pp. 341–359. Blackwell, Oxford.

Mullins, J. J., Peters, J., and Ganten, D. (1990). Fulminant hypertension in transgenic rats har-
bouring the mouse *Ren-2* gene. *Nature* **344**, 541–544.

Mulvany, M. J., and Halpern, W. J. (1977). Contractile properties of small arterial resistance
vessels in spontaneously hypertensive and normotensive rats. *Circ Res* **41**, 19–26.

Mulvany, M. J., Hansen, P. K., and Aalkjaer, C. A. (1978). Direct evidence that the greater contractility of resistance vessels in spontaneously hypertensive rats is associated with a narrowed lumen, a thickened media and an increased number of smooth muscle cell layers.
Circ Res **43**, 854–864.

Mulvany, M. J., and Korsgaard, N. (1983). Correlations and otherwise between blood pressure,
cardiac mass and resistance vessel characteristics in hypertensive, normotensive and hyper-
tensive/normotensive hybrid rats. *J Hypertens* **1**, 235–244.

Mulvany, M. J. (1984). Determinants of vascular haemodynamic characteristics. *Hypertension*
6 (Suppl III), III-13–III-18.

Mulvany, M. J., Baandrup, M. J., and Gundersen, H. J, G. (1985). Evidence for hyperplasia in
mesenteric resistance vessels of spontaneously hypertensive rats using a three-dimensional
disector. *Circ Res* **57**, 794–800.

Mulvany, M. J. (1988). Resistance vessel structure and function in the etiology of hypertension studied in the F2–generation of hypertensive normotensive rats. *J Hypertens* **6**,
655–663.

Mulvany, M. J., and Aalkjaer, C. (1990). Structure and function of small arteries. *Physiol Rev*
70, 921–962.

Mulvany, M., Persson, A., and Andresen, J. (1991). No persistent effect of angiotensin converting enzyme inhibitor treatment in Milan hypertensive rats despite regression of vascular
structure. *J Hypertens* **9**, 589–593.

Mulvany, M. J. (1993). Resistance vessel structure in hypertension: growth or remodeling.
J Cardiovasc Pharmacol **22** (Suppl 5), S44–S47.

Mulvany, M. J. (1994). Resistance vessels in hypertension. In *Textbook of Hypertension*,
Swales, J. D., Ed., pp. 103–119. Blackwell, Oxford.

Mulvany, M. J., Baumbach, G. L., Aalkjaer, C., Heagerty, A. M., Korsgaard, N., Schiffrin, E. L.,
and Heistadt, D. D. (1996). Vascular remodeling. *Hypertension* **28**, 505–506.

Munch, P. A., and Brown, A. M. (1985). Role of vessel wall in acute resetting of aortic baroreceptors. *Am J Physiol* **248**, H843–H852.

Mune, T., Rogerson, F. M., Nikkila, H., Agarwal, A. K., and White, P. C. (1995). Human
hypertension caused by mutations in the kidney isozyme of 11β-hydroxysteroid dehydrogenase. *Nat Gen* **10**, 394–396.

Murakami, E. (1973). Hemodynamics in essential hypertension. *Jpn Circ J* **37**, 717–721.

Mureddu, G. F., de Simone, G., Greco, R., Rosato, G. F., and Contaldo, F. (1997). Left ventricular filling in arterial hypertension: influence of obesity and hemodynamic and structural
confounders. *Hypertension* **29**, 544–550.

Murphy, E. A. (1964). One cause? Many causes? The argument for a bimodal distribution.
J Chronic Dis **17**, 301–324.

Murphy, R. A. (1994). Mechanism of contraction of vascular smooth muscle. In *Textbook of
Hypertension*, Swales, J. D., Ed., pp. 139–145. Blackwell, Oxford.

Murphy, A. M. (1996). Contractile protein phenotypic variation during development. *Cardiovasc
Res* **31**, E25–E33.

Murrell, J. R., Randall, J. D., Rosoff, J., Zhao, J.-l., Jensen, R. V., Gullans, S. R., and Haupert,
G. T. (2005). Endogenous ouabain: upregulation of steroidogenic genes in hypertensive
hypothalamus but not adrenal. *Circulation* **112**, 1301–1308.

Myers, R. D. (1978). Hypothalamic actions of 5–hydroxytryptamine neurotoxins: feeding,
drinking and body temperature. *Ann NY Acad Sci* **305**, 556–578.

Nabika, T., Nara, Y., Ikeda, K., Endo, J., and Yamori, Y. (1991). Genetic heterogeneity of the spontaneously hypertensive rat. *Hypertension* **18,** 12–16.

Nag, S., Papneja, T., Venugopalan, R., and Stewart, D. J. (2005). Increased angiopoietin2 expresssion is associated with endothelial apoptosis and blood brain barrier breakdown. *Lab Invest* **85,** 1189–1198.

Nakamura, K., and Cowley, A. W. (1989). Sequential changes of cerebrospinal fluid sodium during the development of hypertension in Dahl rats. *Hypertension* **13,** 243–249.

Naraghi, R., Geiger, H., Crnac, J., Huk, W., Fahlbusch, R., Engels, G., and Luft, F. C. (1994). Posterior fossa neurovascular anomalies in essential hypertension. *Lancet* **344,** 1466–1470.

Naraghi, R., Schester, H., Toka, H. R., Bahring, S., Toka, O., and Oztekin, O. (1997). Neurovascular compression of the ventrolateral medulla in autosomal dominant hypertension and brachydactyly. *Stroke* **28,** 1749–1754.

Narkiewicz, K., and Somers, V. K. (1997). The sympathetic nervous system and obstructive sleep apnea: implications for hypertension. *J Hypertens* **15,** 1613–1619.

Narkiewicz, K., Pesek, C. A., Kato, M., Phillips, B. G., Davison, D. E., and Somers, V. K. (1998). Baroreflex control of sympathetic nerve activity and heart rate in obstructive sleep apnea. *Hypertension* **32,** 1039–1043.

Navar, L. G., Inscho, E. W., Majid, D. S. A., Imig, J. D., Harrison-Bernard, L. M., and Mitchell, K. D. (1996). Paracrine regulation of the renal microcirculation. *Physiol Rev* **76,** 425–536.

Neil, E., Redwood, C. R. M., and Schweitzer, A. (1949). Effects of electrical stimulation of the aortic nerve on blood pressure and respiration in cats and rabbits under chloralose and nembutal anaesthesia. *J Physiol (Lond)* **109,** 392–401.

Neil, E., and O'Regan, R. G. (1971a). The effects of electrical stimulation of the distal end of the cut sinus and aortic nerves on peripheral arterial chemoreceptor activity in the cat. *J Physiol (Lond)* **215,** 15–32.

Neil, E., and O'Regan, R. G. (1971b). Efferent and afferent impulse activity recorded from few-fibre preparations of otherwise intact sinus and aortic nerves. *J Physiol (Lond)* **215,** 33–47.

Neil, J. J., and Loewy, A. D. (1982). Decreases in blood pressure in response to l-glutamate microinjection into A5 catecholamine cell group. *Brain Res* **241,** 271–278.

Nelson, L., Jennings, G. L., Esler, M. D., and Korner, P. I. (1986). Effect of changing levels of physical activity on blood pressure and haemodynamics in essential hypertension. *Lancet* **ii,** 473–476.

Neyses, L., Nitsch, J., Tüttenberg, H.-P., Korus, H.-C., and Lüderitz, B. (1989). Erhötes atriales natriuretisches Peptid (ANP) bei essentieller Hypertonie: Abhängigkeit vom rechtsatrialen Druckverhalten. *Klin Wochenschr* **67,** 756–761.

Ni, Z., Oveisi, F., and Vaziri, N. D. (1999). Nitric oxide synthase isotype expression in salt sensitive and salt resistant Dahl rats. *Hypertension* **34,** 552–557.

Nichols, W. W., and O'Rourke, M. F. (1997). *McDonald's Blood Flow in Arteries.* Arnold, London.

Nicoletti, A., Heudes, D., Hinglais, N., Appay, M.-D., Philippe, M., Sassy-Prigent, C., Bariety, J., and Michel, J.-B. (1995). Left ventricular fibrosis in renovascular hypertensive rats: effect of losartan and spironolactone. *Hypertension* **26,** 101–111.

Nielsen, M., and Asmussen, E. (1963). Humoral and nervous control of breathing in exercise. In *The Regulation of Human Respiration,* Cunningham, D. J. C., and Lloyd, B. B., Eds., pp. 503–513. Blackwell, Oxford.

Nilsson, H., Ely, D., Friberg, P., Karlström, G., and Folkow, B. (1985). Effects of high and low sodium diets on the resistance vessels and their adrenergic vasoconstrictor fibre control in normotensive (WKY) and hypertensive (SHR) rats. *Acta Physiol Scand* **125,** 323–334.

Nilsson, H., Ljung, B., Sjöblom, N., and Wallin, B. G. (1985). The influence of sympathetic impulse patterns on contractile responses of rat mesenteric arteries and veins. *Acta Physiol Scand* **123**, 303–309.

Nilsson, P. M., Ostergren, P. O., Nyberg, P., Soderstrom, M., and Allebeck, P. (1997). Low birth weight is associated with elevated systolic blood pressure in adolescence a prospective study of a birth cohort of 149,378 Swedish boys. *J Hypertens* **15**, 1627–1631.

Nilsson-Ehle, H. (1909). Kreuzunguntersuchungen an Hafer und Weizen. *Zeitschrift für Induktive Abstammungs-und Vererbungslehre*, **5**, 1–122.

Noble, M. I. M. (1977). Myocardial performance. *Rec Adv Cardiol* **7**, 285–314.

Noble, J. L. M. L. I., Smith, T. L., Hutchins, P. M., and Struyker-Boudier, H. A. J. (1990). Microvascular alterations in adult conscious spontaneously hypertensive rats. *Hypertension* **15**, 415–419.

Nordergraaf, A. (1963). Development of an analog computer for the human circulatory system. In *Circulatory Analog Computers*, Nordergraaf, A., Jager, G. N., and Westerhof, N., Eds., pp. 29–34. North Holland, Amsterdam.

Nordlander, M. (1989). Inhibition of myogenic tone and reactivity by calcium antagonists. *J Hypertens* **7** (suppl 4), S141–S145.

Noresson, E., Ricksten, S.-E., Hallbäck-Nordlander, M., and Thorén, P. (1979). Performance of hypertrophied left ventricle in spontaneously hypertensive rat. Effects of changes in preload and afterload. *Acta Physiol Scand* **107**, 1–8.

Norrelund, H., Christensen, K. L., Samani, N. J., Kimber, P., Mulvany, M. J., and Korsgaard, N. (1994). Early narrowed afferent arteriole is a contributor to the development of hypertension. *Hypertension* **24**, 301–308.

Norusis, M. J. (1986). Predicting cure and credit: discriminant analysis. In *Advanced Statistics SPSS/PC+*, Vol. B, pp. B1–B40. SPSS, Chicago.

Notoya, M., Nakamura, M., and Mizojiri, K. (1996). Effect of lisinopril on the structure of renal arterioles. *Hypertension* **27** (part 1), 364–370.

Nüsslein-Volhard, C., and Wieschaus, E. (1980). Mutations affecting segment number and polarity in *Drosophila. Nature* **287**, 795–801.

Nyengaard, J. R., and Bendtsen, T. F. (1992). Glomerular number and size in relation to age, kidney weight, and body surface in normal man. *Anat Rec* **232**, 194–201.

Oates, J. A., Gillespie, L., Udenfriend, S., and Sjoerdsma, A. (1960). Decarboxylase inhibition and blood pressure reduction by alpha-methyl-3,4–dihydroxy-DL-phenylalanine. *Science* **131**, 1890–1894.

Öberg, B., and White, S. (1970). The role of vagal cardiac nerves and arterial baroreceptors in the circulatory adjustments to hemorrhage in the cat. *Acta Physiol Scand* **80**, 395–403.

Öberg, B., and Thorén, P. (1972). Increased activity in left ventricular receptors during hemorrhage or occlusion of caval veins in the cat—A possible cause of the vaso-vagal reaction. *Acta Physiol Scand* **85**, 164–173.

O'Brien, E. (1994). Blood pressure measurement. In *Textbook of Hypertension*, Swales, J. D., Ed., pp. 989–1008. Blackwell, Oxford.

O'Brien, E. (2003). Ambulatory blood pressure measurement is indispensable to good clinical practice. *J Hypertens* **21** (suppl 2), S11–S18.

Oddie, C. J., Dilley, R. J., and Bobik, A. (1992). Long-term angiotensin II antagonism in spontaneously hypertensive rats: effects on blood pressure and cardiovascular amplifiers. *Clin Exp Pharmacol Physiol* **19**, 392–393.

O'Dea, K., Esler, M., Leonard, P., Stockigt, J., and Nestel, P. (1982). Noradrenaline turnover during under- and over-eating in normal weight subjects. *Metabolism* **31**, 896–899.

O'Donnell, C. P., Tankersley, C. G., Polotsky, V. P., Schwartz, A. R., and Smith, P. L. (2000). Leptin obesity and respiratory function. *Respir Physiol* **119**, 163–170.

Ogawa, N., and Ono, H. (1987). Role of Ca channel in the renal autoregulatory vascular response analysed by the use of BAY K 8644. *Naunyn-Schmiedeberg's Arch Pharmacol* **335,** 189–193.

Ohira, T., Iso, H., Tanigawa, T., Sankai, T., Imano, H., Kiyama, M., Sato, S., Naito, Y., Iida, M., and Shimamotu, T. (2002). The relation of anger expression with blood pressure levels and hypertension in rural and urban Japanese communities. *J Hypertens* **20,** 21–27.

Ohta, K., Kim, S., and Iwao, H. (1996). Role of angiotensin-converting enzyme, adrenergic receptors and blood pressure in cardiac gene expression of spontaneously hypertensive rats during development. *Hypertension* **28,** 627–634.

Okamoto, K., and Aoki, K. (1963). Development of a strain of spontaneously hypertensive rats. *Jpn Circ J* **27,** 282–293.

Okamoto, K. (1969). Spontaneous hypertension in rats. *Int Rev Exp Pathol* **7,** 227–270.

Oldham, P. D., Pickering, G., Fraser Roberts, J. A., and Sowry, G. S. C. (1960). The nature of essential hypertension. *Lancet* **i,** 1085–1093.

Olds, J., and Milner, P. (1954). Positive reinforcement produced by electrical stimulation of septal area and other regions of the rat brain. *J Comp Physiol Psychol* **47,** 419–427.

O'Leary, D. S. (1991). Autonomic mechanisms of muscle metabolic reflex control of heart rate during muscle ischemia in conscious dogs. *Physiologist* **34,** 239.

Oliver, J. R., Korner, P. I., Woods, R. L., and Zhu, J. L. (1990). Reflex release of vasopressin and renin in hemorrhage is enhanced by autonomic blockade. *Am J Physiol* **258,** H221–H228.

Olivetti, G., Lagrasta, C., Quaini, F., Ricci, R., Moccia, G., Capasso, J. M., and Anversa, P. (1989). Capillary growth in anaemia induced ventricular wall remodelling in the rat. *Circ Res* **65,** 1182–1192.

Olson, E. N., and Molkentin, J. D. (1999). Prevention of cardiac hypertrophy by calcineurin inhibition: hope or hype? *Circ Res* **84,** 623–632.

Olsson, R. A., and Bugni, W. J. (1986). Coronary circulation. In *The Heart and Cardiovascular System*, Fozzard, H. A., Haber, E., Jennings, R. B., Katz, A. M., and Morgan, H. E., Eds., Vol. 2, pp. 987–1037. Raven Press, New York.

Oltmans, G. (1983). Norepinephrine and dopamine levels in in hypothalamic nuclei of genetically obese mouse (ob/ob). *Brain Res* **273,** 369–373.

Ono, H., Kokubun, H., and Hashimoto, K. (1974). Abolition by calcium antagonists of the autoregulation of renal blood flow. *Naunyn-Schmiedeberg's Arch Pharmacol* **285,** 201–207.

Oparil, S., and Cutiletta, A. F. (1979). Hypertrophy in the denervated heart: a comparison of central sympatholytic treatment with 6–hydroxydopamine and peripheral sympathectomy with nerve growth factor antiserum. *Am J Cardiol* **44,** 970–978.

Oparil, S., Bishop, S. P., and Clubb, F. J., Jr. (1984). Myocardial hypertrophy or hyperplasia. *Hypertension* **38** (suppl III), III-38–III-43.

Oparil, S., Meng, Q. c., Chen, Y.-F., Yang, R.-H., Jin, H., and Wyss, J. M. (1988). Genetic basis of NaCl-sensitive hypertension. *J Cardiovasc Pharmacol* **12** (suppl 3), S56–S69.

Oparil, S., Chen, Y.-F., Berecek, K. H., Calhoun, D. A., and Wyss, J. M. (1995). The role of the central nervous system in hypertension. In *Hypertension: Pathophysiology, Diagnosis and Management*, Laragh, J. H., and Brenner, B. M., Eds., Vol. 1, pp. 713–740. Raven Press, New York.

Orosz, D. E., and Hopfer, U. (1996). Pathophysiological consequences of changes in the coupling ratio of Na,K-ATPase for renal sodium reabsorption and its implications for hypertension. *Hypertension* **27,** 219–227.

O'Rourke, M. F., and Taylor, M. G. (1966). Vascular impedance in the femoral bed. *Circ Res* **18,** 126–139.

O'Rourke, M. F. (1982a). *Arterial Function in Health and Disease*. Churchill Livingstone, Edinburgh.

O'Rourke, M. F. (1982b). Vascular impedance in studies of arterial and cardiac function. *Physiol Rev* **62**, 571–623.

O'Rourke, M. F. (1995). Mechanical principles in arterial disease. *Hypertension* **26**, 2–9.

O'Rourke, M. F. (2002). From theory into practice: arterial haemodynamics in clinical hypertension. *J Hypertens* **20**, 1901–1915.

Orth, D. N., Kovacs, W. J., and DeBold, C. R. (1992). The adrenal cortex. In *Williams Textbook of Endocrinology*, Wilson, J. D., and Foster, D. W., Eds., pp. 489–620. W.B. Saunders, Philadelphia.

Os, I., Kjeldsen, S. E., Skjoto, J., Westheim, A., Lande, K., Aakesson, I., Fredrichsen, P., Leren, P., Hjermann, I., and Eide, I. K. (1986). Increased plasma vasopressin in low renin essential hypertension. *Hypertension* **8**, 506–513.

Osborn, J., and Provo, B. (1992). Salt-dependent hypertension in the sinoaortic-denervated rat. *Hypertension* **19**, 658–662.

Osol, G., and Halpern, W. (1988). Spontaneous vasomotion in pressurized cerebral arteries from genetically hypertensive rats. *Am J Physiol* **254**, H28–H33.

Osterziel, K. J., Hanlein, D., Willenbrock, R., Eichhorn, C., Luft, F., and Dietz, R. (1995). Baroreflex sensitivity and cardiovascular mortality in patients with mild to moderate heart failure. *Br Heart J* **73**, 517–522.

Owens, G. K. (1987). Influence of blood pressure on development of aortic medial smooth muscle hypertrophy in spontaneously hypertensive rats. *Hypertension* **9**, 178–187.

Owens, G. K. (1989). Control of hypertrophic versus hyperplastic growth of vascular smooth muscle cells. *Am J Physiol* **257**, H1755–H1765.

Owens, G. K. (1995). Regulation of differentiation of vascular smooth muscle cells. *Physiol Rev* **75**, 487–517.

Padfield, P. L., Brown, J. J., Lever, A. F., Schalekamp, M. A., Beevers, D. G., Davies, D. L., Robertson, J. I. S., and Tree, M. (1975). Is low renin hypertension a stage in the development of essential hypertension or a diagnostic entity. *Lancet* **i**, 548–550.

Padfield, P. L., and Edwards, C. R. W. (1993). Mineralocorticoid induced hypertension and the renin-angiotensin system. In *The Renin-Angiotensin System*, Robertson, J. I. S., and Nicholls, M. G., Eds., Vol. 2, pp. 63.1–63.27. Gower, London.

Paffenbarger, R. S., Wing, A. L., Hyde, R. T., and Jung, D. L. (1983). Physical activity and incidence of hypertension in college alumni. *Am J Epidemiol* **117**, 245–257.

Page, I. H. (1939). The production of persistent arterial hypertension by cellophane perinephritis. *JAMA* **113**, 2046–2048.

Page, I. H., and Helmer, O. M. (1939). Crystalline pressor substance, angiotonin, resulting from the reaction between renin and renin activator [Abstract]. *Proc Central Soc Clin Res* **12**, 17.

Page, I. J., and Helmer, O. M. (1940). Crystalline pressor substance (angiotonin) resulting from reaction between renin and renin activator. *N Engl J Med* **71**, 29–43.

Page, I. H. (1949). Pathogenesis of arterial hypertension. *JAMA* **140**, 451–457.

Page, I. H. (1960). The mosaic theory of hypertension. In *Essential Hypertension: An International Symposium*, Bock, K. D., and Cottier, P. D., Eds., pp. 1–29. Springer-Verlag, Berlin.

Page, I. H., and McCubbin, J. W. (1965). The physiology of arterial hypertension. In *Handbook of Physiology, Section 2: Circulation*, Hamilton, W. F., and Dow, P., Eds., Vol. III, pp. 2163–2208. American Physiological Society, Washington, DC.

Page, I. H., and McCubbin, J. W. (1968). *Renal Hypertension*. Year Book, Chicago.

Page, E., and McCallister, L. P. (1973). Quantitative electron microscopy of heart muscle cells. *Am J Cardiol* **31**, 172–181.

Page, I. H. (1987). *Hypertension Mechanisms*. Grune & Stratton, Orlando, FL.

Paintal, A. S. (1971). Cardiovascular receptors. In *Handbook of Sensory Physiology: Enteroceptors*, Neil, E., Ed., Vol. III/1, pp. 1–45. Springer-Verlag, Berlin.

Paintal, A. S. (1973). Vagal sensory receptors and their reflex effects. *Physiol Rev* **53**, 159–227.

Pak, C. H. (1981). Plasma adrenaline and noradrenaline concentrations of the spontaneously hypertensive rat. *Jpn Heart J* **22**, 987–995.

Panza, J. A., Casino, P. R., Badar, D. M., and Quyuumi, A. A. (1993). Effect of increased availability of endothelium-derived nitric oxide precursor on endothelium-dependent vascular relaxation in normal subjects and in patients with essential hypertension. *Circulation* **87**, 1475–1481.

Panza, J. A., Casino, P. R., Kilcoyne, C. M., and Quyyumi, A. A. (1993). Role of endothelium-derived nitric oxide in the abnormal endothelium-dependent vascular relaxation of patients with essential hypertension. *Circulation* **87**, 1468–1474.

Papez, J. W. (1937). A proposed mechanism of emotion. *Arch Neurol Psychiat Chicago* **38**, 725–743.

Pappenheimer, J. R., and Kinter, W. B. (1956). Hematocrit ratio of blood within mammalian kidney and its significance for renal haemodynamics. *Am J Physiol* **183**, 377–390.

Papper, S., Belsky, J. L., and Bleifer, K. H. (1960). The response to the administration of an isotonic sodium chloride lactate solution in patients with essential hypertension. *Circulation* **22**, 876–884.

Parati, G., Castiglioni, P., Di Rienzo, M., Omboni, S., Pedotti, A., and Mancia, G. (1990). Sequential spectral analysis of 24 hour blood pressure and pulse interval in humans. *Hypertension* **16**, 414–421.

Parati, G., Antonicelli, R., Guazzarotti, F., Paciaroni, E., and Mancia, G. (1991). Cardiovascular effects of an earthquake: direct evidence by ambulatory blood pressure monitoring. *Hypertension* **38**, 1093–1095.

Parati, G., Di Rienzo, M., Bonsignore, M. R., Insalaco, G., Marrone, O., Castiglioni, P., Bonsignore, G., and Mancia, G. (1997). Autonomic cardiac regulation in obstructive sleep apnea syndrome: evidence from spontaneous baroreflex analysis during sleep. *J Hypertens* **15**, 1621–1626.

Parlow, J., Viale, J.-P., Annat, G., Hughson, R., and Quintin, L. (1995). Spontaneous cardiac baroreflex in humans. Comparison with drug-induced responses. *Hypertension* **25**, 1058–1068.

Parmley, W. W., and Talbot, L. (1979). Heart as a pump. In *Handbook of Physiology, Section 2: The Cardiovascular System*, Berne, R. M., and Sperelakis, N., Eds., Vol. I, pp. 429–460. American Physiological Society, Bethesda, MD.

Parving, H.-H., and Gyntelberg, F. (1973). Transcapillary escape rate of albumin and plasma volume in essential hypertension. *Circ Res* **32**, 643–651.

Patel, A., Layne, S., Watts, D., and Kirchner, K. A. (1993). L-arginine administration normalises pressure natriuresis in hypertensive Dahl rats. *Hypertension* **22**, 863–869.

Paton, W. D. M., and Zaimis, E. J. (1952). The methonium compounds. *Pharmacol Rev* **4**, 219–253.

Paton, J. F. R., and Spyer, K. M. (1992). Cerebellar cortical regulation of the circulation. *NIPS* **7**, 124–129.

Patzak, A., Lai, E. Y., Persson, P. B., and Persson, A. E. G. (2005). Angiotensin II–nitric oxide interaction in glomerular arterioles. *Clin Exp Pharmacol Physiol* **32**, 410–414.

Paul, M., Wagner, J., and Ganten, D. (1994). Transgenic animals: new models in hypertension research. In *Experimental and Genetic Models of Hypertension, Volume 16: Handbook of Hypertension*, Ganten, D., and de Jong, W., Eds., pp. 606–618. Elsevier, Amsterdam.

Pearson, P. J., and Vanhoutte, P. M. (1993). Vasodilator and vasoconstrictor substances produced by the endothelium. *Rev Physiol Biochem Pharmacol* **122**, 1–67.

Penney, D. G., Dunbar, J. C., and Baylerian, M. S. (1985). Cardiomegaly and haemodynamics in rats with a transplantable growth hormone-secreting tumour. *Cardiovasc Res* **19**, 270–277.

Pepi, M., Alimento, M., Maltagliati, A., and Guazzi, M. D. (1988). Cardiac hypertrophy in hypertension: repolarisation abnormalities elicited by rapid lowering of pressure. *Hypertension* **11**, 84–91.

Peppard, P. E., Young, T., Palta, M., Dempsey, J., and Skatrud, J. (2000). Longitudinal study of moderate weight change and sleep disordered breathing. *JAMA* **284**, 3015–3021.

Peppard, P. E., Young, T., Palta, M., and Skatrud, J. (2000). Prospective study between sleep disordered breathing and hypertension. *N Engl J Med* **342**, 1378–1384.

Perera, G. A. (1955). Hypertensive vascular disease description and natural history. *J Chronic Dis* **1**, 33–42.

Péronnet, F., Nadeau, R. A., De Champlain, J., Magrassi, P., and Chatrand, C. (1981). Exercise plasma catecholamines in dogs: role of adrenals and cardiac nerve endings. *Am J Physiol* **241**, H243–H247.

Persson, P., Ehmke, H., Kirchheim, H., and Seller, H. (1988). Effect of sino-aortic denervation in comparison to cardiopulmonary deafferentation on long-term blood pressure in conscious dogs. *Eur J Physiol* **411**, 160–166.

Persson, P. B., Ehmke, H., Köhler, W., and Kirchheim, H. (1990). Identification of major slow blood pressure oscillations in conscious dogs. *Am J Physiol* **25**, H1050–H1055.

Persson, P. B., Ehmke, H., Kirchheim, H. R., Janssen, B., Bauman, J. E., Just, A., and Nafz, B. (1993). Autoregulation and non-homeostatic behaviour of renal blood flow in conscious dogs. *J Physiol (Lond)* **462**, 261–273.

Persson, M., Mjörndal, T., Carlberg, B., Bohlin, J., and Lindholm, L. H. (2000). Evaluation of a computer-based decision support system for treatment of hypertension with drugs: retrospective, nonintervention testing of cost and guideline adherence. *J Intern Med* **247**, 87–93.

Persson, M., Carlberg, B., Mjörndal, T., Asplund, K., Bohlin, J., and Lindholm, L. (2002). 1999 WHO/ISH Guidelines applied to a 1999 MONICA sample from northern Sweden. *J Hypertens* **20**, 29–35.

Persson, M. (2003). Bring hypertension guidelines into play: guideline-based decision support system for drug treatment of hypertension and epidemiological aspects of hypertension guidelines. Dissertation, No. 837, Umea University, Umea.

Perutz, M. F. (1996). Blood: taking the pressure off. *Nature* **380**, 205–206.

Petersson, M. J., Rundqvist, B., Johannson, M., Eisenhofer, G., Lambert, G., Herlitz, H., Jensen, G., and Friberg, P. (2002). Increased cardiac sympathetic drive in renovascular hypertension. *J Hypertens* **20**, 1181–1187.

Petras, J. M., and Cummings, J. F. (1972). Autonomic neurons in the spinal cord of the rhesus monkey: a correlation of the findings of cytoarchitecture and sympathectomy with fiber degeneration following dorsal rhizotomy. *J Comp Neurol* **146**, 189–218.

Pfeffer, J., Pfeffer, M., Fletcher, P., and Braunwald, E. (1979). Alterations of cardiac performance in rats with established spontaneous hypertension. *Am J Cardiol* **44**, 994.

Pfeffer, J. M., Pfeffer, M. A., Fishbein, M. C., and Frohlich, E. D. (1979). Cardiac function and morphology with ageing in the spontaneously hypertensive rat. *Am J Physiol* **237**, H461–H468.

Pfeffer, M. A., and Pfeffer, J. M. (1985). Left ventricular hypertrophy and pressure generating capacity in aging genetically hypertensive rats. *J Cardiovasc Pharmacol* **7**, S41–S45.

Phelan, E. L. (1970). Genetic and autonomic factors in inherited hypertension. *Circ Res* **26 & 27** (suppl II), II-65–II-74.

Phillips, M. I. (1987). Functions of brain angiotensin in the central nervous system. *Annu Rev Physiol* **49**, 413–435.

Phillips, M. I. (2000). Angiotensin II receptors in central nervous system physiology. In *Drugs, Enzymes and Receptors of the Renin-Angiotensin System: Celebrating a Century of Discovery*, Husain, A., and Graham, R., Eds., Vol. 1, pp. 27–44. Harwood, Amsterdam.

Pickering, G. W., Fraser Roberts, J. A., and Sowry, G. S. C. (1954). The aetiology of essential hypertension. 3. The effect of correcting for arm circumference on the growth rate of arterial pressure with age. *Clin Sci* **13**, 267–271.

Pickering, G. W. (1961). *The Nature of Essential Hypertension*. Churchill, London.

Pickering, G. W. (1968). *High Blood Pressure*. Churchill, London.

Pickering, T. G., Gribbin, B., and Sleight, P. (1972). Comparison of reflex heart rate responses to rising and falling arterial pressure in man. *Cardiovasc Res* **6**, 277–283.

Pickering, T. G., James, G. D., Boddie, C., Harshfield, G. A., Blank, S., and Laragh, J. H. (1988). How common is white coat hypertension? *JAMA* **259**, 225–228.

Pickering, T. G., Gerin, W., James, G. D., Pieper, C., Schlussel, Y. L., and Schnall, P. L. (1992). The effect of occupational and domestic stress on the diurnal rhythm of blood pressure. In *Temporal Variations of the Cardiovascular System*, Schmidt, T. F. H., Engel, B. T., and Bluemchen, G., Eds., pp. 305–317. Springer-Verlag, Berlin.

Pickering, T. G. (1994). Psychosocial stress and hypertension: B. Clinical and experimental evidence. In *Textbook of Hypertension*, Swales, J. D., Ed., pp. 640–654. Blackwell, Oxford.

Pickering, T. G. (1995). White coat hypertension. In *Hypertension: Pathophysiology, Diagnosis and Management*, Laragh, J. H., and Brenner, B. M., Eds., Vol. 2, pp. 1913–1927. Raven Press, New York.

Pickering, T. G., and Mann, S. J. (1995). Renovascular hypertension: Medical evaluation and non-surgical treatment. In *Hypertension: Pathophysiology, Diagnosis and Management*, Laragh, J. H., and Brenner, B. M., Eds., Vol. 2, pp. 2039–2054. Raven Press, New York.

Pickering, T. G., Devereux, R. B., James, G. D., Gerin, W., Landsbergis, P., Schnall, P. L., and Schwartz, J. E. (1996). Environmental influences on blood pressure and the role of job strain. *J Hypertens* **14** (suppl 5), S179–S185.

Pilowsky, I., Spalding, D., Shaw, J., and Korner, P. I. (1973). Hypertension and personality. *Psychosom Med* **35**, 50–56.

Pilowsky, P., West, M., and Chalmers, J. (1985). Renal sympathetic nerve responses to stimulation inhibition and destruction of the ventrolateral medulla in the rabbit. *Neurosci Lett* **60**, 51–55.

Pilowsky, P. (1995). Good vibrations respiratory rhythms in the central control of blood pressure. *Clin Exp Pharmacol Physiol* **22**, 594–604.

Pilowsky, P. M., Minson, J. B., Arnolda, L. F., and Chalmers, J. P. (1995). Brain serotonin and hypertension. In *Hypertension: Pathophysiology, Diagnosis and Management*, Laragh, J. H., and Brenner, B. M., Eds., Vol. 1, pp. 775–787. Raven Press, New York.

Pilowsky, P. M., and Goodchild, A. K. (2002). Baroreceptor reflex pathways and neurotransmitters: 10 years on. *J Hypertens* **20**, 1675–1688.

Pinsky, D. J., Patton, S., Mesaros, S., Brovkovych, V., Kubaszewski, E., Grunfeld, S., and Malinsky, T. (1997). Mechanical tranduction of nitric oxide synthesis in the beating heart. *Circ Res* **81**, 372–379.

Pirpiris, M., Sudhir, K., Yeung, S., Jennings, G., and Whitworth, J. A. (1992). Pressor responsiveness in corticosteroid-induced hypertension in humans. *Hypertension* **19**, 567–574.

Pitts, R. F. (1959). *The Physiological Basis of Diuretic Therapy*. Charles C Thomas, Springfield, IL.

Pitts, R. F. (1963). *Physiology of the Kidney and Body Fluids*. Year Book, Chicago.

Platt, R. (1947). Heredity in hypertension. *Q J Med* **16**, 111–132.

Platt, R. (1959). The nature of essential hypertension. *Lancet* **ii**, 55–57.

Plutchik, R. (1994). *The Psychology and Biology of Emotion*. HarperCollins, New York.

Pollock, D. M., Polakowski, J. S., Divish, B. J., and Opgenorth, T. J. (1993). Angiotensin blockade reverses hypertension during long-term nitric oxide synthase inhibition. *Hypertension* **21**, 660–666.

Pomeranz, B. H., Birtch, A. G., and Barger, A. C. (1968). Neural control of intrarenal blood flow. *Am J Physiol* **215**, 1067–1081.

Popper, K. R. (1959). *The Logic of Scientific Discovery*. Hutchinson, London.

Popper, K. R. (1963). *Conjectures and Refutations*. Routledge & Kegan Paul, London.

Postnov, Y. V., and Orlov, S. N. (1985). Ion transport across plasma membrane in primary hypertension. *Physiol Rev* **65**, 904–945.

Poston, L., Sewell, R. B., Wilkinson, S. P., Richardson, P. J., Williams, R., Clarkson, E. M. et al. (1981). Evidence for a circulating transport inhibitor in essential hypertension. *Br Med J* **282**, 847–849.

Pothos, E., Creese, I., and Hoebel, B. (1995). Restricted eating with weight loss selectively decreases extracellular dopamine response in nucleus accumbens and alters dopamine response to amphetamine, morphine and food intake. *J Neurosci* **15**, 6640–6650.

Potter, E. K. (1982). Angiotensin inhibits action of vagus nerve at the heart. *Br J Pharmacol* **75**, 9–11.

Potter, E. (1988). Neuropeptide Y as an autonomic neurotransmitter. *Pharmacol Ther* **37**, 251–273.

Poulter, N. R., and Sever, P. S. (1994). Low blood pressure populations and the impact of rural-urban migration. In *Textbook of Hypertension*, Swales, J. D., Ed., pp. 22–36. Blackwell, Oxford.

Pravenec, M., Klir, P., Kren, V., Zicha, J., and Kunes, J. (1989). An analysis of spontaneous hypertension in spontaneously hypertensive rats by means of new recombinant inbred strains. *J Hypertens* **7**, 217–222.

Presti, C. F., Jones, L. R., and Lindemann, J. P. (1985). Isoproterenol-induced phosphorylation of a 15–kilodalton sarcolemmal protein in intact myocardium. *J Biol Chem* **260**, 3860–3867.

Prewitt, R. L., Chen, I. I. H., and Dowell, R. (1982). Development of microvascular rarefaction in the spontaneously hypertensive rat. *Am J Physiol* **243**, H243–H251.

Prewitt, R. L., Chen, I. I. H., and Dowell, R. F. (1984). Microvascular alterations in the one-kidney, one-clip renal hypertensive rat. *Am J Physiol* **246**, H728–H732.

Price, R. J., Owens, G. K., and Skalak, T. C. (1994). Immunohistochemical identification of arteriolar development using markers of smooth muscle differentiation: evidence that capillary arterialization proceeds from terminal arteriole. *Circ Res* **75**, 520–527.

Prieto, D., Buus, C., Mulvany, M. J., and Nilsson, H. (1997). Interactions between neuropeptide Y and the adenylate cyclase pathway in rat mesenteric small arteries: role of membrane potential. *J Physiol (Lond)* **502**, 281–292.

Prineas, R. J., and Gillum, R. (1985). U.S. epidemiology of hypertension in blacks. In *Hypertension in Blacks: Epidemiology, Pathophysiology and Treatment*, Hall, W. D., Saunders, E., and Shulman, N. B., Eds., pp. 17–36. Year Book, Chicago.

Prineas, R. J., and Sinaiko, A. R. (1994). Hypertension in children. In *Textbook of Hypertension*, Swales, J. D., Ed., pp. 750–766. Blackwell, Oxford.

Prior, I. A. M., Evans, J. G., Harvey, H. P. B., Davidson, F., and Lindsey, M. (1968). Sodium intake and blood pressure in two Polynesian populations. *N Engl J Med* **279**, 515–529.

PROGRESS Collaborative and Group. (2001). Randomised trial of a perindopril-based blood-pressure lowering regimen among 6105 individuals with previous stroke or transient ischaemic attack. *Lancet* **358**, 1033–1041.

Pugh, L. G. C. E. (1964). Animals in high altitudes: man above 5000 meters—mountain exploration. In *Handbook of Physiology: Adaptation to the Environment*, Dill, D. B., Adolph, E. F., and Wilber, C. G., Eds., pp. 861–868. American Physiological Society, Washington, DC.

Pullan, P. T., Johnston, C. I., Anderson, W. P., and Korner, P. I. (1980). Plasma vasopressin in blood pressure homeostasis and in experimental renal hypertension. *Am J Physiol* **239**, H81–H87.

Quinn, W. G., Harris, W. A., and Benzer, S. (1974). Conditioned behavior in *Drosophila melanogaster*. *Proc Natl Acad Sci, USA* **71**, 708–712.

Quinton, P. M. (1999). Physiological basis of cystic fibrosis. *Physiol Rev* **79** (suppl 1), S3–S22.

Radice, M., Alli, C., Avanzini, F., Di Tullio, M., Mariotti, G., Taioli, E., Zussino, A., and Folli, G. (1986). Left ventricular structure and function in normotensive adolescents with a genetic predisposition to hypertension. *Am Heart J* **111**, 115–120.

Räikkönen, K., Matthews, K. A., and Kuller, L. H. (2001). Trajectory of psychological risk and incident hypertension in middle-aged women. *Hypertension* **38**, 798–802.

Raizada, M. K., Francis, S. C., Wang, H., Gelband, C. H., Reaves, P. Y., and Katovich, M. J. (2000). Targeting of the renin-angiotensin system by antisense gene therapy: a possible strategy for longterm control of hypertension. *J Hypertens* **18**, 353–362.

Rakusan, K., Hrdina, P. W., Turek, Z., Lakatta, E. G., Spurgeon, H. A., and Wolford, G. D. (1984). Cell size and cardiac supply of the hypertensive rat heart: quantitative study. *Bas Res Cardiol* **79**, 389–395.

Ralevic, V., and Burnstock, G. (1995). Neuropeptides in blood pressure control. In *Hypertension: Pathophysiology, Diagnosis and Management*, Laragh, J. H., and Brenner, B. M., Eds., Vol. 1, pp. 801–831. Raven Press, New York.

Rand, M. J., Story, D. F., Allen, G. S., Glover, A. B., and McCulloch, M. W. (1973). Pulse-to-pulse modulation of noradrenaline release through a prejunctional α-receptor autoinhibitory mechanism. In *Frontiers in Catecholamine Research*, Usdin, E., and Snyder, S. H., Eds., pp. 579–581. Pergamon, New York.

Rand, M. J., McCulloch, M. W., and Story, D. F. (1980). Catecholamine receptors on nerve terminals. In *Handbook of Experimental Pharmacology*, Székeres, L., Ed., Vol. 54/1, pp. 223–266. Springer-Verlag, Berlin.

Rao, D. C., Morton, N. E., and Yee, S. (1976). Resolution of cultural and biological inheritance by path analysis. *Amer J Hum Genet* **28**, 228–242.

Rapp, J. P., and Dahl, L. K. (1971). Adrenal steroidogenesis in rats bred for susceptibility and resistance to the hypertensive effect of salt. *Endocrinology* **88**, 52–65.

Rapp, J. P., and Dahl, L. K. (1972a). Mendelian inheritance of 18- and 11-beta-steroid hydroxylase activities in the adrenals of rats genetically susceptible or resistant to hypertension. *Endocrinology* **90**, 1435–1446.

Rapp, J. P., and Dahl, L. K. (1972b). Possible role of 18-hydroxy-deoxycorticosterone in hypertension. *Nature* **237**, 338–339.

Rapp, J. P., and Dahl, L. K. (1976). Mutant forms of cytochrome *P*-450 controlling both 18- and 11-beta-steroid hydroxylation in the rat. *Biochemistry* **15**, 1235–1241 .

Rapp, J. P. (1982). Dahl susceptible and salt resistant rats—a review. *Hypertension* **4**, 753–763.

Rapp, J. P. (1983a). Genetics of experimental and human hypertension. In *Hypertension: Pathophysiology and Treatment*, Genest, J., Kuchel, O., Hamet, P., and Cantin, M., Eds., pp. 582–598. McGraw-Hill, New York.

Rapp, J. (1983b). A paradigm for identification of primary genetic causes of hypertension in rats. *Hypertension* **5** (suppl I), I-198–I-203.

Rapp, J. P. (1987). Use and misuse of control strains for genetically hypertensive rats. *Hypertension* **10**, 7–10.

Rapp, J. P., Wang, S. M., and Dene, H. (1989). A genetic polymorphism in the renin gene of Dahl rats cosegregates with blood pressure. *Science* **243**, 542–544.

Rapp, J. P. (1991). Dissecting the primary causes of genetic hypertension in rats. *Hypertension* **18** (suppl I), I-18–I-28.

Rapp, J. P. (1994). The genetics of hypertension in Dahl rats. In *Handbook of Hypertension, Volume 16: Experimental and Genetics Models of Hypertension*, Ganten, D., and De Jong, W., Eds., pp. 186–201. Elsevier, Amsterdam.

Rapp, J., Dene, H., and Deng, A. (1994). Seven renin alleles in rats and their effects on blood pressure. *J Hypertens* **12**, 349–355.

Rapp, J. P. (1995). The search for the genetic basis of blood pressure variation in rats. In *Hypertension: Pathophysiology, Diagnosis and Management*, Laragh, J. H., and Brenner, B. M., Eds., Vol. 1, pp. 1289–1300. Raven Press, New York.

Rapp, J. P., and Deng, A. Y. (1995). Detection and positional cloning of blood pressure quantitative trait loci: is it possible? *Hypertension* **25**, 1121–1128.

Rapp, J. P., Garret, M. R., Dene, H., Meng, H., Hoebee, B., and Lathrop, G. M. (1998). Linkage analysis and construction of a congenic strain for a blood pressure QTL on chromosome 9. *Genomics* **51**, 191–196.

Rapp, J. P. (2000). Genetic analysis of inherited hypertension in the rat. *Physiol Rev* **80**, 135–172.

Ravussin, E., and Danforth, E. (1999). Beyond sloth—physical activity and weight gain. *Science* **283**, 184–185.

Reader, R., Bauer, G. E., Doyle, A. E., Edmondson, K. W., Hunuyor, S., Hurley, T. H., Korner, P. I., Leighton, P. W., Lovell, R. R. H., McCall, M. G., McPhie, J. M., Rand, M. J., and Whyte, H. M. (1980). The Australian therapeutic trial in mild hypertension: Report by the management committee. *Lancet* **i**, 1261–1267.

Reaven, G. M. (1988). Role of insulin resistance in human disease. *Diabetes* **37**, 1595–1607.

Reaven, G. M. (1991). Insulin resistance, hyperinsulinemia, hypertriglyceridemia, and hypertension: parallels between human disease and rodent models. *Diabetes Care* **14**, 195–202.

Reaven, G. M. (1995). Pathophysiology of insulin resistance in human disease. *Physiol Rev* **75**, 473–486.

Reaves, P. Y., Gelband, C. H., Wang, H., Yang, H., Lu, D., Berecek, K. H., Katovich, M. J., and Raizada, M. K. (1999). Permanent cardiovascular protection from hypertension by the AT_1 receptor antisense gene therapy in hypertensive rat offspring. *Circ Res* **85**, e44–e50.

Rebbeck, T., Turner, S., and Sing, C. (1993). Sodium-lithium countertransport genotype and the probability of hypertension in adults. *Hypertension* **22**, 560–568.

Recordati, G. M., Moss, N. G., and Waselkow, L. (1978). Renal chemoreceptors in the rat. *Circ Res* **43**, 534–543.

Recordati, G. M., Moss, N. G., Genovesi, S., and Rogenes, P. R. (1980). Renal receptors in the rat sensitive to chemical alterations of their environment. *Circ Res* **46**, 395–405.

Reddy, M. M., Light, M. J., and Quinton, P. M. (1999). Activation of the epithelial Na^+ channel (ENaC) requires CFTR Cl channel function. *Nature* **402**, 301–304.

Reeves, T. J., Hefner, L. L., Jones, W. B., Coughlan, C., Prieto, G., and Carroll, J. (1960). The haemodynamic determinants of the rate of change of pressure in the left ventricle during isovolumetric contraction. *Am Heart J* **60**, 745–761.

Reichlin, S. (1992). Neuroendocrinology. In *Williams Textbook of Endocrinology*, Wilson, J., and Foster, D., Eds., pp. 135–219. W.B. Saunders, Philadelphia.

Reid, C. M., Dart, A. M., Dewar, E. M., and Jennings, G. L. (1994). Interactions between the effects of exercise and weight loss on risk factors, cardiovascular haemodynamics and left ventricular structure in overweight subjects. *J Hypertens* **12**, 291–301.

Reis, D. J., Doba, N., and Nathan, M. A. (1975). Neurogenic arterial hypertension produced by brainstem lesions. In *Regulation of Blood Pressure by the Central Nervous System (The Fourth Hahnemann International Symposium on Hypertension)*, Onesti, G., Fernandes, M., and Kim, K. E., Eds. Grune & Stratton, New York.

Reivich, M., Holling, H., Roberts, B., and Toole, J. F. (1961). Reversal of blood flow through the vertebral artery and its effect on the cerebral circulation. *N Engl J Med* **265,** 878.

Remensnyder, J. P., Mitchell, J. F., and Sarnoff, S. J. (1962). Functional sympatholysis during muscular activity. *Circ Res* **11,** 370–380.

Remington, J. W. (1963). The physiology of the aorta and major arteries. In *Handbook of Physiology, Section 2: Circulation*, Hamilton, W. F., and Dow, P., Eds., Vol. II, pp. 799–838. American Physiological Society, Washington, DC.

Rettig, R., Folberth, C. G., Stauss, H., Kopf, D., Waldherr, R., Baldhauf, G., and Unger, T. (1990). Hypertension in rats induced by renal grafts from renovascular hypertensive donors. *Hypertension* **15,** 429–435.

Rettig, R., and Schmitt, B. (1994). Experimental hypertension following kidney transplantation in the rat. In *Handbook of Hypertension, Volume 16: Experimental and Genetic Models of Hypertension*, Ganten, D., and De Jong, W., Eds., pp. 141–157. Elsevier, Amsterdam.

Rettig, R., and Grisk, O. (2005). The kidney as a determinant of genetic hypertension: evidence from renal transplantation studies. *Hypertension* **46,** 463–468.

Reubi, F. C., Weidmann, P., Hodler, J., and Cottier, P. T. (1978). Changes in renal function in essential hypertension. *Am J Med* **64,** 556–563.

Rhodin, J. A. G. (1980). Architecture of the vessel wall. In *Handbook of Physiology, Section 2: The Cardiovascular System, Volume II: Vascular Smooth Muscle,* Bohr, D. F., Somlyo, A. P., and Sparks, H. V., Jr., Eds., pp. 1-31. American Physiological Society, Bethesda, MD.

Richer, C., Doussau, M. P., and Guidicelli, J. F. (1982). Prevention du developpement de l'hypertension genetique par le MK421 chez le SHR. *Arch Mal Coeur* **75,** 55–58.

Richter, D. W., and Spyer, K. M. (1990). Cardiorespiratory control. In *Central Regulation of Autonomic Function*, Loewy, A. D., and Spyer, K. M., Eds., pp. 189–207. Oxford University Press, New York.

Ricketts, J. H., and Head, G. A. (1999). A five parameter logistic equation for investigating asymmetry of curvature in baroreflex studies. *Am J Physiol,* **277** (2, part 2), R441–R454.

Ricksten, S. E., Noresson, E., and Thorén, P. (1981). Renal nerve activity and exaggerated natriuresis in conscious spontaneously hypertensive rats. *Acta Physiol Scand* **112,** 161–167.

Riggs, D. S. (1963). *The Mathematical Approach to Physiological Problems.* Williams & Wilkins, Baltimore, MD.

Riva-Rocci, S. (1896). Un sfigmomanometro nuovo. *Gaz Med Torino* **47,** 981–996; 1001–1017.

Rizzoni, D., Porteri, E., Castellano, M., Bettoni, G., Muiesan, M. L., Muiesan, P., Giulini, S. M., and Agabiti-Rosei, E. (1996). Vascular hypertrophy and remodelling in secondary hypertension. *Hypertension* **28,** 785–790.

Robbins, T. W., and Everitt, B. J. (1995). Arousal systems and attention. In *The Cognitive Neurosciences*, Gazzaniga, M. S., Ed., pp. 703–733. MIT Press, Cambridge, MA.

Roberts, R., and Towbin, J. (1993). Principles and techniques of molecular biology. In *Molecular Basis of Cardiology*, Roberts, R., Ed., pp. 15–111. Blackwell, Boston.

Roberts, C. K., Vaziri, N. D., Wang, X. Q., and Barnard, R. J. (2000). Enhanced NO inactivation and hypertension induced by a high-fat refined-carbohydrate diet. *Hypertension* **36,** 423–429.

Robinson, J., Chidzanja, S., Kind, K., Lok, F., Owens, P., and Owens, J. (1995). Placental control of fetal growth. *Reprod Fertil Dev* **7,** 333–344.

Robinson, R. B. (1996). Autonomic receptor-effector coupling during post-natal development. *Cardiovasc Res* **31**, E68–E76.

Rocchini, A. P., and Barger, A. C. (1979). Renovascular hypertension in sodium-depleted dogs: role of renin and carotid sinus reflex. *Am J Physiol* **236**, H101–H107.

Rocchini, A. P., Key, J., Bondie, D., Chico, R., Moorehead, C., Katch, V., and Martin, M. (1989). The effect of weight loss on the sensitivity of blood pressure to sodium in obese adolscents. *N Engl J Med* **321**, 580–585.

Rocchini, A. P., Moorehead, C., Katch, V., Key, J., and Finta, K. M. (1992). Forearm resistance vessel abnormalities and insulin resistance in obese adolescents. *Hypertension* **19**, 615–620.

Rocchini, A. P., Mao, H. Z., Babu, K., Marker, P., and Rocchini, A. J. (1999). Clonidine prevents insulin resistance and hypertension in obese dogs. *Hypertension* **33** (part II), 548–553.

Rodbard, S. (1975). Vascular caliber. *Cardiology* **60**, 4–49.

Roland, P. E., Kawashima, R., Gulyas, B., and O'Sullivan, B. (1997). Positron emission tomography in cognitive neuroscience: methodological constraints, strategies, and examples from learning and memory. In *The Cognitive Neurosciences*, Gazzaniga, M. S., Ed., pp. 781–788. MIT Press, Cambridge, MA.

Roman, R. J. (1986). Abnormal renal hemodynamics and pressure natriuresis relationship in Dahl salt sensitive rats. *Am J Physiol* **251**, F57–F65.

Roman, R. J., and Alonso-Galicia, M. (1999). P-450 eicosanoids: a novel signaling pathway regulating renal function. *NIPS* **14**, 238–242.

Rosell, S. (1984). Microcirculation and transport in adipose tissue. In *Handbook of Physiology, Section 2: The Cardiovascular System, Volume IV, Microcirculation, Part 2*, Renkin, E. M., and Michel, C. C., Eds., pp. 949–968. American Physiological Society, Bethesda, MD.

Rosen, R. (1967). *Optimality Principles in Biology*. Butterworths, London.

Rosenzweig, M. R., Leiman, A. L., and Breedlove, S. M. (1996). *Biological Psychology*. Sinauer Associates, Sunderland, MA.

Rosmond, R., Dallman, M. F., and Björntorp, P. (1998). Stress-related cortisol secretion in men: relationships with abdominal obesity and endocrine, metabolic and hemodynamic abnormalities. *J Clin Endocrinol Metab* **83**, 1853–1859.

Rosner, B., Hennekens, C. H., Kass, E. H., and Miall, W. E. (1977). Age-specific correlation analysis of longitudinal blood pressure data. *Am J Epidemiol* **106**, 306–313.

Rossant, J. (1996). Mouse mutants and cardiac development. *Circ Res* **78**, 349–353.

Rothe, C. F. (1983). Reflex control of veins and vascular capacitance. *Physiol Rev* **63**, 1281–1342.

Rowe, G. G., Castillo, C. A., Maxwell, G. M., and Crumpton, C. W. (1961). A hemodynamic study of hypertension including observations on coronary blood flow. *Ann Int Med* **54**, 405–412.

Rowell, L. (1974). Human cardiovascular adjustments to exercise and thermal stress. *Physiol Rev* **54**, 75–159.

Rowell, L. B., Hermansen, L., and Blackman, J. R. (1976). Human cardiovascular and respiratory responses to graded muscle ischaemia. *J Appl Physiol* **41**, 693–701.

Rowell, L. B. (1983). Cardiovascular adjustments to thermal stress. In *Handbook of Physiology, The Cardiovascular System: Peripheral Circulation*, Shepherd, J. T., and Abboud, F. M., Eds., pp. 967–1023. American Physiological Society, Bethesda, MD.

Rowell, L. (1986). *Human Circulation during Physical Stress*. Oxford University Press, New York.

Rowell, L. B. (1993). *Human Cardiovascular Control*. Oxford University Press, New York.

Rowlands, D. B., Ireland, M. A., Stallard, T. J., Glover, D. R., McLeay, R. A. B., and Watson, R. D. S. (1982). Assessment of left ventricular mass and its response to antihypertensive treatment. *Lancet* **i,** 467–470.

Roy, C. S., and Brown, J. G. (1879). The blood pressure and its variations in the arterioles, capillaries and smaller veins. *J Physiol (Lond)* **2,** 323–359.

Roy, J. W., and Mayrovitz, H. N. (1982). Microvascular blood flow in normotensive and spontaneously hypertensive rat. *Hypertension (Dallas)* **4,** 264–271.

Rudolph, A. M. (1985). Distribution and regulation of blood flow in the fetal and neonatal lamb [Brief review]. *Circ Res* **57,** 811–821.

Rumantir, M. S., Vaz, M., Jennings, G. L., Collier, G., Kaye, D. M., Seals, D. R., Wiesner, G. H., Brunner-La Rocca, H. P., and Esler, M. D. (1999). Neural mechanisms in human obesity related hypertension. *J Hypertens* **17,** 1125–1133.

Rumantir, M. S., Jennings, G. L., Lambert, G. W., Kaye, D. M., Seals, D. R., and Esler, M. D. (2000). The "adrenaline hypothesis" of hypertension revisited: evidence for adrenaline release from the heart of patients with essential hypertension. *J Hypertens* **18,** 717–723.

Rupp, H., and Jacob, R. (1982). Response of blood pressure and cardiac myosin polymorphism to swimming training in the spontaneously hypertensive rat. *Can J Physiol Pharmacol* **60,** 1098–1103.

Rupp, H., Felbier, H.-R., Buckari, A. R., and Jacob, A. R. (1984). Modulation of myosin isoenzyme populations and activities of monamine oxidase and phenylethanolamine transferase in pressure loaded and normal heart swimming exercise and stress arising from electrostimulation in pairs. *Can J Physiol Pharmacol* **62,** 1209–1218.

Rushmer, R. F. (1961). *Cardiovascular Dynamics.* W.B. Saunders, Philadelphia.

Rutan, G. H., Kuller, L. H., Neaton, J. D., Wentworth, D. N., McDonald, R. H., and McFate-Smith, W. (1988). Mortality associated with diastolic hypertension and isolated systolic hypertension among men screened for Multiple Risk Factor Intervention Trial. *Circulation* **77,** 504–514.

Rutledge, T., and Linden, W. (2000). Defensiveness status predicts 3 year incidence of hypertension. *J Hypertens* **18,** 153–159.

Ruzicka, M., and Leenen, F. H. H. (1994). Experimental renovascular hypertension: methodological aspects and role of renin-angiotensin system. In *Handbook of Hypertension* (D. Ganten and W. de Jong, Eds.), Vol. 16, pp. 49–87. Elsevier, Amsterdam.

Ryuzaki, M., Suzuki, H., Kumagai, K., Kumagai, H., Ichikawa, M., Matsumura, Y., and Saruta, T. (1991). Role of vasopressin in salt-induced hypertension in baroreceptor-denervated uninephrectomized rabbits. *Hypertension* **17,** 1085–1091.

Sachs, F. (1987). Baroreceptor mechanisms at the cellular level. *Fed Proc* **46,** 12–16.

Sacks, F. M., Svetkey, L. P., Volmer, W. M., Appel, L. J., Bray, G. A., Harsha, D., Obarzanek, E., Conlin, P. R., Miller, E. R., Simons-Morton, D. G., Karanja, N., and Lin, P.-H. (2001). Effects on blood pressure of reduced dietary sodium and the Dietary Approaches to Stop Hypertension (DASH) diet. *N Engl J Med* **344,** 3–10.

Sadoshima, J., Jahn, L., Takahashi, T., Kulik, T., and Izumo, S. (1992). Molecular characterization of the stretch-induced adaptation of cultured cardiac cells. *J Biol Chem* **267,** 10551–10560.

Sadoshima, J.-i., and Izumo, S. (1993a). Molecular characterization of angiotensin II-induced hypertrophy of cardiac myocytes and hyperplasia of cardiac fibroblasts: critical role of the AT_1 receptor subtype. *Circ Res* **73,** 413–423.

Sadoshima, J.-i., and Izumo, S. (1993b). Signal transduction pathways of angiotensin II-induced *c-fos* gene expression in cardiac myocytes in vitro. Roles of phospholipid-derived second messengers. *Circ Res* **73,** 424–438.

Sadoshima, J., Qiu, Z., Morgan, J. P., and Izumo, S. (1995). Angiotensin II and other hypertrophic stimuli mediated by G protein-coupled receptors activate tyrosine kinase, miotgen-activated protein kinase and 90–kd S^ kinase in cardiac myocytes. *Circ Res* **76,** 1–15.

Sadoshima, J., Aoki, H., and Izumo, S. (1997). Angiotensin II and serum differentially regulate expressions of cyclins, activity of cyclin-dependent kinases, and phosphorylation of retinoblastoma gene product in neonatal cardiac myocytes. *Circ Res* **80,** 228–241.

Sadoshima, J., and Izumo, S. (1997). The cellular and mechanical responses of cardiac myocytes to mechanical stress. *Annu Rev Physiol* **59,** 551–571.

Safar, M. E., London, G. M., Weiss, Y. A., and Milliez, P. L. (1973). Hemodynamic study of 85 patients with borderline hypertension. *Am J Cardiol* **31,** 315–319.

Safar, M. E., Chau, N. P., Weiss, Y. A., London, G. M., and Milliez, P. L. (1976). Control of cardiac output in essential hypertension. *Am J Cardiol* **38,** 332–336.

Safar, M. E., Lehner, J. P., Vincent, M. I., Plainfosse, M. T., and Simon, A. C. (1979). Echocardiographic dimensions in borderline and sustained hypertension. *Am J Cardiol* **44,** 930–935.

Safar, M. E., Bouthier, J. A., Levenson, J. A., and Simon, A. C. (1983). Peripheral large arteries and the response to antihypertensive treatment. *Hypertension* **5,** III-63–III-68.

Safar, M. (1989). *Clinical Research in Essential Hypertension.* Schattauer, Stuttgart.

Safar, M. E., and London, G. M. (1989). Control of cardiac output in sustained essential hypertension. In *Clinical Research in Essential Hypertension*, pp. 75–87. Schattauer, Stuttgart.

Safar, M. E., Plante, G. E., and London, G. M. (1995). Vascular compliance and blood volume in essential hypertension. In *Hypertension: Pathophysiology, Diagnosis and Management*, Laragh, J. H., and Brenner, B. M., Eds., Vol. 1, pp. 377–388. Raven Press, New York.

Sagawa, K. (1965). Relative roles of the rate sensitive and proportional control elements of the carotid sinus during mild hemorrhage. In *Baroreceptors and Hypertension: Proceedings of an International Symposium held at Dayton, Ohio, 16–17 November, 1965*, pp. 97–105. Pergamon Press, Oxford.

Sagawa, K. (1967). Analysis of ventricular pumping capacity as a function of input and output pressure loads. In *Physical Bases of Circulatory Transport: Regulation and Exchange*, Reeve, E. B., and Guyton, A. C., Eds., pp. 141–149. W.B. Saunders, Philadelphia.

Sagawa, K. (1972). The use of control theory and systems analysis in cardiovascular dynamics. In *Cardiovascular Fluid Dynamics*, Bergel, D. H., Ed., Vol. I. Academic Press, London.

Sagawa, K. (1975). Critique of large-scale organ system model: Guytonian cardiovascular model. *Ann Biomed Eng* **3,** 386–400.

Sakamoto, M., Nishimura, M., and Takahashi, H. (1999). Brain atrial natriuretic peptide family abolishes cardiovascular haemodynamic alterations caused by hypertonic saline in rats. *Clin Exp Pharmacol Physiol* **26,** 684–690.

Sakai, S., Miyauchi, T., Kobayashi, M., Yamaguchi, I., Goto, K., and Sugishita, Y. (1996). Inhibition of myocardial endothelin pathway improves long-term survival in heart failure. *Nature* **384,** 353–355.

Salamone, J., Mahan, K., and Rogers, S. (1993). Ventrolateral striatal dopamine depletions impair feeding and food handling in rats. *Pharmacol Biochem Behav* **44,** 605–610.

Saltin, B. (1985). Haemodynamic adaptations to exercise. *Am J Cardiol* **55,** 42D–47D.

Sample, R. H. B., and DiMicco, J. A. (1987). Localization of sites in the periventricular forebrain mediating cardiovascular effects of GABA agonists and antagonists in anaesthetised cats. *J Pharmacol* **240,** 498–507.

Sanders, B. J., and Lawler, J. E. (1992). The borderline-hypertensive rat as a model for environmentally induced hypertension: a review and update. *Neurosci Biobehav Rev* **16,** 207–217.

Sands, J. M., Kokko, J. P., and Jacobson, H. R. (1992). Intrarenal heterogeneity: vascular and tubular. In *The Kidney: Physiology and Pathophysiology*, Seldin, D. W., and Giebisch, G., Eds., Vol. 1, pp. 1087–1155. Raven Press, New York.

Sannerstedt, R. (1966). Hemodynamic response to exercise in patients with arterial hypertension. *Acta Med Scand* (suppl 458), 1–83.

Sannerstedt, R. (1969). Hemodynamic findings at rest and during exercise in mild arterial hypertension. *Am J Med Sci* **258**, 70–89.

Sannerstedt, R., and Sivertsson, R. (1975). Systemic and peripheral hemodynamics in latent arterial hypertension. In *Symposium on Recent Advances in Hypertension*, Milliez, P., and Safar, M., Eds., pp. 195–203. Boehringer Ingelheim, New York.

Santamore, W. P., and Walinsky, W. P. (1980). Altered coronary flow responses to vasoactive drugs in the presence of cornary arterial stenosis in the dog. *Am J Cardiol* **45**, 276–285.

Santamore, W. P., Walinsky, P., Bove, A. A., Cox, R. H., Carey, R. A., and Spann, J. F. (1980). The effects of vasoconstriction on experimental coronary artery stenosis. *Am Heart J* **100**, 852–858.

Santamore, W. P., Bove, A. A., Carey, R., Walinsky, P., and Spann, J. F. (1981). Synergistic relation between vasoconstriction and fixed epicardial vessel stenosis in coronary artery disease. *Am Heart J* **101**, 428–434.

Santamore, W. P., and Bove, A. A. (1985). A theoretical model of a compliant arterial stenosis. *Am J Physiol* **248**, H274–H285.

Saper, C. B., Scammell, T. E., and Lu, J. (2005). Hypothalamic regulation of sleep and circadian rhythms. *Nature* **437**, 1257–1263.

Sapirstein, L. (1969). Discussion on the paper by Guyton, A. C. and Coleman, T. G., "Quantitative analysis of the pathophysiology of hypertension." *Circ Res* **24**, 1–16.

Sapolsky, R. M. (1998). The stress of Gulf War syndrome. *Nature* **393**, 308–309.

Sapru, H., and Wang, S. (1976). Modification of aortic baroreceptor resetting in the spontaneously hypertensive rat. *Am J Physiol* **230**, 664–674.

Sarnoff, S. J., Mitchell, J. H., Gilmore, J. P., and Remensnyder, J. P. (1960). Homeometric autoregulation in the heart. *Circ Res* **8**, 1077–1091.

Sarnoff, S. J., and Mitchell, J. H. (1962). The control of the function of the heart. In *Handbook of Physiology, Section 2: Circulation*, Hamilton, W. F., and Dow, P., Eds., Vol. I, pp. 489–532. American Physiological Society, Washington, DC.

Sasayama, S., Franklin, D., and Ross, J., Jr. (1977). Hyperfunction with normal inotropic state of the hypertrophied left ventricle. *Am J Physiol* **232**, H418–H425.

Sato, A., Sato, Y., and Schmidt, R. F. (1997). The impact of somatosensory input on autonomic functions. *Rev Physiol Biochem Pharmacol* **130**, 1–328.

Savage, D. D. (1987). Prevalence and evolution of echocardiographic left ventricular hypertrophy. In *The Heart and Hypertension*, Messerli, F. H., Ed., pp. 63–71. Yorke, New York.

Schachter, S., and Singer, J. (1962). Cognitive, social, and physiological determinants of emotional state. *Psych Rev* **69**, 379–399.

Schachter, S. (1971). *Emotion, Obesity and Crime*. Academic Press, New York.

Schadt, J. C., and Gadis, R. R. (1985). Endogenous opiate peptides may limit norepinephrine release during hemorrhage. *J Pharmacol* **232**, 656–660.

Schadt, J. C., and Ludbrook, J. (1991). Hemodynamic and neurohumoral responses to acute hypovolemia in conscious mammals. *Am J Physiol* **260**, H305–H318.

Schalekamp, M. A. D. H., Man in't Veld, A. J., and Wenting, G. J. (1985). What regulates whole body autoregulation? Clinical observations. *J Hypertens* **3**, 97–108.

Schechter, P. J., Horwitz, D., and Henkin, R. I. (1973). Sodium chloride preference in essential hypertension. *JAMA* **225**, 1311–1315.

Scheibel, M., Scheibel, A., Mollica, A., and Moruzzi, G. (1955). Convergence and interaction of afferent impulses on single units of reticular formation. *J Neurophysiol* **18**, 309–331.

Scheibel, M. E., and Scheibel, A. B. (1967). Structural organization of non-specific thalamic nuclei and their projection toward cortex. *Brain Res* **6**, 60–94.

Scher, A. M., and Young, A. C. (1970). Reflex control of heart rate in the unanesthetized dog. *Am J Physiol* **218**, 780–789.

Scher, A. M., O'Leary, D. S., and Sheriff, D. D. (1991). Arterial baroreceptor regulation of peripheral resistance and of cardiac performance. In *Baroreceptor Reflexes*, Persson, P. B., and Kirchheim, H. R., Eds., pp. 75–125. Springer-Verlag, Berlin.

Schiffrin, E. L., Deng, L. Y., and Larochelle, P. (1994). Effects of a β-blocker or a converting enzyme inhibitor on resistance arteries in essential hypertension. *Hypertension* **23**, 83–91.

Schild, L., Canessa, C. M., Shimkets, R. A., Gautschi, I., Lifton, R. P., and Rossier, B. C. (1995). A mutation in the epithelial sodium channel causing Liddle disease increases channel activity in the *Xenopus laevis* oocyte expression system. *Proc Natl Acad Sci, USA* **92**, 5699–5703.

Schlager, G. (1972). Spontaneous hypertension in laboratory animals. A review of the genetic implications. *J Heredity* **63**, 35–38.

Schlaich, M., Lambert, E., Kaye, D. M., Krozowski, Z., Campbell, D. J., Lambert, G., Hastings, J., Aggarwal, A., and Esler, M. D. (2004). Sympathetic augmentation in hypertension: role of nerve firing, norepinephrine reuptake and angiotension neuromodulation. *Hypertension* **43**, 169–175.

Schmid-Schoenbein, G. W., Firestone, G., and Zweifach, B. W. (1986). Network anatomy of arteries feeding the spinotrapezius muscle in normotensive and hypertensive rats. *Blood Vessels* **23**, 34–49.

Schmidt, C. F. (1932). Carotid sinus reflexes to the respiratory centre. *Am J Physiol* **102**, 94–118.

Schmidt, E. M. (1968). Blood pressure responses to aortic nerve stimulation in swine. *Am J Physiol* **215**, 1488–1492.

Schmidt, B., and DiMicco, J. A. (1984). Blockade of GABA receptors in periventricular forebrain of anaesthetised cats: effects on heart rate, arterial pressure and hindlimb vascular resistance. *Brain Res* **301**, 111–119.

Schnall, P. L., Pieper, C., Schwartz, J. E., Karasek, R., Schlussel, Y., Devereux, R., Alderman, M., Warren, K., and Pickering, T. (1990). The relationship between "job strain," workplace diastolic blood pressure and left ventricular mass index. *JAMA* **263**, 1929–1935.

Schnall, P. L., Schwartz, J. E., Landsbergis, P. A., Warren, K., and Pickering, T. G. (1992). Relation between job strain, alcohol and ambulatory blood pressure. *J Hypertens* **19**, 488–494.

Schneider, M., and Parker, T. (1992). Molecular mechanisms of cardiac growth and hypertrophy: myocardial growth factors and proto-oncogenes in development and disease. In *Molecular Basis of Cardiology*, Roberts, R., Ed., pp. 113–134. Blackwell, Oxford.

Schnermann, J., and Briggs, J. P. (1992). Function of the juxtaglomerular apparatus. In *The Kidney: Physiology and Pathophysiology*, Seldin, D. W., and Giebisch, G., Eds., Vol. 1, pp. 1249–1289. Raven Press, New York.

Scholander, P. F., Hammel, H. T., Le Messurier, H., Hemmingsen, E., and Carey, W. (1962). Circulatory adjustments in pearl divers. *J Appl Physiol* **17**, 184–190.

Scholander, P. F. (1964). Animals in aquatic environments: diving mammals and birds. In *Handbook of Physiology, Section 4: Adaptation to the Environment*, Dill, D. B., Adolph, E. F., and Wilber, C. G., Eds., pp. 729–739. American Physiological Society, Washington, DC.

Schramm, L. P., Honig, C. R., and Bignall, K. E. (1971). Active muscle vasodilation in primates homologous with sympathetic vasodilation in carnivores. *Am J Physiol* **221**, 768–777.

Schretzenmayr, A. (1933). Uber kreislaufregulatorische Vorgänge and den grossen Arterien bei der Muskelarbeit. *Pfluegers Arch* **233**, 743–748.

Schull, W. J., Harburg, E., Erfurt, J. C., Schork, M. A., and Rice, R. A. (1970). A family set method for estimating heredity and stress. II. Preliminary results of the genetic methodology in a pilot survey of Negro blood pressure, Detroit, 1966–67. *J Chronic Dis* **23**, 83–92.

Schultz, H. D., Pisarri, T. E., Coleridge, H. M., and Coleridge, J. C. G. (1985). Absence of acute resetting of C-fiber baroreceptors in the carotid sinus of dogs [Abstract]. *Fed Proc* **44**, 103.

Schultz, W. (1992). Activity of dopamine neurons in behaving primates. *Semin Neurosci* **4**, 129–138.

Schultz, W., Dayan, P., and Montague, P. R. (1997). A neural substrate of prediction and reward. *Science* **275**, 1593–1599.

Schulz, R. E., Nava, E., and Moncada, S. (1992). Induction and potential biological relevance of a Ca^{2+} independent nitric oxide synthase in the myocardium. *Br J Pharmacol* **105**, 575–580.

Schuster, H., Wienker, T. F., Bahring, S., Bilginturan, N., Toka, H. R., Neitzel, H., Jeschke, E., Toka, O., Gilbert, D., Lowe, A., Ott, J., Haller, H., and Luft, F. C. (1996). Severe autosomal dominant hypertension and brachydactyly in a unique Turkish kindred maps to human chromosome 12. *Nat Gen* **13**, 98–100.

Schwartz, S. M., Heimark, R. L., and Majesky, M. W. (1990). Developmental mechanisms underlying pathology of arteries. *Physiol Rev* **70**, 1177–1209.

Schwartz, A. R., Gold, A. R., Schubert, N., Stryzak, A., Wise, R. A., Permutt, S., and Smith, P. L. (1991). Effect of weight loss on upper airway collapsibility in obstructive sleep apnea. *Am Rev Respir Dis* **144**, 494–498.

Schwartz, J. H., and Kandel, E. R. (1991). Synaptic transmission mediated by second messengers. In *Principles of Neural Science*, Kandel, E. R., Schwartz, J. H., and Jessel, T. M., Eds., pp. 173–193. Prentice-Hall International, New York.

Schwartz, M. W., Peskind, E., Raskind, M., Boyko, E. J., and Porte, D. (1996). Cerebrospinal fluid levels: relationship to plasma levels and to adiposity in humans. *Nat Med* **2**, 589–593.

Schwartz, M. W., Woods, S. C., Porte, D., Jr., Seeley, R. J., and Baskin, D. G. (2000). Central nervous system control of food intake. *Nature* **404**, 661–671.

Schwartz, M. W. (2002). Keeping hunger at bay. *Nature* **418**, 595–597.

Scotch, N. A. (1963). Sociocultural factors in the epidemiology of Zulu hypertension. *Am J Public Health* **53**, 1205–1213.

Scott, M. J. (1966). Reflex effects of carotid body chemoreceptor stimulation on the heart rate of the rabbit. *Aust J Exp Biol Med Sci* **44**, 393–404.

Scott-Burden, T., Resink, T. J., and Buehler, F. R. (1989). Enhanced growth and growth factor responsiveness of vascular smooth muscle cells from hypertensive rats. *J Cardiovasc Pharmacol* **14** (suppl 6), S16–S21.

Scroop, G. C., and Lowe, R. D. (1968). Central pressor effect of angiotensin mediated by parasympathetic nervous system. *Nature* **220**, 1331–1332.

Scroop, G. C., and Lowe, R. D. (1969). Efferent pathways of the cardiovascular response to vertebral artery infusions of angiotensin in the dog. *Clin Sci* **37**, 605–619.

Seagard, J. L., Van Brederode, J. F. M., Dean, C., Hopp, F. A., Gallenberg, L. A., and Kampine, J. P. (1990). Firing characteristics of single-fiber carotd sinus baroreceptors. *Circ Res* **66**, 1499–1509.

Seagard, J. L., Gallenberg, L. A., Hopp, F. A., and Dean, C. (1992). Acute resetting of two functionally different types of carotid baroreceptors. *Circ Res* **70,** 559–565.

Sealey, J. E., and Laragh, J. H. (1974). A proposed cybernetic system for sodium and potassium homeostasis: coordination of aldosterone and intrarenal physical factors. *Kidney Internat* **6,** 281–290.

Seeliger, E., Wronski, T., Ladwig, M., Rebeschke, T., Persson, P. B., and Reinhardt, H. W. (2005). The 'body fluid pressure control system' relies on the renin-angiotensin-aldosterone system: Balance studies in freely moving dogs. *Clin Exp Pharmacol Physiol* **32,** 394–399.

Segal, M., and Bloom, F. E. (1976). The action of norepinephrine in the rat hippocampus: IV. The effects of locus coeruleus stimulation on evoked hippocampal activity. *Brain Res* **107,** 513–525.

Segal, S. S. (1994). Cell-to-cell communication coordinates blood flow control. *Hypertension* **23** (part 2), 1113–1120.

Segall, H. N. (1985). Quest for Korotkoff. *J Hypertens* **3,** 317–326.

Selig, S. E., Anderson, W. P., Korner, P. I., and Casley, D. J. (1983). The role of angiotensin II in the development of hypertension and in the maintenance of glomerular filtration rate during 48 hours of renal artery stenosis in conscious dogs. *J Hypertens* **1,** 351–355.

Sen, S., Tarazi, R. C., and Bumpus, F. M. (1977). Cardiac hypertrophy and antihypertensive therapy. *Cardiovasc Res* **11,** 427.

Sever, P. S., Gordon, D., Peart, W. S., and Beighton, P. (1980). Blood pressure and its correlates in urban and tribal Africa. *Lancet* **ii,** 60–64.

Shapiro, A. P. (1972). Behavioral approach to the study of cardiovascular disease. In *Neural and Psychological Mechanisms in Cardiovascular Disease*, Zanchetti, A., Ed., pp. 75–83. Casa Editrice Il Ponte, Milano.

Sharma, A. M., and Grassi, G. (2001). Obesity and hypertension: cause or consequence? *J Hypertens* **19,** 2125–2126.

Sharma, A. M., Janke, J., Gorzelniak, K., Engeli, S., and Luft, F. (2002). Hypothesis paper: angiotensin blockade prevents Type 2 diabetes by formation of fat cells. *Hypertension* **40,** 609–611.

Sharpey-Schafer, E. P. (1965). Effect of respiratory acts on the circulation. In *Handbook of Physiology, Section 2: Circulation*, Hamilton, W. F., and Dow, P., Eds., Vol. 3. American Physiological Society, Washington, DC.

Shaw, J., Hunyor, S. N., and Korner, P. I. (1971). Sites of central nervous action of clonidine on reflex autonomic function in the unanaesthetized rabbit. *Eur J Pharm* **15,** 66–78.

Shaw, A. M., and McGrath, J. C. (1996). Initiation of smooth muscle response. In *Pharmacology of Vascular Smooth Muscle*, Garland, C. J., and Angus, J. A., Eds., pp. 103–135. Oxford University Press, Oxford.

Shear, C. L., Burke, G. L., Freedman, D. S., and Berenson, G. S. (1986). Value of childhood measurement and family history in predicting future blood pressure status: results of 8 years of follow-up in the Bogalusa Heart Study. *Pediatrics* **77,** 862–869.

Shek, E. W., Brands, M. W., and Hall, J. E. (1998). Chronic leptin infusion increases arterial pressure. *Hypertension* **31,** 409–414.

Shepherd, R. E., Keuhne, M. L., Kenno, K. A., Durstine, J. L., Balon, T. W., and Rapp, J. P. (1982). Attenuation of blood pressure increases in Dahl salt-sensitive rats by exercise. *J Appl Physiol* **52,** 1608.

Sheridan, D. J. (2000). Regression of left ventricular hypertrophy: do antihypertensive classes differ? *J Hypertens* **18** (suppl 3), S21–S27.

Sherrington, C. (1947). *The Integrative Action of the Nervous System*. Yale University, New Haven, CT. (Original book published 1906)

Sheu, S.-S., and Blaustein, M. P. (1986). Sodium/calcium exchange and regulation of cell calcium and contractility in cardiac muscle, with a note about vascular smooth muscle. In *The Heart and Cardiovascular System: Scientific Foundations*, Fozzard, H. A., Haber, E., Jennings, R. B., Katz, A. M., and Morgan, H. E., Eds., Vol. 1, pp. 509–535. Raven Press, New York.

Shimamatsu, K., and Fouad-Tarazi, F. M. (1986). Basal inotropic state in rats with renal hypertension: influence of coronary flow and perfusion pressure. *Cardiovasc Res* **20**, 269–274.

Shimkets, R. A., Warnock, D. G., Bositis, C. M., Nelson-Williams, C., Hansson, J. H., Schambelan, M. et al. (1995). Liddle's syndrome: heritable human hypertension caused by mutations in the beta-subunit of the epithelial sodium channel. *Cell* **79**, 407–414.

Shore, A. C., and Tooke, J. E. (1994). Microvascular function in human essential hypertension. *J Hypertens* **12**, 717–728.

Short, D. S., and Thompson, A. D. (1959). The arteries of the small intestine in systemic hypertension. *J Path Bact* **78**, 321–334.

Short, D. S. (1966). The vascular fault in chronic hypertension: with particular reference to the role of medial hypertrophy. *Lancet* **i**, 1302–1304.

Shyu, B. C., Andersson, S. A., and Thorén, P. (1984). Circulatory depression following low frequency stimulation of the sciatic nerve in anaesthetized rats. *Acta Physiol Scand* **1121**, 97–102.

Siegel, J. M. (2005). Clues to the functions of mammalian sleep. *Nature* **437**, 1264–1271.

Simchon, S., Manger, W., Golanov, E., Kamen, J., Sommer, G., and Marshall, C. H. (1999). Handling of ^{22}NaCl by the blood-brain barrier and kidney: its relevance to salt-induced hypertension in Dahl rats. *Hypertension* **33** (part II), 517–523.

Simon, E. (1974). Temperature regulation: the spinal cord as a site of extrahypothalamic thermoregulatory functions. *Rev Physiol Biochem Pharmacocol* **71**, 1–76.

Simon, G., Abraham, G., and Altman, S. (1993). Stimulation of vascular glycosaminoglycan synthesis by subpressor angiotensin II in rats. *Hypertension* **23**, I-148–I-151.

Simpson, P., McGrath, A., and Savion, S. (1982). Myocyte hypertrophy in neonatal rat cultures and its regulation by serum and by catecholamines. *Circ Res* **51**, 787–801.

Simpson, P. (1983). Norepinephrine-stimulated hypertrophy of cultured rat myocardial cells is an alpha-1 adrenergic response. *J Clin Invest* **72**, 732–738.

Simpson, P. (1985). Stimulation of hypertrophy of cultured neonatal rat heart cells through an α_1 adrenergic receptor and induction of beating through an α_1 and β_1 adrenergic interaction. *Circ Res* **56**, 884–894.

Simpson, F. O., Phelan, E. L., Ledingham, J. M., and Miller, J. A. (1994). Hypertension in the genetically hypertensive (GH) strain. In *Handbook of Hypertension, Volume 16: Experimental and Genetic Models of Hypertension*, Ganten, D., and De Jong, W., Eds., pp. 228–271. Elsevier, Amsterdam.

Simpson, F. O. (2000). Blood pressure and sodium intake. In *Epidemiology of Hypertension*, Vol. 20, Bulpitt, C. J., Ed., pp. 273–295. Elsevier Science, Amsterdam.

Sing, C. F., Boerwinkle, E., and Turner, S. T. (1986). Genetics of primary hypertension. *Clin Exp Hypertens (Part A)* **A8**, 623–651.

Singer, C. (1928). *A Short History of Medicine*. Clarendon Press, Oxford.

Sinnett, P. F., and Whyte, H. M. (1973). Epidemiology studies in a total Highland population in New Guinea: environment, culture and health status. *Human Ecol* **1**, 245–257.

Sivertsson, R., and Olander, R. (1968). Aspects of the nature of the increased vascular resistance and increased "reactivity" to noradrenaline in hypertensive subjects. *Life Sci* **7**, 1291–1297.

Sivertsson, R. (1970). The hemodynamic importance of structural vascular changes in essential hypertension. *Acta Physiol Scand* **343** (suppl), 1–56.

Sjöblom-Widfeldt, N. (1990). Neuro-muscular transmission in blood vessels: phasic and tonic components. *Acta Physiol Scand* **138** (suppl 587), 1–53.

Skov, K., Mulvany, M. J., and Korsgaard, N. (1992). Morphology of renal afferent arterioles in spontaneously hypertensive rats. *Hypertension* **20**, 821–827.

Skov, K., Nyengaard, J., Korsgaard, N., and Mulvany, M. (1994). Number and size of renal glomeruli in spontaneously hypertensive rats. *J Hypertens* **12**, 1373–1376.

Sleek, G. E., and Duling, B. R. (1986). Coordination of mural elements and myofilaments during arteriolar constriction. *Circ Res* **59**, 620–627.

Sleight, P., Ed. (1974). *Neural Control of the Cardiovascular System*. Butterworths, London.

Sleight, P., Robinson, J. L., Brooks, D. E., and Rees, P. M. (1977). Characteristics of single carotid sinus baroreceptor fibers and whole nerve activity in normotensive and renal hypertensive dogs. *Circ Res* **41**, 750–758.

Sleight, P. (1991). Role of the baroreceptor reflexes in circulatory control, with particular reference to hypertension. *Hypertension* **18** (suppl III), III-31–III-34.

Smallegange, C., Kline, R. L., and Adams, M. A. (2003). Transplantation of enalapril-treated kidneys confers persistent lowering of arterial pressure in SHR. *Hypertension* **42**, 932–936.

Smeda, J. S., Lee, R. M. K. W., and Forrest, J. B. (1988). Structural and reactivity alterations of the renal vasculature of spontaneously hypertensive rats prior to and during established hypertension. *Circ Res* **63**, 518–533.

Smiesko, V., and Johnson, P. C. (1993). The arterial lumen is controlled by flow-related shear stress. *NIPS* **8**, 34–38.

Smirk, F. H. (1957). *High Arterial Pressure*. Blackwell, Oxford.

Smith, O. A., Hohimer, A. R., Astley, C. A., and Taylor, D. J. (1979). Renal and hindlimb vascular control during acute emotion in the baboon. *Am J Physiol* **236**, R198–R205.

Smith, T. L., and Hutchins, P. M. (1979). Central hemodynamics in the developmental stage of spontaneous hypertension in the unanesthetized rat. *Hypertension* **1**, 508–517.

Smith, O. A., Astley, C. A., DeVito, J. L., Stein, J. M., and Walsh, K. E. (1980). Functional analysis of hypothalamic control of the cardiovascular responses accompanying emotional behaviour. *Fed Proc* **39**, 2487–2494.

Smith, O. A., Astley, C. A., Hohimer, A. R., and Stephenson, R. B. (1980). Behavioral and cerebral control of cardiovascular function. In *Neural Control of Circulation*, Hughes, M. J., and Barnes, C. D., Eds., pp. 1–21. Academic Press, New York.

Smith, O. A., and DeVito, J. L. (1984). Central neural integration for the control of autonomic responses associated with emotion. *Annu Rev Neurosci* **7**, 43–65.

Smith, S. H., and Bishop, S. P. (1985). Regional myocyte size in compensated right ventricular hypertrophy in the ferret. *J Mol Cell Cardiol* **17**, 1005–1011.

Smithies, O., and Kim, H. S. (1994). Targeted gene duplication and disruption for analysing quantitative genetic traits in mice. *Proc Natl Acad Sci, USA* **91**, 3612–3615.

Smithies, O. (1997). A mouse view of hypertension. *Hypertension* **30**, 1318–1324.

Smithwick, R. H. (1940). A technique for splanchnic resection for hypertension. Preliminary report. *Surgery* **7**, 1–12.

Smolich, J. J., Weissberg, P. L., Broughton, A., and Korner, P. I. (1988a). Aortic pressure reduction redistributes transmural blood flow in dog left ventricle. *Am J Physiol* **254**, H361–H368.

Smolich, J. J., Weissberg, P. L., Broughton, A., and Korner, P. I. (1988b). Comparison of left and right ventricular blood flow responses during arterial pressure reduction in the autonomically blocked dog: evidence for right ventricular autoregulation. *Cardiovasc Res* **22**, 17–24.

Smolich, J. J., Walker, A. M., Campbell, G. R., and Adamson, T. M. (1989). Left and right ventricular myocardial morphometry in fetal, neonatal and adult sheep. *Am J Physiol* **257**, H1–H9.

Smolich, J. J., Weissberg, P. L., Friberg, P., Broughton, A., and Korner, P. I. (1991). Left ventricular blood flow during aortic pressure reduction in hypertensive dogs. *Hypertension* **18,** 665–673.

Smolich, J. J., Weissberg, P. L., Friberg, P., and Korner, P. I. (1991). Right ventricular coronary blood flow patterns during aortic pressure reduction in renal hypertensive dogs. *Acta Physiol Scand* **141,** 507–516.

Smyth, H. S., Sleight, P., and Pickering, G. W. (1969). Reflex regulation of arterial pressure during sleep in man: a quantitative method of assessing baroreflex sensitivity. *Circ Res* **24,** 109–121.

Snell, J., Korner, P., and Bobik, A. (1986). Differential effects of sino-aortic denervations on cardiac noradrenaline stores, turnover and neuronal re-uptake in normotensive and renal hypertensive rabbits. *J Hypertens* **4,** 413–420.

Sobye, P. (1948). Heredity in essential hypertension. A genetic-clinical study of 200 propositi suffering from nephrosclerosis. *Op Domo Biol Hered Hum, Kbhv* **16,** 1–225.

Sohal, R. S., and Weindruch, R. (1996). Oxidative stress caloric restriction and aging. *Science* **273,** 59–63.

Sokolow, M., and Perloff, D. (1961). The prognosis of essential hypertension treated conservatively. *Circulation* **23,** 697–710.

Sokolow, M., Werdegar, D., Kain, H. K., and Hinman, A. T. (1966). Relationship between level of blood pressure measured casually and by portable recorders and severity of complications in essential hypertension. *Circulation* **34,** 279–291.

Sokolowski, M. B. (2002). Social eating for stress. *Nature* **419,** 893–894.

Somers, V. K., Mark, A. L., and Abboud, F. M. (1988). Potentiation of sympathetic nerve responses to hypoxia in borderline hypertensive subjects. *Hypertension* **11,** 608–612.

Somers, V., Conway, J., Johnston, J., and Sleight, P. (1991). Effects of endurance training on baroreflex sensitivity and blood pressure in borderline hypotension. *Lancet* **337,** 1363–1368.

Somers, V. K., Dyken, M. E., Mark, A. L., and Abboud, F. M. (1993). Sympathetic nerve activity in normal humans. *N Engl J Med* **328,** 303–307.

Somers, V. K., Dyken, M. E., Clary, M. P., and Abboud, F. M. (1995). Sympathetic neural mechanisms in obstructive sleep apnea. *J Clin Invest* **96,** 1897–1904.

Somers, V. K. (1999). Debating sympathetic overactivity as a hallmark of human obesity: an opposing position. *J Hypertens* **17,** 1061–1064.

Somlyo, A. P., and Somlyo, A. V. (1986). Smooth muscle structure and function. In *The Heart and Cardiovascular System: Scientific Foundations*, Fozzard, H. A., Haber, E., Jennings, R. B., Katz, A. M., and Morgan, H. E., Eds., Vol. 2, pp. 845–864. Raven Press, New York.

Somlyo, A. P., and Somlyo, A. V. (1994). Signal transduction and regulation in smooth muscle. *Nature* **372,** 231–236.

Sonnenblick, E. H. (1962). Force-velocity relations in mammalian heart muscle. *Am J Physiol* **202,** 931–939.

Sonnenblick, E. H., Spotnitz, H. M., and Spiro, D. (1964). Role of the sarcomere in ventricular function and the mechanism of heart failure. *Circ Res* **14 & 15** (suppl II), II-70–II-80.

Soubrier, F. (1999). Nitric oxide synthase genes: candidate genes among many others. *Hypertension* **33,** 924–926.

Sowers, J., Tuck, M., Asp, N. D., and Sollars, E. (1981). Plasma aldosterone and corticosterone responses to adrenocorticotrophin, angiotensin, potassium and stress in spontaneously hypertensive rats. *Endocrinology* **108,** 1161–1167.

Sparks, H. V. J. (1980). Effect of local metabolic factors on vascular smooth muscle. In *Handbook of Physiology, Section 2: The Cardiovascular System, Volume II: Vascular Smooth Muscle*, Bohr, D. F., Somlyo, A. P., and Sparks, H. V., Eds., pp. 475–513. American Physiological Society, Bethesda, MD.

Speden, R. N., and Warren, D. M. (1986). The interaction between noradrenaline activation and distension activation of the rabbit ear artery. *J Physiol (Lond)* **375**, 283–302.

Sperry, R. W. (1968). Mental unity following surgical disconnection of the cerebral hemispheres. In *The Harvey Lectures*, Vol. 62, pp. 293–323. Academic Press, New York.

Spirito, P., Pellicia, A., Proschan, M. A., Granata, M., Spataro, A., Bellone, P., Caselli, G., Biffi, A., Vecchio, C., and Maron, B. J. (1994). Morphology of "athletes heart" assessed by echocardiography in 947 elite athletes representing 27 sports. *Am J Cardiol* **74**, 802–806.

Spyer, K. M. (1981). Neural organisation and control of the baroreceptor reflex. *Rev Physiol Biochem Pharmacol* **88**, 23–124.

Spyer, K. M. (1990). The central nervous organisation of reflex circulatory control. In *Central Regulation of Autonomic Function*, Loewy, A. D., and Spyer, K. M., Eds., pp. 168–188. Oxford University Press, New York.

Staessen, J., Amery, A., and Fagard, R. (1990). Isolated systolic hypertension in the elderly [Editorial review]. *J Hypertens* **8**, 393–405.

Staessen, J. A., Poulter, N. R., Fletcher, A. E., Markowe, H. L., Marmot, M. G., Shipley, M. J. et al. and others. (1994). Psycho-emotional stress and salt intake may interact to raise BP. *J Cardiovasc Risk* **1**, 45–51.

Staessen, J. A., Wang, J.-G., Brand, E., Barlassina, C., Birkenhäger, W. H., Herrmann, S.-M., Fagard, R., Tizzoni, L., and Bianchi, G. (2001). Effects of three candidate genes on prevalence and incidence of hypertension in a Caucasian population. *J Hypertens* **19**, 1349–1358.

Stamler, J., Stamler, R., Reidlinger, W. F., Algera, G., and Roberts, R. H. (1976). Hypertension screening of 1 million Americans: Community Hypertension Evaluation Clinic (CHEC) Program, 1973 through 1975. *JAMA* **235**, 2299–2306.

Stamler, J. S., Jia, L., Eu, J. P., McMahon, T. J., Demchenko, I. T., Bonaventura, J., Gernert, K., and Piantadosi, C. A. (1997). Blood flow regulation by S-nitrosohemoglobin in the physiological oxygen gradient. *Science* **276**, 2034–2037.

Stamler, J. S., and Meissner, G. (2001). Physiology of nitric oxide in skeletal muscle. *Physiol Rev* **81**, 209–237.

Stanek, K. A., Neil, J. J., Sawyer, W. B., and Loewy, A. D. (1984). Changes in regional blood flow and cardiac output after L-glutamate stimulation of A5 cell group. *Am J Physiol* **246**, H44–H51.

Starke, K. (1977). Regulation of noradrenaline release by presynaptic receptor systems. *Rev Physiol Biochem Pharmacol* **77**, 1–124.

Stekiel, W. J., Contney, S. J., and Lombard, J. H. (1991). Sympathetic neural control of vascular muscle in reduced renal mass hypertension. *Hypertension* **17**, 1185–1191.

Stella, A., and Zanchetti, A. (1991). Functional role of renal afferents. *Physiol Rev* **71**, 659–682.

Stephens, G., Davis, J., Freeman, R., DeForrest, J., and Early, D. (1979). Hemodynamic, fluid, and electrolyte changes in sodium-depleted, one-kidney renal hypertensive dogs. *Circ Res* **44**, 316–321.

Steptoe, A., Cropley, M., and Joekes, K. (1999). Job strain, blood pressure and response to uncontrollable stress. *J Hypertens* **17**, 193–200.

Steptoe, A., and Cropley, M. (2000). Persistent high job demands and reactivity to mental stress predict future ambulatory blood pressure. *J Hypertens* **18**, 581–586.

St. Lezin, E., Simonet, L., Pravenec, M., and Kurtz, T. W. (1992). Hypertensive strains and normotensive control strains. *Hypertension* **19**, 419–424.

Stokes, G. S., and Korner, P. I. (1964). Effects of posthemorrhagic anemia on the renal circulation of the unanesthetized rabbit. *Circ Res* **14**, 414–425.

Stone, C. A., and Porter, C. C. (1967). Biochemistry and pharmacology of methyldopa and some related structures. *Adv Drug Res* **4**, 71.

Stowasser, M., and Gordon, R. D. (2000). Primary aldosteronism learning from the study of familial varieties. *J Hypertens* **18**, 1165–1176.

Stowasser, M. (2001). Primary aldosteronism: revival of a syndrome. *J Hypertens* **19**, 363–366.

Stradling, J. R. (1996). Sleep-related disorders of breathing. In *Oxford Textbook of Medicine*, Weatherall, D. J., Ledingham, J. G. G., and Warrell, D. A., Eds., Vol. 2, pp. 2906–2918. Oxford University Press, Oxford.

Strandgaard, S. (1976). Autoregulation of cerebral blood flow in hypertensive patients: the modifying influence of prologed antihypertensive treatment on the tolerance to acute, drug-induced hypotension. *Circulation* **53**, 720–727.

Strandgaard, S., and Poulson, O. B. (1994). Hypertension and human cerebrovascular disease. In *Textbook of Hypertension*, Swales, J. D., Ed., pp. 690–697. Blackwell, Oxford.

Strandgaard, S., and Paulson, O. B. (1995). Cerebral blood flow in untreated and treated hypertension. *Neth J Med* **47**, 180–184.

Strauer, B.-E. (1979). Ventricular function and coronary hemodynamics in hypertensive heart disease. *Am J Cardiol* **44**, 999–1007.

Strauer, B. E., Motz, W., Schwartzkopff, B., Vester, E., Leschke, M., and Scheler, S. (1994). The heart in hypertension. In *Textbook of Hypertension*, Swales, J. D., Ed., pp. 712–713. Blackwell, Oxford.

Streeter, D. D., Jr. (1979). Gross morphology and fiber geometry of the heart. In *Handbook of Physiology, Section 2: The Cardiovascular System, Volume 1: The Heart*, Berne, R. M., and Sperelakis, N., Eds., Vol. 1, pp. 61–112. American Physiological Society, Bethesda, MD.

Struijker-Boudier, H. A. J., Le Noble, J. L. M. L., Messing, M. W. J., Huijberts, M. S. P., Le Noble, F. A. C., and Essen, H. v. (1992). The microcirculation in hypertension. *J Hypertens* **10** (suppl 7), S147–S156.

Studer, R., Reinecke, H., Bilger, J., Eschenhagn, T., Boehm, M., Hasenfuss, G. et al. (1994). Gene expression of the cardiac Na^+-exchanger in end-stage human heart failure. *Circ Res* **75**, 443–453.

Stull, J. T., Gallagher, P. J., Herring, B. P., and Kamm, K. E. (1991). Vascular smooth muscle contractile elements. *Cell Regul* **H 17**, 723–732.

Sudhir, K., Woods, R. L., Jennings, G. L., Nelson, L. A., Laufer, E., and Korner, P. I. (1988). Exaggerated atrial natriuretic peptide release during acute exercise in essential hypertension. *J Hum Hypertens* **1**, 299–304.

Sudhir, K., Jennings, G. L., Esler, M. D., Korner, P. I., Blombery, P. A., Lambert, G. A., Scoggins, B. A., and Whitworth, J. A. (1989). Hydrocortisone-induced hypertension in humans: pressor responsiveness and sympathetic function. *Hypertension* **13**, 416–421.

Sudhir, K., and Angus, J. A. (1990). Contractile responses to alpha1–adrenoceptor stimulation during maturation in the aorta of the normotensive and spontaneously hypertensive rat: relation to structure. *Clin Exp Pharmacol Physiol* **17**, 69–82.

Sudhir, K., Angus, J. A., Esler, M. D., Jennings, G. L., Lambert, G. W., and Korner, P. I. (1990). Altered venous responses to vasoconstrictor agonists and nerve stimulation in human primary hypertension. *J Hypertens* **8**, 1119–1128.

Sudhir, K., Smolich, J. J., and Angus, J. A. (1990). Venous reactivity in canine renovascular hypertension. *Clin Exp Hypertens* **A12**, 507–531.

Sudhir, K., Wilson, E., Chatterjee, K., and Ives, H. E. (1993). Mechanical strain and collagen potentiate mitogenic activity of angiotensin II in rat vascular smooth muscle cells. *J Clin Invest* **92**, 3003–3007.

Sudhir, K., Jennings, G. L., Funder, J. W., and Komesaroff, P. A. (1996). Estrogen enhances basal nitric oxide release in the forearm vasculature in perimenopausal women. *Hypertension* **28**, 330–334.

Sudhir, K., Chou, T. M., Chatterjee, K., Smith, E. P., Williams, T. C., Kane, J. P., Malloy, M. J., Korach, K. S., and Rubanyi, G. M. (1997). Premature coronary artery disease associated with a disruptive mutation in the estrogen receptor gene in a man. *Circulation* **96**, 3774–3777.

Sudhir, K., Esler, M. D., Jennings, G. L., and Komesaroff, P. A. (1997). Estrogen supplementation decreases norepinephrine-induced vasoconstriction and total body norepinephrine spillover in perimenopausal women. *Hypertension* **30**, 1538–1543.

Suga, H. (1990). Ventricular energetics. *Physiol Rev* **70**, 247–278.

Sugden, P. H., and Clerk, A. (1998). "Stress-responsive" mitogen-activated protein kinases (c-Jun N-terminal kinases and p38 mitogen-activated protein kinases in the myocardium). *Circ Res* **83**, 345–352.

Sugden, P. H. (1999). Signaling in myocardial hypertrophy: life after calcineurin? *Circ Res* **84**, 633–646.

Sullivan, J. M., Ratts, T. E., Taylor, J. C., Kraus, D. H., Barton, B. R., Patrick, D. R., and Reed, S. W. (1980). Haemodynamic effects of dietary sodium in man: a preliminary report. *Hypertension* **2**, 506–514.

Sullivan, J. M., Prewitt, R. L., and Josephs, J. A. (1983). Attenuation of the microcirculation in young patients with high output borderline hypertension. *Hypertension* **5**, 844–851.

Sullivan, J. M. (1991). Salt sensitivity: definition, conception, methodology and long-term issues. *Hypertension* **17** (suppl I), I-61–I-68.

Sun, D., Messina, E. J., Kaley, G., and Koller, A. (1992). Characteristics and origin of myogenic response in isolated mesenteric arterioles. *Am J Physiol* **263**, H1486–H1491.

Sun, M.-K., Jeske, I. T., and Reis, D. J. (1992). Cyanide excites medullary sympathoexcitatory neurons in rats. *Am J Physiol* **262**, R182–R189.

Sun, D., Huang, A., Smith, C. J., Stackpole, C. J., Connetta, J. A., Shesely, E. G., Koller, A., and Kaley, G. (1999). Enhanced release of prostaglandins contributes to flow-induced arteriolar dilatation in eNOS knockout mice. *Circ Res* **85**, 288–293.

Suwa, N., and Takahashi, T. (1971). *Morphological and Morphometrical Analysis of Circulation in Hypertension and Ischemic Kidney.* Urban & Schwarzenberg, Munich.

Suzuki, H., Zweifach, B. W., and Schmid-Schoenbein, G. W. (1996). Glucocorticoid modulates vasodilator response of mesenteric arterioles in spontaneously hypertensive rats. *Hypertension* **27**, 114–118.

Swales, J. D., Thurston, H., Queiroz, F. P., and Medina, A. (1972). Sodium balance during the development of experimental hypertension. *J Lab Clin Med* **80**, 539–547.

Swales, J. D., and Thurston, H. (1977). Sodium restriction and inhibition of the renin-angiotensin system in renovascular hypertension in the rat. *Clin Sci Mol Med* **52**, 371–375.

Swales, J. D., Bing, R. F., Russel, G. I., Taverner, D., and Thurston, H. (1986). Vasodepressor mechanisms in experimental hypertension: studies using chemical medullectomy. *J Hypertens* **4**, 543–546.

Swales, J. D., Bing, R. F., Edmunds, M. E., Russel, G. I., and Thurston, H. (1987). Reversal of renovascular hypertension: role of the renal medulla. *Can J Physiol Pharmacol* **65**, 1566–1571.

Swales, J. D. (1993). The renin-angiotensin system in essential hypertension. In *The Renin-Angiotensin System,* Robertson, J. I. S., and Nicholls, M. G., Eds., Vol. 2, pp. 62.1–62.12. Gower, London.

Swales, J. D. (1994a). Introduction. Hypertension: the past, the present, and the future. In *Textbook of Hypertension,* Swales, J. D., Ed., pp. 1–7. Blackwell, Oxford.

Swales, J. D., Ed. (1994b). *Textbook of Hypertension*. Blackwell, Oxford.

Swales, J. D. (1994c). Overview of essential hypertension. In *Textbook of Hypertension*, Swales, J. D., Ed., pp.655–660. Blackwell, Oxford.

Swales, J. D. (1994d). Guidelines for treating hypertension. In *Textbook of Hypertension*, Swales, J. D., Ed., pp. 1195–1197. Blackwell, Oxford.

Swales, J. D. (1994e). Hypertension in an unequal world. In *Textbook of Hypertension*, Swales, J. D., Ed., pp. 1263–1266. Blackwell, Oxford.

Swales, J. D. (1995). Dietary sodium restriction in hypertension. In *Hypertension: Pathophysiology, Diagnosis, and Management*, Laragh, J. H., and Brenner, B. M., Eds., Vol. 1. Raven Press, New York.

Swanson, L. W., Sawchenko, P. E., Rivier, J., and Vale, W. (1983). Organization of corticotropin releasing factor (CRF)-immunoreactive cells and fibers in the rat brain: an immunohistochemical study. *Neuroendocrinology* **36**, 165–186.

Tack, C. J., Lutterman, J. A., Verwoort, G., Thien, T., and Smits, P. (1996). Activation of the sodium-potassium pump contributes to insulin-induced vasodilatation in humans. *Hypertension* **28**, 426–432.

Taddei, S., Virdis, A., Mattei, P., and Salvetti, A. (1993). Vasodilatation to acetyl choline in primary and secondary forms of human hypertension. *Hypertension* **21**, 929–933.

Takata, M., Denton, K. M., and Anderson, W. P. (1988). Renal and systemic vascular conductances in renal wrap hypertension in rabbits. *J Hypertension* **6**, 719–722.

Takeda, K., Nakata, T., Takesako, T., Itoh, H., Hirata, M., Kawasaki, S., Hayashi, J., Oguro, M., Sasaki, S., and Nakagawa, M. (1991). Sympathetic inhibition and attenuation of spontaneous hypertension by PVN lesions in rats. *Brain Res* **543**, 296–300.

Takeda, Y., Miyamori, I., Wu, P., Yoneda, T., Furukawa, K., and Takeda, R. (1995). Effects of an endothelin receptor antagonist in rats with cyclosporine induced hypertension. *Hypertension* **26** (part 1), 932–936.

Takeda, Y., Miyamori, I., Yoneda, T., Hurukawa, K., Inaba, S., Ito, Y., and Takeda, R. (1995). Urinary excretion of 19-noraldosterone in the spontaneously hypertensive rat and stroke-prone hypertensive rat. *Clin Exp Pharmacol Physiol* **22** (suppl 1), S20–S22.

Takeshita, A., and Mark, A. (1979). Decreased venous distensibility in borderline hypertension. *Hypertension* **1**, 202–206.

Takeshita, A., Mark, A. L., and Brody, M. J. (1979). Prevention of salt induced hypertension in the Dahl strain by 6-hydroxydopamine. *Am J Physiol* **236**, H48–H52.

Talbott, J. H., Castleman, B., Smithwick, R. H., Melville, R. S., and Pecora, L. J. (1943). Renal biopsy studies correlated with renal clearance observations in hypertensive patients treated by radical sympathectomy. *J Clin Invest* **22**, 387–394.

Tanase, H., Yamori, Y., Hansen, C. T., and Lovenberg, W. (1982). Heart size in inbred strains of rats. Part I. Genetic determinants of the development of cardiovascular enlargement in rats. *Hypertension* **4**, 864–872.

Tarazi, R. C., Frohlich, E. D., and Dustan, H. P. (1968). Plasma volume in men with essential hypertension. *N Engl J Med* **278**, 762–765.

Tarjan, E., Denton, D. A., and Weisinger, R. S. (1988). Atrial natriuretic peptide inhibits water and sodium intake in rabbits. *Regul Pept* **23**, 63–75.

Taubes, G. (1998). The (political) science of salt. *Science* **281**, 898–907.

Taylor, M. G. (1965). Wave travel in a non-uniform transmission line, in relation to pulses in arteries. *Phys Med Biol* **10**, 539–550.

Taylor, M. G. (1966a). The input-impedance of an assembly of randomly-branching elastic tubes. *Biophys J* **6**, 29–51.

Taylor, M. G. (1966b). An introduction to some recent developments in arterial haemodynamics. *Aust Ann Med* **15**, 71–86.

Taylor, M. G. (1966c). Use of random excitation and spectral analysis in the study of frequency-dependent parameters of the cardiovascular system. *Circ Res* **18**, 585–595.

Taylor, R. R., Papadimitriou, J. M., and Hopkins, B. E. (1974). Structure and function in myocardial hypertrophy. In *The Myocardium*, Reader, R., Ed., Vol. 12, pp. 246–255. Karger, Basel.

Thoenen, H., and Barde, Y.-A. (1980). Physiology of nerve growth factor. *Physiol Rev* **60**, 1284–1335.

Thomas, G. D., Hansen, J., and Victor, R. G. (1994). Inhibition of alpha 2-adrenergic vasoconstriction during contraction of glycolytic not oxidative rat hindlimb muscle. *Am J Physiol* **266**, H920–H929.

Thomas, T., Thomas, G., McLendon, C., Sutton, T., and Mullan, M. (1996). Beta amyloid-mediated vasoactivity and vascular endothelial damage. *Nature* **380**, 168–171.

Thomas, G. D., and Victor, R. G. (1997). Nitric oxide mediates contraction-induced attenuation of sympathetic vasoconstriction in rat skeletal muscle. *J Physiol (Lond)* **506.3**, 817–826.

Thomas, G. D., Sander, M., Lau, K. S., Huang, P. L., Stull, J. T., and Victor, R. G. (1998). Impaired metabolic modulation of α_2_adrenergic vasoconstriction in dystrophin-deficient skeletal muscle. *Proc Natl Acad Sci, USA* **95**, 15090–15095.

Thompson, R. F. (1990). Neural mechanisms of classical conditioning in mammals. *Philos Trans R Soc Lond (Biol)* **329**, 161–170.

Thorburn, G. D., Kopald, H. H., Herd, J. A., Hollenberg, M., Morchoe, C. C. C., and Barger, A. C. (1963). Intrarenal distribution of nutrient blood flow determined with krypton-85 in the unanaesthetized dog. *Circ Res* **13**, 290–302.

Thorburn, G. D., and Harding, R. E. (1994). *Textbook of Fetal Physiology.* Oxford University Press, Oxford.

Thorén, P. N., Donald, D. E., and Shepherd, J. T. (1976). Role of heart and lung receptors with nonmedullated vagal afferents in circulatory control. *Circ Res* **38** (supp II), 2–9.

Thorén, P. (1979). Role of cardiac vagal C-fibers in cardiovascular control. *Rev Physiol Biochem Pharmacocol* **86**, 1–94.

Thorén, P., Noresson, E., and Ricksten, S.-E. (1979). Cardiac reflexes in normotensive and spontaneously hypertensive rats. *Am J Cardiol* **44**, 884–888.

Thorén, P., and Ricksten, S.-E. (1979). Recordings of renal and splanchnic sympathetic nervous activity in normotensive and spontaneously hypertensive rats. *Clin Sci* **57**, 197s–199s.

Thorén, P., Andresen, M. C., and Brown, A. M. (1983). Resetting of aortic baroreceptors with non-myelinated afferent fibers in spontaneously hypertensive rats. *Acta Physiol Scand* **117**, 91–97.

Thorén, P., and Lundin, S. (1983). Autonomic nervous system and blood pressure control in normotensive and hypertensive conditions. In *Central Cardiovascular Control*, Ganten, D., and Pfaff, D., Eds., pp. 31–61. Springer-Verlag, Berlin.

Thorén, P., Mark, A. L., Morgan, D. A., O'Neill, T. P., Needleman, P., and Brody, M. J. (1986). Activation of vagal depressor reflexes by atriopeptins inhibits renal sympathetic nerve activity. *Am J Physiol* **251**, H1252–H1259.

Thornburg, K. L., and Morton, M. J. (1994). Development of the cardiovascular system. In *Textbook of Fetal Physiology*, Thorburn, G. D., and Harding, R., Eds., pp. 95–130. Oxford Medical Publications, Oxford.

Thornton, B. S. (1971). Computer aided system design of linked cooperative digital computers for control. *Automatica* **7**, 741–746.

Thrasher, T. N. (2002). Unloading of arterial baroreceptors causes neurogenic hypertension. *Am J Physiol* **282**, R1044–R1053.

Thrasher, T. N. (2005a). Baroreceptors, baroreceptor unloading and long-term control of blood pressure. *Am J Physiol* **288**, R819–R827.

Thrasher, T. N. (2005b). Effects of chronic baroreceptor unloading on blood pressure in dogs. *Am J Physiol* **288,** R863–R871.

Thurau, K. (1964). Renal hemodynamics. *Am J Med* **36,** 698–719.

Thurston, H., Bing, R. F., Pohl, J. E. F., and Swales, J. D. (1978). Renin subgroups in essential hypertension: an analysis and critique. *Q J Med* **47,** 325–337.

Thurston, H. (1994). Goldblatt, coarctation and Page experimental models of renovascular hypertension. In *Textbook of Hypertension*, Swales, J. D., Ed., pp. 477–493. Blackwell, Oxford.

Thybo, N. K., Korsgaard, N., Eriksen, S., Christensen, K. L., and Mulvany, M. J. (1994). Dose-dependent effects of perindopril on blood pressure and small-artery structure. *Hypertension* **23,** 659–666.

Tigerstedt, R., and Bergman, P. G. (1898). Niere und Kreislauf. *Skand Arch Physiol* **8,** 223–270.

Timio, M., Verdecchia, P., Venanzi, S., Gentili, S., Ronconi, M., Francucci, B., Montanari, M., and Bichisao, E. (1988). Age and blood pressure changes: a 20 year follow-up study of nuns in a secluded order. *Hypertension* **12,** 457–461.

Timio, M., Lippi, G., Venanzi, S., Gentili, S., Quintaliani, G., Verdura, C., Monarca, C., Saronio, P., and Timio, F. (1997). Blood pressure trend and cardiovascular events in nuns in a secluded order: a 30 year follow-up study. *Blood Pressure* **6,** 81–87.

Tipton, C. M., Matthes, R. D., Marcus, K. D., Rowlett, K. A., and Leininger, J. R. (1983). Influences of exercise intensity, age, and medication on resting systolic blood pressure of SHR populations. *J Appl Physiol* **55,** 1305–1310.

Tipton, C. M., Sturek, M. S., Oppliger, R. A., Matthes, R. D., Overton, J. M., and Edwards, J. B. (1984). Responses of SHR to combinations of chemical sympathectomy, adrenal demedullation and training. *Am J Physiol* **247,** H109–H118.

Toal, C. B., and Leenen, F. H. H. (1985). Blood pressure responsiveness during the development of hypertension in the conscious spontaneously hypertensive rat. *Can J Physiol Pharmacol* **63,** 1258–1262.

Tobian, L., Lange, J., Azar, S., Iwai, J., Koop, D., Coffee, K., and Johnson, M. A. (1978). Reduction of natriuretic capacity and renin release in isolated, blood-perfused kidney of Dahl-hypertension prone rats. *Circ Res* **43** (suppl I, I-92–I-98).

Tobian, L. (1991). Salt and hypertension: lessons from animal models that relate to human hypertension. *Hypertension* **17** (suppl I), I-52–I-58.

Tomanek, R. J., Wangler, R. D., and Bauer, C. A. (1985). Prevention of coronary vasodilator reserve decrement in spontaneously hypertensive rats. *Hypertension* **7,** 533–540.

Topham, W. S., and Warner, H. R. (1967). The control of cardiac output during exercise. In *Physical Bases of Circulatory Transport: Regulation and Exchange*, Reeve, E. N., and Guyton, A. C., Eds., pp. 77–90. W.B. Saunders, Philadelphia.

Topol, E. J. (1998). *Textbook of Cardiovascular Medicine*. Lippincott-Raven, Philadelphia.

Torgersen, S., and Kringlen, E. (1971). Blood pressure and personality. A study of the relationship between intrapair differences in systolic blood pressure and personality in monozygotic twins. *J Psychosom Res* **15,** 183.

Touw, K. B., Haywood, J. R., Shaffer, R. A., and Brody, M. J. (1980). Contribution of the sympathetic nervous system to vascular resistance in conscious young and adult spontaneously hypertensive rats. *Hypertension* **2,** 408–418.

Traupe, T., Lang, M., Goettsch, M., Muenter, K., Morawietz, H., Vetter, W., and Barton, M. (2002). Obesity increases prostanoid-mediated vaoconstriction and vascular thromboxane gene expression. *J Hypertens* **20,** 2239–2245.

Trimarco, B., and Wikstrand, J. (1984). Regression of cardiovascular changes by antihypertensive treatment. *Hypertension* **6** (suppl III), III-150–III-157.

Trombitas, K., Jin, J.-P., and Granzier, H. (1995). The mechanically active domain of titin in cardiac muscle. *Circ Res* **77**, 856–861.

Trzebski, A., Lipski, J., Majcherczyk, S., Szulczyk, P., and Chruschielewski, L. (1975). Central organization and interaction of the carotid baroreceptor and chemoreceptor sympathetic reflex. *Brain Res* **87**, 227–237.

Trzebski, A., Tafil, M., Zoltowski, M., and Przybylski, J. (1982). Increased sensitivity of arterial chemoreceptor drive in young men with mild hypertension. *Cardiovasc Res* **16**, 163–172.

Tsai, M.-L., Watts, S. W., Loch-Caruso, R., and Webb, R. C. (1995). The role of gap junctional communication in contractile oscillations in arteries from normotensive and hypertensive rats. *J Hypertens* **13**, 1123–1133.

Tschudi, M. R., Mesaros, S., Luscher, T. F., and Malinski, T. (1996). Direct in situ measurement of nitric oxide in mesenteric resistance arteries. Increased decomposition by superoxide in hypertension. *Hypertension* **27**, 32–35.

Tuck, M. L., Sowers, J., and Dornfeld, L. (1981). The effect of weight reduction on blood pressure, plasma renin activity and plasma aldosterone levels in obese patients. *N Engl J Med* **304**, 930–933.

Tuck, M. L. (1994). Obesity. In *Textbook of Hypertension*, Swales, J. D., Ed., pp. 576–592. Blackwell, Oxford.

Tucker, D., and Hunt, R. (1993). Effects of long-term air jet noise and dietary sodium chloride in borderline hypertensive rats. *Hypertension* **22**, 527–534.

Tully, T. (1987). *Drosophila* learning and memory revisited. *Trends Neurosci* **10**, 330–335.

Turkkan, J. S., and Goldstein, D. S. (1991). Stress and sodium hypertension in baboons neuroendocrine and pharmacotherapeutic assessments. *J Hypertens* **9**, 969–975.

Turner, B. H., Mishkin, M., and Knapp, M. (1980). Organization of the amygdalopetal projections from modality-specific cortical association areas. *J Comp Neurol* **191**, 515–543.

Turner, M. E., Johnson, M. L., and Ely, D. L. (1991). Separate sex influenced and genetic components in spontaneously hypertensive rat hypertension. *Hypertension* **17**, 1097–1103.

Turner, M., and Ely, D. (1995). Two Y chromosomes in the SHR strain: polymorphism or interaction? [Abstract]. *FASEB J* **9**, A50.

Tuttle, J. B., Spitsbergen, J. M., Stewart, J. S., McCarty, R. M., and Steers, W. D. (1995). Altered signalling in vascular smooth muscle from spontaneously hypertensive rats may link medial hypertrophy, vessel hyperinnervation and elevated nerve growth factor. *Clin Exp Pharmacol Physiol* **22**, S117–S119.

Uchida, Y., Kamisaka, K., and Ueda, H. (1971). Two types of renal mechanoreceptors. *Jpn Heart J* **12**, 233–241.

Ulfendahl, H. R., and Wolgast, M. (1992). Renal circulation and lymphatics. In *The Kidney: Physiology and Pathophysiology*, Seldin, D. W., and Giebisch, G., Eds., Vol. 1, pp. 1017–1048. Raven Press, New York.

Ulrych, M., Hofman, J., and Hejl, Z. (1971). Cardiac and renal hyperresponsiveness to acute plasma volume expansion in hypertension. *Am Heart J* **68**, 193–203.

Undesser, K. P., Jing-Yun, P., Lynn, M. P., and Bishop, V. S. (1985). Baroreflex control of sympathetic nerve activity after elevations of pressure in conscious rabbits. *AJP* **248**, H827–H834.

Unger, T., and Parati, G. (2005). Acute stress and long-lasting blood pressure elevation: a possible cause of established hypertension? [Editorial comment]. *J Hypertens* **23**, 261–263.

Ungerstedt, U. (1971). Stereotaxic mapping of the monoamine pathways in the rat brain. *Acta Physiol Scand* (suppl 367), 1–48.

Uno, H., Tarara, R., Else, J., Suleman, M., and Sapolsky, R. (1989). Hippocampal damage associated with prolonged and fatal stress in primates. *J. Neurosci.* **9**, 1705–1711.

Urata, H., Tanabe, Y., Kiyonaga, A., Ikeda, M., Tanaka, H., Shindo, M., and Arakawa, K. (1987). Antihypertensive and volume-depleting effects of mild exercise on essential hypertension. *Hypertension* **9,** 245–252.

Urata, H., Healy, B., Stewart, R. W., Bumpus, F. M., and Husain, A. (1990). Angiotensin II-forming pathways in normal and failing human hearts. *Circ Res* **66,** 883–890.

Urata, H., Kinoshita, A., Misono, K. S., Bumpus, F. M., and Husain, A. (1990). Identification of a highly specific chymase as the major angiotensin II-forming enzyme in the human heart. *J Biol Chem* **265,** 22348–22357.

Urata, H., Boehm, K. D., Philip, A., Kinoshita, A., Gabrovsek, J., Bumpus, F. M., and Husain, A. (1993). Cellular localisation and regional distribution of angiotensin II-forming chymase in the heart. *J Clin Invest* **91,** 1269–1281.

Ursin, H., Baade, E., and Levine, S. (1978). *Psychobiology of Stress: A Study of Coping Men.* Academic Press, New York.

U.S. Government National Center for Health Statistics. (1977). *Blood Pressure of Persons 6–74 Years, United States, 1971–1974*, pp. 78–1648. DHEW, Publication No (HRA), Washington, DC.

Uther, J. B., Hunyor, S. N., Shaw, J., and Korner, P. I. (1970). Bulbar and suprabulbar control of the cardiovascular autonomic effects during arterial hypoxia in the rabbit. *Circ Res* **26,** 491–506.

Vallance, P., Collier, J., and Moncada, S. (1989). Effects of endothelium-derived nitric oxide on peripheral arteriolar tone in man. *Lancet* **2,** 997–1000.

VanBavel, E., and Mulvany, M. J. (1994). Role of wall tension in the vasoconstrictor response of cannulated rat mesenteric small arteries. *J Physiol (Lond)* **477,** 103–115.

Van den Bos, G. C., Elzinga, G., Westerhof, N., and Noble, M. I. M. (1973). Problems in the use of indices of contractility. *Cardiovasc Res* **7,** 834–848.

Van den Buuse, M., De Kloet, E. R., Versteeg, D. H. G., and De Jong, W. (1984). Regional brain catecholamine levels and the development of hypertension in the spontaneously hypertensive rat: the effect of 6–hydroxydopamine. *Brain Res* **301,** 221–229.

Van den Buuse, M., Versteeg, D. H. G., and De Jong, W. (1984). Role of dopamine in the development of spontaneous hypertension. *Hypertension* **6,** 899–905.

Van den Buuse, M., Head, G. A., and Korner, P. I. (1991). Contribution of forebrain noradrenaline innervation to the central circulatory effects of L-methyldopa and 6–hydroxydopamine. *Brain Res* **541,** 300–308.

Van den Buuse, M., Head, G. A., and Korner, P. I. (1993). Differential role of brain ascending noradrenergic bundles in the circulatory effects of l-methyldopa and clonidine. *J Cardiovasc Pharmacol* **21,** 112–119.

Vander, A. J. (1967). Control of renin release. *Physiol Rev* **47,** 359–382.

Vandongen, R., and Puddey, I. B. (1994). Alcohol intake and blood pressure. In *Textbook of Hypertension*, Swales, J. D., Ed., pp. 567–575. Blackwell, Oxford.

Vanhoutte, P. M. (1993). Is endothelin involved in the pathogenesis of hypertension? [Invited controversy]. *Hypertension* **21,** 747–751.

Vanhoutte, P. M. (1996). Endothelial dysfunction in hypertension. *J Hypertens* **14** (suppl 5), S83–S94.

van Zwieten, P. A., Safar, M., Laurent, S., Pfaffendorf, M., Hendriks, M. G. C., and Bruning, T. A. (1995). New insights into the role of endothelial dysfunction in hypertension. *J Hypertens* **13,** 713–716.

van Zwieten, P. A. (1999). The renaissance of centrally acting antihypertensive drugs. *J Hypertens* **17** (suppl 3), S15–S21.

Vatner, S. F. (2003). Arthur C. Guyton, MD (1919–2003): in memoriam. *Circ Res* **92,** 1272–1275.

Vaz, M., Turner, A. G., Kingwell, B., Chin, J., Koff, E., Cox, H. S., Jennings, G. L., and Esler, M. D. (1995). Postprandial sympatho-adrenal activity its relation to metabolic and cardiovascular events and to changes in meal frequency. *Clin Sci* **89**, 349–357.

Vaz, M., Jennings, G., Turner, A., Cox, H., Lambert, G., and Esler, M. (1997). Regional sympathetic nervous activity and oxygen consumption in obese normotensive human subjects. *Circulation* **96**, 3423–3429.

Verdecchia, P., Schillaci, G., Guerrieri, M., Gatteschi, C., Benemio, G., Boldrini, F., and Porcellati, C. (1990). Circadian blood pressure changes and left ventricular hypertrophy in essential hypertension. *Circulation* **81**, 528–536.

Vgontzas, A. N., Tan, T. L., Bixler, E. O., Martin, L. F., Shubert, D., and Kales, A. (1994). Sleep apnea and sleep disruption in obese patients. *Arch Int Med* **154**, 1705–1711.

Victor, R. G., and Mark, A. L. (1995). The sympathetic nervous system in human hypertension. In *Hypertension: Pathophysiology, Diagnosis and Manangement*, Laragh, J. H., Ed., Vol. 1, pp. 863–878. Raven Press, New York.

Vincent, M., Kaiser, M. A., Orea, V., Lodwick, D., and Samani, N. J. (1994). Hypertension in the spontaneously hypertensive rat and the sex chromosomes. *Hypertension* **23**, 161–166.

Vogel, F., and Motulsky, A. G. (1997). *Human Genetics: Problems and Approaches*. Springer-Verlag, Berlin.

Volhard, F., and Fahr, T. (1914). *Die Brightsche Nierenkrankheit: Klinik, Pathologie und Atlas*. Springer-Verlag, Berlin.

Wade, O. L., and Bishop, J. M. (1962). *Cardiac Output and Regional Blood Flow*. Blackwell, Oxford.

Wagner, C. D., Nafz, B., and Persson, P. B. (1996). Chaos in blood pressure control. *Cardiovasc Res* **31**, 380–387.

Waldeck, F. (1983). Human physiology. In *Human Physiology*, Schmidt, R. F., and Thews, G., Eds., pp. 587–609. Springer-Verlag, Berlin.

Walgenbach, S., and Donald, D. (1983). Cardiopulmonary reflexes and arterial pressure during rest and exercise in dogs. *Am J Physiol* **244**, H362–H369.

Walker, D. W. (1994). Development of the autonomic nervous system, including adrenal chromaffin tissue. In *Textbook of Fetal Physiology*, Thorburn, G. D., and Harding, R., Eds., pp. 287–300. Oxford University Press, Oxford.

Wall, P. D., and Davis, G. D. (1951). Three cortical systems affecting autonomic function. *J Neurophysiol* **14**, 507–517.

Wall, P. D., and Pribram, K. H. (1951). Trigeminal neurotomy and blood pressure responses from stimulation of lateral cerebral cortex of *Macaca mulatta. J Neurophysiol* **14**, 409–412.

Wallace, A. G., Skinner, N. S., and Mitchell, J. H. (1963). Haemodynamic determinants of maximum rate of rise of left ventricular pressure. *Am J Physiol* **205**, 30–36.

Wallin, B. G., and Sundlof, G. (1979). A quantitative study of muscle sympathetic nerve activity in resting normotensive and hypertensive subjects. *Hypertension* **1**, 67–77.

Wallin, B. G., and Fagius, J. (1988). Peripheral sympathetic activity in conscious humans. *Annu Rev Physiol* **50**, 565–576.

Walsh, J. A., Hyman, C., and Maronde, R. H. (1969). Venous distensibility in essential hypertension. *Cardiovasc Res* **3**, 338–349.

Wang, S. C., and Ranson, S. W. (1939). Autonomic responses to electrical stimulation of the lower brain stem. *J Comp Neurol* **71**, 437–455.

Wang, J., and Morgan, J. P. (1992). Endocardial endothelium modulates myofilament Ca^{2+} responsiveness in aequorin-loaded ferret myocardium. *Circ Res* **70**, 754–760.

Wang, J., Woline, M. S., and Hintze, T. H. (1993). Chronic exercise enhances endothelium-mediated dilatation of epicardial coronary artery in conscious dogs. *Circ Res* **73**, 829–838.

Wang, D., and Strandgaard, S. (1997). The pathogenesis of hypertension in autosomal dominant polycystic kidney disease. *J Hypertens* **15**, 925–933.

Wang, H., and Leenen, F. H. H. (2002). Brain sodium channels mediate increases in brain "ouabain" and blood pressure in Dahl S rats. *Hypertension* **40**, 96–100.

Warber, K. D., and Potter, J. D. (1986). Contractile proteins and phosphorylation. In *The Heart and Cardiovascular System*, Fozzard, H. A., Haber, E., Jennings, R. B., Katz, A. M., and Morgan, H. E., Eds., Vol. 2, pp. 779–788. Raven Press, New York.

Ward, J. E., and Angus, J. A. (1993). Acute and chronic inhibition of nitric oxide synthase in conscious rabbits: role of nitric oxide in the control of vascular tone. *J Cardiovasc Pharmacol* **21**, 804–814.

Ward, R. (1995). Familial aggregation and genetic epidemiology of blood pressure. In *Hypertension: Pathophysiology, Diagnosis and Management*, Laragh, J. H., and Brenner, B. M., Eds., Vol. 1, pp. 67–88. Raven Press, New York.

Warshaw, D. M., Mulvany, M. J., and Halpern, W. (1979). Mechanical and morphological properties of arterial resistance vessels in young and old spontaneously hypertensive rats. *Circ Res* **45**, 250–259.

Wasserman, K., and Mayerson, H. S. (1952). Mechanism of plasma protein changes following saline infusions. *Am J Physiol* **170**, 1–10.

Watson, J. D., and Crick, F. H. C. (1953a). Genetical implications of the structure of deoxyribose nucleic acid. *Nature* **171**, 964–967.

Watson, J. D., and Crick, F. H. C. (1953b). Molecular structure of nucleic acids. A structure for deoxyribose nucleic acids. *Nature* **171**, 737–738.

Watson, R. D. S., Esler, M. D., Leonard, P., and Korner, P. I. (1984). Influence of variation in dietary sodium intake on biochemical indices of sympathetic activity in normal man. *Clin Exp Pharmacol Physiol* **11**, 163–170.

Watt, G. (1986). Design and interpretation of studies comparing individuals with and without a family history of high blood pressure. *J Hypertens* **4**, 1–7.

Watt, G. C. M., Foy, C. J. W., Holton, D. W., and Edwards, H. E. (1991). Prediction of high blood pressure in young people: the limited usefulness of parental blood pressure data. *J Hypertens* **9**, 55–58.

Weber, K., and Brilla, C. (1991). Pathological hypertrophy and cardiac interstitium. Fibrosis and renin-angiotensin-aldosterone system. *Circulation* **83**, 1849–1865.

Weber, K. T., Sun, Y., and Guarda, E. (1994). Structural remodeling in hypertensive heart disease and the role of hormones. *Hypertension* **23** (part 2), 869–877.

Weber, R., Stergiopulos, N., Brunner, H. R., and Hayoz, D. (1996). Contributions of vascular tone and structure to elastic properties of a medium-sized artery. *Hypertension* **27** (part 2), 816–822.

Weder, A. B., Takiyyuddin, M., Sekkarie, M. A., and Julius, S. (1989). Behaviour and hypertension: a pathophysiological puzzle. *J Hypertens* **7** (suppl 1), S13–S17.

Weinberger, M. H., Luft, F. C., Bloch, R., Henry, D. P., Weyman, A. E., and Rankin, L. I. (1981). Blood pressure in sodium fed humans. In *Frontiers in Hypertension Research*, Laragh, J. H., Buehler, F. R., and Seldin, D. W., Eds., pp. 58–61. Springer-Verlag, New York.

Weinberger, M. H., Miller, J. Z., Luft, F. C., Grim, C. E., and Fineberg, N. S. (1986). Definitions and characteristics of sodium sensitivity and blood pressure resistance. *Hypertension* **8** (suppl II), II-127–II-134.

Weinstock, M., and Rosin, A. J. (1984). Relative contributions of vagal and cardiac sympathetic nerves to the reflex bradycardia induced by a pressor stimulus in the conscious rabbit: comparison of "steady-state" and ramp methods. *Clin Exp Pharmacol Physiol* **11**, 133–141.

Weinstock, M., Schorer-Apelbaum, D., and Rosin, A. J. (1984). Endogenous opiates mediate cardiac sympathetic inhibition in response to a pressor stimulus in rabbits. *J Hypertens* **2**, 639–646.

Weinstock, M., Weksler-Zangen, S., and Schorer-Apelbaum, D. (1986). Genetic factors involved in the determination of baroreceptor-heart rate sensitivity. *J Hypertens* **4**, S290–S292.

Weinstock, M., Korner, P. I., Head, G. A., and Dorward, P. K. (1988). Differentiation of cardiac baroreflex properties by cuff and drug methods in two rabbit strains. *Am J Physiol* **255**, R654–R664.

Weiss, L. (1974). Long-term treatment with antihypertensive drugs in spontaneously hypertensive rats (SHR). Effects on blood pressure, survival rate and cardiovascular design. *Acta Physiol Scand* **91**, 393–408.

Weiss, S. M., and Cheresh, D. A. (2005). Pathophysiological consequences of VEGF-induced vascular permeability. *Nature* **437**, 497–504.

Werkö, L., and Lagerlöf, H. (1949). Studies on the circulation in man. IV. Cardiac output and blood pressure in the right auricle, right ventricle and pulmonary artery in patients with hypertensive cardiovascular disease. *Acta Med Scand* **133**, 427–436.

Wesselman, J. P. M., Schubert, R., VanBavel, E., Nilsson, H., and Mulvany, M. J. (1997). K_{Ca} channel blockade prevents sustained pressure-induced depolarization in rat mesenteric small arteries. *Am J Physiol* **272**, H2241–H2249.

West, M. J., and Korner, P. I. (1974). The baroreceptor-heart rate reflex in renal hypertension in the rabbit. *Clin Exp Pharmacol Physiol* **1**, 231–239.

West, M. J., Angus, J. A., and Korner, P. I. (1975). Estimation of non-autonomic and autonomic components of iliac bed vascular resistance in renal hypertensive rabbits. *Cardiovasc Res* **9**, 697–706.

West, D. B., Wehberg, K. E., Kieswetter, K., and Granger, J. P. (1992). Blunted natriuretic response to acute salt load in obese hypertensive dogs. *Hypertension* **19** (suppl I), I-96–I-100.

Wexler, B. C., and Greenberg, B. P. (1978). Pathophysiological differences between paired and communal breeding of male and female Sprague-Dawley Rats. *Circ Res* **42**, 126–135.

Whelan, R. F. (1967). *Control of the Peripheral Circulation in Man*. Charles C Thomas, Springfield, IL.

Whelton, P. K., He, J., and Klag, M. J. (1994). Blood pressure in westernized populations. In *Textbook of Hypertension*, Swales, J. D., Ed., pp. 11–21. Blackwell, Oxford.

Whishaw, I. Q., and Robinson, T. E. (1974). Comparison of anodal and cathodal lesions and metal deposition in eliciting post-operative locomotion in the rat. *Physiol Behav* **13**, 539–551.

White, P. D. (1947). *Heart Disease*, pp. 429–457. Macmillan, New York.

White, S. W., McRitchie, R. J., Porges, W. L., and Korner, P. I. (1972). Respiratory and circulatory effects of hypoxia in the monkey. *Proc Aus Physiol Pharmacol Soc* **3**, 88P.

White, S., Andrew, P., Brown, D., McRitchie, R., Reid, J., and Korner, P. (1973). Arterial hypoxia in the unanaesthetized monkey: role of autonomic and local circulatory mechanisms. *Proc Aus Physiol Pharmacol Soc* **4**, 90P.

White, S. W., and McRitchie, R. J. (1973). Nasopharyngeal reflexes: integrative analysis of evoked respiratory and cardiovascular effects. *Aus J Exp Biol Med Sci* **51**, 17–31.

White, S. W., McRitchie, R. J., and Franklin, D. L. (1974). Autonomic cardiovascular effects of nasal inhalation of cigarette smoke in the rabbit. *Aust J Exp Biol Med Sci* **52**, 111–126.

White, S., McRitchie, R. J., and Korner, P. I. (1975). Central nervous system control of cardiorespiratory nasopharyngeal reflexes in the rabbit. *Am J Physiol* **228**, 404–409.

Whitworth, J. A., Gordon, D., McLachlan-Troup, N., Scoggins, B. A., and Moulds, R. W. F. (1989). Dexamethasone suppression in essential hypertension: effects of cortisol on blood pressure. *Clin Exp Hypertens* **A11**, 323–335.

Whitworth, J. A. (1994). Cushing's syndrome and hypertension. In *Textbook of Hypertension*, Swales, J. D., Ed., pp. 893–903. Blackwell, Oxford.

Whitworth, J. A., Mangos, G. J., and Kelly, J. J. (2000). Cushing cortisol and cardiovascular disease. *Hypertension* **36**, 912–916.

Wicker, P., and Tarazi, R. C. (1985). Right ventricular coronary flow in arterial hypertension. *Am Heart J* **110**, 845–850.

Widimsky, J., Fejfarova, M. H., and Fejfar, Z. (1957). Changes in cardiac output in hypertensive disease. *Cardiologia* **31**, 381–389.

Wiener, N. (1954). *The Human Use of Human Beings*. Sphere Books, London.

Wiener, N. (1961). *Cybernetics or Control and Communication in the Animal and Machine*. Wiley, New York.

Wiggers, C. J. (1928). *The Pressure Pulses in the Cardiovascular System*. Longmans, Green, London.

Wikman-Coffelt, J., Parmley, W. W., and Mason, D. T. (1979). The cardiac hypertrophy process. Analysis of factors determining pathological vs. physiological development. *Circ Res* **45**, 697–707.

Wikstrand, J. (1997). Calculation of left ventricular mass in man—a comment. *J Hypertens* **15**, 811–813.

Wildenthal, K., Mierzwiak, D. S., and Mitchell, J. H. (1969). Effect of sudden changes in aortic pressure on left ventricular dP/dt. *Am J Physiol* **216**, 185–190.

Wilkinson, R. (1994). Renal and renovascular hypertension. In *Textbook of Hypertension*, Swales, J. D., Ed., pp. 831–857. Blackwell, Oxford.

Wilkinson, D. J. C., Thompson, J. M., Lambert, G. W., Jennings, G. L., Schwarz, R. G., Jefferys, D., Turner, A. G., and Esler, M. D. (1998). Sympathetic activity in patients with panic disorder at rest under laboratory mental stress and during panic attacks. *Arch Gen Psych* **55**, 511–520.

Williams, G. H., Dluhy, R. G., Lifton, R. P., Moore, T. J., Gleason, R., Williams, R., Hunt, S. C., Hopkins, P. N., and Hollenberg, N. K. (1992). Non-modulation as an intermediate phenotype in essential hypertension. *Hypertension* **20**, 788–796.

Williams, J. S., Williams, G. H., Raji, A., Jeunemaitre, X., Brown, N. J., Hopkins, P. N., and Conlin, P. R. (2006). Prevalence of primary aldosteronism in mild to moderate hypertension without hypokalaemia. *J Hum Hypertens* **20**, 129–136.

Wilson, C., and Byrom, F. B. (1939). Renal changes in malignant hypertension: experimental evidence. *Lancet* **i**, 136–139.

Wilson, M. F., Ninomiya, I., Franz, G. N., and Judy, W. V. (1971). Hypothalamic stimulation and baroreceptor reflex interaction on renal nerve activity. *Am J Physiol* **221**, 1768–1773.

Wilson, E. O. (1975). *Sociobiology: The New Synthesis*. Harvard University Press, Cambridge, MA.

Winegrad, S. (1982). Mechanism of contraction in cardiac muscle. In *Cardiovascular Physiology IV. International Review of Physiology*, Guyton, A. C., and Hall, J. E., Eds., Vol. 26, pp. 87–117. University Park Press, Baltimore, MD.

Wing, L. M. H., Reid, C. M., Ryan, P., Beilin, L. J., Brown, M. A., Jennings, G. L. R., Johnston, C. I., McNeil, J. J., MacDonald, G. J., Marley, J. E., Morgan, T. O., and West, M. J. (2003). A comparison of outcomes with angiotensin-converting-enzyme inhibitors and diuretics for hypertension in the elderly. *N Engl J Med* **348**, 583–592.

Winternitz, S. R., Katholi, R. E., and Oparil, S. (1982). Decrease in hypothalamic norepinephrine content following renal denervation in the one-kidney, one-clip Goldblatt hypertensive rat. *Hypertension* **4**, 369–373.

Winternitz, S. R., and Oparil, S. (1982). Importance of the renal nerves in the pathogenesis of experimental hypertension. *Hypertension* **4** (suppl III), III-108–III-144.

Wolf, W. A., and Bobik, A. (1988). Effects of 5,6-dihydroxytryptamine on the release, synthesis and storage of serotonin: studies using rat brain synaptosomes. *J Neurochem* **50**, 534–542.

Wolf, W. A., and Bobik, A. (1989). Alpha-methyldopa metabolism in central serotonergic terminals: effects on serotonin levels, synthesis and release. *Eur J Pharm* **163**, 43–53.

Wolinsky, H. (1970). Response of the rat aortic media to hypertension. Morphological and chemical studies. *Circ Res* **26**, 507–522.

Wolk, R., Kara, T., and Somers, V. K. (2003). Sleep-disordered breathing and cardiovascular disease. *Circulation* **108**, 9–12.

Wolk, R., Shamsuzzaman, A. S. M., and Somers, V. K. (2003). Obesity, sleep apnea and hypertension. *Hypertension* **42**, 1067–1074.

Wolny, A., Clozel, J.-P., Rein, J., Vogt, P., Turino, M., Kiowski, W., and Fischli, W. (1997). Functional and biochemical analysis of angiotensin II-forming pathways in the human heart. *Circ Res* **80**, 219–227.

Wolpert, L. (1998). *Principles of Development*. Oxford University Press, London.

Wong, D. M., and Jenkins, L. C. (1975). The cardiovascular effect of ketamine in hypotensive states. *Can Anesth Soc J* **22**, 339–348.

Woods, R. L., Anderson, W. P., and Korner, P. I. (1986). Renal and systemic effects of enalapril in chronic one-kidney hypertension. *Hypertension* **8**, 109–116.

Woods, R. L., Oliver, J., and Korner, P. I. (1989). Direct and neurohumoral cardiovascular effects of atrial natriuretic peptide. *J Cardiovasc Pharmacol* **13**, 177–185.

Woods, R. L., Courneya, C.-A., and Head, G. A. (1994). Nonuniform enhancement of baroreflex sensitivity by atrial natriuretic peptide in conscious rats and dogs. *Am J Physiol* **267**, R678–R686.

Woods, S. C., Seeley, R. J., Porte, D., and Schwartz, M. W. (1998). Signals that regulate food intake and energy homeostasis. *Science* **280**, 1378–1383.

Woods, L. L., Weeks, D. A., and Rasch, R. (2001). Hypertension after neonatal uninephrectomy in rats precedes glomerular damage. *Hypertension* **38**, 337–342.

Woolgar, J. R., and Scott, T. M. (1989). The relationship between innervation and arterial structure in late prenatal and early postnatal development of the rat jejunal artery. *J Anat* **167**, 57–70.

World Health Organization and International Society of Hypertension. (1989). Guidelines for the management of mild hypertension. *Clin Exp Hypertens* **A11**, 1203–1216.

Wright, C. E., Angus, J. A., and Korner, P. I. (1987). Vascular amplifier properties in renovascular hypertension in conscious rabbits. *Hypertension* **9**, 122–131.

Wright, C. E., and Angus, J. A. (1999). Enhanced total peripheral vascular responsiveness in hypertension accords with the amplifier hypothesis. *J Hypertens* **17**, 1687–1696.

Wright, C. E., Angus, J. A., and Korner, P. I. (2002a). The structural factor raises blood pressure through the interaction of resistance vessel geometry with neurohumoral and local factors: estimates in rabbits with renal cellophane-wrap hypertension with intact effectors and during neurohumoral blockade. *J Hypertens* **20**, 471–483.

Wright, C. E., Angus, J. A., and Korner, P. I. (2002b). The interactive vascular resistance amplifier and non-interactive reviewers. *J Hypertens* **20**, 1023–1027.

Wu, J.-N., and Berecek, K. H. (1993). Prevention of genetic hypertension by early treatment of spontaneously hypertensive rats with the angiotensin converting enzyme inhibitor captopril. *Hypertension* **22**, 139–146.

Wyss, J. M., Aboukarsh, N., and Oparil, S. (1982). Sensory denervation of the kidney attenuates renovascular hypertension in the rat. *Am J Physiol* **250**, H82–H86.

Xiao, R.-P., and Lakatta, E. G. (1993). β_1 adrenoceptor stimulation and β_2 adrenoceptor stimulation differ in their effects on contraction, cytosolic Ca^{2+} and Ca^{2+} current in single rat ventricular cells. *Circ Res* **73**, 286–300.

Yagil, Y., Kobrin, I., Leibel, B., and Ben-Ishay, D. (1982). Ischemic changes with initial nifedipine therapy in patients with severe hypertension. *Am Heart J* **103**, 310–311.

Yamada, Y., Mihyjima, E., Tochikubo, O., Matsukawa, T., and Ishii, M. (1989). Age-related changes in muscle sympathetic nerve activity in essential hypertension. *Hypertension* **13**, 870–877.

Yamamoto, S., James, T. N., Sawada, K.-I., Okabe, M., and Kawamura, K. (1996). Generation of new intercellular junctions between cardiocytes: a possible mechanism for compensating for mechanical overload in the hypertrophied human adult myocardium. *Circ Res* **78**, 362–370.

Yamori, Y., and Okamoto, K. (1969). Hypothalamic tonic regulation of blood pressure in spontaneously hypertensive rats. *Jpn Circ J* **33**, 509–519.

Yamori, Y. (1975). Neurogenic mechanisms of spontaneous hypertension. In *Regulation of Blood Pressure by the Central Nervous System*, Onesti, G., Fernandes, M., and Kim, K. E., Eds., pp. 65–76. Grune & Stratton, New York.

Yamori, Y., Igawa, T., Kanbe, T., Kihara, M., Nara, Y., and Horie, R. (1981). Mechanisms of structural vascular changes in genetic hypertension: analyses of cultured vascular smooth muscle cells from spontaneously hypertensive rats. *Clin Sci* **61**, 121s–123s.

Yamori, Y. (1983). Physiopathology of various strains of spontaneously hypertensive rats. In *Hypertension: Physiopathology and Treatment*, Genest, J., Kuchel, O., Hamet, P., and Cantin, M., Eds., pp. 556–581. McGraw-Hill, New York.

Yamori, Y., Igawa, T., Tagami, M., Kanbe, T., Nara, Y., Kihara, M., and Horie, R. (1984). Humoral trophic influence on cardiovascular structural changes in hypertension. *Hypertension* **6** (suppl III), III-27–III-32.

Yamori, Y. (1994). Development of the spontaneously hypertensive rat (SHR), and the stroke-prone SHR (SHRSP) and their various substrain models for hypertension related cardiovascular diseases. In *Handbook of Hypertension, Volume 16: Experimental and Genetic Models of Hypertension*, Ganten, D., and de Jong, W., Eds., pp. 346–364. Elsevier Science, Amsterdam.

Yamori, Y., and Swales, J. D. (1994). The spontaneously hypertensive rat. In *Textbook of Hypertension*, Swales, J. D., Ed., pp. 447–454. Blackwell, Oxford.

Yanagisawa, M., Kurihara, H., Kimura, S., Tomobe, Y., Kobayashi, M., Mitsui, Y., Yazaki, Y., Goto, K., and Masuki, T. (1988). A novel potent vasoconstrictor peptide produced by vascular endothelial cells. *Nature* **332**, 411–415.

Yates, F. E. (1982). Outline of a physical theory of physiological systems (10th J.A.F. Stevenson Memorial Lecture). *Can J Physiol Pharmacol* **60**, 217–248.

Yates, F. E. (1983). Dynamic regulation of mean arterial pressure: special role of renal resistances. *Fed Proc* **42**, 3143–3149.

Yen, T. T., Shaw, W. N., and Yu, P. L. (1977). Genetics of obesity in Zucker rats and Koletsky rats. *Heredity* **38**, 373–377.

Yoran, C., Covell, J. W., and Ross, J. J. (1973). Structural basis for the ascending limb of left ventricular function. *Circ Res* **32**, 297–303.

Young, M. (1963). The fetal and neonatal circulation. In *Handbook of Physiology, Section 2: Circulation*, Hamilton, W. F., and Dow, P., Eds., Vol. II, pp. 1619–1650. American Physiological Society, Washington, DC.

Young, D., Cholvin, N., and Roth, A. (1975). Pressure drop across artificially induced stenoses in the femoral arteries of dogs. *Circ Res* **36**, 735–743.

Young, D., Cholvin, N., Kirkeeide, R., and Roth, A. (1977). Hemodynamics of arterial stenoses at elevated flow rates. *Circ Res* **41**, 99–107.

Young, J. B., and Landsberg, L. (1983). Diminished sympathetic nervous system activity in genetically obese (ob/ob) mouse. *Am J Physiol* **245**, E148–E154.

Young, T., Palta, M., Dempsey, J., Skatrud, J., Weber, S., and Badr, S. (1993). The occurrence of sleep disordered breathing among middle aged adults. *N Engl J Med* **328**, 1230–1235.

Zak, R. (1974). Development and proliferative capacity of cardiac muscle cells. *Circ Res* **34 & 35**, II-17–II-26.

Zanchetti, A., Baccelli, G., and Mancia, G. (1976). Fighting, emotions and exercise: cardiovascular effects in the cat. In *Regulation of Blood Pressure by the Central Nervous System*, Onesti, G., Fernandes, M., and Kim, K. E., Eds., Vol. part 2, pp. 87–103. Grune & Stratton, New York.

Zandi-Nejad, K., Luyckx, V. A., and Brenner, B. M. (2006). Adult hypertension and kidney disease: the role of fetal programming. *Hypertension* **47** (part 2), 502–508.

Zettler, C., Head, R. J., and Rush, R. A. (1991). Chronic nerve growth factor treatment of normotensive rats. *Brain Res* **538**, 251–262.

Zhang, W., Kowal, R. W., Rusnak, F., Sikkink, R. A., Olson, E. N., and Victor, R. G. (1999). Failure of calcineurin inhibitors to prevent pressure-overload left ventricular hypertrophy in rats. *Circ Res* **84**, 722–728.

Zicha, J., and Kuneš, J. (1999). Ontogenetic aspects of hypertension development: analysis in the rat. *Physiol Rev* **79**, 1–56.

Ziegler, D., Laude, D., Akila, F., and Elghozi, J. L. (2001). Time and frequency-domain estimation of early diabetic cardiovascular autonomic neuropathy. *Clin Autonom Res* **11**, 369–376.

Zimmerman, B. G. (1978). Actions of angiotensin on adrenergic nerve endings. *Fed Proc* **37**, 199–202.

Zukowska-Grojec, Z., Dayao, E. K., Karwatowska-Prokopczuk, E., Hauser, G. J., and Doods, H. N. (1996). Stress-induced mesenteric vasoconstriction in rats is mediated by neuropeptide Y Y_1 receptors. *Am J Physiol* **270**, H796–H800.

Zukowska-Grojec, Z. (1998). Neuropeptide Y: an adrenergic cotransmitter, vasoconstrictor and a nerve derived growth factor. In *Catecholamines: Bridging Basic Science with Clinical Medicine*, Goldstein, D. S., Eisenhofer, G., and McCarty, R., Eds., pp. 125–128. Academic Press, San Diego.

Zweifach, B. W. (1983). The microcirculation in experimental hypertension. *Hypertension* **5** (suppl I), I-10–I-16.

Index

Page numbers followed by *f* and *t* indicate figures and tables, respectively. BP, blood pressure; EH, essential hypertension; for other abbreviations see pp. xxiii–xxvi.